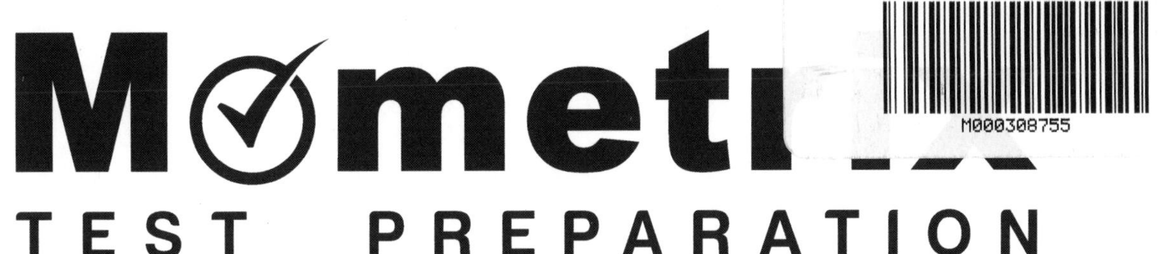

MCAT

Prep Books 2021 & 2022

MCAT Secrets Study Guide

Full-Length Practice Test

Step-by-Step Exam Review Video Tutorials

4th Edition

Written and edited by Mometrix Test Preparation

Printed in the United States of America

This paper meets the requirements of ANSI/NISO Z39.48-1992 (Permanence of Paper).

Mometrix offers volume discount pricing to institutions. For more information or a price quote, please contact our sales department at sales@mometrix.com or 888-248-1219.

Paperback
ISBN 13: 978-1-5167-1470-4
ISBN 10: 1-5167-1470-9

DEAR FUTURE EXAM SUCCESS STORY

First of all, **THANK YOU** for purchasing Mometrix study materials!

Second, congratulations! You are one of the few determined test-takers who are committed to doing whatever it takes to excel on your exam. **You have come to the right place.** We developed these study materials with one goal in mind: to deliver you the information you need in a format that's concise and easy to use.

In addition to optimizing your guide for the content of the test, we've outlined our recommended steps for breaking down the preparation process into small, attainable goals so you can make sure you stay on track.

We've also analyzed the entire test-taking process, identifying the most common pitfalls and showing how you can overcome them and be ready for any curveball the test throws you.

Standardized testing is one of the biggest obstacles on your road to success, which only increases the importance of doing well in the high-pressure, high-stakes environment of test day. Your results on this test could have a significant impact on your future, and this guide provides the information and practical advice to help you achieve your full potential on test day.

Your success is our success

We would love to hear from you! If you would like to share the story of your exam success or if you have any questions or comments in regard to our products, please contact us at **800-673-8175** or **support@mometrix.com**.

Thanks again for your business and we wish you continued success!

Sincerely,
The Mometrix Test Preparation Team

Need more help? Check out our flashcards at:
http://mometrixflashcards.com/MCAT

TABLE OF CONTENTS

Introduction

Thank you for purchasing this resource! You have made the choice to prepare yourself for a test that could have a huge impact on your future, and this guide is designed to help you be fully ready for test day. Obviously, it is important to have a solid understanding of the test material, but you also need to be prepared for the unique environment and stressors of the test, so that you can perform to the best of your abilities.

For this purpose, the first section that appears in this guide is the **Secret Keys**. We've devoted countless hours to meticulously researching what works and what doesn't, and we've boiled down our findings to the five most impactful steps you can take to improve your performance on the test. We start at the beginning with study planning and move through the preparation process, all the way to the testing strategies that will help you get the most out of what you know when you're finally sitting in front of the test.

We recommend that you start preparing for your test as far in advance as possible. However, if you've bought this guide as a last-minute study resource and only have a few days before your test, we recommend that you skip over the first two Secret Keys since they address a long-term study plan.

If you struggle with **test anxiety**, we strongly encourage you to check out our recommendations for how you can overcome it. Test anxiety is a formidable foe, but it can be beaten, and we want to make sure you have the tools you need to defeat it.

Secret Key #1 – Plan Big, Study Small

There's a lot riding on your performance. If you want to ace this test, you're going to need to keep your skills sharp and the material fresh in your mind. You need a plan that lets you review everything you need to know while still fitting in your schedule. We'll break this strategy down into three categories.

Information Organization

Start with the information you already have: the official test outline. From this, you can make a complete list of all the concepts you need to cover before the test. Organize these concepts into groups that can be studied together, and create a list of any related vocabulary you need to learn so you can brush up on any difficult terms. You'll want to keep this vocabulary list handy once you actually start studying since you may need to add to it along the way.

Time Management

Once you have your set of study concepts, decide how to spread them out over the time you have left before the test. Break your study plan into small, clear goals so you have a manageable task for each day and know exactly what you're doing. Then just focus on one small step at a time. When you manage your time this way, you don't need to spend hours at a time studying. Studying a small block of content for a short period each day helps you retain information better and avoid stressing over how much you have left to do. You can relax knowing that you have a plan to cover everything in time. In order for this strategy to be effective though, you have to start studying early and stick to your schedule. Avoid the exhaustion and futility that comes from last-minute cramming!

Study Environment

The environment you study in has a big impact on your learning. Studying in a coffee shop, while probably more enjoyable, is not likely to be as fruitful as studying in a quiet room. It is important to keep distractions to a minimum. You're only planning to study for a short block of time, so make the most of it. Don't pause to check your phone or get up to find a snack. It is also important to **avoid multitasking**. Research has consistently shown that multitasking will make your studying dramatically less effective. Your study area should also be comfortable and well-lit so you don't have the distraction of straining your eyes or sitting on an uncomfortable chair.

The time of day you study is also important. You want to be rested and alert. Don't wait until just before bedtime. Study when you'll be most likely to comprehend and remember. Even better, if you know what time of day your test will be, set that time aside for study. That way your brain will be used to working on that subject at that specific time and you'll have a better chance of recalling information.

Finally, it can be helpful to team up with others who are studying for the same test. Your actual studying should be done in as isolated an environment as possible, but the work of organizing the information and setting up the study plan can be divided up. In between study sessions, you can discuss with your teammates the concepts that you're all studying and quiz each other on the details. Just be sure that your teammates are as serious about the test as you are. If you find that your study time is being replaced with social time, you might need to find a new team.

Secret Key #2 – Make Your Studying Count

You're devoting a lot of time and effort to preparing for this test, so you want to be absolutely certain it will pay off. This means doing more than just reading the content and hoping you can remember it on test day. It is important to make every minute of study count. There are two main areas you can focus on to make your studying count:

Retention

It doesn't matter how much time you study if you can't remember the material. You need to make sure you are retaining the concepts. To check your retention of the information you're learning, try recalling it at later times with minimal prompting. Try carrying around flashcards and glance at one or two from time to time or ask a friend who's also studying for the test to quiz you.

To enhance your retention, look for ways to put the information into practice so that you can apply it rather than simply recalling it. If you're using the information in practical ways, it will be much easier to remember. Similarly, it helps to solidify a concept in your mind if you're not only reading it to yourself but also explaining it to someone else. Ask a friend to let you teach them about a concept you're a little shaky on (or speak aloud to an imaginary audience if necessary). As you try to summarize, define, give examples, and answer your friend's questions, you'll understand the concepts better and they will stay with you longer. Finally, step back for a big picture view and ask yourself how each piece of information fits with the whole subject. When you link the different concepts together and see them working together as a whole, it is easier to remember the individual components.

Finally, practice showing your work on any multi-step problems, even if you're just studying. Writing out each step you take to solve a problem will help solidify the process in your mind, and you'll be more likely to remember it during the test.

Modality

Modality simply refers to the means or method by which you study. Choosing a study modality that fits your own individual learning style is crucial. No two people learn best in exactly the same way, so it is important to know your strengths and use them to your advantage.

For example, if you learn best by visualization, focus on visualizing a concept in your mind and draw an image or a diagram. Try color-coding your notes, illustrating them, or creating symbols that will trigger your mind to recall a learned concept. If you learn best by hearing or discussing information, find a study partner who learns the same way or read aloud to yourself. Think about how to put the information in your own words. Imagine that you are giving a lecture on the topic and record yourself so you can listen to it later.

For any learning style, flashcards can be helpful. Organize the information so you can take advantage of spare moments to review. Underline key words or phrases. Use different colors for different categories. Mnemonic devices (such as creating a short list in which every item starts with the same letter) can also help with retention. Find what works best for you and use it to store the information in your mind most effectively and easily.

Secret Key #3 – Practice the Right Way

Your success on test day depends not only on how many hours you put into preparing, but also on whether you prepared the right way. It is good to check along the way to see if your studying is paying off. One of the most effective ways to do this is by taking practice tests to evaluate your progress. Practice tests are useful because they show exactly where you need to improve. Every time you take a practice test, pay special attention to these three groups of questions:

- The questions you got wrong
- The questions you had to guess on, even if you guessed right
- The questions you found difficult or slow to work through

This will show you exactly what your weak areas are, and where you need to devote more study time. Ask yourself why each of these questions gave you trouble. Was it because you didn't understand the material? Was it because you didn't remember the vocabulary? Do you need more repetitions on this type of question to build speed and confidence? Dig into those questions and figure out how you can strengthen your weak areas as you go back to review the material.

Additionally, many practice tests have a section explaining the answer choices. It can be tempting to read the explanation and think that you now have a good understanding of the concept. However, an explanation likely only covers part of the question's broader context. Even if the explanation makes sense, **go back and investigate** every concept related to the question until you're positive you have a thorough understanding.

As you go along, keep in mind that the practice test is just that: practice. Memorizing these questions and answers will not be very helpful on the actual test because it is unlikely to have any of the same exact questions. If you only know the right answers to the sample questions, you won't be prepared for the real thing. **Study the concepts** until you understand them fully, and then you'll be able to answer any question that shows up on the test.

It is important to wait on the practice tests until you're ready. If you take a test on your first day of study, you may be overwhelmed by the amount of material covered and how much you need to learn. Work up to it gradually.

On test day, you'll need to be prepared for answering questions, managing your time, and using the test-taking strategies you've learned. It is a lot to balance, like a mental marathon that will have a big impact on your future. Like training for a marathon, you'll need to start slowly and work your way up. When test day arrives, you'll be ready.

Start with the strategies you've read in the first two Secret Keys—plan your course and study in the way that works best for you. If you have time, consider using multiple study resources to get different approaches to the same concepts. It can be helpful to see difficult concepts from more than one angle. Then find a good source for practice tests. Many times, the test website will suggest potential study resources or provide sample tests.

Practice Test Strategy

If you're able to find at least three practice tests, we recommend this strategy:

Untimed and Open-Book Practice

Take the first test with no time constraints and with your notes and study guide handy. Take your time and focus on applying the strategies you've learned.

Timed and Open-Book Practice

Take the second practice test open-book as well, but set a timer and practice pacing yourself to finish in time.

Timed and Closed-Book Practice

Take any other practice tests as if it were test day. Set a timer and put away your study materials. Sit at a table or desk in a quiet room, imagine yourself at the testing center, and answer questions as quickly and accurately as possible.

Keep repeating timed and closed-book tests on a regular basis until you run out of practice tests or it is time for the actual test. Your mind will be ready for the schedule and stress of test day, and you'll be able to focus on recalling the material you've learned.

Secret Key #4 – Pace Yourself

Once you're fully prepared for the material on the test, your biggest challenge on test day will be managing your time. Just knowing that the clock is ticking can make you panic even if you have plenty of time left. Work on pacing yourself so you can build confidence against the time constraints of the exam. Pacing is a difficult skill to master, especially in a high-pressure environment, so **practice is vital**.

Set time expectations for your pace based on how much time is available. For example, if a section has 60 questions and the time limit is 30 minutes, you know you have to average 30 seconds or less per question in order to answer them all. Although 30 seconds is the hard limit, set 25 seconds per question as your goal, so you reserve extra time to spend on harder questions. When you budget extra time for the harder questions, you no longer have any reason to stress when those questions take longer to answer.

Don't let this time expectation distract you from working through the test at a calm, steady pace, but keep it in mind so you don't spend too much time on any one question. Recognize that taking extra time on one question you don't understand may keep you from answering two that you do understand later in the test. If your time limit for a question is up and you're still not sure of the answer, mark it and move on, and come back to it later if the time and the test format allow. If the testing format doesn't allow you to return to earlier questions, just make an educated guess; then put it out of your mind and move on.

On the easier questions, be careful not to rush. It may seem wise to hurry through them so you have more time for the challenging ones, but it is not worth missing one if you know the concept and just didn't take the time to read the question fully. Work efficiently but make sure you understand the question and have looked at all of the answer choices, since more than one may seem right at first.

Even if you're paying attention to the time, you may find yourself a little behind at some point. You should speed up to get back on track, but do so wisely. Don't panic; just take a few seconds less on each question until you're caught up. Don't guess without thinking, but do look through the answer choices and eliminate any you know are wrong. If you can get down to two choices, it is often worthwhile to guess from those. Once you've chosen an answer, move on and don't dwell on any that you skipped or had to hurry through. If a question was taking too long, chances are it was one of the harder ones, so you weren't as likely to get it right anyway.

On the other hand, if you find yourself getting ahead of schedule, it may be beneficial to slow down a little. The more quickly you work, the more likely you are to make a careless mistake that will affect your score. You've budgeted time for each question, so don't be afraid to spend that time. Practice an efficient but careful pace to get the most out of the time you have.

Secret Key #5 – Have a Plan for Guessing

When you're taking the test, you may find yourself stuck on a question. Some of the answer choices seem better than others, but you don't see the one answer choice that is obviously correct. What do you do?

The scenario described above is very common, yet most test takers have not effectively prepared for it. Developing and practicing a plan for guessing may be one of the single most effective uses of your time as you get ready for the exam.

In developing your plan for guessing, there are three questions to address:

- When should you start the guessing process?
- How should you narrow down the choices?
- Which answer should you choose?

When to Start the Guessing Process

Unless your plan for guessing is to select C every time (which, despite its merits, is not what we recommend), you need to leave yourself enough time to apply your answer elimination strategies. Since you have a limited amount of time for each question, that means that if you're going to give yourself the best shot at guessing correctly, you have to decide quickly whether or not you will guess.

Of course, the best-case scenario is that you don't have to guess at all, so first, see if you can answer the question based on your knowledge of the subject and basic reasoning skills. Focus on the key words in the question and try to jog your memory of related topics. Give yourself a chance to bring the knowledge to mind, but once you realize that you don't have (or you can't access) the knowledge you need to answer the question, it is time to start the guessing process.

It is almost always better to start the guessing process too early than too late. It only takes a few seconds to remember something and answer the question from knowledge. Carefully eliminating wrong answer choices takes longer. Plus, going through the process of eliminating answer choices can actually help jog your memory.

Summary: Start the guessing process as soon as you decide that you can't answer the question based on your knowledge.

How to Narrow Down the Choices

The next chapter in this book (**Test-Taking Strategies**) includes a wide range of strategies for how to approach questions and how to look for answer choices to eliminate. You will definitely want to read those carefully, practice them, and figure out which ones work best for you. Here though, we're going to address a mindset rather than a particular strategy.

Your chances of guessing an answer correctly depend on how many options you are choosing from.

How many choices you have	How likely you are to guess correctly
5	20%
4	25%
3	33%
2	50%
1	100%

You can see from this chart just how valuable it is to be able to eliminate incorrect answers and make an educated guess, but there are two things that many test takers do that cause them to miss out on the benefits of guessing:

- Accidentally eliminating the correct answer
- Selecting an answer based on an impression

We'll look at the first one here, and the second one in the next section.

To avoid accidentally eliminating the correct answer, we recommend a thought exercise called **the $5 challenge**. In this challenge, you only eliminate an answer choice from contention if you are willing to bet $5 on it being wrong. Why $5? Five dollars is a small but not insignificant amount of money. It is an amount you could afford to lose but wouldn't want to throw away. And while losing $5 once might not hurt too much, doing it twenty times will set you back $100. In the same way, each small decision you make—eliminating a choice here, guessing on a question there—won't by itself impact your score very much, but when you put them all together, they can make a big difference. By holding each answer choice elimination decision to a higher standard, you can reduce the risk of accidentally eliminating the correct answer.

The $5 challenge can also be applied in a positive sense: If you are willing to bet $5 that an answer choice *is* correct, go ahead and mark it as correct.

Summary: Only eliminate an answer choice if you are willing to bet $5 that it is wrong.

Which Answer to Choose

You're taking the test. You've run into a hard question and decided you'll have to guess. You've eliminated all the answer choices you're willing to bet $5 on. Now you have to pick an answer. Why do we even need to talk about this? Why can't you just pick whichever one you feel like when the time comes?

The answer to these questions is that if you don't come into the test with a plan, you'll rely on your impression to select an answer choice, and if you do that, you risk falling into a trap. The test writers know that everyone who takes their test will be guessing on some of the questions, so they intentionally write wrong answer choices to seem plausible. You still have to pick an answer though, and if the wrong answer choices are designed to look right, how can you ever be sure that you're not falling for their trap? The best solution we've found to this dilemma is to take the decision out of your hands entirely. Here is the process we recommend:

Once you've eliminated any choices that you are confident (willing to bet $5) are wrong, select the first remaining choice as your answer.

Whether you choose to select the first remaining choice, the second, or the last, the important thing is that you use some preselected standard. Using this approach guarantees that you will not be enticed into selecting an answer choice that looks right, because you are not basing your decision on how the answer choices look.

This is not meant to make you question your knowledge. Instead, it is to help you recognize the difference between your knowledge and your impressions. There's a huge difference between thinking an answer is right because of what you know, and thinking an answer is right because it looks or sounds like it should be right.

Summary: To ensure that your selection is appropriately random, make a predetermined selection from among all answer choices you have not eliminated.

Test-Taking Strategies

This section contains a list of test-taking strategies that you may find helpful as you work through the test. By taking what you know and applying logical thought, you can maximize your chances of answering any question correctly!

It is very important to realize that every question is different and every person is different: no single strategy will work on every question, and no single strategy will work for every person. That's why we've included all of them here, so you can try them out and determine which ones work best for different types of questions and which ones work best for you.

Question Strategies

Read Carefully

Read the question and answer choices carefully. Don't miss the question because you misread the terms. You have plenty of time to read each question thoroughly and make sure you understand what is being asked. Yet a happy medium must be attained, so don't waste too much time. You must read carefully, but efficiently.

Contextual Clues

Look for contextual clues. If the question includes a word you are not familiar with, look at the immediate context for some indication of what the word might mean. Contextual clues can often give you all the information you need to decipher the meaning of an unfamiliar word. Even if you can't determine the meaning, you may be able to narrow down the possibilities enough to make a solid guess at the answer to the question.

Prefixes

If you're having trouble with a word in the question or answer choices, try dissecting it. Take advantage of every clue that the word might include. Prefixes and suffixes can be a huge help. Usually they allow you to determine a basic meaning. Pre- means before, post- means after, pro - is positive, de- is negative. From prefixes and suffixes, you can get an idea of the general meaning of the word and try to put it into context.

Hedge Words

Watch out for critical hedge words, such as *likely, may, can, sometimes, often, almost, mostly, usually, generally, rarely,* and *sometimes.* Question writers insert these hedge phrases to cover every possibility. Often an answer choice will be wrong simply because it leaves no room for exception. Be on guard for answer choices that have definitive words such as *exactly* and *always.*

Switchback Words

Stay alert for *switchbacks.* These are the words and phrases frequently used to alert you to shifts in thought. The most common switchback words are *but, although,* and *however.* Others include *nevertheless, on the other hand, even though, while, in spite of, despite, regardless of.* Switchback words are important to catch because they can change the direction of the question or an answer choice.

Face Value

When in doubt, use common sense. Accept the situation in the problem at face value. Don't read too much into it. These problems will not require you to make wild assumptions. If you have to go beyond creativity and warp time or space in order to have an answer choice fit the question, then you should move on and consider the other answer choices. These are normal problems rooted in reality. The applicable relationship or explanation may not be readily apparent, but it is there for you to figure out. Use your common sense to interpret anything that isn't clear.

Answer Choice Strategies

Answer Selection

The most thorough way to pick an answer choice is to identify and eliminate wrong answers until only one is left, then confirm it is the correct answer. Sometimes an answer choice may immediately seem right, but be careful. The test writers will usually put more than one reasonable answer choice on each question, so take a second to read all of them and make sure that the other choices are not equally obvious. As long as you have time left, it is better to read every answer choice than to pick the first one that looks right without checking the others.

Answer Choice Families

An answer choice family consists of two (in rare cases, three) answer choices that are very similar in construction and cannot all be true at the same time. If you see two answer choices that are direct opposites or parallels, one of them is usually the correct answer. For instance, if one answer choice says that quantity x increases and another either says that quantity x decreases (opposite) or says that quantity y increases (parallel), then those answer choices would fall into the same family. An answer choice that doesn't match the construction of the answer choice family is more likely to be incorrect. Most questions will not have answer choice families, but when they do appear, you should be prepared to recognize them.

Eliminate Answers

Eliminate answer choices as soon as you realize they are wrong, but make sure you consider all possibilities. If you are eliminating answer choices and realize that the last one you are left with is also wrong, don't panic. Start over and consider each choice again. There may be something you missed the first time that you will realize on the second pass.

Avoid Fact Traps

Don't be distracted by an answer choice that is factually true but doesn't answer the question. You are looking for the choice that answers the question. Stay focused on what the question is asking for so you don't accidentally pick an answer that is true but incorrect. Always go back to the question and make sure the answer choice you've selected actually answers the question and is not merely a true statement.

Extreme Statements

In general, you should avoid answers that put forth extreme actions as standard practice or proclaim controversial ideas as established fact. An answer choice that states the "process should be used in certain situations, if..." is much more likely to be correct than one that states the "process should be discontinued completely." The first is a calm rational statement and doesn't even make a definitive, uncompromising stance, using a hedge word *if* to provide wiggle room, whereas the second choice is a radical idea and far more extreme.

Benchmark

As you read through the answer choices and you come across one that seems to answer the question well, mentally select that answer choice. This is not your final answer, but it is the one that will help you evaluate the other answer choices. The one that you selected is your benchmark or standard for judging each of the other answer choices. Every other answer choice must be compared to your benchmark. That choice is correct until proven otherwise by another answer choice beating it. If you find a better answer, then that one becomes your new benchmark. Once you've decided that no other choice answers the question as well as your benchmark, you have your final answer.

Predict the Answer

Before you even start looking at the answer choices, it is often best to try to predict the answer. When you come up with the answer on your own, it is easier to avoid distractions and traps because you will know exactly what to look for. The right answer choice is unlikely to be word-for-word what you came up with, but it should be a close match. Even if you are confident that you have the right answer, you should still take the time to read each option before moving on.

General Strategies

Tough Questions

If you are stumped on a problem or it appears too hard or too difficult, don't waste time. Move on! Remember though, if you can quickly check for obviously incorrect answer choices, your chances of guessing correctly are greatly improved. Before you completely give up, at least try to knock out a couple of possible answers. Eliminate what you can and then guess at the remaining answer choices before moving on.

Check Your Work

Since you will probably not know every term listed and the answer to every question, it is important that you get credit for the ones that you do know. Don't miss any questions through careless mistakes. If at all possible, try to take a second to look back over your answer selection and make sure you've selected the correct answer choice and haven't made a costly careless mistake (such as marking an answer choice that you didn't mean to mark). This quick double check should more than pay for itself in caught mistakes for the time it costs.

Pace Yourself

It is easy to be overwhelmed when you're looking at a page full of questions; your mind is confused and full of random thoughts, and the clock is ticking down faster than you would like. Calm down and maintain the pace that you have set for yourself. Especially as you get down to the last few minutes of the test, don't let the small numbers on the clock make you panic. As long as you are on track by monitoring your pace, you are guaranteed to have time for each question.

Don't Rush

It is very easy to make errors when you are in a hurry. Maintaining a fast pace in answering questions is pointless if it makes you miss questions that you would have gotten right otherwise. Test writers like to include distracting information and wrong answers that seem right. Taking a little extra time to avoid careless mistakes can make all the difference in your test score. Find a pace that allows you to be confident in the answers that you select.

KEEP MOVING

Panicking will not help you pass the test, so do your best to stay calm and keep moving. Taking deep breaths and going through the answer elimination steps you practiced can help to break through a stress barrier and keep your pace.

Final Notes

The combination of a solid foundation of content knowledge and the confidence that comes from practicing your plan for applying that knowledge is the key to maximizing your performance on test day. As your foundation of content knowledge is built up and strengthened, you'll find that the strategies included in this chapter become more and more effective in helping you quickly sift through the distractions and traps of the test to isolate the correct answer.

Now it is time to move on to the test content chapters of this book, but be sure to keep your goal in mind. As you read, think about how you will be able to apply this information on the test. If you've already seen sample questions for the test and you have an idea of the question format and style, try to come up with questions of your own that you can answer based on what you're reading. This will give you valuable practice applying your knowledge in the same ways you can expect to on test day.

Good luck and good studying!

Biological and Biochemical Foundations of Living Systems

Structure and Function of Proteins and Their Constituent Amino Acids

Amino Acids

Description

ABSOLUTE CONFIGURATION AT THE A POSITION

There are 20 amino acids that cells use to build proteins. An amino acid contains a centrally located stereogenic carbon bonded to four substituents: an amino group (NH_2), a carboxyl group (COOH), a hydrogen atom (H), and a variable R-group. Amino acids that have an amino group bonded directly to the alpha-carbon are referred to as alpha amino acids.

Review Video: Amino Acids
Visit mometrix.com/academy and enter code: 190385

Absolute configuration refers to the spatial orientation of atoms around the asymmetric (chiral) alpha-carbon. Each amino acid (with the exception of glycine, which has two hydrogens bonded to the alpha-carbon) can exist in one of two possible configurations at that carbon and are called stereoisomers. Because these stereoisomers are non-superimposable mirror images (similar to a left and right hand), they are further classified as enantiomers.

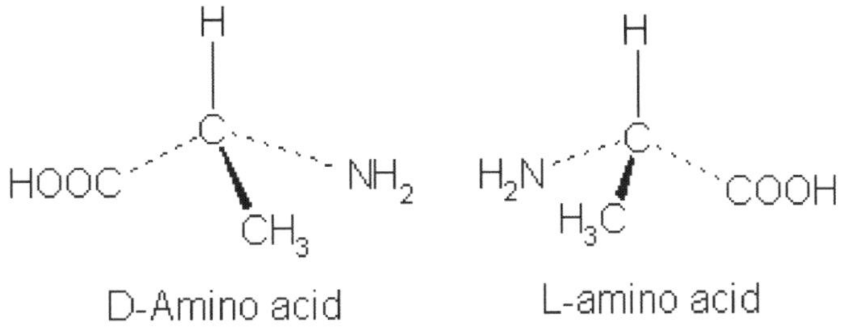

H, C, HOOC, NH_2, CH_3 — D-Amino acid

H, C, H_2N, COOH, H_3C — L-amino acid

There are different methods of specifying the configurations of these enantiomers. Using D/L nomenclature, all the amino acids that make up naturally occurring proteins are of the L-configuration. Using R/S nomenclature, most amino acids are of the S-configuration. Classification of L does not necessarily indicate classification of S.

AMINO ACIDS AS DIPOLAR IONS

In most cellular conditions, the amino group (NH_2) and carboxylic acid group (COOH) of an amino acid are ionized. Each amino acid has a specific pH, known as the isoelectric point (pI), in which it exists as a dipolar ion, or zwitterion. A zwitterion is an electrically neutral molecule with both positive and negative regions. The acidic amino group holds a positive charge that cancels out the negative charge of the basic carboxyl group.

The amino acid can also exist as a positive ion if the aqueous environment has a lower pH than its pI. The excess H ions in the acidic solution protonate the COO-group, neutralizing it. The amino acid becomes a cation.

The amino acid can exist as a negative ion if the aqueous environment has a higher pH than its pI. The NH_3^+ donates a proton, neutralizing it. The amino acid becomes an anion.

Classifications: Acidic or Basic

Amino acids are classified according to the unique chemical properties of each R-group, or side chain. Amino acids with electrically charged side chains will either be acidic or basic. Acidic amino acids have side chains that contain a negatively charged carboxyl group at the pH level of the cell. Basic amino acids have side chains that contain a positively charged amino group at the pH level of the cell.

The acidic amino acids include aspartic acid and glutamic acid. (Note that in anion form they are referred to as aspartate and glutamate.) The basic amino acids include lysine, arginine, and histidine. Because these five amino acids are charged, they are also hydrophilic.

Classifications: Hydrophobic or Hydrophilic

Amino acids can be grouped according to the polarity (or lack thereof) of their side chains. Non-polar side chains (made mostly of carbon and hydrogen) share electrons equally, so there is an even distribution of charge. Because of this property, the side chains cannot form hydrogen bonds with water, hence the classification as hydrophobic, or water fearing.

Polar amino acids have side chains (typically containing an amine, hydroxyl, or carboxyl group) that do not share electrons equally, resulting in a partial positive charge *and* negative charge on that chain. This uneven distribution of charge allows the side chain to form hydrogen bonds with water, hence the classification as hydrophilic, or water loving.

Hydrophilic amino acids include serine, threonine, lysine, asparagine, histidine, aspartate, glutamate, arginine, and glutamine. Hydrophobic amino acids include glycine, alanine, valine, leucine, isoleucine, methionine, phenylalanine, tryptophan, and proline. Cysteine and tyrosine are special exceptions of hydrophobic amino acids with polar side chains.

Reactions

Sulfur Linkage for Cysteine and Cysteine

Cysteine is an amino acid that plays an important role in the stabilization of proteins. The side chain of cysteine contains a thiol group consisting of a sulfur and a hydrogen atom (-SH). Oxidation of this functional group will result in a disulfide bridge (a covalent bond) between the sulfur atoms of two cysteines and the removal of two hydrogen atoms. The product is named cystine, which is the oxidized dimer of cysteine. Disulfide bridges are the strongest bonds found in proteins, and they stabilize both the tertiary and quaternary structure of proteins. Note that sulfur linkages do not form between the sulfur atoms of methionine.

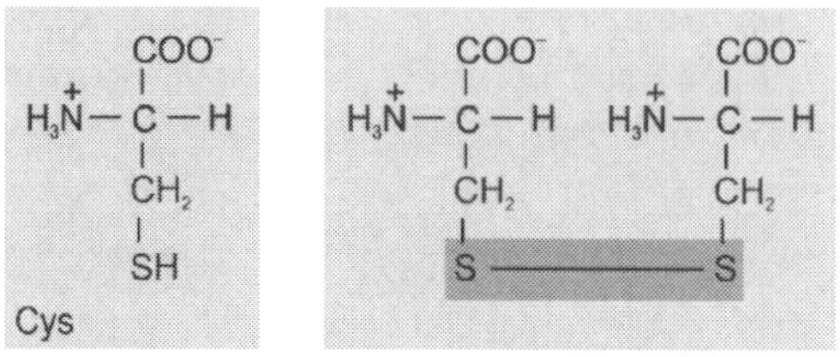

Peptide Linkage: Polypeptides and Proteins

Proteins are made from polypeptides, and polypeptides are unbranched chains of amino acids. The amino acids join together by dehydration synthesis when the lone pair of electrons on the nitrogen of amino group forms a covalent bond with the carbon on the carboxyl group of a second amino acid. A water molecule is released when hydrogen is removed from the amino group and a hydroxyl group is removed from the carboxyl group.

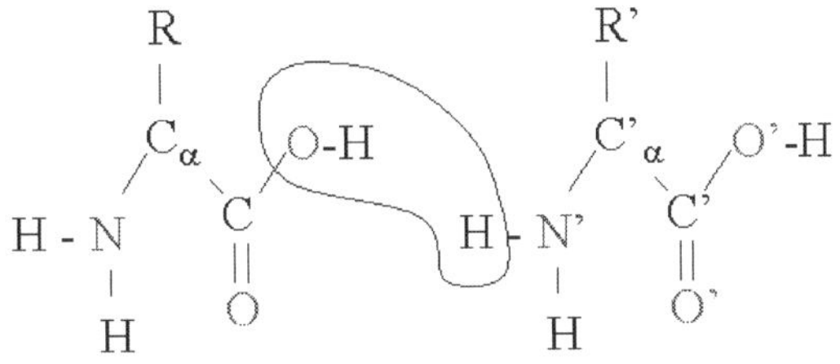

R R'
C_α O-H C'_α O'-H
H - N C H - N' C'
O O'
H H

The resulting bond is called a peptide bond, and two amino acids are collectively called a dipeptide. Amino acids can continue to be added to form a polypeptide that will begin with a nitrogen atom (N-terminal) and end with a carbon atom (C-terminal). Every amino acid within the chain is called a residue. The peptide bonds that hold the residues together are rigid, but the amino acids are free to rotate around the alpha-carbon, and the chain can fold into a three-dimensional configuration.

Hydrolysis

The peptide bond between amino acids is cleaved via a hydrolysis reaction. During this process, a water molecule is split to provide the nitrogen with a hydrogen atom (giving back the amino group) and the carbonyl carbon with a hydroxyl group (giving back the carboxyl group). Hydrolysis of proteins can happen in one of two ways: acid hydrolysis or the use of a proteolytic enzyme, also called protease.

Hydrochloric acid and high temperatures will eventually break all the peptide bonds within a polypeptide, resulting in a stew of individual amino acids.

Proteolytic cleavage is more precise, as certain proteases will only cleave certain bonds. For example, the protease trypsin (produced by the pancreas) acts only on the carboxyl end of lysine or arginine, resulting in shorter chains but not total digestion of the protein.

Protein Structure

Structure

1° Structure of Proteins

Proteins are complex structures made from unbranched chains of amino acids, called polypeptides. The primary level of protein structure is simply the linear sequence of amino acids. The size of a polypeptide can range from 50 to 5,000 residues (amino acids) linked together by peptide bonds. The sequence of nucleotides in a gene determines the specific amino acid sequence, and the amino acid sequence determines the conformation and function of the protein. A mutation in the genetic code can lead to an altered primary structure, which in turn may disrupt subsequent levels of structure.

The primary structure begins with the amino-terminal end and terminates at the carboxyl-terminal end. Typically, each amino acid will be abbreviated with either a three- or one-letter abbreviation as noted below.

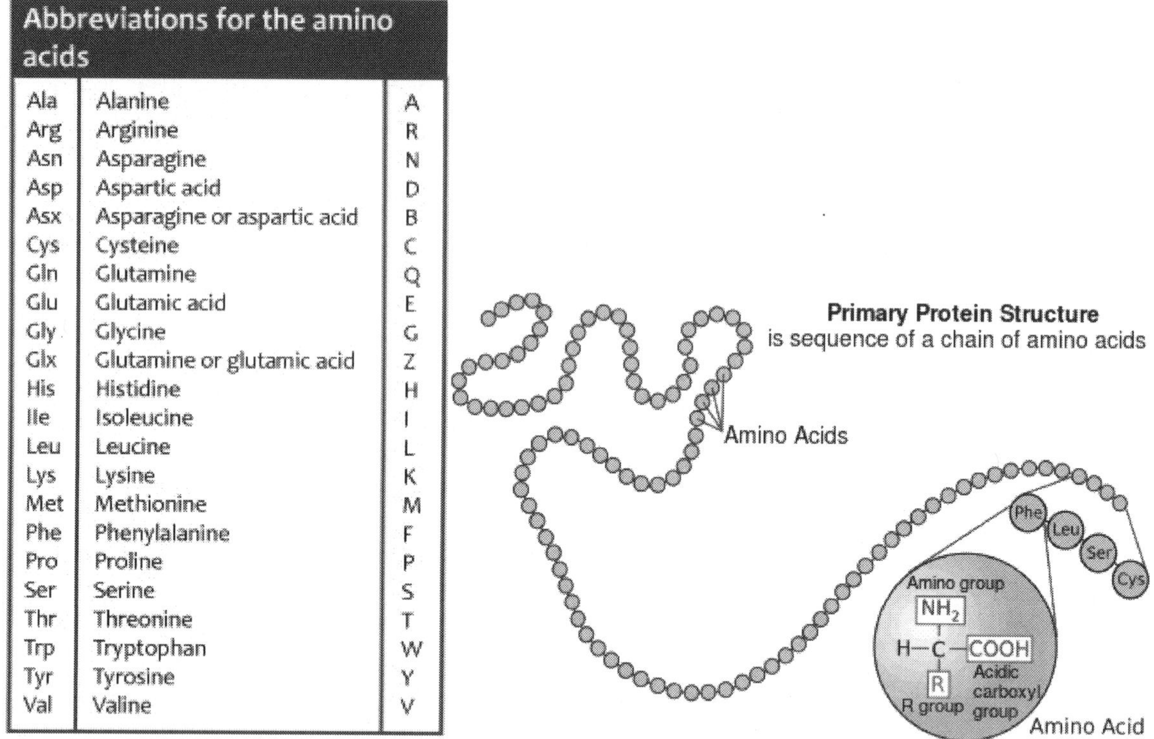

Abbreviations for the amino acids		
Ala	Alanine	A
Arg	Arginine	R
Asn	Asparagine	N
Asp	Aspartic acid	D
Asx	Asparagine or aspartic acid	B
Cys	Cysteine	C
Gln	Glutamine	Q
Glu	Glutamic acid	E
Gly	Glycine	G
Glx	Glutamine or glutamic acid	Z
His	Histidine	H
Ile	Isoleucine	I
Leu	Leucine	L
Lys	Lysine	K
Met	Methionine	M
Phe	Phenylalanine	F
Pro	Proline	P
Ser	Serine	S
Thr	Threonine	T
Trp	Tryptophan	W
Tyr	Tyrosine	Y
Val	Valine	V

2° STRUCTURE OF PROTEINS

The secondary structure of a protein results from hydrogen bonding between the backbone portions of the amino acids. The carbonyl oxygen (C=O) forms a hydrogen bond with the amino hydrogen (N-H) of a different amino acid. Side chains do not participate in secondary structure.

There are two shapes that commonly arise as a result of hydrogen bonding. The first is the alpha-helix. In this case a bond is formed every fourth amino acid. For example, the oxygen of the first amino acid will bond with the hydrogen of the fifth amino acid. The chain coils into a ribbon-like helix with the side chains oriented outward from the spiral.

The second shape commonly seen in secondary structure is the beta-pleated sheet. When strands of a polypeptide lie side by side, hydrogen bonds will stabilize the molecule, and the R-groups will extend above and below the strands. If the strands are antiparallel, then the bonds will be better aligned and more stable than if the strands are parallel.

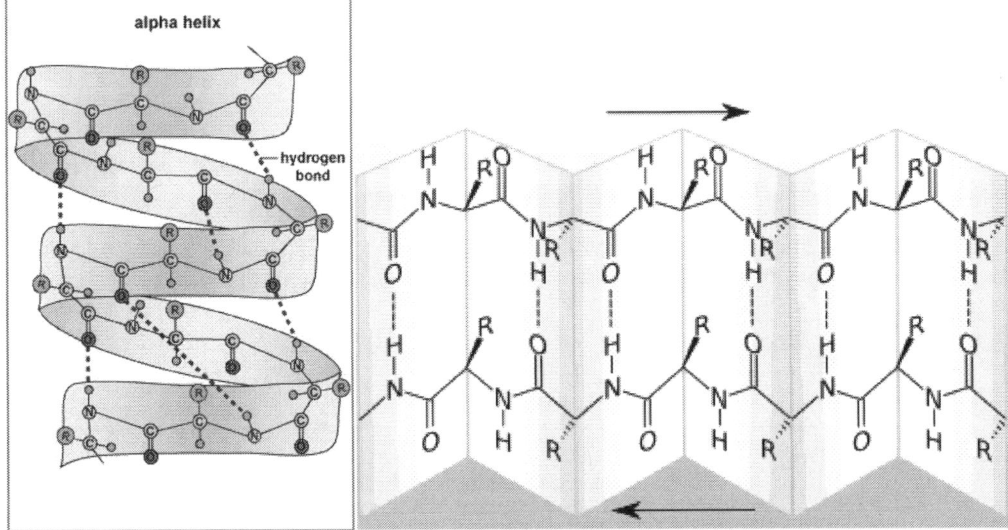

3° Structure of Proteins; Role of Proline, Cystine, and Hydrophobic Bonding

The tertiary structure of a protein results from the interactions of R-groups, and there are many types of bonds and forces between them that hold the protein in its three-dimensional shape.

At cellular pH, hydrophilic side chains of amino acids will orient themselves toward the aqueous environment, whereas hydrophobic chains usually point toward the core of the protein to shield themselves from the cytoplasm. Van der Waals interactions keep these hydrophobic constituents together.

The stability of the protein is further aided by hydrogen bonding between polar side chains. Similarly, disulfide bonds between the sulfur groups on cysteine residues act as bridges to covalently bond two regions of a polypeptide together. Ionic bonds called salt bridges also form between oppositely charged R-groups.

Proline is the only amino acid whose R-group connects to the amino group. It will cause a bend in the polypeptide chain and destabilize both α-helices and β-pleated sheets. However, it does allow for tight turns of the polypeptide chain. By disrupting the secondary structure of a protein, it affects the tertiary structure.

4° Structure of Proteins

Many, but not all, proteins are aggregates of two or more polypeptides. This complex of polypeptides is referred to as the quaternary structure. Each polypeptide within the protein is called a subunit, and these subunits may be identical or combinations of different polypeptides. A protein with two, three or four subunits is known as a dimer, trimer, and tetramer, respectively. Like the tertiary structure, quaternary structure is stabilized by van der Waals, hydrogen, covalent, and ionic bonds.

Proteins are classified according to their three-dimensional conformation. Fibrous proteins are cable-like, without the turns and folds seen in globular proteins. Fibrous proteins are generally insoluble in aqueous solutions and function mainly in the structure of muscle and connective tissue.

Globular proteins play functional roles and participate in reactions. They tend to be water-soluble and more likely to denature (change conformation) if their environment changes.

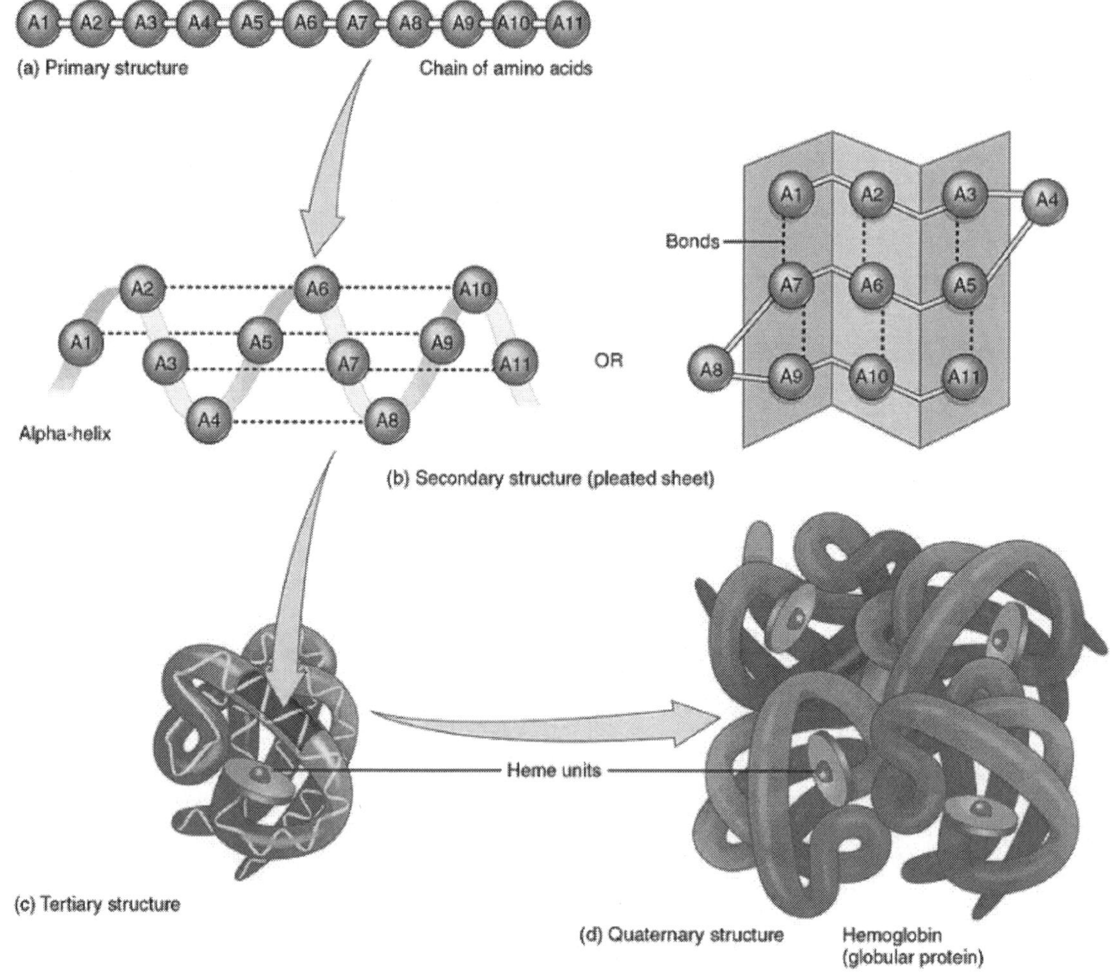

Conformational Stability

Denaturing and Folding

For a protein to function properly, it must fold into a specific conformation (as dictated by its amino acid sequence). Conformation can be altered by misfolding during translation or by denaturation as a result of environmental changes.

Chaperonins are proteins that assist with the folding process by shielding the growing polypeptide from the cytoplasmic environment. They also prevent the N-terminus from aggregating with other polypeptides before translation is finished. Misfolding will occur if the chaperone proteins are not functioning properly or if the conditions of the cytoplasm are not ideal.

Most proteins (particularly globular proteins) are sensitive to changes in the environment. Slight changes in pH, temperature, and salinity can change the native conformation by weakening the bonds that stabilize the protein. Proteins may also denature if they are introduced to a non-polar solvent. In this case the hydrophobic amino acids will reorient themselves to the exterior of the protein.

Note that the *primary* structure is *not* disrupted by the factors described above. In some cases, the protein may return to its native shape when the appropriate environmental conditions are restored.

Hydrophobic Interactions

Hydrophobic interactions play an important role in the tertiary structure of a globular protein by minimizing the interactions of certain amino acids with the solvent. Non-polar side chains of amino acids are hydrophobic (water fearing), and repulsive forces bury them in the core of the protein, whereas dipole-induced dipole interactions (or van der Waals forces) help hold them in place. Charged or polar side chains of amino acids are hydrophilic (water loving) and expose themselves to the aqueous environment to maximize hydrogen bonding. The push and pull to achieve this more ordered conformation is entropy driven. As the protein folds entropy (a measure of the level of disorder in a system) decreases as the entropy of the surroundings increases.

Solvation Layer (Entropy)

The solvation layer refers to the interface of water and the surface area of the protein. Because water molecules in the solvation layer (also known as the hydration shell) are unable to form hydrogen bonds with nonpolar R-groups, the side chains will bury themselves in the interior of the protein. This creates a sort of balancing act as the protein tries to maximize the exposure of polar side chains while minimizing the solvation of nonpolar side chains.

This hydrophobic interaction decreases the surface area of the polypeptide, and the entropy of the solute (protein) decreases as the entropy of the solvent (water) increases. Heat is released as the bonds that stabilize the protein are formed. The folding process is spontaneous because the free energy (ΔG) is negative.

Separation Techniques

Isoelectric Point

Proteins have the ability to be separated according to their properties (such as electrical charge, size, and solubility). One such technique is called isoelectric focusing (IEF). IEF separates molecules by isoelectric point (pI), which is the pH at which the protein is either neutral, or at its lowest ionization. In general, the isoelectric point decreases as the proportion of acidic amino acids increases and vice versa.

The IEF technique spreads the proteins of interest over a medium (usually a gel) with a pH gradient ranging from low to high. A current is passed through the gel, and proteins that carry a positive charge will begin to migrate toward the negative pole (anode), whereas proteins with a negative charge will migrate toward the positive pole (cathode). At some point along the pH gradient, the protein will reach its pI and lose its electric charge to become a zwitterion. Because the protein is now neutral, the electrode will not be able to pull it any further. The result is a banding pattern on the gel, with each band consisting of a species of protein with its unique isoelectric point.

Electrophoresis

Electrophoresis is technique that separates molecules (such as proteins) according to their size or charge. A protein sample is added to a solvent, usually a gel, which behaves like a molecular sieve. The gel is placed in an electrophoresis chamber, which is then connected to a power source. As an electric field is applied, the proteins begin to migrate and separate. The smaller the molecule, the farther it will travel. Because most proteins are charged at any pH, with the exception of their isoelectric point, they will migrate toward the electrode with the opposite charge. The original sample will separate into distinct bands of isolated proteins. The rate at which a protein migrates is dependent on the size of the protein, the net charge, the strength of the electric field, and the viscosity and pore size of the solvent. Two common media used in electrophoresis are agar and polyacrylamide. Polyacrylamide is typically used for proteins because it has the appropriate pore size. SDS-PAGE is a type of electrophoresis that uses polyacrylamide along with a denaturing agent called sodium dodecyl sulfate. Proteins are then separated according to molecular weight.

Non-Enzymatic Protein Function

Binding

Non-enzymatic binding proteins are proteins that bind to ligands but do not catalyze a reaction. The ligand, or substrate, is typically smaller than the protein and will bind to a specific region that is typically concave. Some amino acids are part of the ligand-protein interface, but most of them are responsible for maintaining the tertiary structure. The greater the intermolecular attraction between the protein and ligand, the greater the binding affinity. These forces include non-covalent bonds such as hydrogen bonds, ionic bonds, van der Waals interactions, and hydrophobic interactions. If the conformation of a protein is altered, the ligand may be unable to bind. A change in conformation could also compromise the specificity of the binding site.

Common examples of non-enzymatic binding proteins include the following:

- Receptors, used for communication among cells
- Transport proteins to assist the passage of substances across the plasma membrane
- Antibodies, which play a role in immunity
- Motor proteins, used for cellular motility

Immune System

An antibody, also called an immunoglobulin (Ig), is a glycoprotein secreted by B cells that aids in the immune system's defenses by binding to an antigen (a substance that is foreign or toxic to the body.) Antibodies share a common structure: four polypeptides linked together by disulfide bonds to form a Y-shape. Two of the polypeptides are called "heavy chains" because they are about twice as long as the other "light chains." Regardless of the type of antibody, there are nearly identical regions on the stem of the Y called constant or C-regions. It is the variable, or V-region, that distinguishes one type of antibody from the other. The V-regions on the arms of the Y collectively form a highly specific antigen-binding site. This is where the antibody will lock onto the antigen to disarm it. The non-covalent bonding forces are weak, and therefore the binding is reversible. Antibodies can act by neutralization (rendering the antigen ineffective), precipitation (clumping of soluble antigens so they precipitate out of solution before they are destroyed by phagocytosis), agglutination (clumping of insoluble particle antigens), or complement activation (binding of the antibody to trigger a series of events that will lead to lysis of the pathogen).

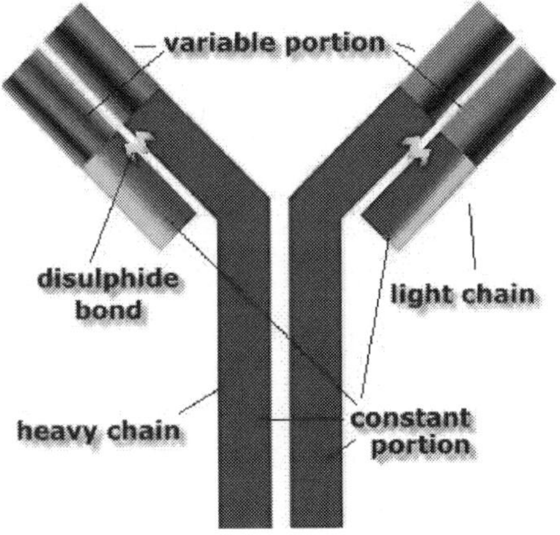

Motors

Motor proteins do mechanical work to move structures within the cell and aid in the movement of the cell itself. They accomplish this by undergoing a conformational change powered by the hydrolysis of ATP. There are three major classes of motor proteins: myosins, kinesins, and dyneins.

Myosin plays a role in muscle contraction by interacting with the protein actin. Thick myosin filaments bind to thinner actin filaments and then release. This causes the filaments to slide over each other during muscle contraction.

Kinesins are involved in the shuttling of vesicles and other cellular components within the cell. The proteins appear to "walk" along microtubules of the cytoskeleton, carrying their cargo toward the plus end of the microtubule (usually away from the center of the cell). They are also essential to the formation of the mitotic spindle and the alignment and separation of sister chromatids.

Dyneins are the largest motor proteins and assist in the transport of cargo within the cell. Unlike kinesins, they move in the direction of the minus end of the microtubule (usually toward the center of the cell). Dyneins are also responsible for the beating of cilia and flagella. They achieve this by sliding microfilaments over each other.

Enzyme Structure and Function

Function of Enzymes in Catalyzing Biological Reactions

An enzyme is a protein catalyst that increases the rate of chemical reactions. Each enzyme has an active site that interacts with a substrate or substrates (also called reactants). Because the active site has a highly specific structure, it can bind only to certain reactants. As the enzyme interacts with its substrate, the activation energy is lowered either by weakening the chemical bonds of the substrate or bringing substrate molecules together in an orientation that allows them to react more efficiently. Lowering the activation energy accelerates the reaction. When the reaction is complete, the enzyme will release the reactant(s) and return to its original conformation to be used again. Without enzymes, the reactions of the body would occur slowly to sustain life.

Enzyme Classification by Reaction Type

Identify the major classes of enzymes, and describe the reactions in which they participate.

Enzymes can be classified into six major classes based on the type of reaction that they catalyze.

1. Oxidoreductases involve the transfer of electrons, usually in the form of a hydrogen atom. This reaction is known as an oxidation-reduction, or redox, reaction. The molecule that donates electrons is "oxidized," and the molecule that accepts them is "reduced."
2. Transferases catalyze the transferring of a functional group (such as an amino or phosphate group) from a donor molecule (usually a coenzyme) to the acceptor.
3. Hydrolases are similar to transferases because they transfer a functional group, but this reaction always involves hydrolysis, and the group is donated to water.
4. Lyases catalyze the breaking of bonds via elimination reaction, forming a double bond or ring structure. They are unique in that they need only one substrate for the reaction in the forward direction but two for the reverse.
5. Isomerases transfer functional groups within the substrate to create an isomer. The chemical formula does not change—only the arrangement of the atoms.
6. Ligases use the hydrolysis of ATP to power a condensation reaction between two molecules.

Review Video: Enzymes
Visit mometrix.com/academy and enter code: 656995

Reduction of Activation Energy

Activation energy is the minimum amount of energy needed to break the bonds of a reactant. More precisely it is the difference between the free energy of the reactants and the free energy of the transition state. The transition state (represented by the peak on an energy graph) occurs when the bonds of the substrate are partially broken and the potential energy is at a maximum. This energy is lowered when the enzyme attracts the reactant(s) and then alters its configuration to orient the reactants in a way that promotes the transfer of electrons. The change in shape puts a strain on the bonds within the substrate, making the covalent bonds easier to break. The stabilization of the transition state and subsequent reduction in activation energy allows the reaction to proceed more rapidly.

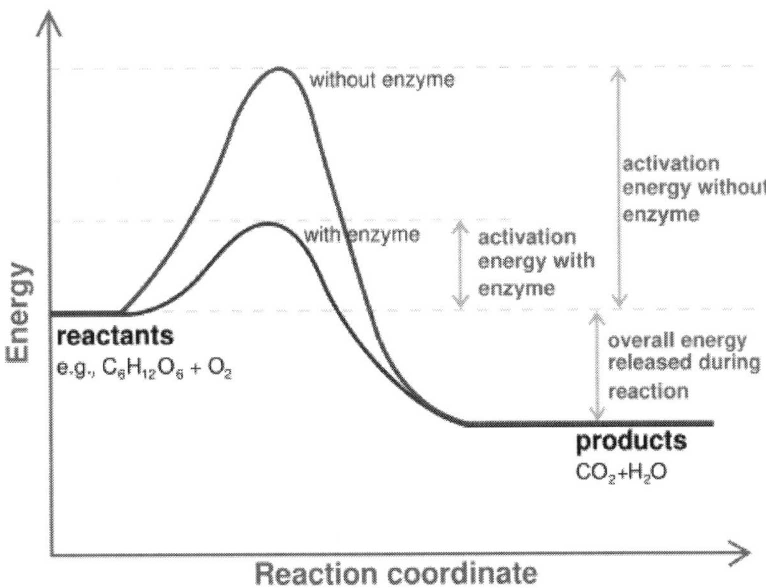

Substrates and Enzyme Specificity

Enzyme specificity refers to the ability of an enzyme to bind to a target substrate. The part of the enzyme to which the substrate binds is called the active site. The amino acids within this region are responsible for the complementary shape and chemical properties of the active site. There are varying degrees of molecular recognition; some enzymes are specific to only one reactant, whereas others work on a range of molecules. As such the specificity of enzymes can be sorted into the following categories:

- Absolute specificity: the enzyme will only bind to one particular substrate.
- Group specificity: the enzyme will bind to substrates that share the same functional groups.
- Linkage specificity: the enzyme will hydrolyze a specific type of bond.
- Stereochemical specificity: the enzyme is specific to a steric or optical isomer.

Active Site Model

The active site is a relatively small folded region on an enzyme that interacts with a substrate. The sequence of amino acids found in this region determines the unique folded shape, and therefore the specificity, of this region. Note, however, that the amino acids found at the active site are not necessarily in the same linear sequence as the primary structure of the protein. The folds of the tertiary structure will bring amino acids from various portions of the polypeptide together to form a binding site that is complementary to the shape of the substrate. The enzyme will "recognize" the substrate, bind to it (forming an enzyme-substrate complex), and bring it to the transition state. The chemical bonds within the substrate are modified as the enzyme changes its configuration, the activation energy is lowered, and the reaction proceeds more rapidly.

Induced-Fit Model

The induced-fit model of enzyme activity explains how the enzyme interacts with its substrate. It is an updated version of the "lock and key" model in which the substrate fits perfectly into the active site without any modification of the enzyme. In the induced fit model, the enzyme is more like a flexible baseball glove than a rigid puzzle piece. A substrate with an imperfect fit will bind to the enzyme, causing a slight conformational change in that enzyme. The affinity for the substrate will increase, "inducing" a more perfect fit. As such the enzyme is complementary to the transition state, not the initial form of the substrate. As the enzyme and substrate mold together into a complex, the enzyme stabilizes the transition state and converts it into a product. This model describes a more dynamic process rather than the static binding of two perfectly matched puzzle pieces. Molecules can be "flexible" because of the ability for single covalent bonds to rotate.

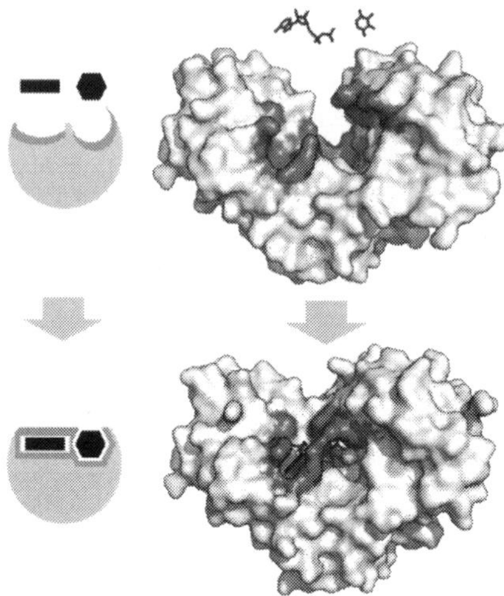

Mechanism of Catalysis

There are many mechanisms by which an enzyme carries out catalysis:

- General acid or general base hydrolysis: the transition state is stabilized when a reactive group on an enzyme receives or donates a proton.
- Approximation: the enzyme assists in bringing the reactants together in the proper orientation, similar to (but more effective than) the effects achieved by increasing the concentration of the reactants. The closeness of proximity reduces entropy.
- Metal ion catalysis: enzymes use electrophilic metal ions such as copper, iron, or zinc to catalyze a reaction by binding to the substrate and stabilizing the charges on the transition state.
- Covalent catalysis: a temporary covalent bond is formed between a nucleophilic reactive group on the enzyme and substrate. Electrons are withdrawn from the substrate before the reactive group is removed and the enzyme returns to its original state.

Cofactors

Cofactors are chemical compounds (not proteins) that are required for some enzymes to perform their catalytic function. They are sometimes referred to as "helper compounds" as they help regulate the rate at which reactions occur. Cofactors may be classified as organic (and include coenzymes and tightly bound prosthetic groups) or inorganic (typically metallic ions). In some classifications all cofactors are assumed to be inorganic. Examples of inorganic cofactors include iron, magnesium, manganese, and zinc. These ions increase the energy for the chemical reaction by acting as a bridge between the enzyme and substrate. Hemoglobin is an example of a protein that requires a cofactor because iron is needed for it to bind to oxygen. An enzyme in the absence of a required cofactor is called an apoenzyme. If the cofactor is present, the enzyme is referred to as a holoenzyme.

Coenzymes

Coenzymes are organic non-protein molecules that are necessary for certain enzymes to function. They bind to the enzyme covalently and serve as intermediate carriers of atoms or functional groups. They help catalyze the conversion of substrate to products, but unlike enzymes they are not specific to the substrate, and they can be chemically altered by the reaction. One example of a coenzyme includes nicotinamide adenine dinucleotide (NAD^+), which is an electron acceptor in the redox reactions of metabolic pathways, such as glycolysis and the citric acid cycle. It is regenerated during the electron transport chain of cellular respiration. Another important example is adenosine triphosphate (ATP), which powers cellular work by phosphorylating another molecule. Many water-soluble vitamins serve as coenzymes or precursors to coenzymes.

Water-Soluble Vitamins

Vitamins are organic molecules that are required for many enzymes to function. Few vitamins are synthesized by the body and must be obtained through diet. Vitamins are classified as either fat-soluble (which do not function as coenzymes) or water-soluble. The water-soluble vitamins form hydrogen bonds with water and include beta-carotene (which is actually a form of the fat-soluble vitamin A), vitamin C (ascorbic acid), and the vitamin B series. The ionized version of vitamin C (ascorbate) is an antioxidant and neutralizes free radicals but does not function as a coenzyme. The vitamin B series includes B1 (thiamin), B2 (riboflavin), B3 (niacin), B5 (pantothenic acid), B6 (pyridoxine), B7 (biotin), B9 (folic acid), and vitamin B12. These vitamins function as coenzymes that help catalyze many vital reactions in the body. Vitamins B2 and B3, for example, are involved in the making of ATP, and vitamin B12 is required for DNA synthesis.

Effects of Local Conditions on Enzyme Activity

The most common factors that affect enzyme activity are temperature, pH, and salinity.

If the temperature is below the optimal range, the number of collisions between the enzyme and substrate will decrease, as will the energy of those collisions. The reaction rate may be too slow to be effective, or it may halt altogether. Increasing the temperature increases the rate of reaction but only to a point. Eventually the bonds that hold together the tertiary structure of the protein will begin to weaken and break, and the enzyme will denature.

If salinity is too low, then charged R-groups of the amino acids will attract one another. If it is too high, the charged side chains will not be able to interact at all. Both cases may result in the loss of native shape of the enzyme.

Changes in pH will affect the ionization of certain amino acids. As pH increases, the enzyme will lose hydrogen ions, and as pH decreases, it will gain hydrogen ions. This may break the non-covalent bonds responsible for its structure.

Because fluctuations in the conditions surrounding an enzyme can lead to a change in conformation, the activity of the enzyme will either decrease or halt altogether.

Control of Enzyme Activity

Kinetics

General (Catalysis)

Kinetics is the study of the rate of reactions, and reactions can be accelerated in a process known as catalysis. In biological systems, enzymes are often responsible for catalyzing reactions. They do this by binding to the reactant, stabilizing the transition state, and lowering the activation energy (the minimum amount of energy needed to jumpstart a reaction). The lower the activation energy, the more rapid the reaction. The equilibrium of the reaction is not affected, meaning that the addition of an enzyme will not shift the equilibrium concentration to favor either the substrate or product. ΔG (change in Gibbs free energy) and K_{eq} (equilibrium constant) remain the same.

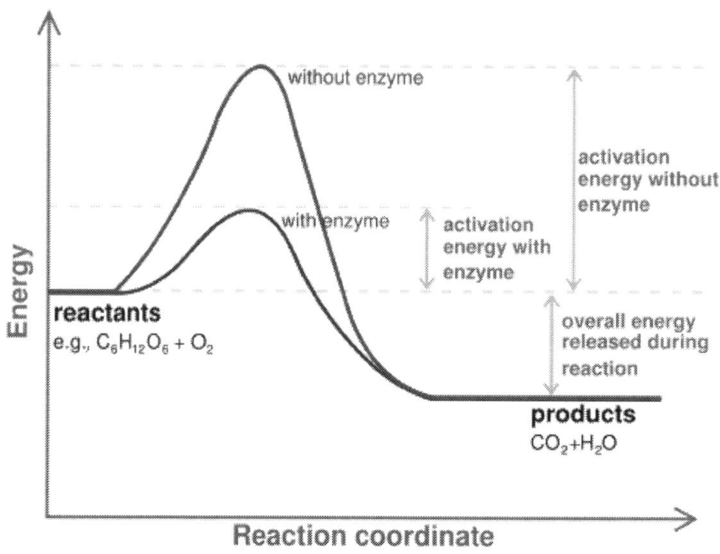

MICHAELIS–MENTEN

Michaelis-Menten equation:

$$V = \frac{V_{max}[S]}{K_m + [S]}$$

The Michaelis-Menten equation calculates the rate of reaction, or amount of product formed over time, by relating it to the concentration of the substrate. Variables in the equation include maximum reaction rate (v_{max}), the concentration of the substrate ([S]), and the Michaelis-Menten constant (K_m). The Michaelis-Menten constant is a loose measure of binding affinity—more specifically, the concentration of substrate that is required for the reaction to reach half of its maximum velocity. The higher the K_m, the weaker the affinity of an enzyme for its target substrate (or "catalytic efficiency"), and the higher the concentration of substrate needed for the reaction to reach v_{max}. Below is a graph of reaction velocity as a function of substrate concentration. Note that as the concentration of substrate increases, the rate of reaction begins to plateau as some of the product is lost to the reverse reaction.

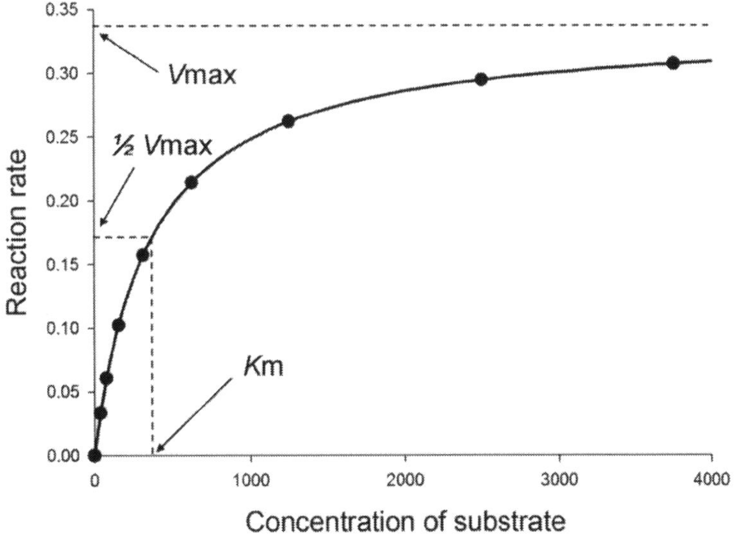

COOPERATIVITY

Some enzymes with quaternary structure have more than one binding site, and the binding of one substrate may influence the binding of subsequent substrates. The influence could be positive (the binding of the first substrate increases affinity for subsequent ligands) or negative (affinity for subsequent ligands decreases). If the enzyme has multiple binding sites, but substrate binding has no influence on the other sites, then this is called non-cooperativity. Cooperativity may also be classified by substrate type. Homotropic cooperativity occurs when the substrate affects its own affinity, and heterotropic cooperativity occurs when a third ligand is involved.

Not all binding sites are active (sites where the catalytic reaction takes place). Ligands may bind to alternate sites called allosteric sites, which influence the activity of the enzyme by changing its conformation. A ligand that decreases the efficiency of an enzyme is called an allosteric inhibitor, and a ligand that increases enzyme activity is called an allosteric activator.

FEEDBACK REGULATION

Feedback refers to the process by which an enzyme is regulated by the product it produces. Typically, as the product accumulates and binds to an allosteric site on the enzyme, the activity of the enzyme is inhibited by decreasing the affinity of the enzyme for the reactant(s). This negative feedback mechanism seeks to restore balance and is known as feedback inhibition. In the rarer case of positive feedback, the product increases the rate of reaction by increasing the affinity of the enzyme for the substrate. Neither form of feedback is by definition beneficial or harmful.

INHIBITION – TYPES

COMPETITIVE

Competitive inhibition occurs when a molecule that resembles the enzyme's normal substrate "competes" for the active site. If the active site is occupied by a competitive inhibitor, the enzyme will not catalyze the reaction, and the intended product will not be formed. Most inhibitory ligands have a greater affinity for the active site than the substrate does, and as concentrations of the inhibitor increase, so does the chance they will bind to the enzyme and block the reaction. The maximum velocity (v_{max}) is not affected by competitive inhibition. However, more substrate will be required to achieve ½ v_{max}, so the apparent Michaelis constant K_m (a rough measure of binding affinity) increases. The higher the K_m, the lower the binding affinity. Once the inhibitor is released from the active site, the enzyme is free to interact with another inhibitor or with its intended substrate.

Noncompetitive

Noncompetitive inhibition occurs when a molecule binds to an allosteric site on an enzyme, that is, a binding site other than the active site. Because it is not competing with the substrate for the same region on the enzyme, the process in noncompetitive. The inhibitor does not block the substrate. The inhibitor can bind to an enzyme even if the substrate is bound, and the inhibitor does not favor one state over the other. When the inhibitor molecule binds to an allosteric site, the conformation of the enzyme changes, and the product cannot be formed. The affinity for the substrate hasn't changed (and therefore there is no change in K_m), but the enzyme is unable to catalyze the reaction. Therefore, increasing the concentration of the substrate will not affect the rate of reaction, and the maximum velocity (v_{max}) is decreased by noncompetitive inhibition.

Mixed

Like noncompetitive inhibition (which is often classified as a special case of mixed inhibition), mixed inhibition will decrease the maximum rate of reaction. However, the binding affinity *will* vary in mixed inhibition. Because this type of feedback can behave like competitive inhibition when it increases the apparent K_m, or uncompetitive inhibition when it decreases the apparent K_m, it is called "mixed." The mixed inhibitor binds to an allosteric site on the enzyme, whether or not the substrate has already bound. Note that in noncompetitive inhibition, the inhibitor (I) has no greater affinity for the enzyme (E) than the enzyme-substrate complex (ES); it is equally attracted to the enzyme with or without the substrate. But in mixed inhibition, the inhibitor will favor one state over the other. When the inhibitor binds the conformation of the enzyme is changed, and the reaction is inhibited.

Uncompetitive

Uncompetitive inhibition (sometimes referred to as anticompetitive inhibition) occurs when the inhibitor molecule (I) binds to the enzyme-substrate complex (ES) to form the ESI complex. It is the only type of feedback in which the inhibitor *requires* a bound substrate to bind to an allosteric site. This indicates that the binding of the substrate is what makes the allosteric site available to the inhibitor. Unlike competitive inhibition increasing the concentration of the substrate will not overcome the inhibitory process. In fact, uncompetitive inhibition is more effective when substrate concentration is high because the enzyme is only inhibited after the substrate is bound to the active site. Uncompetitive inhibition decreases both the K_m and the maximum velocity of the reaction. It would seem counterintuitive that an increased affinity for reactants would result in the decreased production of product, but more substrate binding leads to more inhibitor binding.

Regulatory Enzymes

Cells must be able to regulate their metabolic processes, and one way to achieve this is by controlling the production and/or activity of the enzymes that assist in these processes. These regulatory enzymes vary the rate of their catalytic activity in response to certain biomolecules and are essential in maintaining homeostasis. If a product is in high demand, enzyme regulation can stimulate the biochemical pathway that produces that product. Conversely, if there is an ample supply of product, enzyme regulation can inhibit the production of that product. Enzymes respond to signals. *Activators* are molecules that increase enzymatic activity, whereas i*nhibitors* reduce activity. Two important classes of regulatory enzymes include allosteric enzymes and covalently modified enzymes.

Allosteric Enzymes

Allosteric regulation refers to any form of regulation in which a regulatory molecule binds non-covalently and reversibly to an allosteric site: a binding region that is *not* an active site. Note that the majority of allosteric proteins have more than one active site. When the regulatory molecule (also called an effector or a modulator) binds to the allosteric site, the conformation of the enzyme is changed, which in turn affects the activity of the enzyme. The binding of an allosteric activator may turn the enzyme "on" or simply increase its activity. In some cases, the binding of the substrate can increase the effectiveness of a second or third active site. This is known as homotropic cooperativity. There are also allosteric inhibitors that cause the active site(s) to change in such a way that the reaction is slowed or ceases altogether. Nearly all forms of noncompetitive inhibition involve allosteric enzymes.

Covalently Modified Enzymes

Enzymes can be activated or deactivated by the addition or removal of a molecular group such as a phosphate, methyl, uridine, adenine, or adenosine diphosphate ribose group. The making or breaking of these covalent bonds is achieved by the action of other enzymes and is usually reversible. The modification of the enzyme will affect the conformation of the enzyme and the affinity of the enzyme for the substrate. The most frequent type of covalent modification is the addition or removal of a phosphate group. The enzymes that are responsible for phosphorylation reactions are called kinases, and those that dephosphorylate are called phosphatase enzymes.

Zymogen

A zymogen (also known as a proenzyme) is a protein that is a precursor to an enzyme. Zymogens cannot catalyze reactions because they are either not in the correct conformation, or the active site is shielded by an extra region (or prosegment) of the protein. The zymogen can be irreversibly activated by the cleavage of a peptide bond (allowing the protein to "spring" into shape) or the revealing of the active site by removal of the inactivating prosegment of the protein. The activation process may be achieved by digestive enzymes called proteases or by changes in the environment (usually pH). One example of a zymogen is trypsinogen. Trypsinogen is inactive until it reaches the small intestine, where a protease known as enterokinase hydrolyzes a specific peptide bond, forming the enzyme trypsin.

Transmission of Genetic Information from the Gene to the Protein

Nucleic Acid Structure and Function

Description

Nucleic acids are one of four major classes of organic biomolecules, the rest being carbohydrates, lipids, and proteins.

The monomers (subunits) of nucleic acids are called nucleotides: three-part structures consisting of a nitrogenous base, a pentose sugar, and a phosphate group. Nucleotides are covalently bonded to one another by phosphodiester linkages.

There are two types of nucleic acids: deoxyribonucleic acid (DNA) and ribonucleic acid (RNA). DNA consists of two polynucleotide strands that bond together in a double helix formation. The nucleotides found in DNA contain the pentose sugar **2-deoxyribose**, and there are four possible nitrogenous bases: adenine, guanine, cytosine, and thymine. The order of the bases is sometimes called the "genetic code" because it holds instructions for the production of proteins. DNA is the hereditary information that is passed from parent to offspring.

RNA is single stranded, and much shorter in length. Its nucleotides contain the sugar **ribose**, and it has all the bases found in DNA, with the exception of thymine. Instead, it has uracil. RNA is made using a DNA template, and is directly involved in the synthesis of proteins.

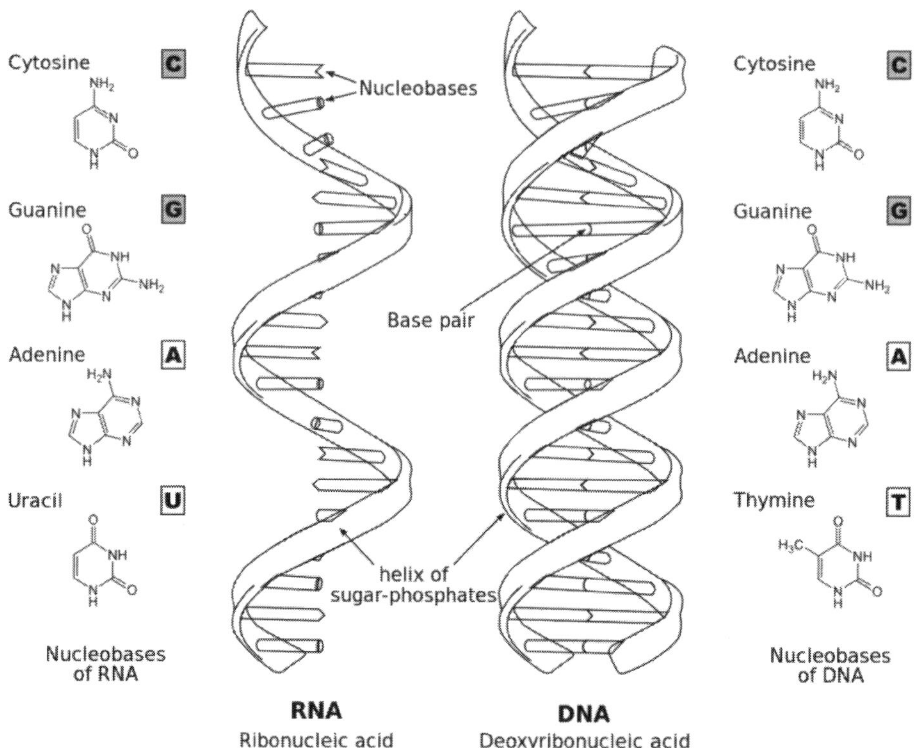

NUCLEOTIDES AND NUCLEOSIDES

A **nucleoside** is a compound composed of a nitrogenous base (adenine, thymine, guanine, cytosine, or uracil) bonded to a pentose sugar (ribose or deoxyribose) by a glycosidic linkage. Nucleosides that contain ribose are called ribonucleosides, while those that contain deoxyribose are called deoxyribonucleosides. Nucleosides can be synthesized from smaller molecules in the cell, but they are usually the result of breakdown of nucleic acids (polymers of nucleotides) in the diet.

A **nucleotide** is formed when one or more phosphate groups are linked to the sugar component of the nucleoside. The bond between the sugar and phosphate on a nucleotide is an ester linkage, and the bonds between any additional phosphate groups are anhydrous bonds. A nucleotide with one, two, or three phosphate groups is called a nucleoside monophosphate, nucleoside diphosphate, or nucleoside triphosphate, respectively. Nucleotides that are incorporated into a chain have only one phosphate group.

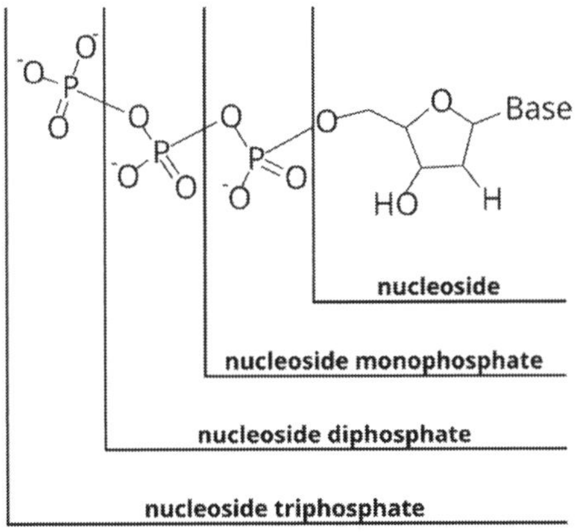

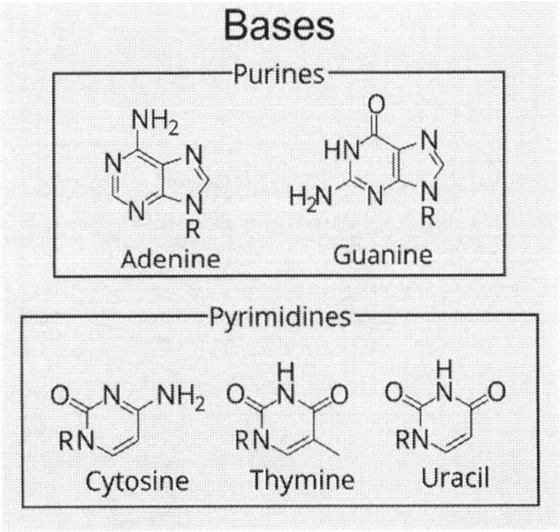

SUGAR PHOSPHATE BACKBONE

Nucleic acids are chains of nucleotides that are held together by strong covalent bonds known as phosphodiester bonds. These bonds involve the phosphate groups and sugars of the nucleotides, but not the bases. In a nucleotide, an ester linkage exists between the phosphate group and the 5' carbon of the sugar. When the nucleotide is incorporated into a chain, it forms a second ester bond to the 3' carbon of the sugar on the adjacent nucleotide. Any additional phosphate groups in unincorporated nucleotides (as seen in nucleoside diphosphates and nucleoside triphosphates) are removed before they are added to a growing polynucleotide. The repeating phosphate-sugar-phosphate-sugar sequence is the backbone of a nucleic acid.

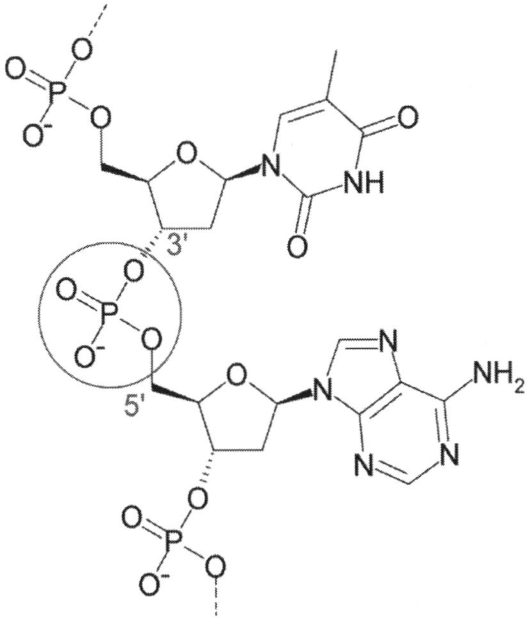

PYRIMIDINE, PURINE RESIDUES

Pyrimidines and purines are types of nitrogenous bases that make up the nucleotides found in nucleic acids. **Pyrimidines** have a single carbon-nitrogen ring, while **purines** have a double ring. More specifically, purines consist of a pyrimidine that is fused to an imidazole ring ($C_3N_2H_4$). There are three pyrimidines found in nucleic acids: thymine (DNA only), uracil (RNA only) and cytosine (both DNA and RNA.) The two purines (found both in DNA and RNA) are adenine and guanine.

Purines (double ringed bases)	Adenine	DNA and RNA
	Guanine	DNA and RNA
Pyrimidines (single ringed bases)	Cytosine	DNA and RNA
	Thymine	DNA only
	Uracil	RNA only

Purine

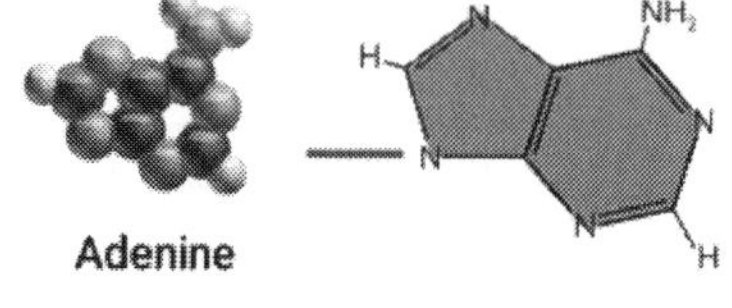

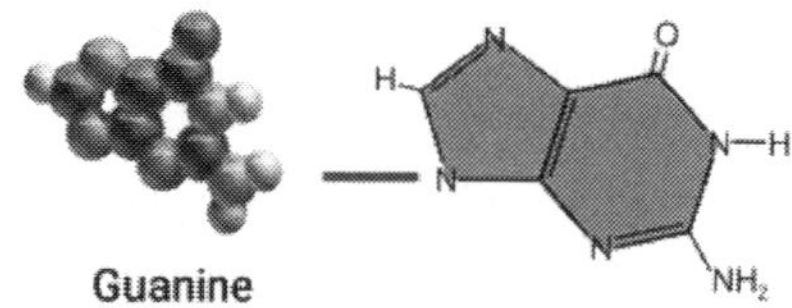

Pyrimidine

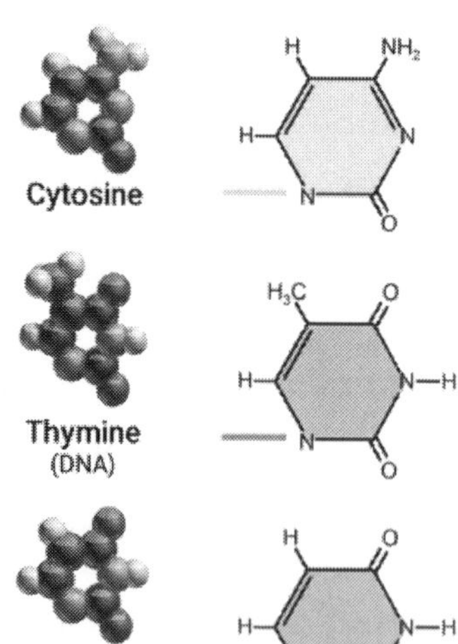

Deoxyribonucleic Acid (DNA): Double Helix, Watson–Crick Model of DNA Structure

James Watson and Francis Crick were the first to build an accurate model of deoxyribonucleic acid. The molecule consists of two polynucleotide chains that spiral around an invisible axis to make a twisted ladder shape, or **double helix**. The repeating sugar-phosphate units form the strong "backbone" on the exterior of the molecule, with nitrogenous base pairs forming the interior "rungs" of the ladder. Adenine always forms two hydrogen bonds with thymine, and guanine forms three hydrogen bonds with cytosine (note that purines bond with pyrimidines.) Each turn of the helix has about 10.5 base pairs, and each pair is spaced 0.34 nanometers (or 3.4 angstroms) apart. The diameter of the molecule is about 2.0 nanometers (or 20 angstroms).

Each polynucleotide strand has a distinct end. The 5' end terminates with a phosphate group that stems from the 5' carbon of the sugar. The 3' end terminates with a hydroxyl group off of the 3' carbon of the sugar. The strands are antiparallel, meaning they run in opposite directions.

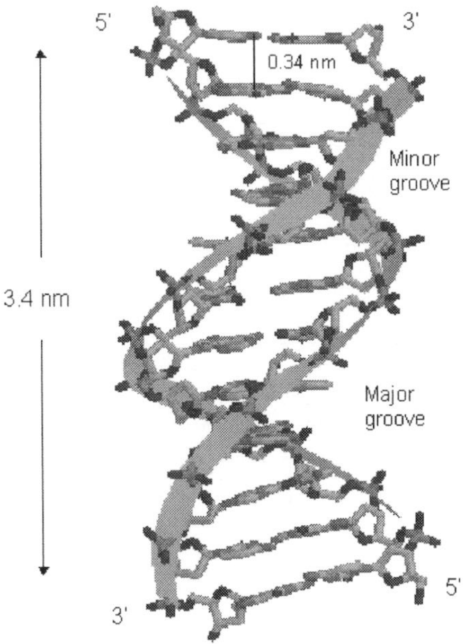

BASE PAIRING SPECIFICITY: A WITH T, G WITH C

Before the structure of DNA was known, it was observed that the proportion of guanine in a sample of DNA matched that of cytosine. The same was true of adenine and thymine. This information helped lead to the complementary base pair rules: adenine bonds specifically with thymine, and cytosine bonds specifically with guanine.

Pyrimidines (single ringed bases) must bond with purines (double ringed bases) to fit properly within the 2.0 nanometer diameter of the double helix. If purines tried to bond together, they would extend beyond this constraint, and pyrimidine pairs would be too far apart from each other to form hydrogen bonds at all. This explains why purines must bond with pyrimidines, but it does not explain why a purine cannot bond with *any* pyrimidine. The reason for the specific rules (A-T and G-C) is seen in the hydrogen bonds that form between base pairs. The hydrogen bond donors on adenine match up with the hydrogen bond acceptors on thymine. The same is true for guanine and cytosine. Two hydrogen bonds form between A-T and three form between G-C.

If the sequence on one strand is 5'-TAGCAGG-3', then the complementary sequence will be 5'-CCTGCTA-3' (or 3'-ATCGTCC-5'.)

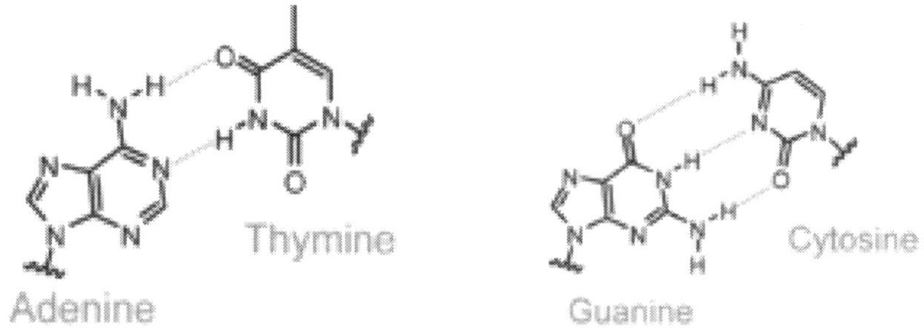

Function in Transmission of Genetic Information

Nucleic acids store genetic information in the order of their nitrogenous bases. Each sequence of three bases corresponds to one of twenty **amino acids**: the building blocks of proteins. DNA holds the *instructions* to build proteins, and RNA (which is made from a DNA template) is responsible for *assembling* the proteins.

Each time a cell divides, the DNA molecule must replicate itself so that each daughter cell receives a complete set of genetic material. The complementary base pairing allows for an exact copy of the genetic material to be made through semiconservative replication. The hydrogen bonds between the base pairs are broken, and nucleotides added to each unzipped strand. The result is two identical molecules of DNA, each with an original strand and a new strand.

DNA Denaturation, Reannealing, Hybridization

DNA **denaturation** is the unwinding and separation of the two polynucleotide strands. The breaking of hydrogen bonds between base pairs can be achieved by certain chemicals, sonication, or high temperatures. Denaturation as a result of high temperatures is also called DNA "melting." When normal conditions are restored, the single strands may recombine into a double stranded molecule in a process called **reannealing**.

Hybridization is the binding of two single DNA strands; usually these are strands that were not previously bonded together. If one strand is perfectly complementary to the other, it will anneal readily. The more mismatches in base pairing, the less likely that hybridization will be successful.

DNA Replication

Mechanism of Replication: Separation of Strands, Specific Coupling of Free Nucleic Acids

DNA replication is the process by which a molecule of DNA is copied to produce two identical molecules. For replication to begin, the hydrogen bonds between the two strands must be broken to form a **replication fork**: the site of strand separation where bases are exposed. The unzipping of the double strand is accomplished by enzymes called helicases. Each original strand serves as a template for the daughter strand. The enzyme that adds free nucleotides to each parent strand is called DNA polymerase. But polymerase cannot add nucleotides to a single strand, so an RNA primer must be created before DNA synthesis can proceed. Free nucleotides are added to each parent strand by polymerase enzymes according to the complementary base pair rules (A-T, G-C), and in the 5' to 3' direction of the elongating strand (the parent strand is read from 3' to 5'). Since DNA is antiparallel, each side is copied in opposite directions. On the *leading* strand, nucleotides are added continuously, but on the *lagging* strand, nucleotides must be added in short segments called Okazaki fragments. Each fragment begins with an RNA primer which is later removed.

In the image below:

a: parent strands
b: leading strand
c: lagging strand
d: replication fork
e: RNA primer
f: Okazaki fragment

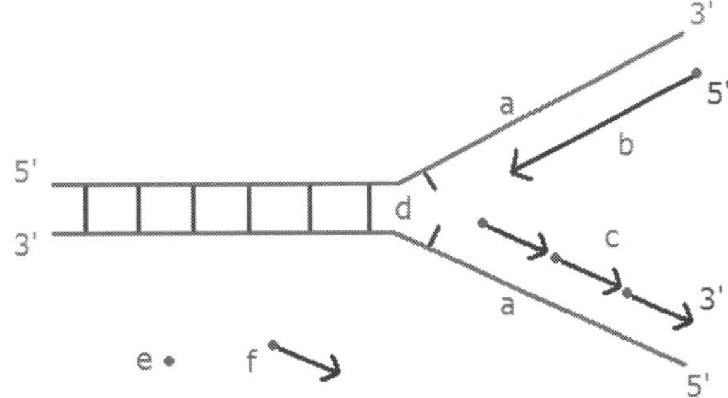

Semi-Conservative Nature of Replication

Following the discovery of DNA's structure in 1953, different models of replication were considered. If replication was "**conservative**," the original strands would remain together, and two new polynucleotides would be synthesized and bonded together to form a new, but genetically identical, DNA molecule. If replication was "**dispersive**," each new DNA molecule would have mixed segments of the parent and daughter strands.

Evidence from an experiment performed by Matthew Meselson and Franklin Stahl in 1958 supported the more common hypothesis that DNA replication was "semi-conservative". In this experiment, original strands of bacterial DNA were marked with nitrogen isotopes, and then traced in subsequent generations to discover that replication is indeed semi-conservative. In this accepted model, the original DNA strands serve as a template for the growing daughter strands. The result is two identical DNA molecules, each with one original and one new strand of nucleotides.

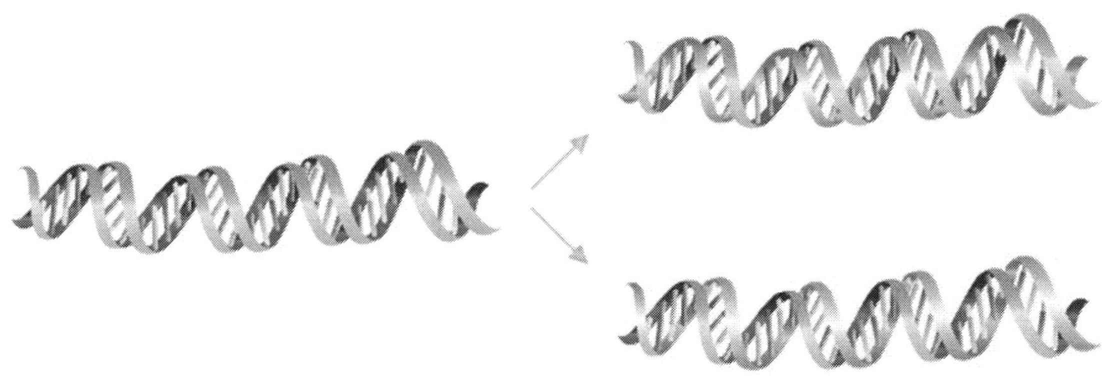

Specific Enzymes Involved in Replication

Helicase – breaks the hydrogen bonds between complementary base pairs, separating the strands and forming a replication fork.

Topoisomerase / DNA gyrase – helps reduce the tension that builds up when the double helix unwinds.

SSB proteins (single stranded binding proteins) – prevent the double helix from reforming at the replication fork by keeping the template strands apart.

Primase – adds an RNA primer that serves as an attachment point for DNA polymerase (which cannot add nucleotides to a single strand.)

DNA polymerase – adds complementary nucleotides to the exposed bases of the unzipped template strands in a 5' to 3' direction (or 3' to 5' as compared to the parent strand.) Some polymerases also play a role in proofreading and repair of mismatched nucleotides.

Telomerase – helps to counteract the shortening of telomeres (repeating DNA sequences at the extreme ends of the DNA molecule) by adding nucleotides where no other enzyme can.

Ligase – binds Okazaki fragments together, as well as any portions of the molecule that needed to be repaired.

Exonuclease – removes the RNA primers.

Origins of Replication, Multiple Origins in Eukaryotes

An **origin of replication** is the site along a DNA molecule where replication is initiated. Helicase binds to this region, and uses the energy from ATP hydrolysis to break the hydrogen bonds between bases. The nucleotide sequence at an origin of replication will often have a high proportion of A–T base pairs, because they are easier to separate than G–C base pairs. (Adenine and thymine have two hydrogen bonds between them while guanine and cytosine have three.)

Most prokaryotes have a single circular chromosome with only one origin of replication. But eukaryotic cells have multiple linear chromosomes that carry far more genetic material. Multiple origins of replication per chromosome help to increase the rate of replication. The human genome (which consists of around three billion base pairs) has approximately a hundred thousand origins of replication per cell.

Replicating the Ends of DNA Molecules

Each time a linear DNA molecule is replicated, there is a segment at the end of the lagging strand that cannot be synthesized. Recall that replication must proceed in the 5' → 3' direction (with respect to the growing strand) because DNA polymerase can only attach nucleotides to the 3' hydroxyl group on the sugar. This means that one strand (the lagging strand) has to be replicated in short discontinuous segments called Okazaki fragments, each which begins with an RNA primer which provides the necessary hydroxyl group. But when the final primer is removed, DNA polymerase cannot fill in that last gap. As a result, the DNA molecule is shortened more and more with each replication. This can lead to cell **senescence**: the loss of ability to divide.

Each end of the chromosome has a non-coding repeated sequence called a **telomere** that helps prevent the loss of coding regions. They are often compared to plastic shoelace ends because telomeres help prevent deterioration of the molecule. The enzyme **telomerase** can halt the shortening of the telomere by adding more repeating segments to the parent strand. When the parent strand is elongated, a missing segment at the end of the growing strand will not be problematic.

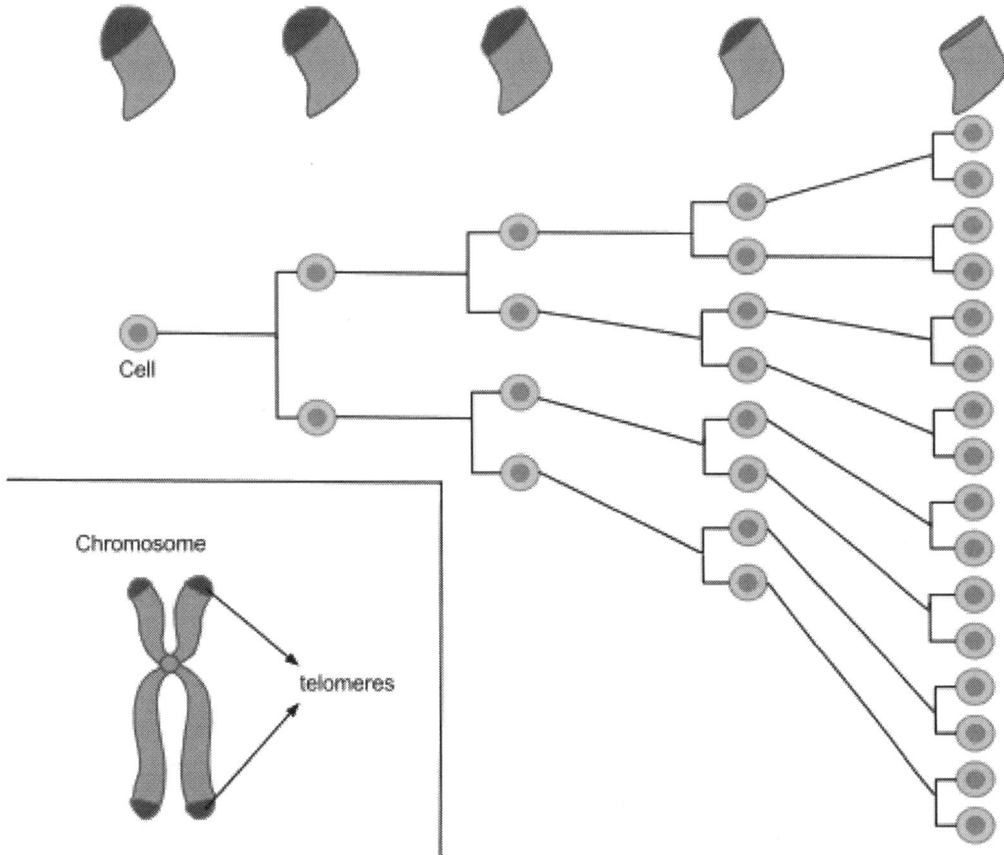

Repair of DNA

Repair During Replication

DNA polymerase is a highly accurate enzyme that incorporates nucleotides onto a template strand of DNA according to the base pair rules (A-T, G-C). However, a mismatch will occur approximately 1 out of 100,000 nucleotides, often because of **tautomerization**. A tautomer of a nitrogenous base has a different arrangement of electrons than its non-tautomeric form, which may "confuse" DNA polymerase. For example, a tautomer of guanine could mistakenly be paired with thymine.

The same DNA polymerase that elongates the daughter strand can proofread its work. If an error is detected, the enzyme can back up in the 3' → 5' direction and use its ability as an exonuclease to cleave off a single incorrect nucleotide and replace it with the proper one. Polymerase can also work in the direction of elongation (5' → 3') to remove short sequences of misincorporated nucleotides and also RNA primers.

Repair of Mutations

While many replication errors are repaired during the replication process, there are some that are not fixed until after replication is complete. Such mutations include mismatched pairs, as well as insertions and deletions (due to polymerase slippage). The post-replication repair pathway is complex, involving multiple proteins that correct most of the mutations missed during replication.

First, the repair proteins must be able to distinguish the original strand from the daughter strand in order to know which one to fix. Many of the bases on the parent strand have methyl groups (CH_3) attached to them as a way to control gene expression. The newly synthesized strand will not yet be methylated. A protein complex binds to the site of mutation, and a second complex cuts out a short sequence that includes the error. The gap in the daughter strand is filled in by polymerase and sealed with ligase. Once repair mechanisms are complete, the error rate is reduced to only one in ten billion nucleotides, on average.

Genetic Code

Central Dogma: DNA → RNA → Protein

The **central dogma** of biology describes the flow of genetic information in a cell, and is summarized as follows: *DNA → RNA → Protein*. DNA is the inherited genetic material inside the nucleus that stores information in the sequence of its four bases: adenine, guanine, cytosine, and thymine. The genes within the DNA hold instructions to build the proteins that are responsible for the activities of a cell.

For the information in a gene to be expressed, it must first be rewritten into a molecule of messenger RNA. This process (DNA → RNA) is called **transcription**, and takes place in the nucleus. Transcription can be compared to copying a recipe out of an enormous genetic cookbook. The mRNA transcript carries the instructions from a gene out of the nucleus to a ribosome: the site of protein synthesis. Here, the transcript is decoded, and amino acids linked together to form a protein. This process (RNA → protein) is called **translation**. To continue the cookbook example, translation would be analogous to the adding of ingredients in the correct order as indicated by the copied recipe.

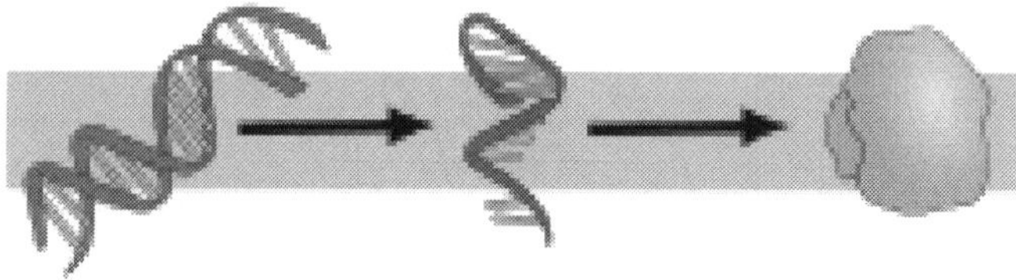

The Triplet Code

The sequence of nucleotides in a gene determines the structure and function of the final product: the protein. More specifically, each **triplet**, or set of three DNA nucleotides, codes for one of twenty amino acids. The triplets are read sequentially, and do not overlap. Because there are four nitrogenous bases, there are sixty-four combinations that either code for an amino acid or are one of three stop codons which mark the end of translation. All amino acids except tryptophan and methionine can be encoded by more than one triplet combination.

In order for this information to be translated into a protein, it must first be transcribed into a molecule of mRNA. Each DNA triplet is rewritten as an mRNA codon, which is directly involved in the assembly of the protein. For example, if a DNA triplet is TAC, then the mRNA codon will be AUG, and the amino acid that is incorporated into the growing protein will be methionine. This code is nearly universal among all species, meaning the same triplet/codons correspond to the same amino acids (or a stop codon).

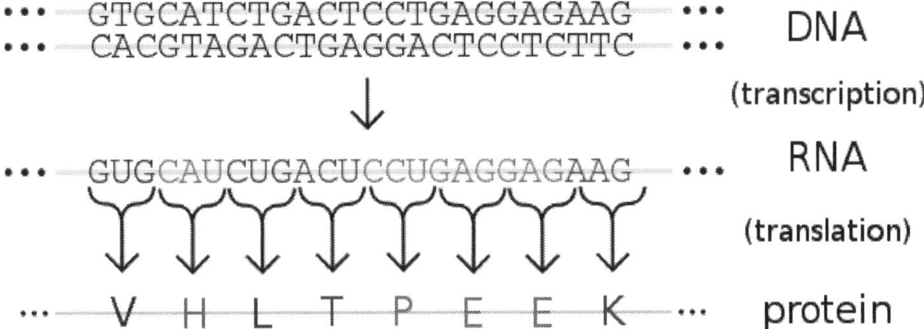

Codon–Anticodon Relationship

A **codon** is a three-nucleotide sequence on messenger RNA that either specifies an amino acid or signals the end of translation. When an amino acid is called for, it is **transfer RNA** that delivers it. Transfer RNA is a folded, cloverleaf-shaped molecule made of approximately 75 to 90 nucleotides. At one end is the **anticodon**: a three-nucleotide sequence that recognizes mRNA's codon and binds to it according to the complementary base pair rules (with some exceptions as seen in wobble pairing). For example, if the codon is 5' GCC 3', then the anticodon on tRNA will be 3' CGG 5'. At the other end of tRNA is the amino acid. In this example, the amino acid carried by tRNA that is specified by mRNA is alanine. The binding of an anticodon to a codon happens on a ribosome: the site of protein synthesis.

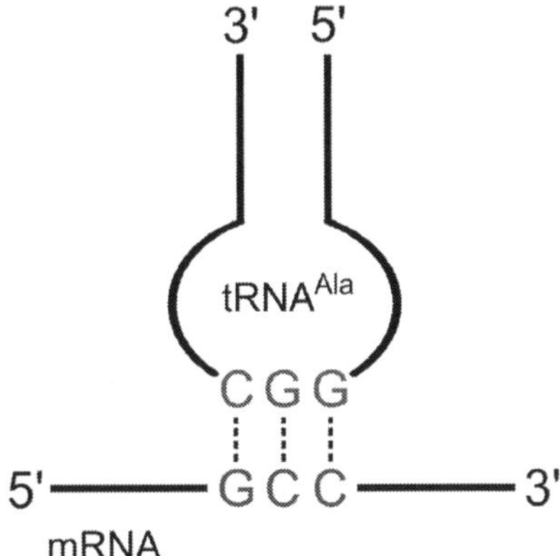

Degenerate Code, Wobble Pairing

The genetic code is **degenerate** because there are several different nucleotide combinations that all code for one amino acid. For example, the codons GCU, GCA, GCC, and GCG all specify alanine. This reduced specificity helps to eliminate the effects of some point mutations. If the intended codon was GCU, and a point substitution resulted in GCA, then the incorporated amino acid would still be alanine.

Not all anticodons bond to codons according to the classic base pair rules. There are "allowable" variations in pairing, called **wobble pairs**. Transfer RNA has a base not commonly found in other nucleic acids called hypoxanthine. It is abbreviated "I" after inosine, the nucleoside that it is a part of. Hypoxanthine is unique in that it can form base pairs with multiple bases: adenine, cytosine, and uracil. The most common wobble pairs are I-A, I-C, I-U, and G-U. In the standard base pair rules, an anticodon sequence of 3'-CGU-5' would bond with a codon sequence of 5'-GCA-3'. Wobble pairing, for example, allows for this same anticodon to bond to a codon sequence of '5-GCG-3'.

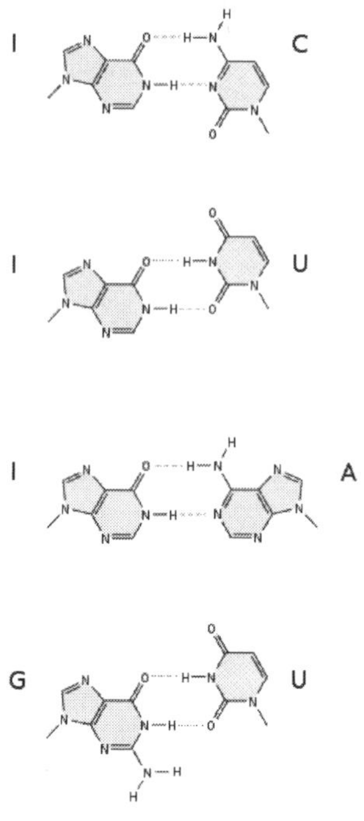

I C

I U

I A

G U

Missense, Nonsense Codons

A **missense** mutation occurs when a base substitution in a DNA triplet causes the corresponding mRNA codon to code for the wrong amino acid. The effects of such codon mutations can be minimal if the incorrect amino acid shares the chemical properties of the intended amino acid. But often the change in primary structure results in a conformational and functional change in the protein.

In a **nonsense** mutation, a base substitution in a DNA triplet changes the corresponding codon to a stop codon, and translation is cut short. Only part of the polypeptide will be built.

Example of a missense codon: the intended codon of GAG is changed to GUG and valine is incorporated instead of glutamic acid.

Example of a nonsense codon: the intended codon of CAG is changed to UAG and where glutamine should be added, there is nothing. Translation simply ends.

Initiation, Termination Codons

The first AUG toward the 5' end of a eukaryotic mRNA transcript is the **initiation site**, or start codon, of translation. A transfer RNA molecule carries the amino acid methionine to the P-site of a ribosome and binds it to the start codon. Methionine is found at the N-terminus of nearly every growing polypeptide chain. Sometimes it is removed during post-translational modification as a way to stabilize the protein.

Translation ends when one of three **termination codons** (UAG, UAA, or UGA) occupies the A-site on a ribosome. Transfer RNA molecules do not bind to stop codons; rather proteins called **release factors** bind to these sites and release the protein from the P-site. They do this by hydrolyzing the ester bond between the last amino acid and its associated tRNA.

MESSENGER RNA (MRNA)

Messenger RNA (mRNA) is a single strand of nucleotides made during transcription that encodes the information from a gene. Transcription first produces a molecule of *pre*-mRNA which is then modified to cut out non-coding regions and to add certain groups to each end. Each modified eukaryotic mRNA molecule begins with a 5' cap and ends with a poly-A tail. The 5' cap attaches to the first mRNA nucleotide by a triphosphate linkage, and consists of a modified guanine-containing nucleotide. The cap helps the mRNA to interact with the ribosome, and also protects the transcript from being broken down by exonuclease enzymes. At the 3' end of the molecule is a series of up to 200 adenine-containing nucleotides which, like the 5' cap, prevents degradation of the coding regions of mRNA. Between the cap and the tail are the codons which specify the amino acids needed to build the protein dictated by the gene sequence.

TRANSCRIPTION

TRANSFER RNA (TRNA); RIBOSOMAL RNA (RRNA)

Transfer RNA, or tRNA, is the nucleic acid responsible for delivering amino acids to the site of protein synthesis - the ribosome. It is transcribed by the enzyme RNA polymerase II, and is typically made of fewer than 90 nucleotides that are arranged in a cloverleaf shape (secondary structure). At one end of the strand is a 3' CCA tail to which the amino acid is bound. The enzyme **aminoacyl-tRNA synthetase** assists in the formation of an ester bond between the amino acid and the 3' OH group on the last nucleotide.

At the tip of the tRNA molecule is a three-nucleotide anticodon sequence that is complementary to an mRNA codon (with the exception of wobble pairs, in which one anticodon can bind to more than one specific codon). The tertiary structure of tRNA resembles an "L" shape, which fits into the binding sites on the ribosome. When a tRNA binds to mRNA, it transfers its amino acid to the growing polypeptide chain.

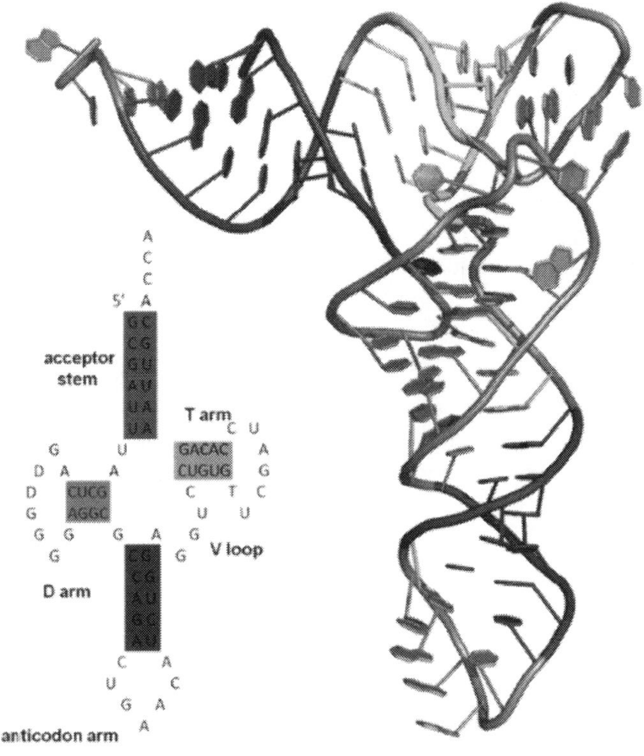

Ribosomal RNA, or rRNA, is the nucleic acid that makes up the bulk of a ribosome (about 60%). The rest of the ribosome is made up of proteins. Ribosomal RNA is transcribed in a region of the nucleus called the **nucleolus** before it migrates to the cytoplasm to form a ribosome. A ribosome is composed of two parts: the large subunit (LSU) and the small subunit (SSU). The LSU contains around 5000 rRNA nucleotides and 46 proteins, and the SSU contains fewer than 2000 nucleotides and 33 proteins. During translation, these subunits come together with the start codon of an mRNA transcript trapped in between. The ribosome then slides down mRNA one codon at time. The small subunit ensures that codons and anticodons pair up properly during translation, and the large subunit has an active site that catalyzes the formation of a peptide bond between adjacent amino acids.

Mechanism of Transcription

Transcription is the synthesis of RNA using the information encoded in DNA and occurs in three main stages: initiation, elongation, and termination.

Transcription is **initiated** by the binding of RNA polymerase to the promoter: the segment of DNA which (in eukaryotes) contains the TATA box and lies upstream (or toward the 5' end) of the gene to be transcribed. When it binds, it unwinds the helix and breaks the hydrogen bonds between the two DNA strands. It then moves along the DNA template in the 3' → 5' direction, adding RNA nucleotides during **elongation**. Since RNA polymerase can add nucleotides to a single strand, no primer is needed as in DNA replication. If a sequence of the template DNA strand is 3' GAATCCAAA 5', then the RNA strand will read 5' CUUAGGUUU 3'. The method of **termination** differs depending on which type of RNA polymerase is involved (I, II, or III), and the type of RNA that is being synthesized (mRNA, tRNA, or rRNA). Usually, there is a sequence on DNA called the terminal signal that has a relatively weak attraction to RNA, causing the transcript to slide off the template.

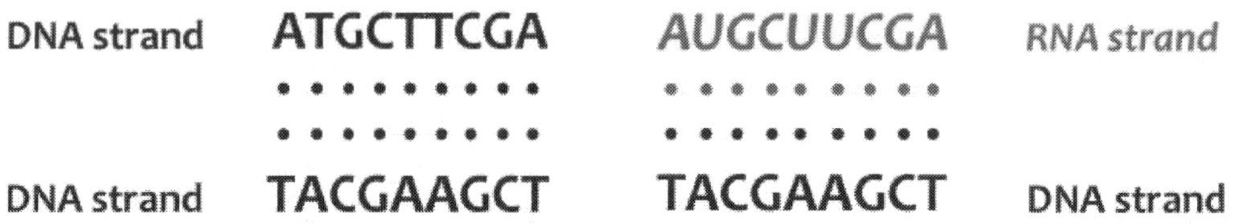

DNA strand	ATGCTTCGA	AUGCUUCGA	RNA strand
DNA strand	TACGAAGCT	TACGAAGCT	DNA strand

mRNA Processing in Eukaryotes, Introns, Exons

The messenger RNA that is translated on a ribosome is an abridged version of the original RNA that is transcribed in the nucleus. The transcribed gene contains intermittent non-coding segments called **introns** that are not part of the instructions for the protein. These introns interrupt the coding regions (called **exons**), and for this reason the RNA must be processed to remove these introns before translation can proceed. The editing process takes place in the nucleus, and is achieved by the action of small nuclear ribonucleoproteins (**snRNPs**) that bind to each end of an intron. These ends are brought together, and the snRNPs combine into a larger structure called a spliceosome which cuts out the intron in the form of a lariat (or loop), which is later broken down. The exons are spliced together through the action of the enzyme ligase, a 5' cap is added to one end, and a poly-A tail is added to the 3' end. These help to protect the coding information within the mature mRNA.

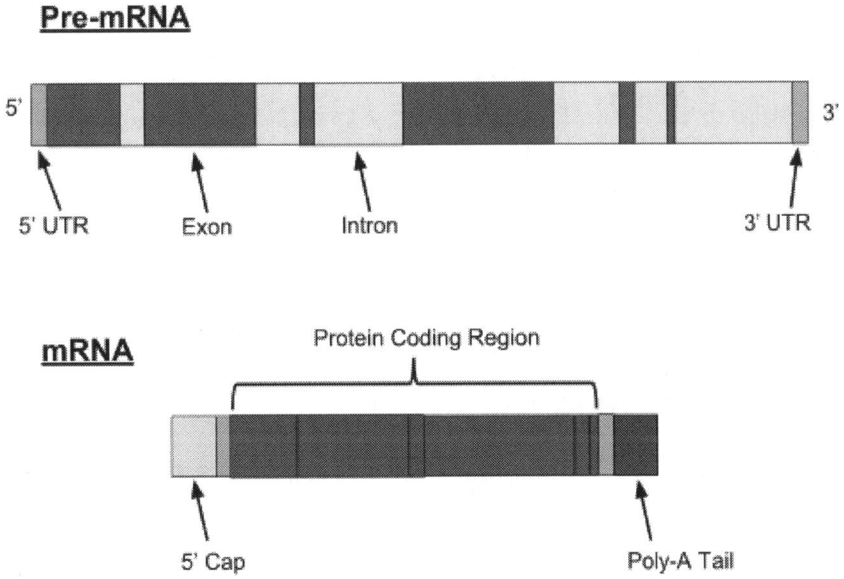

Pre-mRNA

5' 3'

5' UTR Exon Intron 3' UTR

mRNA

Protein Coding Region

5' Cap Poly-A Tail

RIBOZYMES, SPLICEOSOMES, SMALL NUCLEAR RIBONUCLEOPROTEINS (SNRNPS), SMALL NUCLEAR RNAS (SNRNAS)

Ribozymes are molecules of ribonucleic acid (RNA) that act as non-protein enzymes by catalyzing certain reactions. Some ribozymes are part of a ribosome, and aid in the formation of peptide bonds between amino acids during translation. Other ribozymes are involved in the splicing of pre-mRNA, or the modification of pre-tRNA to produce functional tRNA.

Spliceosomes are large protein-RNA complexes that cut out non-coding portions of pre-mRNA called introns, before the coding regions (exons) are spliced together. Spliceosomes are made of several smaller complexes called small nuclear ribonucleoproteins (also called snRNPs or "snurps") which are themselves made of small nuclear RNA molecules (snRNA) and proteins. The RNA portions of the snRNPs bind to each end of an intron by complementary base pairing, and then more snRNPs help to bring each end together. The snRNPs gather into a large complex (the spliceosome) and the intron forms a loop before being cut out by the spliceosome.

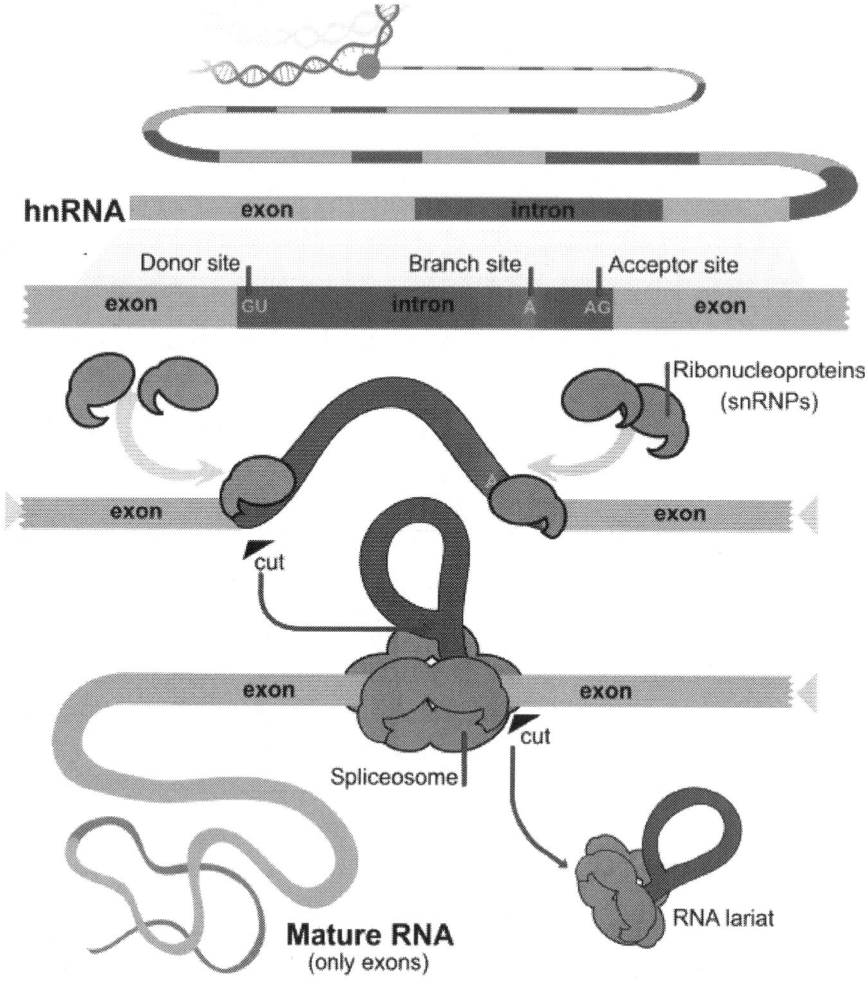

Functional and Evolutionary Importance of Introns

Introns (or intragenic regions) are intermittent non-coding regions of DNA that produce corresponding introns in messenger RNA that are removed from the mRNA during splicing. While introns do not code for proteins *directly*, it is hypothesized that they play a role in gene expression. The presence of introns also allows the shuffling of exons to produce a greater variety of proteins. The human genome has approximately 20,000 genes, but there are far more than 20,000 proteins in the proteome because of the mixing and matching of the separated coding regions within the gene. It is unclear whether introns (which are not found in prokaryotes) have always been a part of the genome of eukaryotes, or whether they have been inserted into the genome over the course of evolution. It is possible that introns may once have coded for proteins, or they may have simply been the mechanism for the shuffling of exons.

Translation

Roles of mRNA, tRNA, rRNA

Messenger RNA, transfer RNA, and ribosomal RNA all play an important role in protein synthesis. Messenger RNA (mRNA) transcribes the information from a gene and delivers it from the nucleus to a ribosome. Each mRNA molecule encodes the sequence of amino acids for a particular protein in a series of codons. Transfer RNA (tRNA) carries the amino acids specified by the mRNA transcript. The anticodon on tRNA binds to the codon, and the amino acid that is attached to the tail of the tRNA molecule is transferred to the growing polypeptide chain. Ribosomal RNA (rRNA) combines with proteins to form ribosomal subunits. During translation, a large and small subunit sandwich together around mRNA and catalyze the formation of peptide bonds between amino acids.

Role and Structure of Ribosomes

Ribosomes are the sites of translation, and they can be free-floating in the cytosol or bound to the rough endoplasmic reticulum. Each ribosome is made of two **subunits** that assemble together around the first AUG sequence (start codon) that is downstream from the 5' cap on mRNA. Both subunits are made of ribosomal RNA and proteins. In eukaryotes, the small subunit is called the 40S subunit (which is based on its sedimentation coefficient). It contains 33 proteins and a single rRNA strand of about 1900 rRNA nucleotides. The small subunit reads the mRNA transcript and monitors the pairing of codons and anticodons. The large subunit, or 60S, contains 46 proteins and 3 strands of rRNA with around 4700, 160, and 120 nucleotides. This subunit has an active site made from the rRNA that assists in the linking of amino acids. It has three binding sites for tRNA: the A-site which acts as the acceptor for the polypeptide chain, the P-site which holds the chain, and the E-site which is the exit site for tRNA. The two subunits together form an 80S ribosome (or 70S in eukaryotes).

Initiation, Termination Co-Factors

Initiation of translation in eukaryotes is a complex process involving a variety of proteins called initiation factors. The initiation process begins with the binding of eukaryotic initiation factor 3 (eiF-3) to the small ribosomal subunit, inhibiting the binding of the large subunit. EiF-1 also binds to the small subunit to stabilize the conformational change that creates a channel for the mRNA transcript. Meanwhile, initiation factor eiF-2 binds to a specific Met-tRNA that only binds to the AUG start codon (and no other AUG sequences within the transcript). This is called the initiator tRNA, or Met-$tRNA_i^{Met}$. EiF-2 is bound to GTP – guanosine triphosphate. The complex of eiF-2 and tRNA is called a ternary complex, and it binds to the small 40S subunit. Another initiation factor, eiF-4F, binds to the 5' cap of the mRNA transcript, allowing the 40S subunit to bind to the end of the strand. It then slides down the transcript until it reaches the first AUG sequence (the start codon). Finally, initiation factor eiF-5 catalyzes the hydrolysis of GTP, allowing the release of all initiation factors, and the large 60S subunit associates with the small 40S subunit to form the 80S ribosome. The initiator tRNA (carrying methionine) slides into the P-site of the ribosome, and the elongation stage commences. Note that in prokaryotic initiation, there are only three initiation factors.

Termination of translation occurs when one of three stop codons (UAA, UAG, or UGA) enters the A-site of the ribosome. Transfer RNA does not bind to the A-site; instead, proteins called termination factors cause the polypeptide chain to be released. First, eukaryotic release factor 1 (eRF-1) forms a complex with the GTP-binding protein eRF-3. This complex binds to the ribosome and breaks the ester bond between the last tRNA molecules and its amino acid. All termination factors are released as a result of the hydrolysis of GTP to form GDP.

Post-Translational Modification of Proteins

Post-translational modification greatly increases the diversity of the **proteome**: all the proteins expressed by a genome. Modifications that occur during or immediately after translation may assist in the proper folding of proteins, stabilization of the structure, or labeling the protein's destination (called localization). Further modifications may occur to activate or deactivate the protein, or to mark the protein. Most modifications occur in the rough endoplasmic reticulum and/or Golgi apparatus.

There are a variety of ways in which a protein may be modified. Common types of modification are summarized in the table below.

Modification	Action	Purpose
Methylation	Addition of CH_3 group.	Makes protein more hydrophobic, and aids in epigenetic regulation.
Phosphorylation	Addition of PO_3^- group to certain amino acids.	Plays a role in gene expression.
N-acetylation	Replacement of the N-terminal methionine with an acetyl group.	Aids in signal transduction and cell cycle regulation.
Glycosylation	Addition of a sugar component.	May assist in protein folding, stability, and activity.
Proteolysis	Cleavage of certain peptide bonds.	Turns an inactive protein (zymogen) into an active form
Lipidation	Addition of a lipid component.	Increases the hydrophobic nature of a protein; common in proteins that are incorporated into plasma membranes.

Eukaryotic Chromosome Organization

Chromosomal Proteins

Chromatin is the mass of genetic material and associated proteins within the nucleus of the cell. There are two main classifications of chromosomal proteins: histones and nonhistones. **Histone** proteins account for approximately 50% of the mass of chromosomes. They help to organize DNA into chromosomes by providing a structure for DNA to wrap around, like thread around a spool. They are positively charged (and therefore attracted to the negatively charged phosphate groups in DNA) and alkaline in nature.

Nonhistone chromosomal proteins play a role in regulation and enzymatic activity. They are acidic, and tend to be negatively charged. While they are less common in chromatin than histone proteins, they have many important roles. They aid histones in the coiling of DNA, and assist in the movement of chromosomes during cell division. Enzymes involved in DNA replication, transcription, and gene expression are also nonhistone proteins.

Single Copy vs. Repetitive DNA

Single copy DNA refers to sequences in DNA that do not repeat. These nonrepetitive sequences contain **exons**: portions of a gene that are transcribed and translated. Single copy DNA has a low mutation rate.

Repetitive DNA accounts for the majority of the human genome, and consists of copy after copy of the same sequence. There are different classifications of repeating elements, and they all have a higher mutation rate than single copy DNA. **Transposable elements**, such as transposons and retrotransposons, change locations in the genome. While some transposable elements are translated into proteins, these repeating sequences are considered non-coding because the proteins have no known function. Other repeating elements are called **tandem repeats**, which consist of back-to-back repeating sequences. These are found near the centromeres, and also within the telomeres.

SUPERCOILING

Supercoiling is the manner in which chromatin condenses into chromosomes. It may also play a role in gene expression by allowing or denying access to certain genes. Supercoiling begins when negatively charged DNA wraps around positively charged histone proteins. There are four main varieties of histone proteins (H2A, H2B, H3, and H4), and DNA wraps twice around a complex of eight histones to form a nucleosome; each nucleosome has two of each type of histone. This stage of coiling resembles beads on a string; each bead representing a nucleosome strung together by a strand of DNA. The tails of the histones interact with other nucleosomes, and also with the DNA between the nucleosomes, to further compact the chromatin into thicker fibers. These fibers twist into loops, which in turn coil into a chromosome. The width of DNA before coiling is 2 nanometers, and each nucleosome is 10 nm, followed by a coiled 30 nm fiber, then 300 nm, and finally each chromatid of the chromosome has a width of 700 nm.

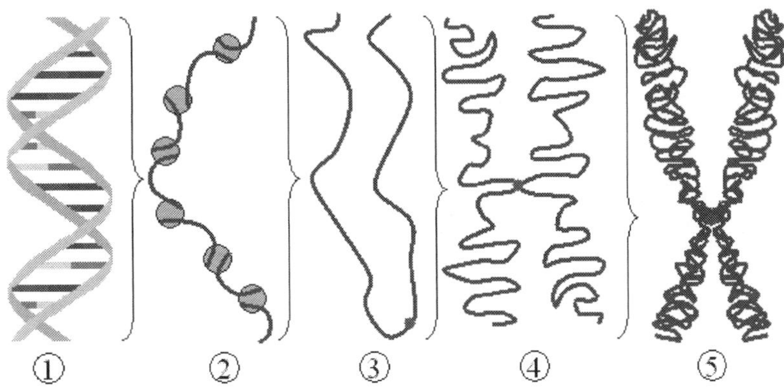

HETEROCHROMATIN VS. EUCHROMATIN

Chromatin is the complex of DNA and proteins that is found in the nucleus. It comes in two forms, euchromatin and heterochromatin. **Euchromatin** is less tightly packed than heterochromatin, and resembles beads on a chain. Each bead represents a nucleosome, and the string represents "linker" DNA (the uncoiled portion of DNA). DNA at this level of packaging is accessible for transcription and therefore gene expression.

Heterochromatin displays a higher level of packaging and stains darker than euchromatin, and the two forms of chromatin can therefore be distinguished under a microscope. The enzymes involved in transcription cannot transcribe DNA in such a tightly wound form. Both forms of chromatin exist during interphase.

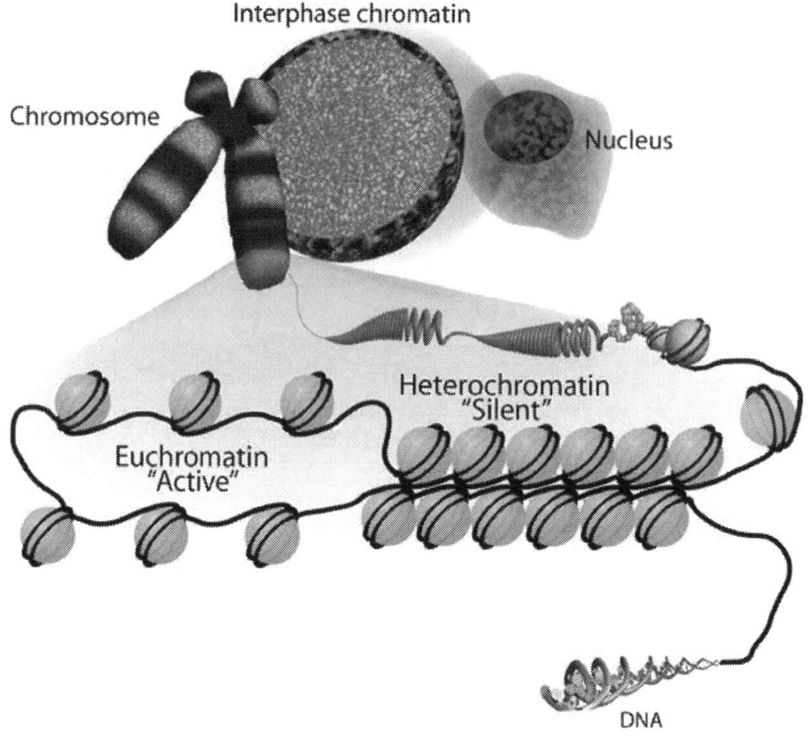

TELOMERES, CENTROMERES

Telomeres are the end portions of eukaryotic chromosomes that consist of noncoding repeating sequences that function as buffers. In humans, the sequence TTAGGG repeats approximately 2,500 times. With each replication, the DNA strand shortens due to the inability of DNA polymerase to add nucleotides to the last portion on the lagging strand. Since the repetitive DNA in the telomere does not produce proteins, the loss is inconsequential—that is, unless the molecule shortens beyond the telomere region into important genes. In this case, the cell could become senescent or cancerous, or could undergo apoptosis. Telomeres also prevent the ends of chromosomes from fusing together.

The **centromere** is the region that joins the two sister chromatids of a duplicated chromosome together. Depending on the chromosome number, the centromere may be nearer to one end of the chromosome than the other, resulting in a short and long arm of each chromatid, or it could be metacentric (centrally located). The centromere contains chromatin called centromeric (or cen) chromatin which provides the foundation for a protein structure called a kinetochore to which microtubules attach during cell division. Without the centromere, there would be no way to segregate and distribute the chromatids to daughter cells.

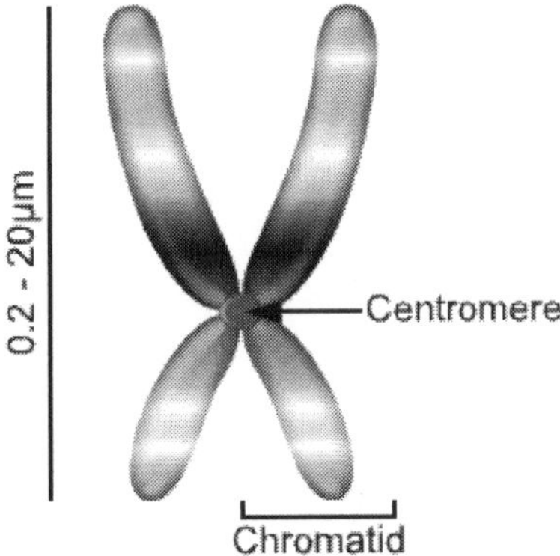

Control of Gene Expression in Prokaryotes

Operon Concept, Jacob–Monod Model

The **Jacob-Monod Model** describes how gene expression is controlled in prokaryotes. Francois Jacob and Jacques Monod studied sugar metabolism in *E. coli*, and they used their data to create a model of an operon. An **operon** is a unit of DNA that contains a group of genes that are transcribed as a whole and are regulated by the same operator. The components of an operon are as follows (from upstream to downstream):

- **Promoter**: signals the beginning of the region to be transcribed by RNA polymerase.
- **Operator**: acts as the switch to control the activity of a gene.
- **Structural genes**: a group of genes that produce proteins involved in a similar function or metabolic pathway.

Upstream from the operon is the **regulator gene**, which produces one of two types of regulatory enzymes. The binding of a repressor protein will block transcription, while the binding of an activator protein stimulates transcription.

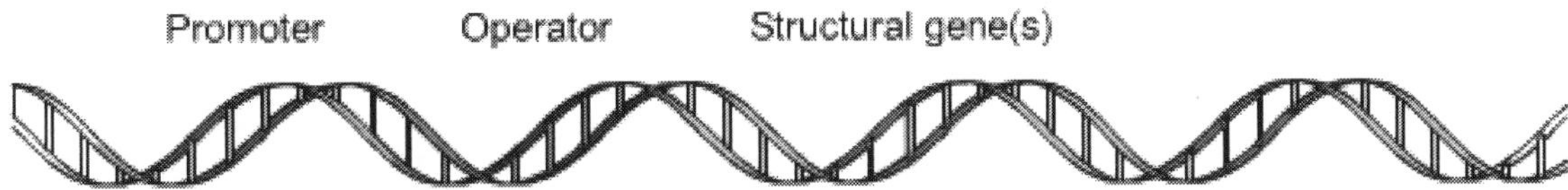

Gene Repression in Bacteria

Bacteria are able to control gene expression in response to changes in their environment. **Gene repression** is the inhibition of gene activity as a result of a regulatory protein. Some operons are "on" by default, and are only turned off if a repressor protein binds to the operator region of an operon. When a repressor binds, RNA polymerase cannot proceed past the operator to transcribe the structural genes that lie downstream.

A classic example of a repressible operon is the **trp operon** that is found in many species of bacteria. This operon contains five genes that produce the proteins responsible for synthesizing tryptophan. The trpR gene continually produces the repressor protein that controls the expression of these genes. When tryptophan is present in the environment, it binds to the repressor, causing a conformational change that allows it to bind to the operator. This prevents the bacteria from making a product that is already supplied by the surroundings. In the absence of tryptophan, the repressor is still produced by the trpR gene, but since there is no tryptophan to cause the conformational change, it cannot bind to the operator. RNA polymerase transcribes the structural genes, and tryptophan will be synthesized.

Positive Control in Bacteria

Some genes operate under **positive control**. This means that they are "off" by default, and can only be transcribed when a regulatory protein called an activator binds to the DNA. An example of this can be seen in the **lac operon**, which contains the structural genes that code for the enzymes needed for lactose metabolism (but note that in some environments the *lac* operon is under negative control). When bacteria are in the presence of both lactose and glucose, it is more efficient for the cell to metabolize the glucose first. As glucose levels drop, concentrations of cyclic AMP (cAMP) rise. Cyclic AMP forms a complex with the catabolite activator protein (CAP), which then binds to a region adjacent to the promoter called the cap site. Only when this cAMP-CAP complex binds does RNA polymerase have a high affinity for the promoter of the *lac* operon. Since gene activation is dependent on an activator, this operon demonstrates positive control under the described conditions.

Control of Gene Expression in Eukaryotes

Transcriptional Regulation

Gene expression, or the production of a protein from the information encoded in DNA, is controlled largely by **transcriptional regulation**. Eukaryotic gene expression differs from prokaryotic gene expression in that eukaryotic RNA polymerase can only transcribe a gene with the help of proteins called **transcription factors**. These proteins are responsible for turning genes on and off at the right time, in the appropriate type of cell. Transcription factors called activators increase the affinity of RNA polymerase for the promoter, but there are also transcription factors called repressors that block it. Transcription factors can also control gene expression by causing changes in the arrangement of chromatin. When DNA takes the form of tightly coiled heterochromatin, the genes are inaccessible to the proteins required for transcription. The less-condensed euchromatin allows for the binding of transcription factors.

DNA Binding Proteins, Transcription Factors

DNA binding proteins are proteins that are attracted to DNA. The affinity may be for a specific sequence or simply for the nucleic acid in general. These proteins have a region called a DNA-binding domain that interacts with the grooves of DNA (usually the major groove). Common examples of DNA binding proteins include histones, polymerases, nucleases, and transcription factors.

Transcription factors mediate gene expression. Turning a eukaryotic gene "on" involves the binding of transcription factors called activators to a region far upstream or downstream from the promoter called an enhancer. DNA-bending proteins then fold the DNA into a hairpin shape as the activator proteins are brought toward the promoter. The activator proteins assemble with general transcription factors and mediator proteins to form an initiation complex. This complex increases the affinity of RNA polymerase for the promoter, and the gene is transcribed. Repressor proteins, on the other hand, prevent transcription by binding to a sequence on DNA known as a silencer. This prevents the binding of RNA polymerase to the promoter, and the gene is not transcribed.

GENE AMPLIFICATION AND DUPLICATION

Gene duplication is the process that results in multiple copies of the same coding region of DNA. It is also referred to as gene amplification. There are many ways that duplication can happen, and it commonly occurs during meiosis. When homologous chromosomes swap portions of DNA during crossing-over, the exchange is sometimes unequal. This results in duplicated genes on one chromosome, and deleted genes on the other. It is also possible for a cell to receive an extra copy of a chromosome (and therefore a duplicate copy of every gene on that chromosome) as a result of nondisjunction during meiosis. Duplication can also arise as a result of **retrotransposition**: slippage of DNA polymerase during replication. Retrotransposition produces extra copies of a gene when the transcribed RNA is reverted back into DNA by viral proteins and then inserted back into the genome.

Duplicate copies of a gene can lead to overexpression of that gene, meaning more copies of the protein are produced. The consequences of duplication range from deleterious to favorable. Overexpression of proto-oncogenes (which are involved in cell cycle regulation) can produce an oncogene and lead to cancer. But having a "backup" copy of other types of genes can be beneficial in some circumstances. For example, if one of the copies is mutated, the original sequence will continue to produce the intended protein. Since gene duplication can lead to new alleles, it plays a key role in the evolution of a species.

POST-TRANSCRIPTIONAL CONTROL, BASIC CONCEPT OF SPLICING (INTRONS, EXONS)

Gene expression is usually regulated by transcription factors that control the binding of RNA polymerase, but it can also be regulated *after* RNA is made. This is called **post-transcriptional control**. One way that genes are regulated in eukaryotes is through **alternative splicing**. When RNA is first transcribed, it is called pre-mRNA because it contains non-coding regions called introns that must be removed before translation. These introns interrupt the regions that code for proteins, called exons. While still in the nucleus, complexes of RNA and proteins called spliceosomes remove the introns, and the exons are spliced together by ligase. However, exons within a single gene can produce more than a single type of protein by alternative splicing. Consider a gene with 4 exons: A, B, C, and D, separated by introns. After splicing, one mRNA might have the sequence ACD. The same transcript could be modified to produce ABC, ABD, etc. This non-random process is controlled by regulatory proteins and based on the type and/or needs of the cell. Mature mRNA can also be regulated after it leaves the nucleus by small regulatory RNAs that lead to the breakdown of mRNA, or prevent it from ever binding to a ribosome.

CANCER AS A FAILURE OF NORMAL CELLULAR CONTROLS, ONCOGENES, TUMOR SUPPRESSOR GENES

Cancer is characterized by uncontrolled cell division and is caused by mutations in the genes that help to regulate the cell cycle. Cancer cells are able to proliferate in conditions that would lead to senescence or apoptosis in normal cells and continue to divide in the absence of growth factors, even when crowded by other cells. They can also survive without anchorage to tissues.

One way that a cancer cell arises is by the mutation and/or overexpression of a positive cell cycle regulator called a proto-oncogene. This type of gene (such as the SRC gene) normally helps a cell to grow and divide, but it can mutate into an **oncogene** and cause the cell to divide uncontrollably.

Cancer may also result from a mutation of a **tumor repressor gene**: a gene that helps to suppresses cell division. A common example is the TP53 gene. TP53 produces the p53 protein which inspects the cell early during the cell cycle to ensure there is no damage to the DNA. If damage is detected, p53 will either signal for repair enzymes or trigger apoptosis. But if a mutated p53 protein cannot put the brakes on cell division, the damaged DNA will be inherited by the daughter cells. Mutations will accumulate over generations to produce a cancer cell.

Regulation of Chromatin Structure

One mechanism for gene control involves regulation of chromatin structure. Euchromatin is more relaxed than heterochromatin, and therefore more accessible to transcription factors. When DNA condenses, it wraps tightly around positively charged histone octamers to form nucleosomes. The octamers consist of eight histone proteins, each with an N-terminal tail that is oriented outward from the core. Acetylation of the histone tails neutralizes the charge, thereby reducing the attraction between the histone octamers and negatively charged DNA. Acetylation occurs when the enzyme **histone acetyltransferase**, or HAT, transfers an acetyl group (C_2H_3O) from acetyl-coenzyme A to a lysine residue within the tail of a histone. This action can be reversed (deacetylation) to restore the positive charge on the histone, and DNA will condense into heterochromatin.

Methylation of histones can also influence the organization of chromatin, but it can go either way; some forms of methylation relax DNA and others condense it. Methylation does not directly affect the charge on a histone.

DNA Methylation

Methylation of DNA (the addition of CH_3) is one of the many regulatory mechanisms of gene expression. It is important to distinguish between methylation of a *histone* and methylation of the *DNA molecule* itself.

Methylation of histones can elicit opposite results. The DNA may coil more tightly around the histones, or loosen so that genes can be activated. The effect of methylation depends on the part of the histone to which the enzyme **histone methyltransferase**, or HMT, adds the methyl group(s) and how many groups are added.

When the DNA molecule is methylated, the enzyme **DNA methyltransferase**, or DNMT, adds a methyl group to the fifth carbon of a cytosine base. The methyl group extends into the major groove of DNA, suppressing transcription and silencing the gene. These methyl "tags" are heritable, and provide the mechanism for epigenetics: a change in phenotype as a result of gene *expression*, not a change in the gene *sequence*.

Role of Non-Coding RNAs

Non-coding RNAs, or **ncRNAs**, are molecules synthesized during transcription that do not encode proteins. In fact, the majority of transcribed RNA molecules are not translated. Many of these ncRNAs participate either directly or indirectly in the regulation of gene expression. There are many types of ncRNAs, notably transfer RNA (or tRNA, which delivers amino acids to the ribosome during translation) and ribosomal RNA (or rRNA, which combines with proteins to make the ribosome).

Other examples of ncRNAs include but are not limited to microRNA, small nuclear RNA, and PIWI-interacting RNA. MicroRNAs (**miRNAs**) are short ncRNAs that bind to mRNA via complementary base pairing. This could interfere with translation, or it could mark the mRNA for degradation by enzymes. Small nuclear RNA (**snRNA**) plays a role in post-transcriptional modification by combining with proteins to form a spliceosome, which then removes an intron from the mRNA transcript before translation. PIWI interacting RNA (or **piRNA**) combines with proteins to inhibit the movement of **transposons**, segments of DNA that change positions in the genome.

RECOMBINANT DNA AND BIOTECHNOLOGY

GENE CLONING

Gene cloning is a process by which multiple copies of a gene of interest are produced. A common method of gene cloning involves the insertion of a target gene into a vector (often a circular piece of bacterial DNA known as a plasmid). First, the gene is cut from its source by a restriction enzyme. (Restriction enzymes are proteins that cleave DNA at specific sites.) The same restriction enzyme that cut the DNA is used to cut the plasmid, and the gene is pasted in place by the enzyme ligase. This "recombinant" plasmid can then be placed into host cells such as bacteria to be replicated.

There are many applications of gene cloning. Having many copies of a gene makes it easier to study. It may be possible to determine the function of a gene, or how it is affected by certain mutations. It can also be used to mass produce a desired protein, such as insulin, when the gene is expressed by a host cell.

Review Video: Cloning
Visit mometrix.com/academy and enter code: 289634

RESTRICTION ENZYMES

Restriction enzymes are often referred to as molecular scissors because they cut DNA at a specific site. They are also called restriction *endo*nucleases because they cleave a region *within* the DNA molecule rather than at the end. These enzymes exist in prokaryotes (possibly as a defense against foreign DNA) and are harvested for use in biotechnology.

A restriction enzyme works by scanning the DNA molecule until it recognizes a short sequence, usually four to six nucleotides long. It cuts the DNA at or near this sequence by hydrolyzing the phosphodiester bond that forms the sugar-phosphate backbone. Sometimes restriction enzymes cut in such a way that one strand overhangs the other, leaving a few nucleotides without a pair. These are called "sticky ends" because they easily stick to a complementary sequence. This is useful when inserting a gene into a cloning vector. Other enzymes cut straight across to produce "blunt ends" with no overhangs. Blunt ends are less likely to adhere to each other.

G|AATTC
Restriction enzyme producing sticky ends → CTTAA|G

CCC|GGG
Restriction enzyme producing blunt ends → GGG|CCC

DNA LIBRARIES

DNA libraries are collections of either plasmids or another type of vector called bacterial artificial chromosomes (BACs), each containing a different fragment from a foreign source of DNA. BACs are useful in DNA libraries because they can store larger sequences than plasmids (up to 300 kilobase pairs, compared to plasmids which can only store up to 10 kb).

There are two types of DNA libraries: genomic libraries and complementary DNA (or cDNA) libraries. **Genomic libraries** contain the entire genome of an organism, including regulatory elements, introns, all other non-coding regions, and exons. The clones are organized and stored in multi-well plates; each well contains one clone. An entire genome library would require many of these trays. Genomic libraries are useful when studying gene regulation, or when sequencing a full genome.

cDNA libraries do not store entire genomes. The inserted DNA fragments are synthesized in vitro from mature mRNA, and therefore do not contain the non-coding sequences seen in genomic libraries. These libraries are useful in studying specific proteins because the genes are easily expressed.

Generation of cDNA

The generation of complementary DNA begins with the extraction and purification of mRNA. There are different ways to purify mRNA, but a common method is column purification. After the mRNA is isolated, the enzyme **reverse transcriptase** is added to the sample. This enzyme (which is extracted from retroviruses) is able to synthesize a single strand of DNA from mRNA; the product is called a reverse transcript. Before reverse transcriptase can add nucleotides, a short strand of thymine deoxynucleotides called **oligo-dT** binds to the poly-A tail to make a primer. Reverse transcriptase then extends the single-stranded DNA from this primer at the 3' end of mRNA. Once the strand is complete, enzymes break down the mRNA transcript. A primer binds to the single stranded DNA, and DNA polymerase synthesizes the complementary strand. The cDNA can then be ligated into a vector, such as a plasmid. If the library of cDNA is complete, all the messenger RNA within the genome of an organism will be present.

Hybridization

Hybridization is the annealing of two separate sources of single-stranded DNA to each other (or sometimes RNA to DNA). Hybridization can be used to detect the location of a gene or sequence of interest. First, a **probe** is synthesized. A probe is a fragment of nucleic acid (either RNA or DNA) that is complementary to the target gene. It is tagged with either a fluorescent or a radioactive marker and added to the sample of DNA where it will hydrogen bond with its complementary sequence. Various imaging techniques can be used to identify where the probe annealed.

Hybridization can also be used to determine the relatedness of different species. DNA from two species is added to a tube which is then heated to separate the strands (this is called DNA "melting"). When the sample is cooled, some of the strands from one species will hybridize with the strands of the other. These strands will not be perfectly complementary, and there will be fewer hydrogen bonds formed between them. As a result, hybridized strands will melt at lower temperatures. The more dissimilar the DNA sequence, the lower the melting temperature.

Expressing Cloned Genes

A cloned gene is first inserted into a specially designed plasmid. The plasmid must have an origin of replication so that it can replicate within a host cell (usually a bacterium), and it must also have an antibiotic resistance gene. This gene is not required for expression of the cloned gene, but it provides a way for the researcher to eliminate any host cells that do not harbor the foreign gene. The plasmid is cut with a restriction enzyme (the same enzyme that was used to remove the foreign gene) and the gene is inserted. Only some of the host cells will absorb the plasmid, so antibiotics are applied to kill any bacteria that have not been transformed. The surviving bacteria can then transcribe and translate the cloned gene.

Polymerase Chain Reaction

Polymerase chain reaction, or PCR, is a process that amplifies a targeted sequence of DNA to billions of copies in a few hours. This technology, often called "molecular photocopying," allows scientists to locate and replicate a short section of DNA within a much larger sequence. First, the following reagents are added to a tube:

- the DNA sample
- DNA nucleotides (dNTPs)
- primers
- buffer
- Taq polymerase (a polymerase that can withstand high temperatures)

The tube is then placed in a machine called a thermocycler where it is repeatedly heated and cooled in a 3-stage cycle:

1. (95 °C) Denaturation – DNA strands separate.
2. (55 °C) Primer Annealing – primers hybridize to the beginning and end of the desired DNA sequence to provide a starting point for replication while limiting the length of the copied DNA to the target sequence.
3. (75 °C) Extension – Taq polymerase adds nucleotides between the two primers in a 5' → 3' direction.

At the completion of each cycle, the sequence is doubled resulting in an exponential production of the original sequence. Applications of this technology can be found in DNA fingerprinting, diagnosis of hereditary diseases, identification of pathogens, and DNA sequencing.

Gel Electrophoresis and Southern Blotting

Gel electrophoresis is a lab technique used to separate charged molecules based on their size. A sample of nucleic acids or proteins is inserted into wells at the end of a gel matrix made of polyacrylamide or agar. An electric field is applied to the gel, causing negatively charged molecules to migrate toward the positive electrode. The smaller the molecule, the further it will travel, resulting in a series of bands arranged according to size. The gel can be stained afterwards to visualize the banding pattern.

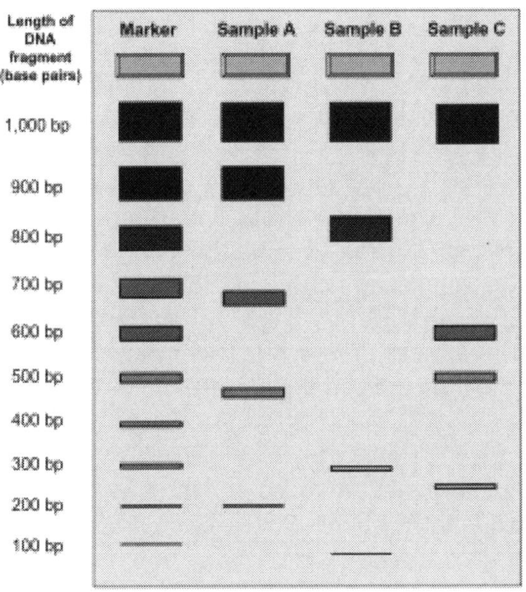

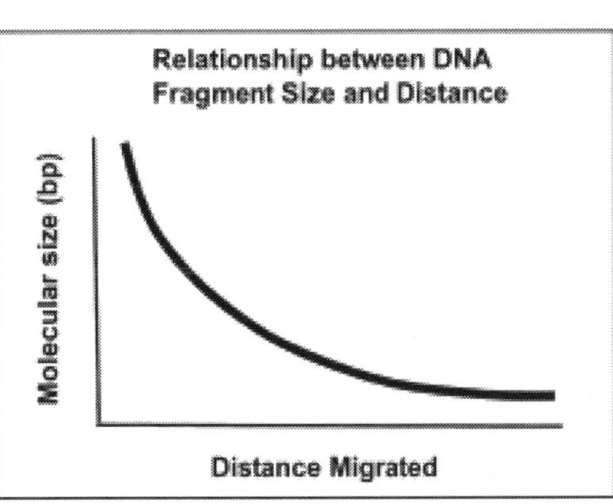

Southern blotting combines gel electrophoresis and hybridization to locate a specific nucleotide sequence. First, a restriction enzyme digests the sample of DNA into fragments of different size. Gel electrophoresis is used to separate the fragments, producing many invisible bands. The gel is placed atop an alkaline solution which moves up through the gel by capillary action, denaturing the double-stranded fragments and blotting them onto a nitrocellulose membrane that is resting over the gel. The membrane is bathed in a solution that contains radioactive or fluorescent probes which hybridize to the target sequence. X-ray imaging can be used to see only the bands that contain the sequence of interest.

DNA SEQUENCING

DNA sequencing is the process of determining the order of the four types of nucleotides that make up DNA. There are several ways that DNA can be sequenced. The **Sanger method**, also called the chain termination method, is slower than some of the latest technology, but it is far from obsolete. In this method, the DNA sample is mixed with all the factors needed for DNA replication: dNTPs (deoxynucleotide triphosphates, or "normal" free nucleotides), DNA polymerase, and primers. Special nucleotides called dideoxyribonucleotides (or ddNTPs) are added as well: ddATP, ddGTP, ddTTP, ddCTP. All of these ddNTPs are missing the hydroxyl group on the 3' carbon of the sugar, making it impossible for another nucleotide to be added after the ddNTP is incorporated into the growing chain. They are also tagged with a fluorescent dye. The DNA mixture is placed through a series of temperature changes to promote DNA replication. Replication stops anytime a ddNTP is added, resulting in DNA fragments of different sizes. These fragments are separated by gel electrophoresis and a laser detects the wavelengths at which each ddNTP fluoresces. Since each type of ddNTP has a different "tag," the sequence can be read.

ANALYZING GENE EXPRESSION

Gene expression can be detected using a variety of techniques. One common method is called **northern blotting**. This is very similar to the procedure for southern blotting, except it detects RNA instead of DNA. The RNA is extracted from the cell, separated using gel electrophoresis, and then blotted onto a nitrocellulose membrane. Specific probes are applied to the membrane, and they will hybridize if a gene is expressed in the cell.

Another way to analyze gene expression is through **RT-PCR** (reverse transcriptase polymerase chain reaction). The extracted mRNA is transcribed back into cDNA by the enzyme reverse transcriptase, and the cDNA can then be amplified by PCR and run on a gel. Any gene that is identified on the gel is a gene that is being expressed.

A **microarray analysis** is a technique that analyzes gene expression by comparing isolated mRNA from two different sources: the experimental source and a control source. Each sample is reverse transcribed into cDNA and color-coded with a fluorescent probe to distinguish between the sources; the experimental sample is often red, and the reference sample green. The two sources of mRNA are combined before hybridizing to a microarray slide. Any red spots that appear on the microarray indicate greater expression in the experimental sample, while green spots indicate greater expression in the control sample. Yellow spots indicate equal expression.

DETERMINING GENE FUNCTION

The function of a gene can be studied using a strategy known as **reverse genetics**. With reverse genetics, the activity of a gene is altered in some way, and the effects on the phenotype are observed. One example method is called **genetic knockout**. The target gene is "knocked out" by silencing it in some way, perhaps by replacing it with a mutated version that will not make the intended product, or by mutating the promoter. It is also possible to interfere with the activity of messenger RNA through the binding of microRNA (miRNA) or small interfering RNA (siRNA). The expression of the gene of interest will be reduced, and the effect on the phenotype will indicate the function of the gene. Since there is still *some* gene expression, this method is sometimes called **gene knock*down***. Sometimes a gene can be *over*expressed to determine its function, or even transferred into an organism that does not have the gene.

Stem Cells

Stem cells are undifferentiated cells that have the potential to become specialized. They have the ability to self-renew through mitosis, while maintaining their differentiation capabilities. Stem cells are aptly named, because all cell types "stem" from them. These cells give rise to specialized tissues during development, and repair and replenish tissues throughout the life of an organism.

Stem cells have varying degrees of **potency**: the ability to produce other cell types. Embryonic cells are **pluripotent** and can develop into any type of cell as a result of selective gene expression. Adult stem cells, also called somatic stem cells, are usually **multipotent** because their ability to differentiate is more limited.

There are many potential applications of stem cells. The differentiation process can be controlled to produce specialized cells, tissues, and even organs as a treatment for certain diseases or injuries. Some stem cell therapies are in current use, but many are still in development. Progress is being made in reversing the differentiation process to induce pluripotent cells from differentiated somatic cells.

Practical Applications of DNA Technology

Some practical applications of DNA technology to the medical field:

- Vaccines such as hepatitis B are developed by using DNA technology to synthesize only a protein-based portion of the virus, a safer alternative to using a live weakened virus.
- Hormones such as insulin and growth hormones are made by inserting the hormone-producing gene into bacteria and harvesting the products.
- Diseases, or predisposition for diseases, can be identified through DNA sequencing and other technologies.
- Human gene therapy seeks to treat genetic diseases by introducing a normal copy of a defective gene. The vector that delivers the gene is usually a virus which inserts the normal gene into the cells of an affected individual. Sometimes the cells are removed from the patient and reinserted, or the vector may be injected directly into the diseased tissue.

Some practical applications of DNA technology to evidence, environmental cleanup, and agriculture:

- Forensics: DNA evidence is often used to solve crimes. Each person has a unique DNA profile which can be visualized using PCR and gel electrophoresis. This is called DNA fingerprinting.
- Environmental Cleanup: bacteria can be bioengineered with genes that allow them to metabolize toxic substances (such as hydrocarbons from an oil spill) in a process known as bioremediation.
- Agriculture: Crops can be genetically modified with genes that change their properties. Examples of modifications include resistance to pests, herbicides, or certain diseases. Some crops are modified to be more nutritious, or to have a longer shelf life. Livestock can be vaccinated against diseases.

Safety and Ethics of DNA Technology

The Food and Drug Administration (FDA) and National Institutes of Health (NIH) help to regulate the products of DNA technology and ensure their safety. However, many important questions are raised regarding the safety and ethics of DNA technology.

- Could GMOs hybridize with non-GMOs, and disrupt the ecosystem?
- What are the long-term effects of GMO modification and/or consumption?
- Will gene therapy introduce foreign genes to the gene pool?
- Can a person be discriminated against by insurance companies or employers if genetic testing reveals a disease-carrying gene?
- Will our ability to manipulate genes lead to eugenics, designer babies, and genetic enhancement?

Transmission of Heritable Information

Evidence That DNA Is Genetic Material and Mendelian Concepts

Phenotype and Genotype

The genotype of an organism refers to the alleles that have been inherited for a certain trait. Alleles are alternate forms of the same gene that are located at the same locus (location) on a particular chromosome. Organisms that reproduce sexually inherit chromosomes from each parent, resulting in homologous pairs. Homologous chromosomes are similar in size and centromere position, and they carry the same genes, but not necessarily the same alleles for those genes. The combination of inherited alleles is the genotype.

Phenotype refers to observable characteristics that exist mostly as a result of the expression of the genotype. For example, a pea plant might inherit two dominant alleles for purple flower color. Its genotype for that trait is "PP," and the phenotype is purple flower color. Phenotype is not limited to outward appearances; it also includes behavioral traits, diseases, and more. Phenotype may also be influenced by environmental factors. For example, flower color might be influenced by the pH of the soil. For many traits genotype gives an organism a range of possible phenotypes, and environment narrows that range to produce the given phenotype.

Gene

A gene defined as a unit of heredity. It consists of a segment of DNA nucleotides, and the sequence of these nucleotides encodes instructions for a protein. DNA is double stranded, but the gene is almost always found on only one strand. The length of a sequence can vary greatly, but the average size of a human gene is between 10,000 and 15,000 base pairs (kbps). This is relatively short given the 3 billion base pairs that make up the human genome.

Each gene contains sequences that help regulate the expression of that gene. During transcription, complementary RNA nucleotides are added to the unzipped DNA strand. A promoter (found at the 5' end of the gene) signals the beginning of the sequence to be transcribed, and the terminator (at the 3' end) signals transcription to end. There are also segments on this RNA transcript that are noncoding (called introns), which are removed, leaving continuous coding regions (exons) that are ligated together. This sequence is used during translation to link specific amino acids together and make the protein specified by the gene.

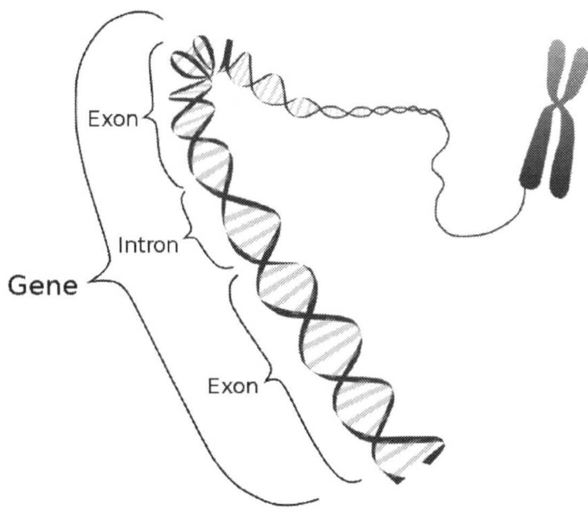

Locus

A locus is often described as a gene's address on a chromosome. The address consists of a sequence of numbers and letters that narrow down the location from (in humans) 46 possible chromosomes to a specific band on one chromosome. These bands only appear if the chromosome is stained; some regions are darker because the DNA coils more tightly.

The "address" begins with a number that represents the chromosome number. The 46 human chromosomes are arranged in order of size (with the sex chromosomes last), so the number 1 would indicate the largest chromosome.

Next will be a letter, either "p" or "q." The p indicates the short arm of the chromosome, and the q represents the long arm.

After the letter will be two numbers. The first is the region on the arm, and the second is the band number. Sometimes there will be a decimal followed by another digit or digits that indicates sub-bands.

Example of cystic fibrosis locus: 7q31.2

Chromosome #7, long arm, region 3, band 1, sub-band 2.

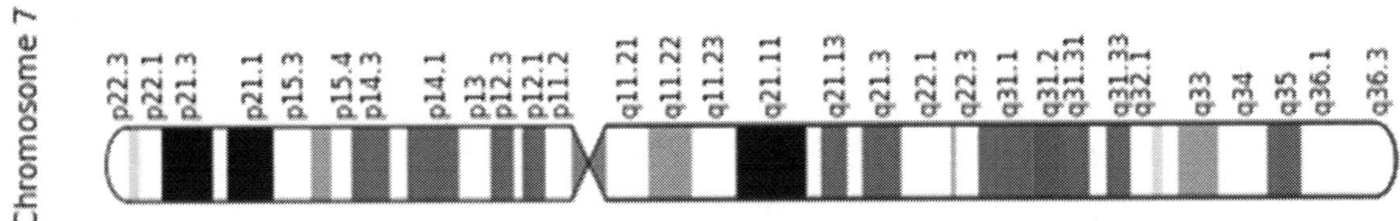

Allele: Single and Multiple

An organism can only inherit two alleles for a gene (one from each parent). In rare cases there may only be one version of that gene, which would mean there would be no variability among the population for that trait. It is much more common for at least two versions of a gene to exist. Oftentimes three or more alleles for a single gene exist in the population. This phenomenon is known as multiple alleles. The individual can still only inherit two, but there will be greater variability at the level of the population due to the many possible combinations.

A common example of multiple alleles occurs with blood type. There is only one gene that determines blood type, but that gene has three alleles, abbreviated I^A (A), I^B (B), and i (O). Six possible genotypes can exist in the population.

HOMOZYGOSITY AND HETEROZYGOSITY

Organisms that reproduce sexually have body cells (or somatic cells) that are diploid. Diploid cells contain pairs of chromosomes called homologous chromosomes; one member of the pair is inherited from the mother and the other from the father.

Homologous pairs have the same genes, but the alleles at the same locus on each homolog may differ. If the alleles are the *same*, the individual is said to be homozygous, or "pure," for a given trait. If both alleles are recessive, then it is further classified as homozygous-recessive. If both alleles are dominant, the individual is homozygous-dominant.

If the alleles are *different*, then the individual is heterozygous for that trait. For example, BB = homozygous-dominant, bb = homozygous-recessive, Bb = heterozygous.

The phenotype of a heterozygous genotype may vary depending on the form of dominance displayed by that trait. The dominant allele may achieve full expression, both alleles could appear in the phenotype, or the alleles may blend to produce a new phenotype.

WILD-TYPE

A wild-type allele is the allele that is responsible for producing the most prevalent phenotype in a population. This allele is often considered the "standard" or "normal" variant of a gene and may be denoted with a "+" superscript when abbreviated. The non-wild-type allele is more commonly referred to as the mutant allele and may refer to any allele that is *not* the wild-type. Mutant alleles may be beneficial but are more commonly neutral or deleterious.

A changing environment may cause a shift in allelic frequencies. For example, the wild-type allele for the peppered moth produces pale wings. But during the Industrial Revolution, the mutant allele that produced dark wings increased in the population and temporarily became the wild-type. It is also important to note that wild-type alleles are not always dominant. Huntington's disease is rare (and therefore not the wild-type phenotype), but the disease is caused by a dominant allele.

RECESSIVENESS

A recessive trait can be expressed only in the absence of a dominant allele. In other words two copies of the same allele must be inherited from each parent (homozygous recessive) for the phenotype to show. It would be impossible for a parent with a homozygous dominant genotype to produce offspring of the recessive phenotype. Most, but not all, diseases follow a recessive inheritance pattern. For example, individuals affected by cystic fibrosis must inherit both recessive alleles. If a single dominant allele is inherited, the heterozygous carrier will not show symptoms. But dwarfism is a dominant trait, and therefore carriers do not exist; the presence of a dominant allele will result in the disease. A trait that is recessive is not necessarily less common in a population. Examples of recessive traits that are more common than dominant traits include type O blood and five-fingered hands.

COMPLETE DOMINANCE

Complete dominance refers to a type of dominance in which the dominant allele completely masks the effects of the recessive allele. In this case an individual that is heterozygous for a trait has the same phenotype as a homozygous dominant individual. There are no intermediates between the dominant and recessive phenotype. An example of this can be seen in Mendel's pea plants. Plants with a heterozygous phenotype for flower color (Pp) are just as purple as the plants with a homozygous dominant genotype (PP), and the white allele has no expression. It is important to note that inheritance and expression of alleles is usually more complex than these simple rules. Traits are often influenced by both versions of a gene or may even be controlled by multiple genes.

CO-DOMINANCE

Co-dominance is a phenomenon in which a heterozygote expresses *both* alleles simultaneously. The effects of one allele is no greater than the other; there is no recessiveness. Nor do the phenotypes blend together. Roan coloring in cattle is an example of co-dominance. If one parent passes on an allele for red coat and the other parent passes on the white allele, the offspring will have a red *and* white phenotype known as roan. Another common example can be seen in blood type inheritance. Blood cells may carry two different antigens on their surface: antigen A and antigen B. If both A and B alleles are inherited, then heterozygous individual will have genotype AB and a blood type (phenotype) AB. Type O indicates a lack of an antigen and is therefore recessive to the allele for A and the allele for B.

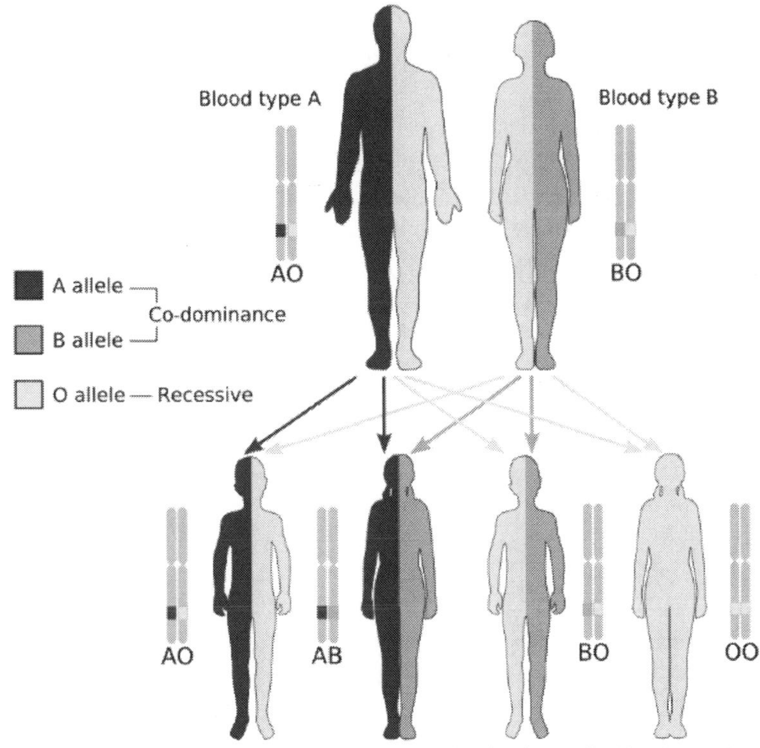

INCOMPLETE DOMINANCE, LEAKAGE, PENETRANCE AND EXPRESSIVITY

Incomplete dominance, sometimes called partial dominance, is observed when a heterozygote expresses a phenotype that is a blend of the two different alleles. As in codominance, there is no recessiveness because both alleles achieve expression. However, the new phenotype is an intermediate between the two variant forms of the gene. The commonly used example of incomplete dominance is flower color in snapdragons. Snapdragons may be red, white, or different shades of pink. There is no "pink" allele; this phenotype indicates a heterozygous phenotype. Incomplete dominance should not be confused with the refuted idea of "blending inheritance," which indicates the blending of the alleles themselves (not the phenotypes) to make a new allele.

Genetic leakage is the flow of alleles from one species to another. In most cases members of two different species cannot interbreed either because of physical barriers or because of their genetic differences (such as a different number of chromosomes). If mating between members of separate species produces offspring, the hybrid offspring are usually sterile. But occasionally the hybrids can successfully reproduce with one of the parent species to produce fertile offspring. In this way alleles from one species can be introduced to another and "leak" into the population.

Penetrance is a measure of the percentage of individuals who carry a given allele that expresses the phenotype associated with that allele. It is a term commonly used in the medical field to describe the likelihood that a carrier will develop symptoms of a disease. If every individual who inherits the allele also displays the phenotype for that allele, then the penetrance is complete, or 100 percent. An example of penetrance can be seen in the mutation in the BRCA1 gene (which is known to be a factor in developing breast cancer). Since 80 percent of women with this mutation develop breast cancer, the penetrance is 80 percent. This is considered incomplete penetrance.

Penetrance is rarely determined by genetics alone. Environment is likely to be a contributing factor. Individuals with the BRCA1 mutation who smoke and have poor dietary habits will be more likely to develop breast cancer than carriers with healthy lifestyles.

Expressivity is often confused with penetrance. Whereas penetrance is a measure of the proportion of carriers that expresses the phenotype associated with an allele, expressivity describes the manifestation of the phenotype or the *level* of phenotype expression. A disease might show 100 percent penetrance in a population, but there could be a range of phenotypes. For example, all individuals with sickle cell anemia share the same genotype (both alleles that code for the protein hemoglobin are mutated). However, there are varying degrees of symptoms. Anemia may be mild, moderate, or life-threatening. Pain may frequent the legs for some individuals but the chest in others. Like penetrance, the spectrum of expressivity may be accounted for by environmental factors or differences in the rest of the genome.

Hybridization: Viability

Individuals that belong to two separate species are rarely able to interbreed either because of prezygotic reproductive isolation (there is no fertilization of the egg) or postzygotic reproductive isolation (the egg *is* fertilized, but there is rarely further gene flow). Fertilization of an egg is not enough to ensure reproductive success. The genes that are passed on to the hybrid zygote are often incompatible. If the number of chromosomes is different between the two species, there will be problems with gene expression, and this will result in a range of potential outcomes. The zygote may not be viable, and it is highly probable that it will die during its development. If the hybrid is viable and survives, it may continue to experience abnormal development. It may be weak, infertile, or never reach sexual maturity. Even if the hybrid reproduces with one of the parent species, the third-generation offspring will have reduced fitness compared to the "pure" population, and the alleles will be unlikely to spread.

Gene Pool

A gene pool is the collection of all the alleles in a given population. The larger the gene pool, the greater the genetic variability within the group, and the greater the chance of the population's survival. A wide range of phenotypes is bound to produce favorable traits to select in the presence of certain environmental pressures. Smaller populations tend to have smaller gene pools as compared to larger groups. Such reduced variability puts the population at risk of extinction; there may not be a favorable trait shared by a subset of the population that allows that subset to survive under pressure. Populations with small gene pools are also more susceptible to genetic diseases. Too many members could be carriers of a deleterious recessive disorder, leading to an increased probability of disease expression. Random mutations are the main source of new alleles in a gene pool, although leakage may introduce new alleles as well.

Meiosis and Other Factors Affecting Genetic Variability

Significance of Meiosis

Meiosis is the process by which sexually reproducing organisms create gametes, or sex cells, from a single diploid cell. The events of meiosis ensure that these gametes have half the number of chromosomes (haploid) and that each gamete has a unique combination of genes. In the first stage of meiosis (prophase I), chromatin condenses into chromosomes, and each chromosome pairs up with its homolog in a process called synapsis. One homolog then exchanges genetic material with the other. This process, known as crossing-over, results in chromosomes with new, reshuffled alleles. Sister chromatids are no longer identical, and each member of a homologous pair now has DNA from the other.

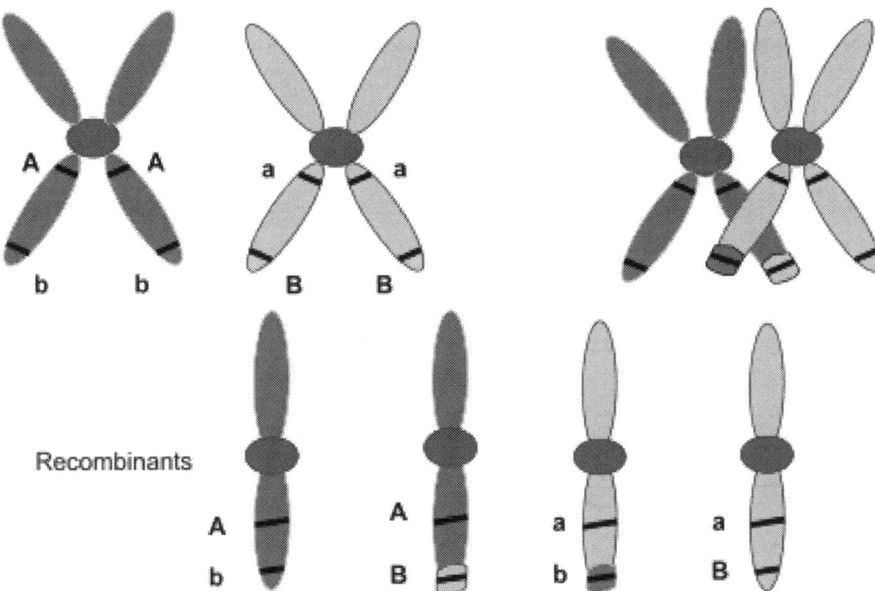

In the second stage of meiosis (metaphase I), chromosomes line up in pairs, and the orientation of the pairs is random every time. This means that gametes receive a random assortment of maternal and paternal chromosomes when homologous are split and distributed to each daughter cell in anaphase II. The events described above allow for a nearly infinite amount of genetically unique gametes.

Important Differences Between Meiosis and Mitosis

Mitosis is the mechanism by which a fertilized egg (zygote) grows into an adult and also the process that repairs tissues. Mitosis involves a single division of the nucleus and includes these stages: prophase, prometaphase, metaphase, anaphase, and telophase. During these stages, the chromatin condenses into chromosomes that then line up in a single line along the equator of the cell. Sister chromatids (with identical alleles) are split at the centromere and pulled toward each pole of the cell by the mitotic spindle, and a nuclear envelope forms around each group of chromosomes. Each nucleus has a complete set of DNA with the same number of chromosomes as the original cell.

Meiosis is a type of cell division that makes gametes. The process involves two divisions: meiosis I (prophase I, prometaphase I, metaphase I, anaphase I, and telophase I) and meiosis II (prophase II, etc.). During prophase I, homologous chromosomes pair up to form a tetrad and exchange genetic material before lining up in pairs along the equator of the cell during metaphase I. (Synapsis does not happen in mitosis.) These pairs are separated during anaphase I, and by the end of the first division, there are two genetically different daughter cells with half the number of chromosomes as the parent cell. These cells undergo a second division (similar to the stages of mitosis) to split the sister chromatids and produce four genetically different haploid daughter cells.

Segregation of Genes

Independent Assortment

The law of segregation states that alleles are separated during meiosis; therefore, each gamete receives only one allele from each pair. This law explains why genetic material is not doubled with each generation.

The law of independent assortment states that allele pairs separate independently of each other. The inheritance of a particular gene does not usually influence the inheritance of another. This principle arises from the random lineup of homologous pairs during metaphase I of meiosis. There is a 50 percent chance that a gamete will receive a maternal chromosome and a 50 percent chance it will receive a paternal chromosome. There are more than 8 million (2^{23}) possible combinations of chromosomes that a gamete could be dealt. There are exceptions to this principle. Genes that are in close proximity to each other are likely to be inherited together.

Linkage

Genetic linkage is a phenomenon seen in genes that are in close proximity on the same chromosome. Most genes are inherited independently of each other. The inheritance on a gene on one chromosome will never influence the inheritance of a gene on a different chromosome. However, if the genes are located near one another on the same chromosome, it is likely that they will be inherited together, or "linked." The closer they are to one another, the higher the probability that they will be linked. This principle can be seen in the process of crossing-over, also known as homologous recombination. During the formation of gametes, homologous chromosomes pair up to form a tetrad, and random segments of the chromosome are exchanged between them. A series of consecutive genes can easily be inherited together, whereas genes that are far apart are more likely to be separated. Genes on nonhomologous chromosomes are never linked.

Recombination: Single Crossovers and Double Crossovers

Crossing-over is the swapping of DNA between homologous chromosomes. A single crossover occurs when the exchange happens once, resulting in two non-sister chromatids that have new alleles at the same locus. With a double crossover, there are two exchanges, and these exchanges may happen in various ways. There may be chiasmata (points of contact between non-sister chromatids) at more than one locus. Another case may involve the exchange of genes at one chiasma and then swapping them back. Although a double crossover has occurred, the chromosomes have regained their original genetic content. Another possibility involves an exchange between two non-sister chromatids and a second exchange between sister chromatids on one of those chromosomes. Because three strands are involved, this is called a three-strand double crossover. If DNA is swapped between two non-sister chromatids, and then further exchanged between the sister chromatids of both chromosomes, it is called a four-strand double crossover.

Recombination: Synaptonemal Complex

The synaptonemal complex is a protein-based structure that is required for synapsis and recombination of homologous chromosomes in nearly all species. The complex is comprised of three parts: two parallel elements (often called "cores") and a central horizontal element made of filaments that span horizontally between the two cores, connecting them together. The chromatin that makes up the chromosomes can be seen as a series of thread-like loops that connect to the lateral elements.

The synaptonemal complex is formed in the zygotene phase of prophase I (the second of five phases of prophase I) and disassembled during the diplotene stage (the fourth phase of prophase I). The synaptonemal complex provides a framework that aligns and stabilizes the chromosomes during synapsis. It is also required for the formation of chiasmata where crossing-over occurs.

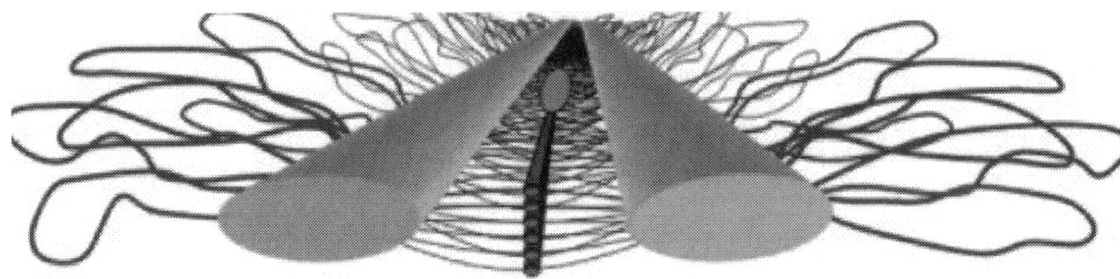

Recombination: Tetrad

A tetrad (sometimes called a bivalent) is a four-part structure that is formed during synapsis when two homologous chromosomes are paired up. This event occurs during prophase I of meiosis. The chromatids of the homologous chromosomes, with the help of the synaptonemal complex, are held together at one or more points called chiasmata, where crossing-over takes place. Without the formation of tetrads, the stages of meiosis would resemble those of mitosis. The homologs would not exchange DNA, nor would they be separated to form haploid cells. It remains unclear *how* one member of a pair finds the other, although there must be some basis for recognition in the similarity of nucleotide sequences.

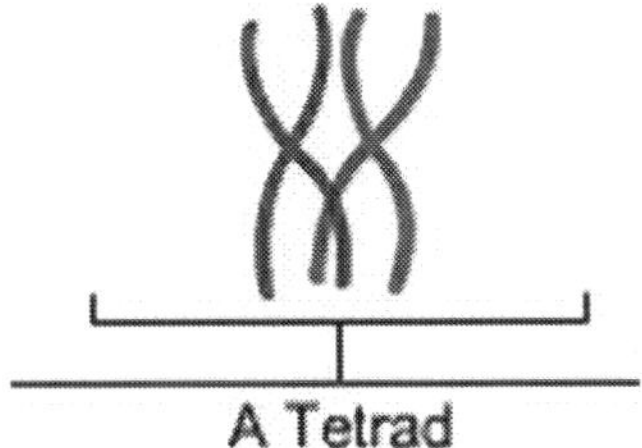

Sex-Linked Characteristics

Sex-linked genes are found on the sex chromosomes (X or Y). The X and Y chromosomes are not homologous; they are different in size, centromere position, and genetic content (with the exception of small regions that are required for synapsis during meiosis). Females inherit two X-chromosomes (which *are* homologous), and males inherit an X and a Y-chromosome. Any gene on the X-chromosome is said to be X-linked, and any gene on the Y-chromosome is Y-linked. These Y-linked genes are responsible for male sex determination and development.

Unlike Y-linked genes, X-linked genes are inherited by both males and females. Recessive X-linked traits are seen in both sexes but are far more common in males. Because females carry two X-chromosomes, the effects of the recessive allele can easily be masked by a dominant allele on the second X-chromosome. However, because males do not have homologous X-chromosomes, inheritance of a single recessive allele will always result in expression of that allele. Examples of recessive x-linked disorders include hemophilia, Duchene muscular dystrophy, and colorblindness. If the X-linked trait is dominant, then it will not necessarily affect males more than females. Traits that are *not* sex-linked are referred to as autosomal.

VERY FEW GENES ON Y CHROMOSOME

The Y-chromosome is one of two sex-chromosomes, the other being the X-chromosome. Females inherit two homologous X-chromosomes, and males inherit one X- and one Y-chromosome. The Y-chromosome is not homologous to the X; it is smaller with different (and far fewer) genes. (Note that there are two homologous *regions* called pseudo-autosomal regions that recombine during meiosis.)

The human X-chromosome has more than 150 million base pairs and carries more than 800 genes. The Y-chromosome has less than 60 million base pairs with approximately 70 genes. It is sometimes referred to as a "gene desert" owing to the scarcity of protein-coding genes within lengthy non-coding DNA sequences. The Y-linked genes are not required for survival but are required for normal male development and fertility. The SRY gene is arguably the most important Y-linked gene because it produces a protein that stimulates the development of testes and suppresses the development of female reproductive organs. Lack of a Y chromosome will result in a female embryo, even in the absence of a second X-chromosome.

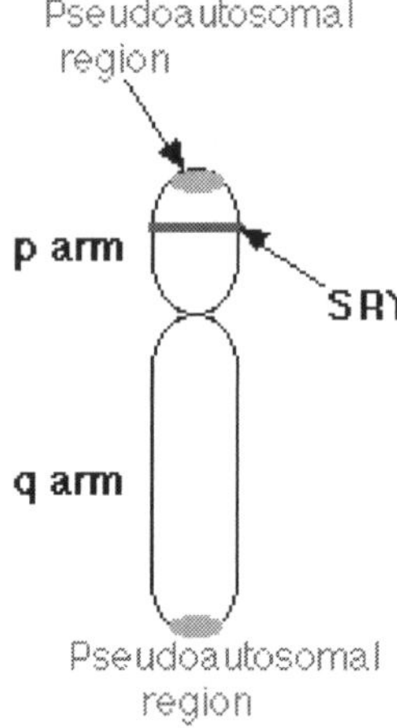

Y chromosome

SEX DETERMINATION

Sex is determined by the sex chromosomes present in the fertilized egg (zygote). The sex cells are haploid, meaning that they have half the chromosomes as a somatic cell. An ovum, or egg, will always have an X-chromosome because females have two X-chromosomes. Sperm cells on the other hand will have either an X or a Y chromosome because males have both and X and a Y, which are then separated during meiosis. Thus, it is the chromosome inherited from the father that determines the sex of the offspring.

Sometimes the wrong number of sex chromosomes can be inherited because of nondisjunction during meiosis. Females with only a single X-chromosome (XO) have a condition called Turner Syndrome. Affected individuals are usually sterile and experience a range of physical abnormalities. Sometimes one or more extra X-chromosomes are inherited with relatively few side effects.

Males with Klinefelter syndrome inherit an extra X chromosome (XXY) and are often sterile with development of secondary female characteristics. In the case of an extra Y-chromosome (XYY) males appear to develop normally but produce high amounts of testosterone.

Cytoplasmic/Extranuclear Inheritance

Cytoplasmic inheritance, also called extranuclear inheritance, is the inheritance of genes that are not contained within the nucleus. Sources of such DNA could be mitochondria, chloroplasts (in autotrophs), or parasites such as HIV. However, it is mitochondria that are of most significance in humans.

Mitochondria are organelles that likely evolved from independently living prokaryotes that were engulfed by ancestral eukaryotic cells. Mitochondria are able to transform the energy in food into adenosine triphosphate (ATP) through the process of cellular respiration. The mitochondrial genome contains 37 genes, 13 of which code for enzymes that are involved in the reactions of cellular respiration. The remaining 24 produce RNA transcripts that aid in translation (two ribosomal RNAs, and 22 transfer RNAs). Mitochondrial DNA (mtDNA) rarely changes because it does not recombine the way that nuclear DNA does.

mtDNA is passed on only by the mother because none of the mitochondria present in sperm are taken inside the egg during fertilization. All mtDNA originates from the ovum.

Mutation: General Concept of Mutation or Error in DNA Sequence

A mutation is a change in the sequence of DNA. Mutations range from the alteration of a single nucleotide to entire segments of chromosomes. Mutations are not always deleterious; they are sometimes neutral or even advantageous. In fact, mutations are the source of new alleles and therefore are the mechanism for genetic diversity and evolutionary change.

Some mutations are inherited, meaning that they are passed on from a parent in either the sperm or egg. As such, every cell in the body will have this mutation. Others are somatic, or acquired after fertilization. These types of mutations are usually the result of errors in DNA replication.

Environmental factors such as exposure to radiation or tobacco can also cause somatic mutations. Not all cells in the body will harbor these mutations.

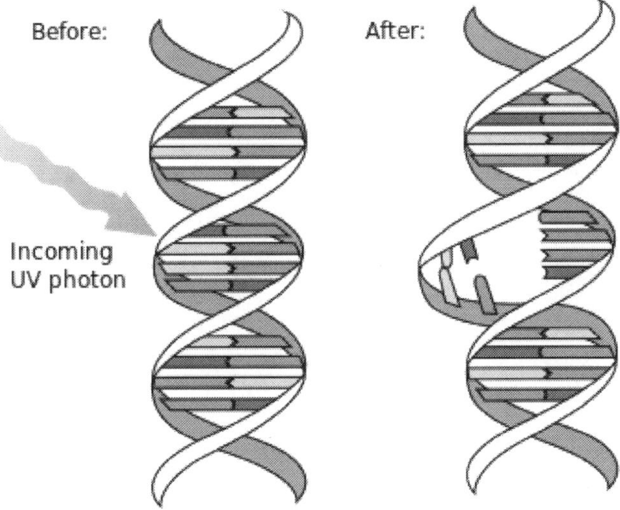

MUTATION: TYPES OF MUTATIONS

Mutations are permanent changes in the genetic sequence of an organism. These changes can be harmful, neutral, or beneficial and are the source of new alleles in a population. Evidence shows that mutations are random, not directed. A mutation does not occur as a way to help an organism survive; it is not a response to an environmental pressure. This is not to say that the rates of mutation are unaffected by the environment. For example, exposure to toxic chemicals could mutate the DNA of exposed individuals but not in a directed way that would allow the mutants to survive in that environment. More likely some individuals harbored a mutation *before* exposure that, by chance, helped them survive. The mutation might have been inherited or arisen as a result of previous environmental factors or errors in DNA replication. Most of these replication errors (such as the mispairing of DNA nucleotides) are repaired by proofreading enzymes, but some are missed.

It is possible that a random mutation may provide a selective advantage and become a "favorable" allele, but harmful effects are more likely than advantageous. It is most probable that random mutations will be neutral and have no significant effect on the organism at all.

Protein synthesis begins with the transcription of a gene sequence into a molecule of messenger RNA (mRNA). An enzyme called RNA polymerase uses complementary base pairing (A-U and G-C) to synthesize a strand of mRNA. Even if the DNA template has the correct sequence, it is possible for the RNA transcript to contain errors. The wrong nucleotide could be added, or transcription could terminate prematurely. There could also be an error in exon splicing; a process in which the introns (non-coding regions) of pre-mRNA are cut out and exons (coding regions) ligated together. A faulty RNA transcript can sometimes be repaired, but it can also be targeted by surveillance mechanisms and destroyed to avoid translation into a faulty protein.

Errors can also occur during translation: the process by which amino acids are linked together using the code carried by mRNA. Amino acids may be misincorporated, which will affect the folding of the protein into its native shape.

Mispairing refers to an error of DNA replication in which the wrong nucleotide is added to the template strand. Adenine should bond with thymine and guanine with cytosine. If the wrong nucleotide is added and not repaired, it is referred to as a base substitution. Whereas this mutation will only affect a single mRNA codon, it can have serious, even lethal, consequences depending on its location in the genome.

A *missense* mutation occurs when a base substitution alters one amino acid in the protein, while the rest are unaffected. If the new amino acid has properties similar to the intended amino acid, the effect may be minimal. A more serious consequence can be seen in sickle cell anemia. The DNA triplet GAG is changed to GTG, and the amino acid valine is added to the polypeptide chain instead of glutamic acid. This causes the protein hemoglobin to fold into the wrong shape.

If the sequence of DNA changes such that a codon that originally specified an amino acid is changed to a stop codon, the polypeptide will be cut short. This is called a *nonsense* mutation.

A *silent* mutation occurs if the base substitution causes a change in the codon but not the amino acid. For example, if GCC is mutated to GCT, there will be no change in the amino acid sequence because both DNA triplets produce an RNA codon that specifies arginine.

Point mutations

	No mutation	Silent	Nonsense	Missense: conservative	Missense: non-conservative
DNA level	TTC	TTT	ATC	TCC	TGC
mRNA level	AAG	AAA	UAG	AGG	ACG
protein level	Lys	Lys	STOP	Arg	Thr

basic
polar

An inversion is a chromosomal mutation in which a chromosome breaks in two places, and the free segment flips in reverse orientation and reattaches. If the broken piece originates from only one arm of the chromosome, it is called a *paracentric* inversion. If both arms break and the centromere is included in the free portion, then it is a *pericentric* inversion. Because there is rarely a loss or addition of DNA, these mutations are often harmless unless a vital gene is interrupted by the break.

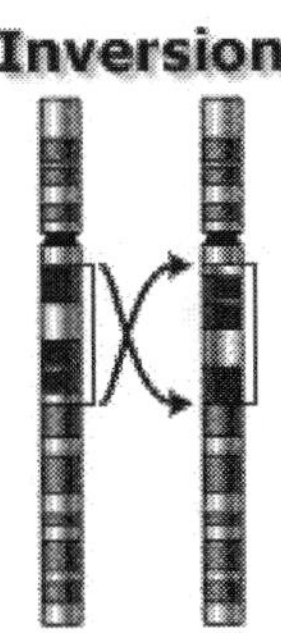

Translocations occur when a segment of a chromosome breaks free and attaches to a nonhomologous chromosome. Like inversions, this type of mutation is likely to be "balanced" because DNA is rarely deleted or added to the genome.

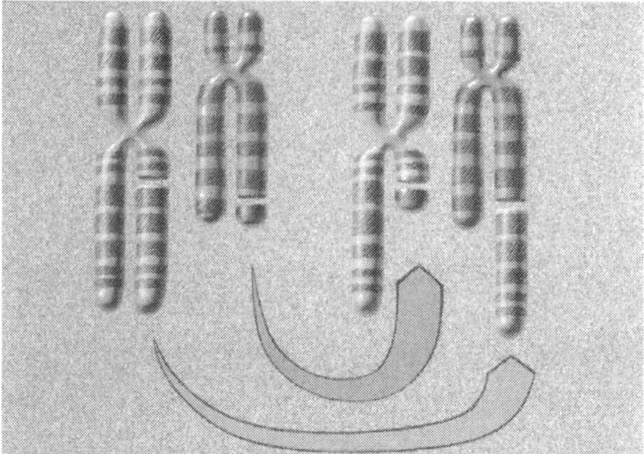

An insertion is a type of mutation in which one or more nucleotides are added to a sequence of DNA. Sometimes the inserted DNA consists of a series of repeated triplets. For example, Huntington's disease is caused by too many repeated CAG sequences in the gene that produces the Huntingtin protein. This is called trinucleotide repeat expansion.

A deletion is a mutation in which one or more nucleotides are removed from a genetic sequence. An inserted or deleted sequence that is not in a multiple of three nucleotides will cause a *frameshift mutation*: the shifting of a genetic sequence such that the codons are changed from that point on. An analogy can be made by deleting a letter from the sentence, "THE BIG BAT HAS RED FUR." Deletion of the letter "I" would change the sentence to "THE BGB ATH ASR EDF UR."

The earlier in the sequence that the insertion or deletion (indel) mutation occurs, the greater the effects on the protein. Short sequence insertions or deletions are usually caused by strand slippage during DNA replication. Insertion or deletion of longer sequences is more likely the result of an error of crossing-over during meiosis.

Mutation: Advantageous Versus Deleterious Mutation

Mutations are the driving force behind evolution because they are the original source of variation within a population. An advantageous mutation produces an allele that is favored by natural selection, and the individuals that inherit this allele will have greater fitness. The mutation that gave rise to lactose tolerance in some adults is an example of an advantageous mutation. It is more common for a mutation to be harmful than beneficial. Deleterious mutations cause a decrease in fitness and in extreme cases are responsible for fatal diseases such as Tay Sachs and cystic fibrosis. In most cases mutations are neutral and have no measurable effect on the individual.

There are factors that can influence the effects of a mutation; notably, environment. A mutation that is deleterious in one environment may be neutral or even advantageous in another. A mutation that produces short wings in a fruit fly, for example, may be harmful in most environments but helpful in geographical regions that experience high winds.

Mutation: Inborn Errors of Metabolism

Inborn errors of metabolism (IEMs) belong to a class of genetic diseases in which a protein (usually an enzyme) involved in a metabolic pathway is faulty. These diseases are congenital and result from the inheritance of a defective gene that would normally play a role in the conversion of nutrients to products. If the metabolic pathway becomes blocked, materials will accumulate in the body that either interfere with normal function or are themselves toxic. An example of an IEM is phenylketonuria (PKU): a disease in which the enzyme phenylalanine hydroxylase is not able to fully metabolize the amino acid phenylalanine. Newborns are commonly screened for this disease because the effects can be minimized by eliminating phenylalanine from the diet. The severity of IEMs depends on many factors. Sometimes other functional enzymes or cofactors can help compensate for the defective enzyme. Environment can play a role in the onset and severity of symptoms. Also, the earlier the position of the enzyme on the metabolic pathway, the more likely it is that the disease will be severe.

Mutation: Relationship of Mutagens to Carcinogens

A mutagen is a substance or agent that permanently changes a genetic sequence. (Natural errors in replication or recombination are not caused by mutagens.) Radiation (depending on the type) can either directly break the bonds in DNA or cause a change in the cell that leads to a change in the genetic code. Similarly, chemicals can mutate DNA either indirectly by interfering with the cell's metabolic activities or directly. Viruses can also act as mutagens if their DNA is incorporated into a host cell.

Not all mutagens are carcinogens (cancer-causing agents), but many are. (Sodium azide is an example of a toxic mutagen that is not linked to cancer.) There are also carcinogens that increase rates of mitosis without causing mutations. Exposure to a carcinogen increases the risk of cancer, but development of the disease depends on the time, duration, and level of exposure as well as other environmental and genetic factors.

Genetic Drift

Genetic drift is an unpredictable shift in allele frequency as a result of chance, not selection. It is independent of the effects of advantageous or harmful alleles. Instead the shift happens as a result of the random "sampling" of alleles that are passed on to the next generation. Consider a population in which 40 percent of the members reproduce. Unless that sample shares the exact same allele frequency as the entire population, the allele frequency of the next generation will change.

The smaller the population, the more likely genetic drift will happen because smaller populations are more likely to be influenced by chance events. To illustrate, imagine a population of ten individuals with only two that carry a given allele. It is possible that for reasons unrelated to the effects of that allele, those two individuals will not reproduce. The allele would be eliminated, and the more common variant would reach fixation (100 percent frequency.) Now imagine a similar population with 10,000 members, 2,000 of which carry the allele. It is unlikely that *none* of those

2,000 will reproduce. A random sample of a large population will better represent the allele frequencies of the whole population.

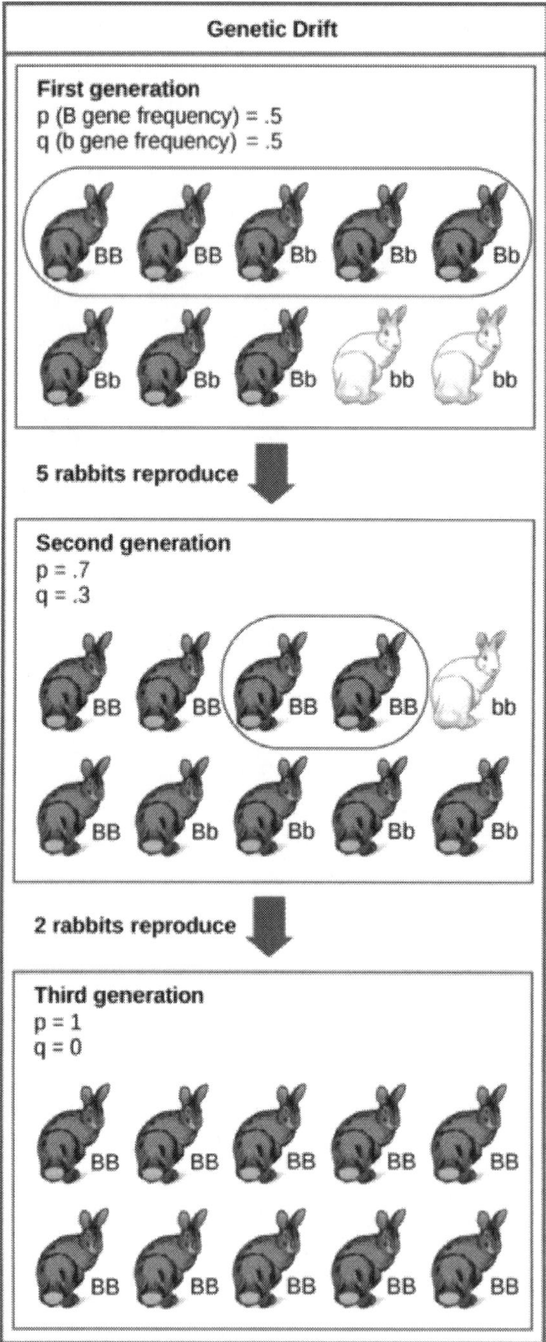

SYNAPSIS OR CROSSING-OVER MECHANISM FOR INCREASING GENETIC DIVERSITY

Synapsis and crossing-over are processes that take place during prophase I of meiosis. Without these events, genetic diversity would be greatly reduced. Synapsis is the pairing of homologous chromosomes to form a tetrad. One chromosome consists entirely of maternal DNA, and the other consists entirely of paternal DNA. The sister chromatids on each chromosome are identical to each other. During synapsis, the homologs are arranged by the synaptonemal complex so that the loci on the maternal chromosome are perfectly aligned with the same loci on the paternal chromosome.

The homologs join at regions called chiasmata, and segments of each homolog are switched. As a result, the chromosomes that are distributed to each gamete will no longer be completely maternal or paternal; they will have unique combinations of alleles. If synapsis were to occur without crossing-over, the gametes would still be genetically different due to independent assortment but to a much lesser degree.

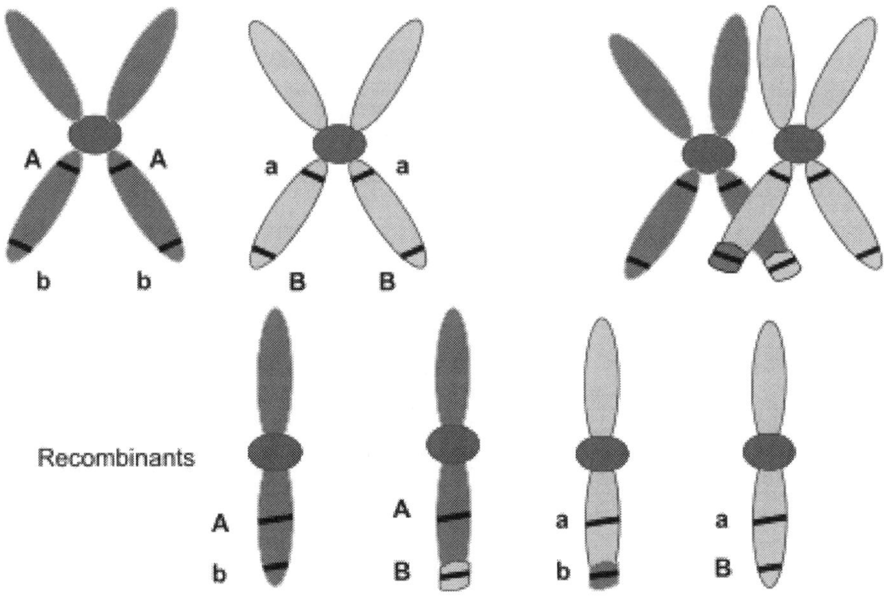

Analytic Methods

Hardy–Weinberg Principle

The Hardy-Weinberg Principle states that allele and genotype frequencies remain constant from generation to generation, assuming the population is not evolving. Only if the conditions below are met can a population remain in equilibrium:

- The population must be very large (preferably infinite) to eliminate genetic drift.
- There must be no selection; all alleles are "equal" in terms of favorability.
- Mating is random.
- There is no flow of genes between other populations, that is, no immigration or emigration.
- There are no mutations; new alleles are not created

It is nearly impossible for a real population to be in this state of equilibrium, but the model does allow predictions to be made using the Hardy-Weinberg equation:

$$p^2 + 2pq + q^2 = 1$$

p = dominant allele

q = recessive allele

Derivation of equation $(p + q) = 1$ (always):

To predict *genotype* frequency (and not individual alleles), then $(p + q) = 1$ is squared to give:

$$p^2 + 2pq + q^2 = 1$$

p^2 = the frequency of individuals with the homozygous dominant genotype

$2pq$ = the frequency of individuals with the heterozygous genotype

q^2 = the frequency of individuals with the homozygous recessive genotype

(Note that the same method can be used to derive an equation when multiple alleles exist. Three alleles would begin with the equation $p + q + r = 1$.)

This equation can be used to predict genotypic frequencies of a population that is not evolving.

Testcross (Backcross; Concepts of Parental, F1, and F2 Generations)

First, some terminology is necessary:

- The parental generation (P) is the "starting" generation—the first parents.
- The first filial generation (F1) is the offspring of the P generation.
- The second filial generation (F2) is the offspring of the F1 generation.

A backcross is the mating of a heterozygous F1 individual with one of its parents (or an individual with the same genotype as one of the parents) as a way to create offspring with a genotype that resembles the chosen parent. The F1 hybrid is also called a BC1 hybrid (BC = back cross), and the F2 individuals (the offspring of the F1 hybrid and a chosen parent) are referred to as the BC2 generation.

A testcross is used to determine the unknown genotype of an individual with a dominant phenotype by mating them with a homozygous recessive individual. By examining the phenotypes of the offspring, it is possible to identify the unknown genotype of the parent. If roughly 50 percent of the offspring display the recessive phenotype, then the parent must be a carrier of the recessive allele (it is heterozygous). If 100 percent of the offspring show the dominant phenotype, then it can be assumed* that the parent was homozygous dominant.

*The offspring generation would need to be somewhat large to increase the certainty because there is a 50-50 chance of a heterozygote passing on the dominant allele.

Gene Mapping: Crossover Frequencies

Gene mapping is a process that identifies the order and relative distances between genes. One approach used in gene mapping involves the use of recombination frequencies. Data that is collected by examining pedigrees and/or conducting test crosses can be used to calculate these frequencies and generate a linkage map. The distance between genes on a chromosome is proportional to the probability that they will be separated during crossing-over. The maximum recombination frequency involving two genes on the same chromosome is 50 percent. Genes that are this far apart are as "unlinked" as genes on separate chromosomes. As the distance between genes decreases, so does the likelihood of crossing-over, and the recombination frequency will approach 0 percent. Using these frequencies, the "neighborhood" of a gene can be found. The exact distances between genes cannot be calculated this way, but the relative distances can. Analysis of the data can also determine the order of the genes on the chromosome. Other methods such as DNA sequencing must be used to pinpoint the precise locus of a gene.

Biometry: Statistical Methods

Biometry is the application of statistics and mathematics to solve problems and make predictions relating to biological phenomena. Fields that use biometry include agriculture, medicine, ecology, genetics, and any area of science that has a biological component. Biometry is useful in predicting appropriate sample sizes, examining correlation relationships, calculating population standard deviation, estimating gene location, and so on. One of the most indispensable tools is the chi-square test: a nonparametric test that determines whether an observed distribution is due to chance. It is sometimes called the "goodness-of-fit test." A low chi-square test value indicates the distribution is not caused by chance and that the observed values closely match the expected values. A high value indicates that the observed results are due to chance. This test is often used to compare the genotypic frequencies predicted by the Hardy-Weinberg equation with the observed frequencies.

Evolution

Natural Selection

Natural selection is the process by which individuals that are better suited to their environment survive and reproduce. It is often described as "survival of the fittest," but this description leaves out a key component: reproduction. Differential reproductive success is a driving force behind evolution, that is, a change in allele frequencies in a population over time. However, it is important to note that it is *phenotypes*, not genotypes, that are selected. For example, deer that carry the allele for albinism have the same phenotype as those that are homozygous dominant. Because both genotypes produce the same phenotype, one will not be selected over the other. But the dominant allele (which is the basis for phenotype) may increase in frequency if brown deer survive and reproduce at greater rates than white deer.

There are certain conditions that must be met for natural selection to occur: heritable variation within the population, reproduction within the population, and changing environmental conditions that lead to pressure.

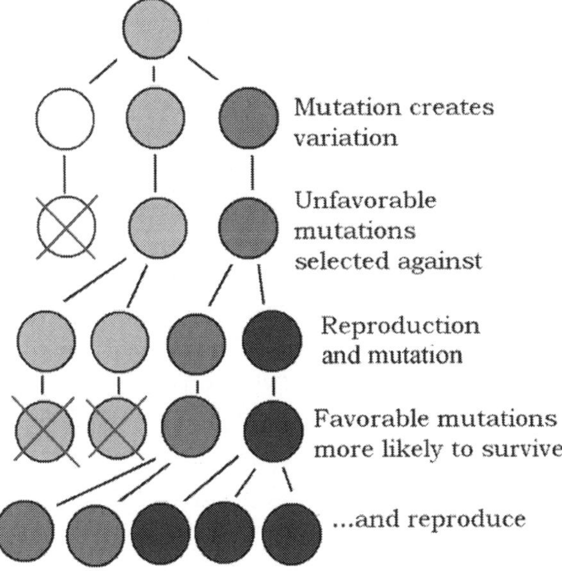

Fitness Concept

Fitness is a measure of reproductive success. The term is commonly associated with strength, agility, and speed, but *any* heritable trait that increases reproductive success will contribute to fitness. In a hot climate rabbits with oversized ears climate may be more "fit" than those with smaller ears because they can release excess heat more readily, which in turn may allow them to survive and reproduce at greater rates. Even if the long-eared rabbits have shorter life spans, they are still more fit; it is reproductive success alone that determines fitness.

There are two ways of measuring fitness. "Absolute fitness" compares the genotypic ratio before and after selection. However, "relative fitness" is more valuable when looking at natural selection because it measures the *competitive* ability of an allele. In other words, it measures the allele contribution to the next generation *relative* to others. Two forms of a gene may (in an absolute sense) both be favorable, but if one appears in greater frequency in the next generation, then it is the "fitter" of the two. At the level of the organism, an individual that produces more offspring with the favorable inherited trait is more fit than an individual that produces less.

Selection by Differential Reproduction

Differential reproduction describes the varying degrees of reproductive success that are found in a population. Individuals with a favorable phenotype have a selective advantage; they are more likely to survive and reproduce than individuals who don't share the phenotype. This is called differential reproduction. The more "fit" individuals will produce the most offspring and (assuming the trait is heritable) transmit the alleles that contribute to the desirable phenotype. The traits that are selected by the environment will spread throughout the population, and over time that population will evolve to resemble the members with the greatest reproductive success.

Concepts of Natural and Group Selection

Natural selection is normally described as acting at the level of the individual; the classic description is often as follows: "individuals with favorable traits are more likely to survive and reproduce." But it is believed by many that selection can happen at the group level as well. Whereas some argue that individuals act for self-preservation alone, others claim that altruistic behaviors may increase the reproductive success of a group, thereby favoring the fitness of the group over the individual. For example, an individual behaves altruistically when defending the group against a predator. Such action puts the individual at risk but protects the group. Other types of behaviors that may lead to group selection include maternal instincts, cooperative hunting, and predatory alert systems.

Evolutionary Success as Increase in Percent Representation in the Gene Pool of the Next Generation

Evolutionary success is measured by the change in the frequency of an allele in a gene pool. If an allele's frequency in the population increases, then evolutionary success has been achieved. As alleles responsible for beneficial traits spread throughout the population, they may become fixed and lead to adaptation. Natural selection is the nonrandom mechanism by which these allele frequencies change. Members of a population that express a favorable phenotype will be more likely to survive to sexual maturity and pass their genes on to the next generation.

Speciation

A species is a group of genetically similar individuals that are able to breed naturally and produce viable and fertile offspring. Speciation is the formation of a new species, and this process occurs through various pathways. Anagenesis is the process by which a species changes as a single group until it is too genetically different from the original species to be considered the same. The new species completely "replaces" the original.

The more common mechanism for speciation is called cladogenesis: the process by which one species diverges into two. Cladogenesis occurs as a result of reproductive isolation. In *allopatric speciation*, the reproductive barrier is a physical separation of a population (geographic isolation). Selection and genetic drift act differently on each subpopulation, and they diverge.

If the population is not geographically isolated, but a subset of the population occupies a new niche, a new species may form in a process called *parapatric speciation*. Rarely a new species may arise from a group that occupies the same niche. This is called *sympatric speciation* and is the result of mutations that stop certain members of the population from breeding.

POLYMORPHISM

Polymorphism describes the existence of two or more alleles at the same locus within a population. Polymorphisms are distinguished from mutations because they are considered "normal" variants and are inherited (they do not arise spontaneously). Their origins, however, can be traced back to a mutation. They are not responsible for traits that have a continuous spectrum of phenotypes, such as height or hair color. Human blood groups are an example of polymorphism because the trait is controlled by a single gene with A, B, and O alleles. If the sequence of DNA at the given locus varies by only one nucleotide, then it is called a single nucleotide polymorphism (SNP). Other polymorphisms arise from deletions, insertions, duplications, and tandem repeats.

ADAPTATION AND SPECIALIZATION

Adaptation is the dynamic process by which a population changes due to natural selection. It can also refer to the result of that process, that is, the inherited feature that increases reproductive success. Adaptations are not always structural traits. Certain behaviors and abilities can be adaptations as long as they are heritable and increase fitness. They also must have arisen by natural selection for the purpose that they currently serve. Feathers, for instance, are not adaptations for flight because their original function was not flight related. Adaptations are also not the result of genetic drift (chance), even if the trait eventually proves advantageous.

Specialization is the use of an adaptation to better fill a specific niche. For example, the different species of finches that inhabit the Galapagos Islands each have a beak shape that is suited to the food sources unique to each island. But the adaptation of a nonvenomous king snake to resemble the venomous coral snake is not an example of specialization because it does not help it better fill a niche.

INBREEDING AND OUTBREEDING

Inbreeding is the mating of relatives, whereas outbreeding is the mating of nonrelatives within a species. Closely related individuals collectively have more similar genetic sequences than members who are less related. Inbreeding will produce a higher proportion of homozygous genotypes than outbreeding because there are comparatively more "like" alleles in a closely related group. Because heterozygosity is reduced, genetic diversity becomes limited. Inbred populations are more likely to express recessive disorders because relatives have a greater chance of being carriers of the same deleterious allele than a group with a robust gene pool. Outbreeding has the opposite effect of inbreeding; heterozygosity increases.

BOTTLENECKS

The bottleneck effect describes a drastic reduction in population size as a result of an environmental event such as a natural disaster, habitat destruction, or overhunting. The remaining population is unlikely to have the same proportion and variety of alleles as the original population. The population may rebound, but its gene pool will be more limited than it was. It is important to note the distinction between bottlenecking and natural selection. The survivors of a bottleneck event survived by chance, not their genetic makeup. As such, there is no improved "fitness," and the new population is unlikely to be better suited to its environment. The random change in allele frequency is known as genetic drift, and bottleneck events increase the effect of this phenomenon.

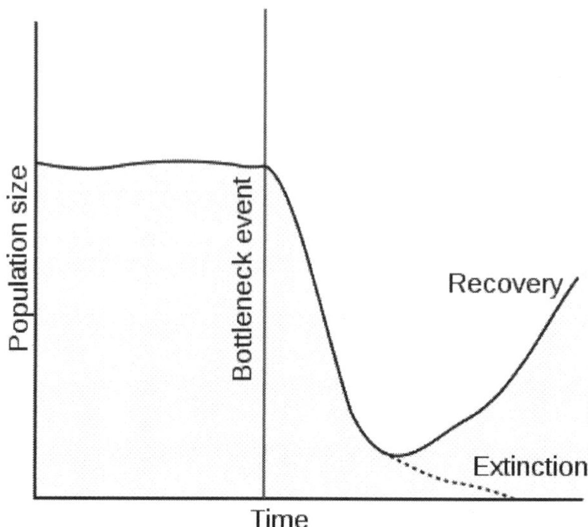

Evolutionary Time as Measured by Gradual Random Changes in Genome

Random mutations that are neutral (not selected by the environment) can be used as "molecular clocks" to estimate when two species diverged. DNA sequences (unless acted on by natural selection) change at a rate that is relatively constant, and therefore the number of base changes is proportional to the amount of time that has passed since a species diverged from the common ancestor.

In reality the rate of mutation is not constant. Different sections of a genome may change at different rates, or natural selection may favor one mutation over another. Nevertheless, the effects can be averaged out to approximate elapsed time. First, the molecular clock is "calibrated" by using an absolute time (as known by a historical event or fossil record) and the mutation rate of a particular gene. Once the number of mutations is graphed as a function of time, the information can be used to give estimated dates of events outside of what is directly measured.

Principles of Bioenergetics and Fuel Molecule Metabolism

Principles of Bioenergetics

Bioenergetics/Thermodynamics

Bioenergetics is the study of energy flow through biological systems. The first law of thermodynamics is a restatement of the law of conservation of energy. According to the law of conservation of energy, the total amount of energy in an isolated system remains constant. When applied to thermodynamics, the change in the internal energy of a system is equal to the amount of heat supplied to the system minus the work done by the system on the surroundings. Organisms are open systems because they are always exchanging both matter and energy with their surroundings; they are never at equilibrium. They take free energy from the surroundings either through sunlight or nutrients, and do work on the surroundings by moving, breathing, etc. Any energy that is taken in is returned to the surroundings as heat, resulting in an increase in entropy/disorder of the surroundings.

Free Energy/Keq: Equilibrium Constant

Equilibrium describes a state of maximum stability where the rate of the forward reaction is equal to the rate of the reverse reaction. This does not mean that the concentrations of products and reactants are equal; rather there is no net change in the concentrations of the reactants or products. The equilibrium constant can predict whether the products or the reactants will be in higher concentration at equilibrium, and which direction of the reaction is favored. In other words, it relates the concentration of products to reactants.

The following equation can be used to calculate the equilibrium constant:

$$K_{eq} = \frac{[\mathrm{C}]^c[\mathrm{D}]^d}{[\mathrm{A}]^a[\mathrm{B}]^b}$$

- **C** and **D** are equilibrium product concentrations
- **A** and **B** are equilibrium reactant concentrations
- **a**, **b**, **c** and **d** are stoichiometric constants (the numbers in front of each reactant and product in the chemical equation)

When $K_{eq} = 1$, the reactants and products are equal in concentration. When $K_{eq} > 1$, the concentration of products exceeds that of the reactants, and when $K_{eq} < 1$ the concentration of products is less than that of the reactants.

Free Energy/Keq: Relationship of the Equilibrium Constant and ΔG°

Free energy, often called Gibbs free energy (G), is the energy available to do work at a constant temperature and pressure. The notation G^0 indicates "standard" free energy, or the free energy at standard state conditions. The relationship between K_{eq} and standard Gibbs free energy is as follows:

$$\Delta G^0 = -RT\ln(K_{eq})$$

- G^0 = standard free energy
- R = gas constant
- T = absolute temperature in Kelvins
- $\ln(K_{eq})$ = natural log of the equilibrium constant

When $K_{eq} = 1$, then ΔG is zero and reactants and products are favored equally. When $K_{eq} > 1$, then ΔG is negative and products are favored. When $K_{eq} < 1$, then ΔG is positive and the reactants are favored at equilibrium.

Concentration

Increasing the concentration of reactants will lead to more collisions per unit time between those reactants, and therefore the rate of the forward reaction increases as concentration increases. When there is a high concentration of reactants, the free energy of the reactants is greater than that of the products. As the concentration of the products increases, the rate of the reverse reaction increases. When the concentrations of the reactants and products become stable (not necessarily equal), the rate of the forward and reverse reactions are the same, and the reaction is at equilibrium.

CONCENTRATION: LE CHÂTELIER'S PRINCIPLE

According to **Le Châtelier's Principle**, when the equilibrium of a system is disrupted, the system will shift to restore equilibrium. For this reason, it is sometimes referred to as the equilibrium law. Factors that can disrupt equilibrium include changes in concentration, volume and pressure, and temperature. Le Châtelier's Principle can be observed in biological systems, for example the metabolism of glucose. When glucose levels rise, insulin will facilitate the uptake of glucose into the cells, and stimulate glycolysis.

Variable	Change	System's response to restore equilibrium
Concentration	Reactants or products are added	The added reactants / products are consumed
	Reactants or products are removed	More reactants / products are produced to replace those that were removed
Volume	Increase (with decrease in pressure)	Shifts to the side with more moles of gas
	Decrease (with increase in pressure)	Shifts to the side with fewer moles of gas
Temperature	Increase	Endothermic reaction is favored
	Decrease	Exothermic reaction is favored

ENDOTHERMIC/EXOTHERMIC REACTIONS

An **endothermic reaction** is a reaction that absorbs heat from the surroundings, meaning the heat content of the products is greater than the reactants. An **exothermic reaction** releases heat into the surroundings; the heat content of the products is less than the reactants. These reactions cause a change in **enthalpy**, a measure of the heat content of a thermodynamic system. The change in enthalpy (ΔH) is negative for an exothermic reaction and positive for an endothermic reaction. Endothermic reactions will often cause the surroundings to decrease in temperature, as they require the addition of energy to proceed. These reactions are usually non-spontaneous. On the other hand, exothermic reactions will increase the temperature of the surroundings, and are usually spontaneous. Photosynthesis is an example of a biological endothermic process; the energy from the sun is used to build carbon dioxide into molecules of glucose. The glucose can then be oxidized during cellular respiration to produce ATP and heat. Cellular respiration is an example of an exothermic process because the bonds in glucose hold more energy than those of the products.

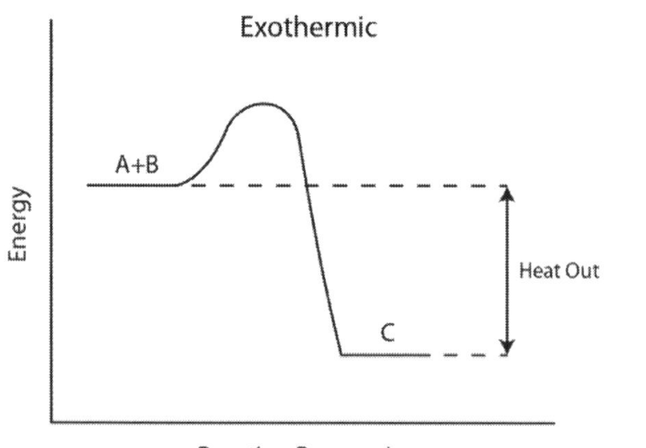

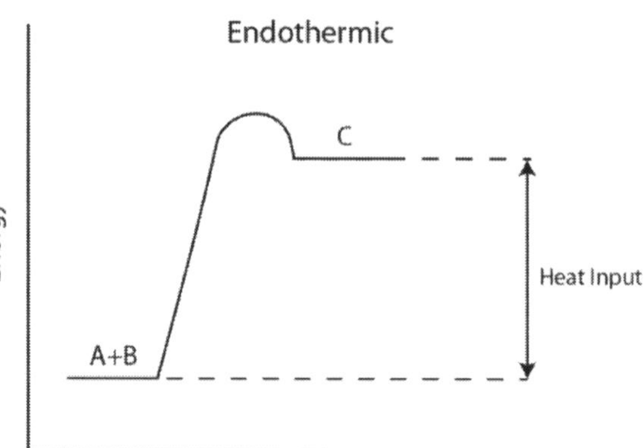

Free Energy: G

Free energy is a measure of the energy within a system that is available to do work. The change in Gibbs free energy (ΔG) is the usable energy that is either absorbed or released during the reaction. ΔG can be calculated using the following equation:

$$\Delta G = \Delta H - T\Delta S$$

- ΔG = change in Gibbs free energy; SI units: Joules
- ΔH = change in enthalpy
  - Enthalpy is the total heat content of a system, and the *change* in enthalpy measures the difference between the energy stored in the bonds of the reactants and the products, assuming a constant pressure. If ΔH is positive, heat is absorbed, and if ΔH is negative, heat was released.
- T = absolute temperature
  - Always positive (because it is expressed in units of Kelvins)
- ΔS = change in entropy
  - Entropy is a measure of the disorder of a system. A positive change in entropy means that the system is more disordered. If ΔS is negative, the system becomes more ordered.

Spontaneous Reactions and $\Delta G°$

When ΔG^0, or the change in free energy at standard conditions (1.0 atm, 298 Kelvin), is negative, the reaction will be exergonic and favor the formation of products. These reactions are always spontaneous. It is important to note that spontaneous reactions do not always happen quickly; it simply means that the change in free energy is negative.

When ΔG^0 is positive, the reaction will be non-spontaneous and endergonic, and favor the reactants. While all non-spontaneous reactions are endergonic, they are not always endothermic. When the entropy increases by more than ΔH, the reaction will be non-spontaneous and exothermic.

When ΔG^0 is zero, the reaction is in equilibrium; neither the reactants nor products are favored.

Phosphoryl Group Transfers and ATP

ATP, or **adenosine triphosphate**, is an adenine-containing RNA nucleotide. Adenine (the nitrogenous base) is covalently bonded to the sugar ribose, which has a chain of three phosphate groups that stems from its 5' carbon. The closest phosphate group is termed "alpha," followed by "beta," and terminating with "gamma," and they are all linked by phosphoanhydride bonds. Because these groups are negatively charged, they repel each another. ATP is sometimes called "energy currency" because it drives most of the reactions in a cell, often by transferring of one of its phosphate groups to another molecule. When a molecule is phosphorylated, its function will change; it may be activated or deactivated as a result of a change in conformation.

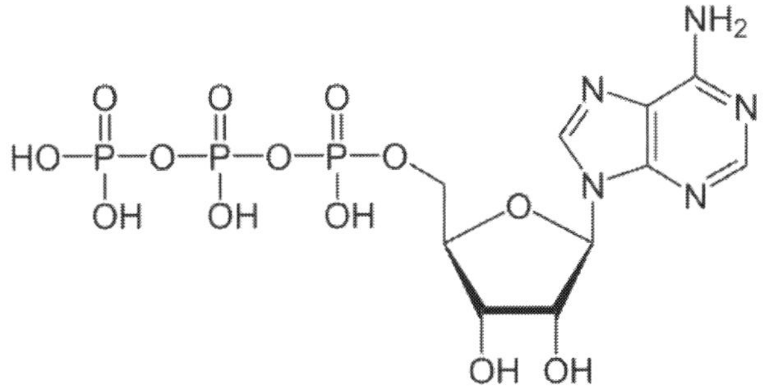

ATP Hydrolysis ΔG << 0

ATP is hydrolyzed to produce adenosine diphosphate (ADP) and an inorganic phosphate group in the following reaction:

$ATP + H_2O \rightarrow ADP + P_i$

Less commonly, two phosphate groups are removed to produce adenosine monophosphate (AMP). The free energy released by the hydrolysis of ATP is used to drive cellular work. The phosphoanhydride bonds between the phosphate groups are often described as "high energy bonds" but it is the difference in free energy between the products and the reactants that explains the output of energy, not the breaking of the bond itself.

The Gibbs free energy change (ΔG) associated with the hydrolysis of ATP (which is highly exergonic) is dependent on the surrounding conditions. Under standard conditions, it is −30.5 kJ/mol (or −7.3 kcal /mol). But under typical cellular conditions, the concentration of ATP is far below the standard 1.0 M. Also, Mg^{2+} ions in the cytosol bind to ATP and stabilize it. For this reason, ΔG can be much greater than the value at standard conditions, even double or more.

ATP Group Transfers

The hydrolysis of ATP without a coupled reaction and/or group transfer is unlikely, because it would result in simply the release of heat. Usually, the hydrolysis of ATP is coupled with a less energetically favorable reaction to help drive cellular work. ATP participates in the reaction that it is driving, usually by the covalent binding of one or more of its phosphate groups to an intermediate molecule, which is then used in the next reaction. Sometimes, part of an ATP molecule will bind to another molecule in order to change its conformation and function. The sodium potassium pump, for example, is only able to shuttle sodium ions out of the cell when a phosphate group binds to it. AMP (the molecule that remains after the removal of two phosphates from ATP, or one phosphate from ADP) can also bind to a protein to change its function.

Biological Oxidation-Reduction

Reactions that involve the transfer of electrons are called **oxidation-reduction reactions**, or **redox reactions**. Oxidation is the process of losing electrons, and reduction is the process of gaining electrons. One reaction must be accompanied by the other; they cannot occur independently. The electron acceptor, or **oxidizing agent**, is reduced by the electron donor, or **reducing agent**. Biological redox reactions are essential to all living organisms. Both photosynthesis and cellular respiration are driven by these reactions. During photosynthesis (a non-spontaneous endergonic process), electrons are transferred from water (which is oxidized) to carbon dioxide (which is reduced). During cellular respiration (a spontaneous exergonic process), glucose is oxidized, and oxygen is reduced. In both these processes, electrons are not moved directly from the starting reactants to the end products. They are transferred along intermediates via a series of enzyme-catalyzed reactions.

Reduction

$\text{Oxidant} + e^- \xrightarrow{\quad} \text{Product}$

(Electrons **gained**; oxidation number **decreases**)

Oxidation

$\text{Reductant} \xrightarrow{\quad} \text{Product} + e^-$

(Electrons **lost**; oxidation number **increases**)

Half-Reactions

In a redox reaction, one agent is oxidized while another is reduced. A **half reaction** is only one part of a redox reaction; it is either the oxidation component (in which the agent accepts electrons) or the reduction component (in which the agent loses elections). These are called half reactions because they are always coupled together. Separating these redox reactions into their half components allows one to determine how many electrons are being transferred. Electrons should be balanced on either side, and will cancel out to give the complete redox reaction.

Generalized format:

Complete redox reaction	$X + Y \rightarrow X^+ + Y^-$
Half reaction (X is oxidized)	$X \rightarrow X^+ + e^-$
Half reaction (Y is reduced)	$Y + e^- \rightarrow Y^-$

Specific example:

Complete reaction	Acetaldehyde + NADH + $H^+ \rightarrow$ Ethanol + NAD^+
Half reaction (acetaldehyde is reduced)	Acetaldehyde + 2 H^+ + $2e^- \rightarrow$ Ethanol
Half reaction (NADH is oxidized)	NADH $\rightarrow NAD^+ + H^+ + 2e^-$

Soluble Electron Carriers

There are many molecules that function as electron carriers in the cell; some are water-soluble and some are lipid-soluble. The list below describes some of the common electron carriers that participate in metabolic pathways.

Nicotinamide adenine dinucleotide (**NAD**): accepts two electrons and a proton during glycolysis and the citric acid cycle, and donates them to establish the proton motive force that leads to the production of ATP during oxidative phosphorylation. **NADP** is a similar molecule that is used in the pathways of photosynthesis.

Flavin adenine dinucleotide (**FAD**): accepts one or two electrons and two protons. It accepts electrons during the citric acid cycle, and donates them to oxidative phosphorylation.

Ubiquinone (also called coenzyme Q): lipid soluble, accepts one or two electrons, and helps to move electrons across phospholipid bilayers.

Cytochrome c: a protein with an electron-accepting iron atom inside it called the heme group. It participates in the final stage of cellular respiration. (Cytochrome c is water soluble, but most cytochromes are lipid soluble.)

Flavoproteins

Flavoproteins are proteins that contain a prosthetic group, either flavin adenine dinucleotide (FAD) or less commonly flavin mononucleotide (FMN). FAD and FMN are derived from riboflavin, and are essential to many cellular processes, including cellular respiration, photosynthesis, fatty acid oxidation, and the activation of vitamin B. They can catalyze the transfer of either one or two electrons, and this characteristic allows them to act as cofactors for many types of enzymes. These cofactors are tightly bound, but only rarely by covalent bonds.

Carbohydrates

Description

Carbohydrates are the most abundant class of organic compounds found in nature, and the most accessible source of energy for most organisms. Each gram of carbohydrate releases around 17 kJ, or 4 kcal, of energy. Carbohydrates serve other roles as well, including cell-cell recognition, structural components in cell walls and the exoskeletons of arthropods, and intermediates in metabolic pathways.

All carbohydrates contain predictable ratios of carbon, hydrogen, and oxygen. Nearly all simple sugars have a 1:2:1 ratio of C, H, and O. Each additional sugar that is added will result in the removal of a water molecule via dehydration synthesis reaction. As such, the empirical formula for carbohydrates is $C_n(H_2O)_m$.

Review Video: Carbohydrates
Visit mometrix.com/academy and enter code: 601714

Nomenclature and Classification, Common Names

Carbohydrates can be classified by the number of substituent sugar units, their functional groups, and stereochemistry (L / D, R / S nomenclature).

- **Monosaccharide**: a simple sugar made of one sugar unit. These can be classified further according to the number of carbons.
  - **Triose**: Three carbons (ex: glyceraldehyde)
  - **Tetrose**: Four carbons (ex: erythrulose)
  - **Pentose**: Five carbons (ex: deoxyribose, ribose)
  - **Hexose**: Six carbons (ex: glucose, fructose, galactose)
- **Disaccharide**: a double sugar consisting of two monosaccharides (ex: sucrose, lactose, maltose)
- **Oligosaccharide**: a carbohydrate usually made of three to ten monosaccharides (ex: raffinose)
- **Polysaccharide**: a long chain (sometimes branched) of monosaccharides (ex: glycogen, starch, chitin)
- **Aldose**: contains an aldehyde functional group (ex: glucose, glyceraldehyde)
- **Ketose**: contains a ketone functional group (ex: fructose, dihydroxyacetone)

Absolute Configuration

Absolute configuration refers to the three-dimensional arrangement of the atoms that are bonded to a chiral carbon. A **chiral carbon** is an asymmetrical carbon with four different ligands. There are different ways of designating absolute configuration.

The **L / D designation** compares the configuration of the carbohydrate to glyceraldehyde, and is determined by examining the chiral carbon that is furthest from the carbonyl group. When depicted in a Fischer projection, an L enantiomer will have the OH group (hydroxide) on the left, and a D enantiomer will have the hydroxide pointing to the right. (+) enantiomers rotate plane-polarized light in the clockwise direction, and (−) enantiomers rotate it counterclockwise.

The **R / S designation** examines each ligand on a chiral carbon and assigns it a priority number, based on atomic number (1 = highest atomic number and priority, 4 = least). When the lowest priority substituent points away from the viewer, the remaining ligands will decrease either in the clockwise direction (R) or the counterclockwise direction (S).

Cyclic Structure and Conformations of Hexoses

A monosaccharide with more than four carbons will usually arrange itself into a cyclic conformation in aqueous solution. A five-membered ring is a furanose, and a six-membered ring is a pyranose. An aldose is a monosaccharide that contains an **aldehyde**: a functional group composed of a carbon with a single bond to hydrogen and a double bond to oxygen. A ketose is a sugar that contains a **ketone group**, which has an R group in place of the hydrogen. The carbon of the aldehyde or keto group interacts with a nucleophilic hydroxyl group, and the double bond between carbon and oxygen is eliminated resulting in a more energetically favorable arrangement. Aldose sugars form hemiacetals, and ketose sugars form hemiketals. Fischer projections are commonly used to portray open-chain carbohydrates, but monosaccharides that can form rings are usually translated into Haworth projections and/or chair conformations to give a more realistic depiction of the stereochemistry and structure.

Epimers and Anomers

Epimers are specific types of diastereomers that differ from each other at only one of the chiral carbons. D-glucose and D-mannose are epimers because they share the same chemical formula ($C_6H_{12}O_6$) but differ in the orientation of the OH group on carbon 2.

```
    CHO
     |
  H—C—OH
     |
 HO—C—H
     |
  H—C—OH
     |
  H—C—OH
     |
    CH2OH

 D-Glucose
```

```
    CHO
     |
 HO—C—H
     |
 HO—C—H
     |
  H—C—OH
     |
  H—C—OH
     |
    CH2OH

 D-Mannose
```

Anomers are specific types of epimers. The difference in configuration occurs at the **anomeric carbon**: the carbonyl carbon that rotates to become a chiral center and form a cyclic structure. There are two conformations that can emerge as a result of the rotation: alpha (α) and beta (β). In the α-form, the OH group is on the opposite side of the ring from CH_2OH, and in the β-form, it is on the same side. (See the example below of α-D-glucose and β-D-glucose.)

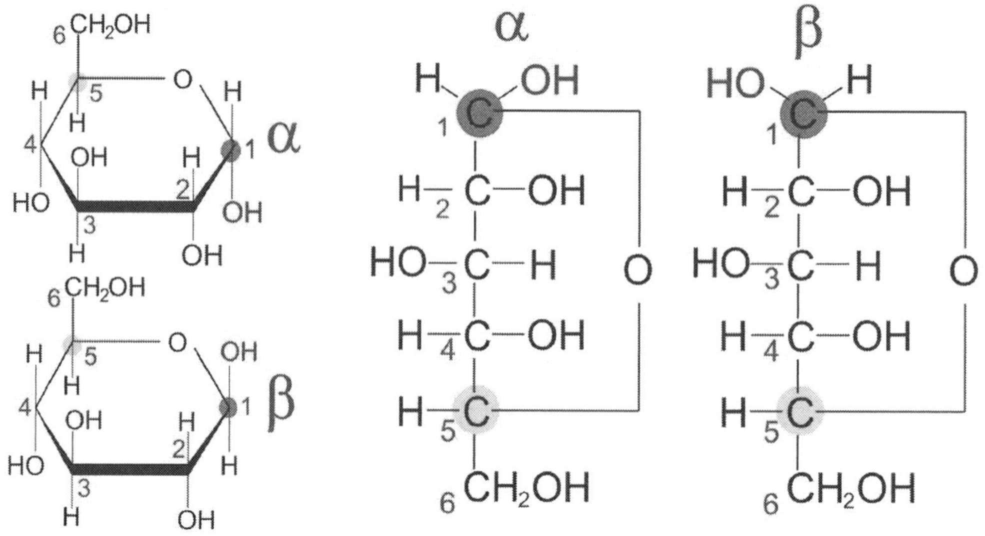

Hydrolysis of the Glycoside Linkage

A **glycosidic linkage** is a covalent bond formed between the anomeric hydroxyl and the hydroxyl group of another compound (often another sugar). These bonds link individual sugar units together to form disaccharides and polysaccharides, and also link a nitrogenous base to the pentose in a nucleotide. When an anomeric center participates in a glycosidic bond, it can no longer revert back and forth between the α and β form as it did when it was free. These bonds are stable, but they can be broken in an acidic aqueous environment. Water is split to give a hydrogen back to one unit and an OH back to the other. Enzymes called **hydrolases** can help to cleave these bonds. They are specific, in that a particular enzyme can only act on α-linkages *or* β linkages. For example, the hydrolase known as α-amylase can break the α(1→4) linkages between glucose subunits of starch, but not the β(1→4) linkages of cellulose. This explains why humans cannot digest cellulose. Other animals rely on microbes to hydrolyze these bonds. Another enzyme called glycosylase assists in the cleavage of the nitrogen base from the sugar in a nucleotide.

Monosaccharides

Monosaccharides are the simplest sugars. They cannot be broken down into smaller carbohydrates, but they can bond together via glycosidic linkage to form larger ones. Nearly all monosaccharides share the same general formula $(CH_2O)_n$, where n is greater than or equal to three. (The notable exception is deoxyribose ($C_5H_{10}O_4$), which lacks an oxygen on the 2' carbon.) Monosaccharides differ in the number of carbons, and how the atoms are arranged. Below are some common monosaccharides.

- Trioses: glyceraldehyde, dihydroxyacetone
- Tetroses: erythrose, erythrulose
- Pentoses: deoxyribose, ribose, arabinose
- Hexoses: glucose, mannose, fructose, galactose
- Heptoses: glucoheptose, mannoheptulose

Monosaccharides can be oxidized to release energy (as seen in the oxidation of glucose during cellular respiration). In fact, all monosaccharides are considered "reducing sugars" because they either have aldehyde groups that are oxidized, or they can tautomerize to form aldehyde groups in solution. Non-reducing sugars lack a hydroxyl group on the anomeric carbon. Reducing sugars can be detected by various reagents. Benedict's solution oxidizes the aldehyde to produce an orange precipitate, Cu_2O. Tollens' reagent contains Ag^+ ions which are reduced by the aldehyde to produce a silver color.

Disaccharides

Disaccharides are composed of two monosaccharides linked by a glycosidic bond. The general formula for a disaccharide is $C_n(H_2O)_m$. While monosaccharides almost always have a 1:2:1 ratio of carbon, hydrogen, and oxygen (respectively), disaccharides are formed via dehydration synthesis, and therefore a water molecule is subtracted from the formula. The formula for nearly all disaccharides is $C_{12}H_{22}O_{11}$.

The glycosidic linkage between monosaccharides can vary, even when both of the sugar subunits are the same. This is because the linkage can stem from any OH group, and be in the α or β form. For example, maltose, cellobiose, and trehalose are each made of two glucoses linked together in different ways to give rise to sugars with different properties. An $\alpha(1 \rightarrow 4)$ linkage produces maltose, $\beta(1 \rightarrow 4)$ produces cellobiose, and $\alpha,\alpha(1 \rightarrow 1)$ produces trehalose.

Some disaccharides, such as maltose, lactose, and cellobiose, are reducing sugars because only one anomeric carbon participates in the glycosidic bond. This allows one of the subunits to take an open chain form and free up an aldehyde, which can then be oxidized. Other disaccharides, such as trehalose and sucrose, are nonreducing sugars because both anomeric carbons are involved in the glycosidic linkage.

Polysaccharides

Polysaccharides are large carbohydrates with at least ten monosaccharides, but they typically contain hundreds to thousands of monosaccharides. Like disaccharides, the sugar subunits are joined by glycosidic bonds, and the general formula for the whole unit is $C_n(H_2O)_m$. The most common polysaccharides include starch, glycogen, cellulose, and chitin, all of which are polymers of glucose. Since they are composed of only one type of monosaccharide, they are all homopolysaccharides. Heteropolysaccharides have more than one type of monosaccharide, and are less common.

Some polysaccharides (ex: starch, glycogen) function as a source of fuel, and others form structural components (ex: cellulose, chitin). Starch is a storage polysaccharide in plants, and is an important part of the human diet. It is made up of two polymers: **amylose** and the branched polymer **amylopectin**. Glycogen is a storage polysaccharide in animals and fungi. Like amylopectin, it a branched polymer of glucose, but the branches are shorter and more frequent. Most of the bonds between the subunits of these storage polysaccharides are $\alpha(1 \rightarrow 4)$, with the exception of branch points which are $\alpha(1 \rightarrow 6)$. Cellulose is a structural polysaccharide found in the cell walls of plants. The glucose monomers are joined by $\beta(1 \rightarrow 4)$ linkages. Chitin is a component in fungal cell walls and the exoskeleton of arthropods. It is structurally similar to cellulose, but each glucose has a nitrogen-containing appendage.

Glycolysis, Gluconeogenesis, and the Pentose Phosphate Pathway

Glycolysis (Aerobic), Substrates and Products

Glycolysis is a process that metabolizes glucose to produce pyruvate and ATP. The process is inefficient, producing only two net ATP per glucose. However, the breakdown of glucose can continue with the citric acid cycle and oxidative phosphorylation if oxygen is present. In the absence of oxygen, pyruvate is reduced into lactate (or in some cells, ethanol). The overall reaction for glycolysis is:

$C_6H_{12}O_6$ (Glucose) + 2 NAD^+ + 2 P_i + 2 ADP → 2 $C_3H_4O_3$ (pyruvate) + 2 NADH + 2 ATP + 2 H^+ + 2 H_2O

Glycolysis can be divided into three main stages:

- Stage 1: Two ATP are invested to convert glucose into fructose 1,6-biphosphate.
- Stage 2: Fructose 1,6-biphosphate is split into two phosphorylated 3-carbon compounds called glyceraldehyde-3-phosphate, or G3P.
- Stage 3: G3P is oxidized, resulting in two 3-carbon compounds called pyruvate. Four ATP and two NADH are made during this stage. Since two ATP were invested in stage 1, there is a net production of two ATP.

The ten steps of glycolysis:

Step of Glycolysis	Substrate	Catalyzed by	Product
1 (irreversible)	Glucose	Hexokinase	Glucose 6-phosphate
2	Glucose 6-phosphate	Phosphoglucoisomerase	Fructose 6-phosphate
3 (irreversible)	Fructose 6-phosphate	Phosphofructokinase	Fructose 1, 6-biphosphate
4	Fructose 1, 6-biphosphate	Aldolase	Dihydroxyacetone phosphate
5	Dihydroxyacetone phosphate	Triose phosphate isomerase	Glyceraldehyde 3-phosphate (isomer of dihydroxyacetone phosphate)
6	Glyceraldehyde 3-phosphate	Triose phosphate dehydrogenase	1,3-Biphosphoglycerate
7	1,3-Biphosphoglycerate	Phosphoglycerokinase	3-Phosphoglycerate
8	3-Phosphoglycerate	Phosphoglyceromutase	2-Phosphoglycerate
9	2-Phosphoglycerate	Enolase	Phosphoenolpyruvate
10 (irreversible)	Phosphoenolpyruvate	Pyruvate kinase	Pyruvate

Feeder Pathways: Glycogen, Starch Metabolism

A **feeder pathway** for glycolysis describes the entrance of glucose or another reactant into glycolysis. Glucose is not the only carbohydrate that can enter glycolysis. Other hexoses such as fructose and galactose can enter the pathway as well. Fructose is phosphorylated by the enzyme hexokinase to produce fructose 1,6-bisphosphate, which is an intermediate in glycolysis and the process continues from there. In the liver, fructose is metabolized in a different pathway. It is phosphorylated by fructokinase and then cleaved to produce glyceraldehyde 3-phosphate and dihydroxyacetone phosphate, which are intermediates in glycolysis.

Not all non-glucose hexoses are converted to intermediates. A series of reactions can convert galactose into glucose 1-phosphate, which is then converted into glucose 6-phosphate for entry into glycolysis. Disaccharides can be cleaved, and their substituents fed into glycolysis in the manner described above. The polysaccharides, glycogen and starch, can be catabolized into their substituents to feed glucose into glycolysis. Phosphorylase breaks the $\alpha(1 \rightarrow 4)$ bond between the last glucose in a branch to produce glucose 1-phosphate, before the enzyme phosphoglucomutase converts it to glucose 6-phosphate.

Fermentation (Anaerobic Glycolysis)

Anaerobic respiration is one way in which certain organisms can metabolize sugar in the absence of oxygen. It is similar to aerobic respiration, but the final electron acceptor is not oxygen. (Often, it is sulfate or nitrate). Other organisms rely on fermentation to break down sugar when oxygen is not available. In **fermentation**, glycolysis is the only pathway that releases some of the energy stored in glucose; it is not followed by the citric acid cycle or the electron transport chain as in anaerobic respiration. Instead, the pyruvate that is made at the end of glycolysis is reduced to either lactate or ethanol, depending on the type of cell.

Both types of fermentation occur in the cytosol and produce two ATP per molecule of glucose and two NAD^+. NAD^+ is important because it is recycled back into glycolysis to act as an electron acceptor, allowing glycolysis to continually operate in the absence of oxygen. Fermentation is only about 2% efficient, releasing 14.6-kcal from the 686-kcal stored in a mole of ATP.

Lactic acid fermentation occurs in animal cells, often during exertion when the supply of oxygen is too low to keep up with the expenditure of ATP. It also occurs in some types of bacteria, and can be used to make products such as yogurt and cheese. The reversible reaction (beginning with pyruvate) is catalyzed by the enzyme lactate dehydrogenase.

Pyruvate ($C_3H_4O_3$) + NADH + H^+ $\leftrightarrow$ Lactic Acid ($C_3H_4O_3$) + NAD^+

Alcoholic fermentation occurs in yeast cells, and some types of bacteria. This form of fermentation is used in the production of alcoholic beverages and bread-making. There are two steps in this process: the formation of acetaldehyde by pyruvate decarboxylase (irreversible), followed by the reduction of acetaldehyde by alcohol dehydrogenase to form ethanol (reversible). The reactions are summarized below. Note that in the first reaction, CO_2 is produced as a waste product.

Pyruvate ($C_3H_4O_3$) $\rightarrow$ Acetaldehyde (C_2H_4O) + NADH + H^+ + CO_2 $\leftrightarrow$ Ethanol (C_2H_6O) + NAD^+

Gluconeogenesis

Gluconeogenesis (GNG) is the biosynthesis of glucose from non-carbohydrate substrates; i.e. not from glycogen or starch. It is essentially the reverse of glycolysis. This valuable but energetically expensive metabolic pathway occurs when glucose levels are low. In humans it occurs mostly in the liver, but also occurs in the small intestine, kidneys, and muscle. Precursors to glucose include lactate, pyruvate, glycerol, and glucogenic amino acids. In fact, all amino acids except lysine and leucine (which are purely ketogenic) can be converted to glucose, and alanine and glutamine are the most commonly used. The net reaction of gluconeogenesis is as follows:

2 pyruvate + 4 ATP + 2 GTP + 2 NADH + 2 H^+ + 6 H2O $\rightarrow$ Glucose + 4 ADP + 2 GDP + 2 NAD^+ + 6 P_i.

Gluconeogenesis is described as the reverse of glycolysis, but three of the ten steps of glycolysis are highly energetically favorable (large negative ΔG) and therefore irreversible.

The steps of glycolysis that must be bypassed are:

- Step 1: the phosphorylation of glucose to form glucose 6-phosphate.
  *Bypass accomplished by the use of the enzyme glucose 6-phosphatase.

- Step 3: the phosphorylation of fructose-6-phosphate to form fructose 1,6-bisphosphate
  *Bypass accomplished by the use of the enzyme fructose 1,6-bisphosphatase.
- Step 10: the transfer of a phosphate from phosphoenolpyruvate (PEP) to ADP to form pyruvate.
  *Bypass accomplished through a series of reactions that convert pyruvate to oxaloacetate to PEP.

Pentose Phosphate Pathway

The **pentose phosphate pathway** is an alternative pathway to glycolysis that occurs in the cytosol of certain cells. It is sometimes referred to as the hexose monophosphate shunt. This pathway degrades glucose to generate NADPH and ribose 5-phosphate. NADPH is used in reductive reactions within the cell, and is necessary for the anabolism of fatty acids and steroidogenesis. It also donates electrons to antioxidants. Ribose 5-phosphate is required for the synthesis of nucleotides.

This pathway consists of two phases: the oxidative phase and the non-oxidative phase. The oxidative phase is irreversible and produces CO_2, NADPH, and ribulose 5-phosphate from glucose 6-phosphate. The nonoxidative phase is reversible and generates ribose 5-phosphate, as well as fructose 6-phosphate and glyceraldehyde 3-phosphate which can be used in glycolysis. Note that no ATP are produced or expended during either phase.

Net (Maximum) Molecular and Energetic Results of Respiration Processes

Glycolysis requires the investment of energy in order to produce a net amount of ATP. One ATP is needed to power step 1 of glycolysis, where glucose is phosphorylated to produce glucose 6-phosphate. ATP is also utilized in step 3, where phosphofructokinase catalyzes the phosphorylation of fructose 6-phosphate to produce fructose 1,6-bisphosphate. Step 6 produces two NADH molecules when two molecules of glyceraldehyde 3-phosphate are oxidized to give way to 1,3-biphosphoglycerate. ATP is produced during step 7 when a phosphate group is removed from each of two molecules of 1,3-biphosphoglycerate and transferred to ADP, producing two ATP and two 3-phosphoglycerate. Two more ATP are made during step 10, when a phosphate group from each of two molecules of 1,3-biphosphoglycerate is transferred to ADP, forming pyruvate.

To summarize, two ATP are invested, and four ATP are produced, resulting in a net output of two ATP, two NADH, and two pyruvate per glucose. This process is only about 2% efficient, assuming the standard free energy change of −7.3 kcal/mol for the hydrolysis of ATP, and −686 kcal/mol for the complete oxidation of glucose. However, under cellular conditions, the efficiency may be as high as 4%.

The chemical equation for glycolysis is as follows:

$C_6H_{12}O_6$ (Glucose) + 2 NAD^+ + 2 P_i + 2 ADP → 2 $C_3H_4O_3$ (pyruvate) + 2 NADH + 2 ATP + 2 H^+ + 2 H_2O

Principles of Metabolic Regulation

Regulation of Metabolic Pathways

Maintenance of a Dynamic Steady State

A **metabolic pathway** is a series of connected reactions that result in the synthesis or breakdown of molecules. The product of one reaction is used as a substrate in the next reaction. These pathways must be monitored and regulated so that the immediate demands of a cell can be met. Enzymes play a critical role in this process by increasing the rate of these reactions. Furthermore, activators and inhibitor molecules can control the activity of the enzyme as a way to turn a reaction on or off.

Dynamic steady state is a condition in which a system remains constant as a result of the work being done to maintain that condition. Free energy enters and leaves biological systems, and the system has a higher energy level than its surroundings. This is in contrast to static equilibrium, in which there *is* a stable condition, but no input of energy is required to keep it that way. A cell's metabolism is a steady state condition because the concentrations of reactants and products remains constant, but new substrates are entering the pathway as products are removed.

Regulation of Glycolysis and Gluconeogenesis

During glycolysis, glucose is used to form pyruvate, and during gluconeogenesis, pyruvate is used to form glucose. These processes are reciprocally regulated so that when one pathway is operating, the other is inhibited. The reason for this becomes clear when examining the production and expenditure of ATP in each process. In glycolysis, 2 ATP are *produced*, while in gluconeogenesis, 4 ATP and 2 GTP are *used*. If both processes occurred at the same time, then the effects of glycolysis would be negated.

Allosteric enzymes are responsible for coordinating these processes. If the cell has high amounts of ATP (relative to AMP) there is no need for glycolysis, and phosphofructokinase is inhibited. High amounts of GTP will inhibit hexokinase. Without these enzymes, glycolysis will not proceed. The surplus of ATP is then used in gluconeogenesis to make glucose, which is then built up into glycogen for later use. Gluconeogenesis is inhibited when AMP builds up in a cell. AMP inhibits the activity of fructose 1,6-bisphosphatase, and ADP inhibits pyruvate carboxylase and phosphoenolpyruvate carboxykinase.

Metabolism of Glycogen

Glycogenolysis is the breakdown of glycogen. It begins with the action of the enzyme **glycogen phosphorylase**, which catalyzes the hydrolysis of the terminal $\alpha(1\rightarrow4)$ glycosidic linkage, releasing glucose 1-phosphate. This process continues until a branch point within the glycogen macromolecule is reached. Glycogen phosphorylase cannot hydrolyze the $\alpha(1\rightarrow6)$ linkage at the branch point, so **glycogen debranching enzyme** (GDE) breaks the bond. The glucose 1-phosphates that are clipped from glycogen must then be converted to glucose 6-phosphates for further breakdown. This is achieved by the enzyme **phosphoglucomutase**, which transfers a phosphate to carbon 6 of glucose 1-phosphate to produce glucose 1,6-bisphosphate. The phosphate on carbon 1 is then transferred to phosphoglucomutase, and glucose 6-phosphate is formed. (Note that these processes do not require the hydrolysis of ATP.) Glucose 6-phosphate can be converted to glucose in the liver, kidneys, and small intestine, but not the skeletal muscles.

Glycogenesis, or the synthesis of glycogen, begins with the phosphorylation of glucose to form glucose 6-phosphate (G6P). ATP provides the phosphate, and the reaction is catalyzed by **hexokinase** (in the muscle) or **glucokinase** (in the liver). G6P is then converted to glucose 1-phosphate by **phosphoglucomutase**. The enzyme **UDP-glucose phosphorylase** (UGPP) attaches glucose-1-phosphate with uridine triphosphate (UTP) to form uridine diphosphate glucose (UDP glucose). The enzyme **glycogenin** then attaches carbon 1 of UDP glucose to one of its tyrosine residues via $\alpha(1\rightarrow4)$ glycosidic linkage to begin the formation of a primer. Once the primer has around eight UDP-glucose residues, the enzyme **glycogen synthase** takes over, linking carbon 1 UDP-glucose to carbon 4 of the non-reducing end of glycogen via $\alpha(1\rightarrow4)$ bonds. Branch points are handled by **glycogen branching enzyme** (GBE). This metabolic pathway occurs in the liver and muscle cells.

Regulation of Glycogen Synthesis and Breakdown

Glycogenesis and glycogenolysis must be coordinated so that both processes do not occur simultaneously and cancel each other out. This complex process is achieved through both allosteric control (which acts at the level of the cell) and hormonal control (which acts at the level of the organism). Enzymes such as glycogen synthase and glycogen phosphorylase are allosterically activated or inhibited by molecules that signal the needs of the cell. For example, both glucose-6 phosphate and ATP inhibit glycogen phosphorylase, which is the primary enzyme involved in the degradation of glycogen. It can be also be controlled by the hormones glucagon, epinephrine, and insulin. Glucagon and epinephrine activate glycogen phosphorylase (and therefore glycogenolysis) while insulin deactivates it. This is accomplished through second messenger systems in which the hormone binds to receptors in the cell membrane, causing a cascade of events that affect the concentrations of cAMP. cAMP plays a role in the activation of protein kinase A (PKA) which in turn plays a role in activating the enzymes directly involved in glycogenesis and glycogenolysis by phosphorylation or dephosphorylation.

Analysis of Metabolic Control

Metabolic control analysis (MCA) quantifies the control of a specific enzyme over the flux (the rate of the pathway as a whole) and concentration of metabolites. "Control" in this context refers to the degree that an enzyme can alter a pathway. This analysis calculates the effects of the enzyme quantitatively, rather than describing it qualitatively in terms of rate limitation or rate determining steps. For example, instead of labeling a step along the pathway as simply rate-limiting, MCA is used to determine the *amount* that flux varies in response to a change in enzyme activity, and to study the relationship between the *control coefficient* of an enzyme and its *elasticity*. The **control coefficient** is a measure of the effects of flux or concentration on the system as a whole. **Elasticity** measures the effect of metabolite concentration on a local reaction. Elasticity is positive for metabolites that increase the reaction rate, and negative for metabolites that inhibit it. If the flux control coefficient is multiplied by the elasticity for every enzyme in the pathway, they will add up to zero, as stated by the connectivity theorem.

Citric Acid Cycle

Acetyl-CoA Production

There are various ways in which acetyl coenzyme A (acetyl-CoA) is produced, including the β-oxidation of fatty acids, the breakdown of amino acids, and the oxidative decarboxylation of the pyruvate that was made during glycolysis. Oxidative decarboxylation occurs in the matrix of the mitochondria through the action of the pyruvate dehydrogenase complex. This complex consists of the enzymes pyruvate dehydrogenase, dihydrolipoyl transacetylase, and dihydrolipoyl dehydrogenase. The main events of oxidative decarboxylation occur as follows. First, a carboxyl group is removed from 3-carbon pyruvate in the form of carbon dioxide. The resulting two-carbon acetyl group is oxidized, as NAD^+ accepts two electrons and two hydrogens to form NADH. The acetyl group combines with a derivative of pantothenic acid called coenzyme A, resulting in acetyl-

CoA (two acetyl-CoA molecules per glucose). Acetyl-CoA is then catabolized in the citric acid cycle. The overall reaction for the production of acetyl-CoA via oxidative decarboxylation is:

$$\text{pyruvate} + \text{CoA} + NAD^+ \rightarrow \text{acetyl-CoA} + NADH + CO_2$$

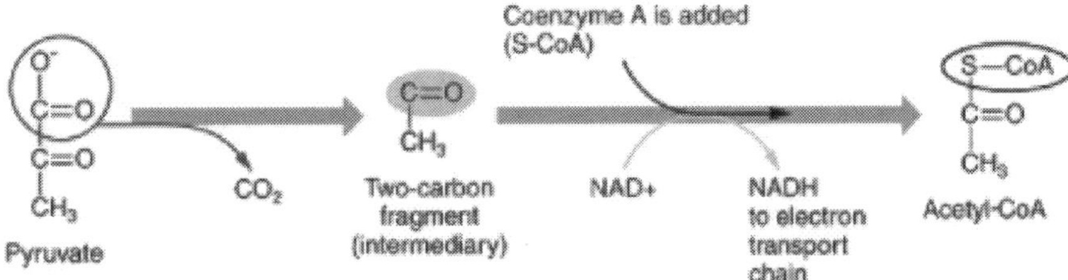

Reactions of the Cycle, Substrates and Products

The **citric acid cycle** (also called the Krebs cycle) occurs in the mitochondrial matrix and transfers the energy stored in acetyl-CoA into molecules that are used in oxidative phosphorylation. Some of the important products are 3 NADH, 1 $FADH_2$, and 1 ATP (per molecule of acetyl-CoA).

The cycle begins when the enzyme citrate synthase combines acetyl-CoA with 4-carbon oxaloacetate to form 6-carbon **citric acid**. A hydroxyl group changes location on the citric acid molecule by the enzyme aconitase to form **isocitrate**. The enzyme isocitrate dehydrogenase oxidizes isocitrate to produce 5-carbon **α-ketoglutarate**, as a carbon is released in the form of carbon dioxide. NAD^+ accepts the electrons to make NADH. A similar reaction occurs through the action of α-ketoglutarate dehydrogenase, except when carbon is removed, it is replaced by coenzyme A. NADH and 4-carbon **succinyl** *CoA* are formed. The enzyme succinyl-CoA synthetase catalyzes the next reaction in which a phosphate group replaces coenzyme A on succinyl CoA, before being transferred to GDP to make GTP, and then transferred again from GTP to ADP to form ATP. **Succinate** is produced during the reaction. The transfer of two hydrogens to FAD (forming $FADH_2$) is catalyzed by succinate dehydrogenase, yielding **fumarate**. Fumarase adds water to fumarate to form **malate**, which is then oxidized to regenerate **oxaloacetate**. NAD^+ accepts the electrons and forms NADH.

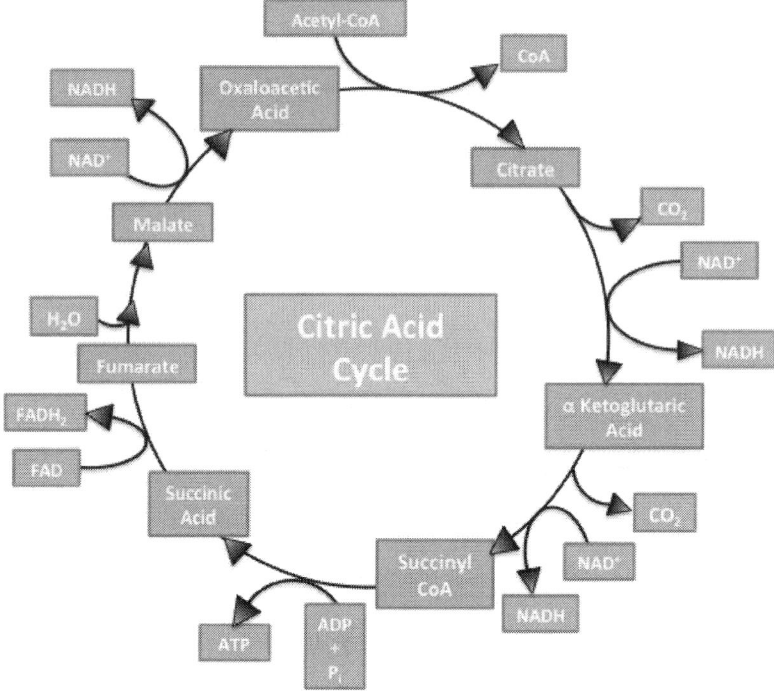

Regulation of the Cycle

The citric acid cycle is regulated at many levels. The production of acetyl-CoA can be controlled before the cycle begins, and then there are different control points within the cycle itself that can be regulated.

The production of acetyl-CoA (the initiator of the citric acid cycle) is catalyzed by the pyruvate dehydrogenase complex. Pyruvate dehydrogenase can be activated or deactivated in response to levels of NADH, ATP, and acetyl-CoA. High concentrations of these molecules promote phosphorylation of the enzyme, effectively turning it off when energy-rich molecules are in abundance. The enzyme can be activated by high levels of calcium.

Three enzymes within the citric acid cycle also serve as regulation points: citrate synthase, isocitrate dehydrogenase, and α-ketoglutarate dehydrogenase. When NADH is in high concentration, these enzymes are inhibited. They are further regulated by other factors. Both ATP and Succinyl-CoA (an intermediate of the citric acid cycle) inhibit citrate synthase and α-ketoglutarate dehydrogenase. High levels of calcium, ADP and NAD^+ promote the citric acid cycle.

Net (Maximum) Molecular and Energetic Results of Respiration Processes

The citric acid cycle alone produces 3 NADH, 1 $FADH_2$, and 1 GTP (later converted to ATP) per cycle. Since two cycles run per glucose molecule, these numbers can be doubled when considering the molecular and energetic results of the cycle. Half of the reactions of the cycle are oxidation reactions, and the energy is conserved in NADH and $FADH_2$. These molecules are used during the next stage (oxidative phosphorylation) to produce more ATP. The maximum ATP yield per NADH and $FADH_2$ is 3 and 2, respectively, but actual yields are closer to 2.5 ATP per NADH and 1.5 per $FADH_2$. Using the maximum values, one acetyl CoA will give rise to 12 ATP when NADH and $FADH_2$

are considered. 2 CO_2 molecules (per molecule of acetyl-CoA) are released as waste products during the cycle. The overall reaction for the citric acid cycle is:

Acetyl-CoA + 3 NAD^+ + FAD + GDP + P_i + 2 $H_2O \rightarrow$ 2 CO_2 + CoA-SH + 3 NADH + $FADH_2$ + GTP + $3H^+$

Metabolism of Fatty Acids and Proteins

Description of Fatty Acids

A **fatty acid** is a carboxylic acid with a hydrophobic hydrocarbon chain. The carboxyl group (COOH) is the component that participates in chemical reactions. Dehydration synthesis results in an ester linkage between the carboxyl group and a hydroxyl group of an alcohol, often glycerol.

The aliphatic (non-aromatic) chain can be saturated or unsaturated. Saturated fatty acids contain only single bonds, and are therefore "saturated" with hydrogens at every position. Unsaturated fatty acids have at least one double bond. In a **cis** configuration, both hydrogens on either side of the double bond point in the same direction, resulting in a kink in the chain. In a **trans** configuration, the adjacent hydrogens point in opposite directions and the chain has little to no bend.

Chains also vary in the number of carbons, and they are almost always even numbers.

- Short-chain fatty acids (SCFA): fewer than six carbons
- Medium-chain fatty acids (MCFA): 6–12 carbons
- Long-chain fatty acids (LCFA): 13–21
- Very long chain fatty acids (VLCFA) more than 22 carbons

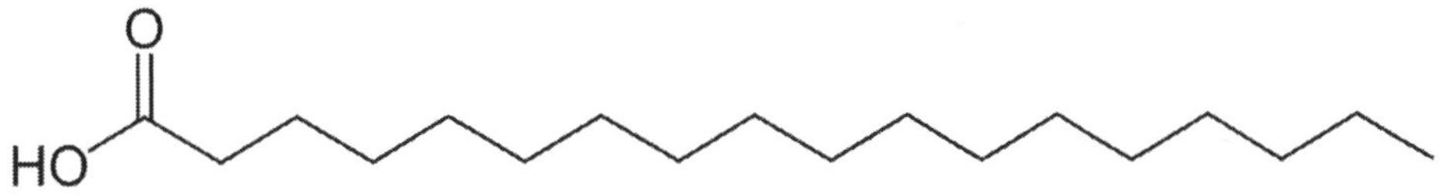

O
HO

Fatty acids have many important roles in the body. They can be built up into triglycerides to store energy, and serve as a source of fuel when oxidized. They also make up phospholipids, the main components of plasma membranes. The nonpolar nature of the fatty acids prevents the passage of certain substances across the membrane. The outer leaflets of membranes also contain glycolipids, which aid in cell recognition and membrane stability. Intracellular proteins are often tagged with a lipid to help direct them to their destinations in the membrane. Fatty acids can also act as signaling molecules. For example, some fatty acids regulate transcription factors, and thereby play a role in gene expression.

Digestion, Mobilization, and Transport of Fats

Triacylglycerols (or TAGs) are the most common source of fat in the body. They are insoluble in aqueous solution, and group together to form droplets. The liver secretes bile to break down these droplets into micelles so that enzymes have more surface area to act on. Lipases are secreted mainly by the pancreas and empty into the small intestine. These enzymes break the ester linkages within a TAG, producing a free glycerol molecule and 3 fatty acid chains. The subunits are then small enough to be absorbed by the cells of the small intestine. Once in the intestinal wall, they can recombine into TAGs again. These hydrophobic fats must then be transported by a specialized lipoprotein called a chylomicron which carries fats within its core. Since the proteins are too large to enter the blood capillaries directly, they are taken up by lymphatic capillaries before draining into thoracic ducts, which in turn drain into veins. Enzymes known as lipoprotein lipases break down the chylomicron and the TAGs within, which are then taken up by various tissues within the body. Adipose tissue stores fat in large droplets, and can release fatty acids in response to hormonal signals. Other tissues, with the exception of cells of the central nervous system and red blood cells, extract the energy by oxidation of the fatty acids. First, the fatty acids are activated by combining with coenzyme A to form fatty acyl-CoA. This activated form can be transported into the mitochondria via the carnitine carrier system for oxidation.

Oxidation of Fatty Acids

Saturated Fats

The β-oxidation of saturated fatty acids begins with the oxidation of α and β carbons (C2 and C3) via acyl-CoA-dehydrogenase to form a trans double bond between those carbons. The accompanying reduction reaction produces $FADH_2$ from FAD, and the resulting molecule is called trans-Δ^2-enoyl CoA. In the next reaction, enoyl-CoA hydratase catalyzes the hydration of the double bond to produce L-3-hydroxyacyl CoA. The newly added hydroxyl group on the β-carbon is then oxidized by 3-hydroxyacyl CoA dehydrogenase to form 3-ketoacyl CoA, and NAD+ is reduced to NADH. In the final reaction, the bond between the α and β carbon is cleaved when the thiol group of coenzyme A is added between the α and β carbons via β-ketothiolase, releasing acetyl-CoA which can then enter the citric acid cycle. The remaining shortened fatty acid will then be put through the same set of reactions repeatedly until all the carbons have been released as acetyl-CoA. An 18-C fatty acid, for example, would eventually give rise to nine molecules of acetyl-CoA. Nine citric acid cycles (at 12 ATP per cycle), plus 9 NADH (3 ATP max, per NADH), plus 9 $FADH_2$ (2 ATP max, per $FADH_2$), would produce a theoretical maximum of 153 ATP for a fatty acid of this length.

Unsaturated Fats

The β-oxidation of unsaturated fatty acids is a similar pathway to that of saturated fatty acids, but additional enzymes are required any time a double bond is encountered. The double bonds of most unsaturated fatty acids are **cis** bonds, meaning the hydrogen atoms on either side of the double bond are on the same side. If there is an odd number of double bonds, as in a monounsaturated fat such as palmitoleate, the enzyme enoyl CoA isomerase converts the cis double bond to a trans double bond to produce **trans-Δ^2-enoyl CoA**: a normal substrate in the β-oxidation pathway that can be acted on by enoyl-CoA hydratase. In the case of an even number of bonds, an intermediate called 2,4 dienoyl-CoA is formed that requires an additional enzyme (2,4 dienoyl CoA reductase) before it can be acted on by enoyl CoA isomerase. 2,4 dienoyl-CoA is reduced (and NADPH is oxidized) to form trans-Δ3-enoyl CoA. Isomerase can now act on this molecule, allowing it to be fed into the β-oxidation pathway.

Ketone Bodies

Ketone bodies are byproducts of the breakdown of fatty acids that can be used as sources of energy when carbohydrates are scarce (as in starvation). Acetoacetate, β-hydroxybutyrate, and acetone are all ketone bodies, but only acetoacetate and β-hydroxybutyrate are catabolized for energy; acetone is simply excreted from the body. The production of ketone bodies (ketogenesis) occurs in the mitochondria of liver cells when acetyl-CoA begins to accumulate. Two acetyl-CoA molecules combine to form acetoacetyl-CoA, which combines with another acetyl-CoA molecule via HMG-CoA synthase to form HMG-CoA. The enzyme HMG-CoA lyase then breaks down HMG-CoA to produce acetoacetate, which can give rise to both β-hydroxybutyrate and acetone. Ketoacidosis will occur when high amounts of ketone bodies bring the pH of the body to dangerously low levels. The liver cannot use the ketone bodies it produces because it lacks the enzyme thiophorase (also known as succinyl CoA-acetoacetate CoA transferase) which oxidizes β-hydroxybutyrate to form acetoacetate. This active form can be metabolized in the mitochondria to yield energy.

Anabolism of Fats

Fatty acids are constructed from acetyl-CoA, mainly in the cytoplasm of liver and fat cells. Acetyl-CoA cannot cross the mitochondrial membrane into the cytoplasm, but citrate can. Once citrate is in the cytoplasm, it is split apart by the enzyme **citrate lyase** into acetyl-CoA and oxaloacetate. Acetyl-CoA can now be incorporated into a fatty acid. It is activated by the enzyme **acetyl-CoA carboxylase** by adding CO_2 to produce malonyl-CoA. This process requpass-throughenditure of ATP, and the cofactor biotin. The enzyme complex **fatty acid synthase** (which requires vitamin B_5) then catalyzes a series of reactions, including the reduction of the carboxyl group, as NADPH is oxidized. Water is removed, creating a double bond which is reduced by a second NADPH. The 2-carbon compound is incorporated into the elongating fatty acid chain until it is 16 carbons in length. This compound is known as **palmitate**, and is the only fatty acid produced by humans from simple starting materials. To form a triacylglycerol, three fatty acid chains must form ester linkages to glycerol 3-phosphate. As with fatty acid synthesis, triacylglycerol formation occurs mostly in the liver and adipose tissue.

Overall reaction for fatty acid synthesis:

8 Acetyl CoA + 7 ATP + 14 NADPH + 14 H^+ → Palmitate + 7 CO2 + 7 ADP + 7 P_i + 8 CoA + 14 $NADP^+$ + $6H_2O$

Metabolism of Proteins

When proteins are digested, the amino acids are usually incorporated into new proteins (during translation), but they can be metabolized for energy as a last resort.

Protein digestion begins in the stomach with the enzyme pepsin, which denatures the protein and begins hydrolyzing some of the peptide bonds. Polypeptides and free amino acids will stimulate the secretion of cholecystokinin (CCK), which in turn stimulates the release of pancreatic proteases trypsin, chymotrypsin, and carboxypeptidases, each with its own specificity. They are activated in the small intestine with the help of enteropeptidase and continue to hydrolyze the peptide bonds. Aminopeptidase is an enzyme found in the plasma membrane of the cells of the small intestine that finishes the degradation of the protein into units no longer than a tripeptide. The amino acids, dipeptides, and tripeptides are actively transported into the cells and then released into the blood.

Proteins are only metabolized as a source of energy in extreme circumstances when carbohydrates and lipids are not available. For this to happen, the amino group must be removed from the amino acid in a process called deamination. The amino group is converted to ammonia (which is then converted to urea and excreted), and the remaining molecule (a keto acid) can be used as a source of fuel.

Oxidative Phosphorylation

Electron Transport Chain and Oxidative Phosphorylation, Substrates and Products, General Features of the Pathway

Oxidative phosphorylation refers to the combined processes of the electron transport chain and chemiosmosis. This pathway produces more ATP than any other stage of cellular respiration. In the electron transport chain (located in the cristae), a series of redox reactions helps to generate a proton gradient. NADH and $FADH_2$ (products of previous stages) are oxidized, and their electrons passed along a chain of four enzyme complexes: NADH dehydrogenase (I), succinate dehydrogenase (II), Q-cytochrome *c* oxidoreductase (III), and cytochrome *c* oxidase (IV). Electrons from NADH enter the chain at complex I (more specifically to a prosthetic group on the complex called flavin mononucleotide or FMN), while electrons from $FADH_2$ enter at complex II. Electrons from both

NADH and $FADH_2$ are passed onto a carrier called ubiquinone (also called coenzyme Q) which transports them to complex III. Cytochrome C carries the electrons to complex IV, where oxygen (the final electron acceptor) is reduced to form water. The energy that is lost by the moving electrons is used by complexes I, III, and IV to pump protons from the mitochondrial matrix to the intermembrane space. This establishes an electrochemical gradient, and the protons re-enter the matrix through an enzyme called ATP synthase. As they flow through the enzyme, they turn a portion of it like a water wheel, allowing it to add a phosphate to ADP, forming ATP (1 ATP per 3 protons).

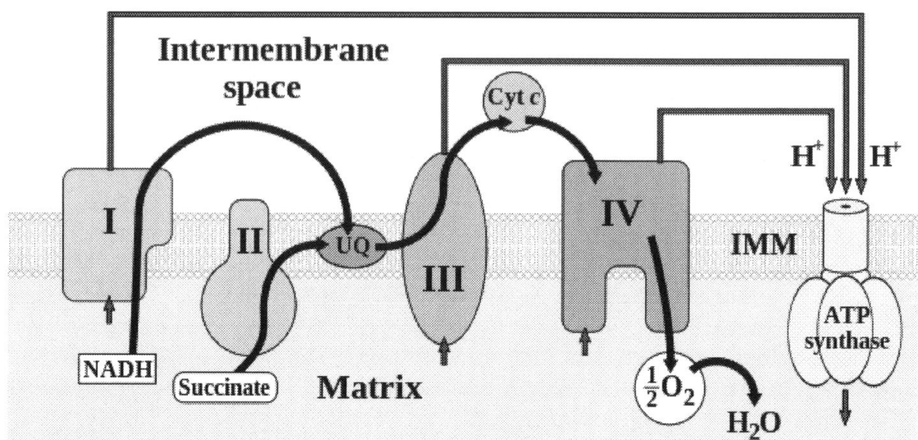

Electron Transfer in Mitochondria

First, NADH is oxidized to NAD^+, donating two electrons to complex I. The electrons are passed to ubiquinone (which becomes ubiquinol, or QH_2 in its reduced form). Complex 1 pumps four protons out of the matrix into the intermembrane space. $FADH_2$ donates two electrons to complex II, which also passes them onto ubiquinone. The electrons then travel from ubiquinone to complex III (which pumps out another four protons), where they are carried by cytochrome C to complex IV (which pumps out two protons). The final electron acceptor is oxygen, which splits apart and combines with hydrogen ions to form water.

NADH, NADPH

Nicotinamide adenine dinucleotide (NADH) is a coenzyme that can switch back and forth between its reduced form (NADH) and its oxidized form (NAD^+). Its role in oxidative phosphorylation is vital, as it shuttles electrons to the electron transport chain, where the energy of those electrons is harvested to synthesize ATP. NADH donates two electrons to complex I of the electron transport chain within the inner mitochondrial membrane. Each subsequent complex (II, III, and then IV) is more electron-hungry than the last, so the electrons are transferred through a series of redox reactions before being accepted by O_2.

Nicotinamide adenine dinucleotide phosphate $NADP^+$ is another coenzyme that can cycle between its reduced (NADPH) and oxidized ($NADP^+$) forms. While NADH is often employed in catabolic reactions, NADPH is a reducing agent in many anabolic reactions. In photosynthesis, it is produced in the redox reactions of the electron transport chain of the thylakoid membrane, and used to reduce intermediates within the Calvin cycle (where sugars are made).

Flavoproteins and Cytochromes

Flavoproteins are one of the many types of electron carriers found in the electron transport chain. They contain a flavin nucleotide such as flavin adenine dinucleotide (FAD) or flavin mononucleotide (FMN). These prosthetic groups transfer electrons and protons during many cellular processes, including cellular respiration. Both NADH dehydrogenase (complex I) and succinate-dehydrogenase (complex II) contain flavoproteins. NADH donates two electrons to FMN of complex 1, reducing it to $FMNH_2$. The flavoprotein within complex II contains FAD, which is reduced to $FADH_2$. There is also an electron transfer flavoprotein complex within the mitochondrial membrane that accepts electrons from primary dehydrogenases.

Cytochromes are electron carriers that contain a heme group (with a central iron atom) that allows it to transfer electrons. They are found in complexes III and IV. When electrons are transferred to complex III (Q-cytochrome *c* oxidoreductase), they are passed to cytochrome c, and then to complex IV (cytochrome *c* oxidase). Complex IV accepts one electron at a time, but transfers four electrons to oxygen at once.

ATP Synthase, Chemiosmotic Coupling

Proton Motive Force

ATP synthase is an enzyme that uses a proton motive force to form ATP from ADP and an inorganic phosphate. It is often referred to as the world's smallest motor. This protein complex is integrated into the inner mitochondrial membrane. The proton motive force is established by pumping protons from the matrix into the intermembrane space using the energy from the electrons traveling along the electron transport chain. Complex 1 (the first of the enzyme complexes in the ETC) pumps four protons out of the matrix into the intermembrane space. Complex III pumps out four more protons and complex IV pumps out two, for a total of ten protons. The protons accumulate, and the energy stored in this electrochemical gradient is used to drive **chemiosmosis**: the process that couples the reactions of the electron transport chain to the production of ATP.

The protein complex ATP synthase consists of two main coupled regions, F_O and F_1. The proton motive force causes the accumulated H^+ ions to move down the gradient into the F_O portion of the enzyme. This flow of protons causes the F_O portion to spin like a rotor, similar to the way that water turns a water wheel. Each proton completes one full revolution and is released on the opposite side of the membrane. The torque created by the rotation of the F_O complex is transferred to the F_1 region by a shaft. The rotating shaft does not turn the F_1 region, but it does cause a conformational change, which in turn catalyzes the formation of ATP from ADP and a phosphate group. One ATP molecule is produced for every three H^+ ions that pass through ATP synthase.

Net (Maximum) Molecular and Energetic Results of Respiration Processes

Oxidative phosphorylation yields more ATP than any other pathway of cellular respiration, though it is dependent on the products of the previous reactions. The exact amount of ATP can vary depending on environmental conditions and cell type. Each NADH is capable of producing 3 ATP, however 2.5 is often used in calculations to account for suboptimal conditions and the active transport of NADH. Each $FADH_2$ can generate a maximum of 2 ATP, but 1.5 is more likely in normal conditions. To summarize the important products of each stage (per molecule of glucose):

Glycolysis: 2 ATP, 2 NADH, and 2 pyruvate

The **link reaction** (pyruvate decarboxylation): 2 NADH, 2 acetyl-CoA, and 2 CO_2 (waste)

The **citric acid cycle**: 2 ATP, 6 NADH, 2 $FADH_2$, and 4 CO_2 (waste)

Oxidative phosphorylation generates a maximum of 34 ATP, though the actual amount may be closer to 28 when using the more realistic yields per NADH and $FADH_2$. It also produces water when oxygen accepts electrons at the end of the electron transport chain.

Under the most ideal conditions, a eukaryotic cell could generate a maximum of 38 ATP per glucose. Using this number, the efficiency of aerobic respiration would be about 40%, assuming the standard free energy change of −7.3 kcal/mol for the hydrolysis of ATP, and −686 kcal/mol for the complete oxidation of glucose. However, it is probably closer to 34% when accounting for normal conditions.

Regulation of Oxidative Phosphorylation

Oxidative phosphorylation is regulated mainly by O_2 and ADP, and is directly tied to the energy requirements of the cell. If oxygen levels are depleted, electrons will have nowhere to go at the end of the electron transport chain, and the redox reactions come to a halt. The electron carriers NADH and $FADH_2$ accumulate, inhibiting the citric acid cycle. If oxygen *is* present, then oxidative phosphorylation is further regulated by ADP. As ATP is consumed, the levels of ADP rise. ADP allosterically stimulates the activity of isocitrate dehydrogenase, the enzyme that catalyzes the third step of the citric acid cycle (the oxidative decarboxylation of isocitrate into alpha-ketoglutarate). The rate of the citric acid cycle increases, which in turn increases the rate of oxidative phosphorylation. If ATP is in abundance, it acts as an allosteric inhibitor of cytochrome *c* oxidase (complex IV of the electron transport chain). Complex IV can also be inhibited by carbon monoxide, cyanide, and azide. When the complex is deactivated, the proton motive force will not be established, and chemiosmosis will not occur.

Mitochondria, Apoptosis, Oxidative Stress

Mitochondria play a critical role in inducing apoptosis in response to oxidative stress. **Apoptosis** is programmed cell death. This mechanism targets cells that, for one reason or another, need to be eliminated, and does not refer to the demise of cells that are exposed to extreme conditions or infection. Cells singled out for apoptosis include those that have lost their anchorage to adjacent cells, have damaged DNA, or experience oxidative stress.

Oxidative stress is the loss of balance between the production of reactive oxygen species (ROS) and the antioxidants that defend against them. ROS are results of the incomplete reduction of O_2 during the processes of the electron transport chain. They are highly reactive and unstable, and include superoxide anions, peroxides, and hydroxyl radicals. Antioxidants and certain enzymes seek to neutralize them, but sometimes apoptosis is required.

To initiate apoptosis, the permeability of the outer mitochondrial membrane increases as a result of proapoptotic Bcl-2 proteins. This allows cytochrome c (part of the electron transport chain) to move into the cytoplasm and activate enzymes known as caspases. These enzymes begin the breakdown of specific intracellular components, while activating other enzymes to do the same.

Hormonal Regulation and Integration of Metabolism

Higher Level Integration of Hormone Structure and Function

Hormones are responsible for the integration of energy metabolism. Metabolism is regulated on the cellular level, but it is important that it be regulated at a higher level, the level of the organism. The endocrine system produces hormones that work to maintain homeostasis by responding to changes in activity, food intake, or other events. They act as chemical messengers, traveling through body fluids and binding to receptors on or inside target cells. Hormones are involved with many essential functions including growth and development, reproduction, and metabolism (such as carbohydrate, lipid, and protein metabolism).

Hormones come in a variety of structures that can be grouped into three main classes: lipid-based, amino acid-derived, and peptides. Lipid hormones (such as cortisol) are usually derived from cholesterol to form steroids, and they are insoluble in water. Most amino-acid derived and peptide hormones (such as epinephrine and insulin, respectively) are water-soluble, and cannot diffuse across the plasma membrane. Water-soluble hormones act relatively quickly through second-messenger systems, while lipid-soluble hormones tend to regulate transcription and act more slowly (but with a more prolonged effect).

Tissue Specific Metabolism

The metabolic reactions that occur in various tissues can change depending on whether the body is in an absorptive state (well-fed, energy-storing) or post-absorptive state (fasting, energy-utilizing).

Liver: In the absorptive state, insulin facilitates the synthesis of glycogen and/or fatty acids from glucose. Fatty acids will be built into triglycerides and sent to adipose tissue. In the fasting state, glycogen is broken down into glucose and released in the blood. Amino acids are converted to keto acids, which the liver can metabolize for energy.

Adipose tissue: When the body is well fed, fat cells take up glucose and use it to make triglycerides. During the post-absorptive state, low levels of insulin stimulate the breakdown of triglycerides so that fatty acids can be released.

Skeletal muscle: In the absorptive state, glucose can be made into glycogen or oxidized if needed for energy, and amino acids are built into proteins. In the fasting state, glycogen is broken down into glucose, and proteins are broken down into amino acids which are taken up by the liver to form keto acids and glucose.

Cardiac muscle: In both the absorptive and post-absorptive states, fatty acids are oxidized for fuel.

Brain: The brain does not store energy. In the absorptive state, it oxidizes glucose. In a prolonged fasting state, it oxidizes both ketones and glucose.

Hormonal Regulation of Fuel Metabolism

The main hormones involved in the regulation of fuel metabolism include insulin, glucagon, epinephrine, glucocorticoids, and thyroid hormones.

During the absorptive state, insulin facilitates the uptake of glucose from the blood, and stimulates the synthesis of glycogen while inhibiting glycogenolysis. Insulin is opposed by many counterregulatory hormones, as described below.

Glucagon (in the fasting state) signals the cell to mobilize its glucose reserves, breaking down glycogen and increasing the levels of glucose in the blood.

Epinephrine stimulates glycogenolysis. Furthermore, an increase in epinephrine (and therefore a decrease in insulin) causes cells to release amino acids from muscle cells and fatty acids and glycerol from adipose tissue. The liver will use amino acids and glycerol to synthesize glucose during gluconeogenesis so that the body has a source of glucose during longer episodes of fasting. (Glycogenolysis releases glucose into the blood more quickly than gluconeogenesis.) Epinephrine is also known to raise the basal metabolic rate.

Glucocorticoids inhibit the uptake of glucose, and stimulate gluconeogenesis in response to stress by stimulating the release of amino acids and glycerol into the blood.

Thyroid hormones increase the basal metabolic rate.

OBESITY AND REGULATION OF BODY MASS

When caloric intake is equal to the energy expended, the body mass of an individual will not change. Excess calories result in the storage of fat in adipose tissue and an increase in body mass. Hormones such as leptin and ghrelin help to balance the intake and output of energy. Leptin is produced by adipose tissue, and binds to receptors in the hypothalamus to suppress appetite when full. Obesity can result if leptin is not produced, or if it cannot bind to the leptin receptors. Ghrelin is sometimes called the "hunger hormone" because it (like leptin) acts on the cells of the hypothalamus. But unlike leptin, ghrelin enhances hunger. It is secreted by the stomach when it is empty, but the secretion stops as the stomach stretches with food. It can also be secreted in response to stimuli such as the scent or sight of a good meal.

Assemblies of Molecules, Cells, and Groups of Cells Within Single Cellular and Multicellular Organisms

PLASMA MEMBRANE

GENERAL FUNCTION IN CELL CONTAINMENT

While the plasma membrane is involved in many functions (such as the regulation and transportation of materials, cell to cell recognition, and cell signaling), its most basic function is cell containment. The cell membrane is composed of a double layer of phospholipids that surrounds the cytoplasm of virtually all types of cells. The phospholipids form a fluid-like barrier that is reinforced by cholesterol and protein molecules. This barrier helps to contain the structures and molecules within the cell's interior, and also helps to maintain the desired concentrations of substances on either side of the membrane. Since the phospholipids orient themselves with their fatty acid chains pointed inward, the interior of the membrane is hydrophobic. This property causes the membrane to remain intact in its aqueous environment, while being somewhat impermeable to substances that are soluble in water (with the notable exception of nonpolar gases such as oxygen and carbon dioxide).

Review Video: Plasma Membrane
Visit mometrix.com/academy and enter code: 943095

COMPOSITION OF MEMBRANES

LIPID COMPONENTS: PHOSPHOLIPIDS (AND PHOSPHATIDS)

A phospholipid consists of two nonpolar fatty acid chains bonded to a polar head made of glycerol, a phosphate group, and an organic R-group. (Phosphatids are the simplest phospholipids and lack the functional group on the phosphate.) Phospholipids are amphipathic, meaning that they have both hydrophilic (polar head) and hydrophobic (nonpolar tails) components. Because of this property, they arrange themselves into micelles or bilayers. A micelle is a small spherical structure made of a single layer of phospholipids with the tails pointed inward to form a hydrophobic core. They are used to transport lipid soluble materials. A bilayer is formed when the phospholipids assemble into parallel layers with the tails pointed in toward each other and the heads pointed out. Phospholipid bilayers surround liposomes and other vesicles, and also enclose the organelles in a eukaryotic cell. These bilayers also form cell membranes, which regulate the passage of materials into and out of all types of cells.

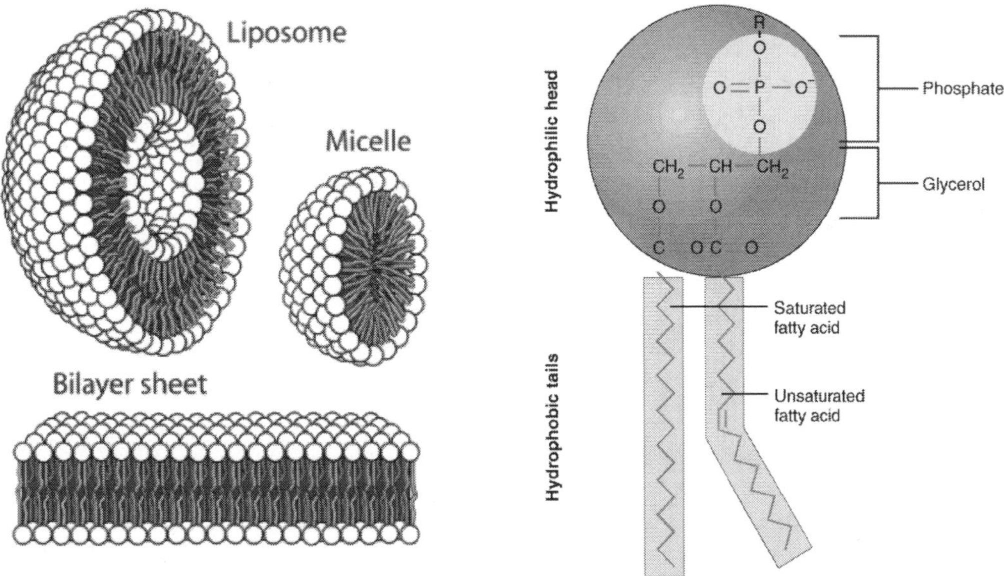

LIPID COMPONENTS: STEROIDS AND WAXES

Steroids are lipids that are derived from cholesterol. Cholesterol has a hydrophilic hydroxyl group and a hydrophobic region consisting of four fused hydrocarbon rings and a hydrocarbon chain. The hydrophilic region interacts with the polar heads of the phospholipids, and the hydrophobic regions interact with the nonpolar tails. Its role in the membrane is to maintain stability and proper membrane viscosity by restraining phospholipids from spreading too far apart, or packing too close together (as can occur with fluctuations in temperature).

Cholesterol: HO

Waxes are lipids that are offer stability to some types of cell membranes, usually in plants. They are composed of a long fatty acid chain bonded to an alcohol with a long carbon chain. Because of their highly hydrophobic property, they interact only with the tails of the phospholipids. Waxes can be used as a water repellant in many plants and some animals.

PROTEIN COMPONENTS

The proteins associated with the membrane enable most of the membrane's functions, such as the shuttling of various ions and molecules through the membrane, catalyzing reactions, joining of adjacent cells, cell signaling, cellular support and stability, and cell recognition. Some of these proteins penetrate into the hydrophobic interior of the membrane, and are called **integral** proteins. **Glycoproteins** are integral proteins with an attached sugar chain that aid in cell recognition. When integral proteins extend completely through the membrane, they are called **transmembrane** proteins, and these are often used as receptors for cell signaling. A signal molecule (like a hormone) will bind to the receptor from the extracellular side, and relay a message to the cytoplasmic side. Transmembrane proteins are also required for transport across the membrane. Some transport proteins (called **channel** proteins) have a tunnel-like conformation that allows materials to move passively, while others (**carrier** proteins) change conformation to move materials either by active or passive transport. **Peripheral proteins** are loosely bound to either side of the membrane, and often act as enzymes or receptor proteins. (Note that both of these can also be integral proteins).

Fluid Mosaic Model

The currently accepted model of the plasma membrane, proposed by S.J. Singer and G.L. Nicolson in 1972, is called the **fluid mosaic model** and it describes the membrane as a fluid bilayer of phospholipids with a mosaic of proteins, cholesterol and carbohydrates associated with it. Phospholipids arrange themselves in a sandwich-like formation, with the fatty acids pointed inward and the polar heads pointed outward. They move rapidly within their layer (or "leaflet"), but only rarely flip to the opposite layer. Higher temperatures increase the fluidity and permeability of the membrane as phospholipids spread apart. (Additionally, a higher proportion of unsaturated fatty acid chains will increase fluidity; conversely saturated chains will decrease fluidity.) Proteins that extend into the hydrophobic interior of the membrane are called integral proteins, while those that are bound to either surface of the membrane are called peripheral proteins. Most proteins can drift slowly in the membrane, but some are fixed in place. Carbohydrates are only found on the exterior of the membrane, and they play a role in cell-cell recognition. They are either bound to a protein (glycoprotein) or a phospholipid (glycolipid). Cholesterol, which is found in the hydrophobic interior of the membrane, acts as a sort of fluidity buffer, restraining phospholipids from spreading or clustering.

Membrane Dynamics

The plasma membrane is not a rigid, static structure; nearly all of the molecules within it are in motion. Phospholipids can change locations without assistance, but certain movements are catalyzed by an enzyme. They can move very rapidly, switching places with adjacent (lateral) phospholipids without the aid of an enzyme. Uncatalyzed transbilayer diffusion (or flip-flopping from one leaflet to the other) is rarer, and occurs at a slow rate. Flippase is an enzyme that catalyzes the transfer of a phospholipid from the extracellular layer to the cytoplasmic layer, and floppase translocates it from the cytoplasmic layer to the extracellular layer. Both enzymes require the expenditure of ATP. Scramblases translocate phospholipids in either direction, and do not require ATP.

Proteins can move laterally, but not transversally, within the membrane. Integral proteins are kept within the membrane by hydrophobic interactions, but most can drift slowly within the membrane. (Some are held to the cytoskeleton and do not move.) Peripheral proteins can drift as well, as they are only loosely (and temporarily) bound to either the lipid bilayer or an integral protein.

Solute Transport Across Membranes

Thermodynamic Considerations

When solutes are transported across the membrane, they can move up or down their concentration gradients. The diffusion of solutes down the electrochemical gradient (passive transport) is a spontaneous and thermodynamically favorable process that results in a negative free energy change ($\Delta G < 0$). Diffusion will continue to occur until a state of dynamic equilibrium has been reached and the concentrations on each side of the membrane are the same. Diffusion illustrates the second law of thermodynamics, as the direction of movement is entropy-driven. Solutes move from high to low concentration, increasing entropy (ΔS). Active transport is the thermodynamically unfavorable process in which solutes are moved up their electrochemical gradients, decreasing entropy as they accumulate on one side of the membrane. Only when it is paired with an exergonic process such as the hydrolysis of ATP can active transport occur. Since energy is consumed, the free energy change is positive ($\Delta G > 0$).

Osmosis

Osmosis is the diffusion of water across a semipermeable membrane. The net movement of water is down its concentration gradient, meaning it will move from an area of higher water concentration to lower, or lower solute concentration to higher. Osmosis can help to restore balance when the solute cannot cross the membrane (or if it can't cross fast enough to maintain homeostasis). When the extracellular fluid has a higher solute concentration as compared to the cytoplasm, the fluid is described as **hypertonic**. Since there are fewer free water molecules surrounding the cell, the net flow of water will be *out* of the cell. When the extracellular fluid has a lower solute concentration as compared to the cytoplasm, the fluid is described as **hypotonic**. Since there are more free water molecules on the extracellular side of the membrane, the net flow of water will be *into* the cell, causing it to swell and in some cases burst. When the extracellular fluid has the same solute concentration as the cytoplasm, the fluid is described as **isotonic**, and water will move in and out of the cell at equal rates.

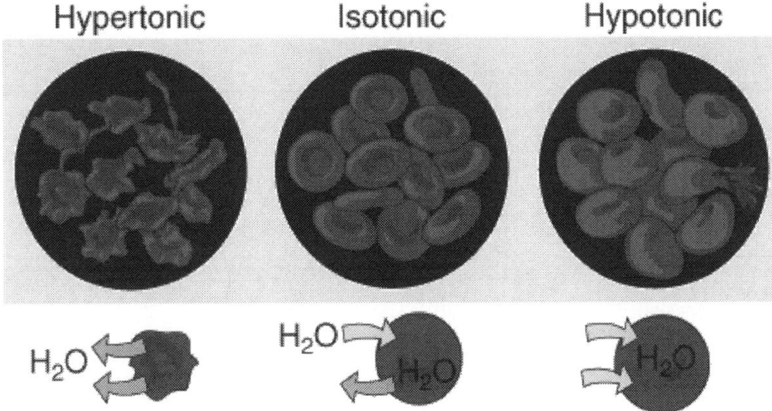

Osmosis: Colligative Properties; Osmotic Pressure

A **colligative property** is a property of a solution that depends only on the *amount* of solute, and not the size, mass, or chemical nature of the solute. Osmotic pressure, the minimum amount of pressure required to stop the diffusion of pure water across the membrane, is a colligative property because it is determined by the concentration of solute, as can be seen in the equation:

$$\pi = iMRT$$

- π = osmotic pressure (in atmospheres)
- i = van't Hoff factor (the number of particles formed from one unit of solute)
- M = molar concentration
- R = ideal gas constant
- T = temperature (in Kelvins)

If a vessel is divided into two chambers by a semipermeable membrane, and pure water placed into one chamber while a solution (such as sugar water) is placed in the other chamber, the water level will rise on the side of greater solute concentration. The diffusion of water will continue in this direction until the osmotic pressure becomes too great. The solute concentration will not have changed, but water will have moved from high to low water concentration.

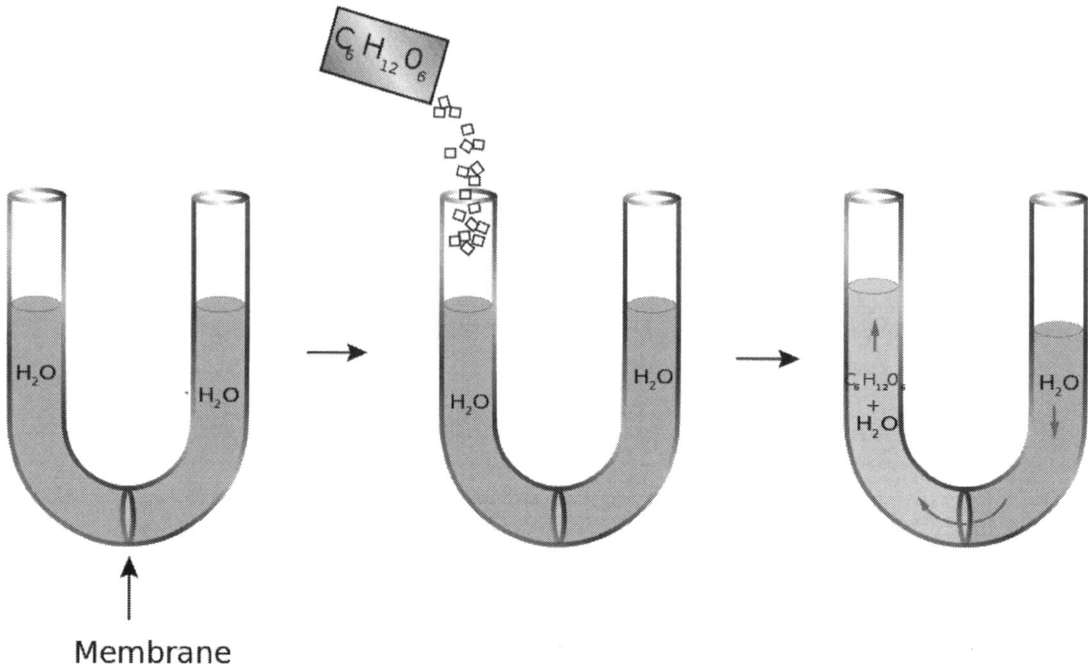

Passive Transport

Passive transport is the movement of substances across a cell membrane without the input of energy. Random motion of particles will lead to the net movement of substances down their concentration gradients in a spontaneous process that leads to an increase in entropy. Simple diffusion, osmosis, and facilitated diffusion are all forms of passive transport. In simple diffusion, substances cross the membrane directly, without the aid of a transport protein. Small, nonpolar molecules such as oxygen gas, carbon dioxide, and uncharged lipids are not repelled by the hydrophobic interior of the membrane.

Osmosis is the passive transport of water across the membrane. Most polar molecules cannot use simple diffusion, but water molecules are small enough to slowly squeeze between the phospholipids. Water can also use channel proteins called aquaporins to increase the rate of osmosis. When proteins are used to transport substances down their concentration gradients, this is called **facilitated diffusion**. Large, polar, and/or charged substances require shielding from the interior of the membrane, and they may use channel or carrier proteins to assist in their transport. None of these processes require ATP, and are driven by the difference in solute concentration.

Review Video: Passive Transport: Diffusion and Osmosis
Visit mometrix.com/academy and enter code: 642038

Active Transport

In **active transport**, energy is used to move solutes into or out of the cell. In most forms of active transport, substances are pumped against their concentration gradients from areas of low to high concentration. Active transport is required for processes such as the maintenance of a membrane potential, and the uptake of glucose by intestinal cells even between meals. In **primary active**

transport, the pumping of solutes by a carrier protein is directly coupled to the hydrolysis of ATP. In this process, the binding of a phosphate group causes a conformational change in the protein, allowing it to transport solutes across the membrane. **Secondary active transport** relies on ATP to generate an electrochemical gradient, and it is this gradient that directly drives the active transport of a different solute. As one solute moves down its gradient, another is pumped up its gradient. When both solutes move in the same direction, it is called **symport**, and when they move in opposite directions, it is called **antiport**.

Endocytosis and **exocytosis** are types of active transport that employ vesicles to import or export substances. While these processes require ATP, they do not necessarily move solutes up their concentration gradients.

ACTIVE TRANSPORT: SODIUM/POTASSIUM PUMP

The **sodium/potassium pump** is a carrier protein that establishes a membrane potential by pumping three sodium ions (Na^+) out of the cell for every two potassium ions (K^+) that are pumped inside. The pump is an ATPase (an enzyme that hydrolyzes ATP) and the binding of a phosphate group causes a conformational change that allows the ions to be transported. Before it is phosphorylated, the pump is open to the cytoplasm and three sodium ions from the inside of the cell bind to it. Phosphorylation of the pump causes it to open to the extracellular side, and the sodium ions are released. The pump now has an affinity for potassium ions. Two potassium ions bind to the pump, stimulating the release of the phosphate group. This causes the protein to return to its original conformation, and the potassium ions are released inside the cell. The pump once again has an affinity for sodium ions and the process repeats. Since three positive ions are removed for every two positive ions that enter, the intracellular space is relatively negative compared to the outside. This contributes to the negative resting membrane potential of the cell. The membrane potential can be thought of as a battery that drives cellular work. It also aids in the functioning of neurons, which rely on a membrane voltage to transmit messages.

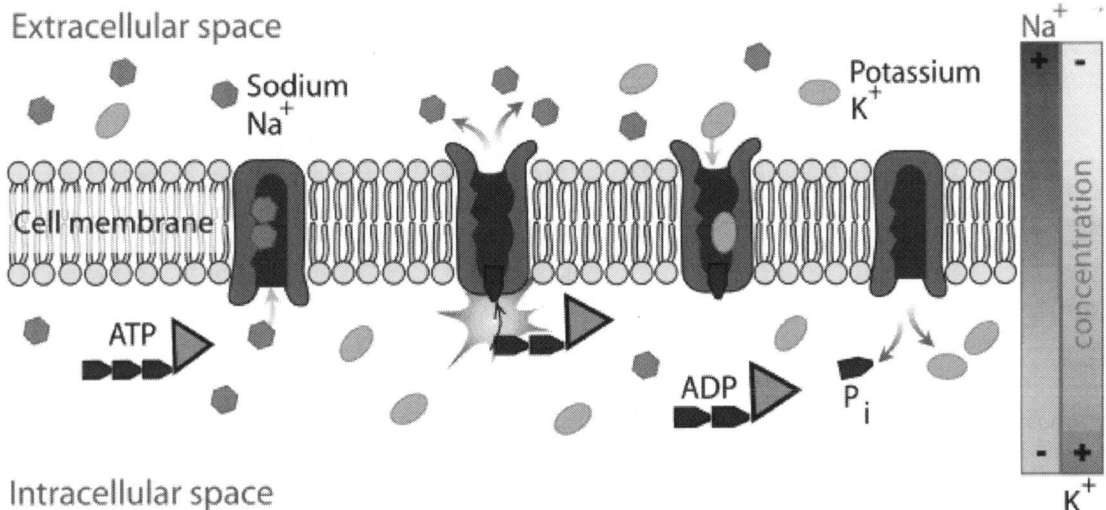

MEMBRANE CHANNELS

Membrane channels belong to a class of transport proteins that form pores to allow the passage of small, charged particles. They are specific to the solutes they transport, and act as a sort of tunnel for particles of a certain size and charge. All channels move substances down their concentration gradient by facilitated diffusion, and therefore do not require energy. Unlike carrier proteins, channels interact very weakly with the solutes they transport, allowing them to move rapidly across the membrane. Channel proteins that allow the passage of water are called aquaporins, and they are always open. Without them, osmosis would occur too slowly to accommodate the needs of the cell. Ion channels, on the other hand, are usually gated; they open and close in response to various stimuli. Voltage-gated channels respond to changes in membrane potential. These types of ion channels are vital to generating electrical impulses in nerve and cardiac cells. Ligand-gated ion channels open in response to the binding of a ligand, such as a hormone or neurotransmitter. Mechanically-gated ion channels respond to a physical stimulus, such as the stretching of the membrane, and are useful in sensory tissues.

Membrane Potential

The **membrane potential** (abbreviated *V* or *E*) is the voltage across a membrane that is determined by the relative concentrations of ions on each side of the membrane, and the permeability of the membrane to those ions. More precisely, it is the electrical potential difference between the inside and outside of a cell. Active transport mechanisms such as the sodium/potassium pump are required to maintain the membrane potential because ions use **leak channels** in an attempt to restore equilibrium. The sodium potassium pump uses ATP to pump three sodium ions out of the cell for every two potassium ions that it pumps into the cell. Most cells have a resting potential of anywhere between −30 and −90 millivolts, depending on cell type. In this state, a cell is polarized. If the inside of the cell becomes relatively positive, the membrane is said to be "depolarized", and if it becomes more negative than its resting potential, it is "hyperpolarized". Membrane potential can be calculated using the Nernst equation:

$$V = \frac{RT}{zF} \ln \frac{[K^+]_o}{[K^+]_i}$$

- V (or E) = membrane potential
- R = ideal gas constant (8.314 $JK^{-1}\,mol^{-1}$)
- T = temperature (Kelvin)
- z = charge on the ion
- F = Faraday's constant (96485 C mol^{-1})
- ln = natural log
- $[K^+]o$ = ion concentration outside the cell
- $[K^+]i$ = ion concentration inside the cell

Membrane Receptors

Membrane receptors are proteins (usually transmembrane) that bind extracellular molecules such as hormones and neurotransmitters. When a ligand binds, it causes a conformational change in the protein. In **ligand-gated ion channels**, the "gate" of the ion channel is opened, allowing ions to cross the membrane. **Enzyme-linked receptors** are receptor proteins that (as the name suggests) act as both receptors and enzymes. When a ligand binds, it stimulates the enzymatic activity of the receptor itself, or an associated protein. **G protein-coupled receptors** (GPCRs) are involved in a process known as signal transduction. When the GPCR changes conformation in response to the binding of a ligand, it triggers a signaling cascade in which a chemical message is passed along from molecule to molecule within the cytoplasm, until the desired response is elicited. For example, when insulin binds to its receptor, it sends a message to the cell to activate the glucose transporter, GLUT4, which aids in the uptake of sugar from the blood. Receptors are highly specific to the ligands they bind.

EXOCYTOSIS AND ENDOCYTOSIS

Endocytosis and exocytosis are types of vesicular transport that are used for the transport of very large particles, or bulk quantities of smaller particles. Both processes are examples of active transport because the transportation and pinching off of vesicles requires energy. (Note that particles are not necessarily moving up their concentration gradients as in other forms of active transport.) During **exocytosis**, cellular products and wastes are transported via vesicle to the cell membrane where the vesicle fuses, releasing its contents into the extracellular environment. Exocytosis is also the means by which certain membrane components (such as glycoproteins and glycolipids) become incorporated into the cell membrane. **Endocytosis** involves the ingestion of fluid, large particles, or target molecules. During this process the cell membrane folds inward, engulfing the material and pinching off into a vesicle. The ingestion of fluids is called **pinocytosis**, and it is non-specific, meaning it takes in any enzymes and nutrients that happen to be available. **Phagocytosis** is the engulfing of particles, sometimes even entire cells. Immune system cells ingest harmful bacteria by phagocytosis before destroying them. **Receptor-mediated endocytosis** is a form of endocytosis that targets certain molecules (such as LDLs, or low-density lipoproteins) that are in low concentration outside the cell. These molecules bind to receptors on the cell membrane, which then invaginates to form a vesicle.

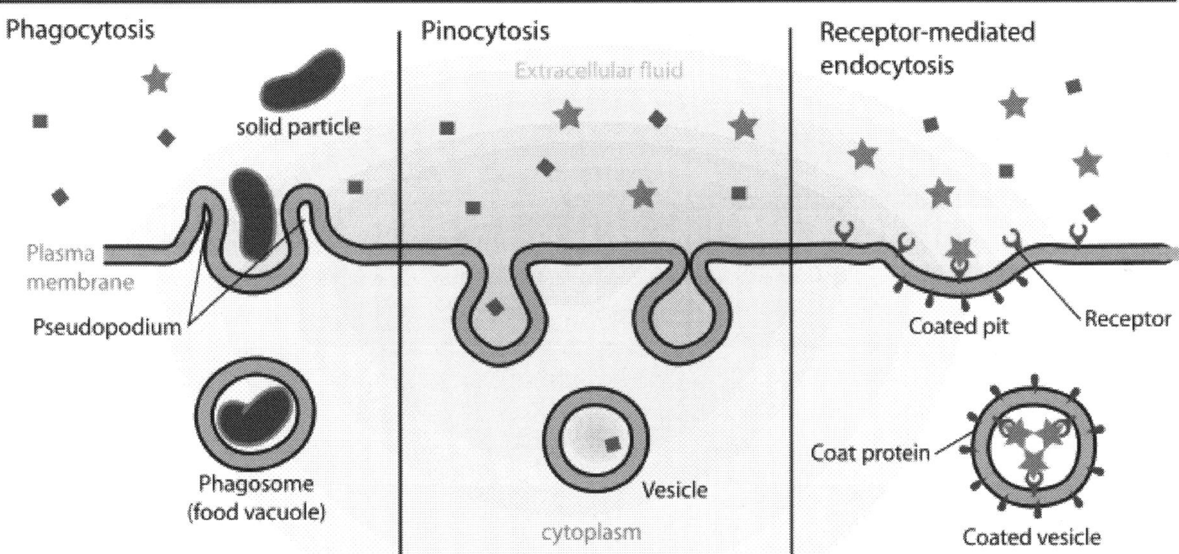

INTERCELLULAR JUNCTIONS

Intercellular junctions are structures that connect adjacent cells within a tissue. There are three main types of cell junctions found in animal tissues: gap junctions, tight junctions, and desmosomes, all of which are made of special proteins called cell adhesion molecules (CAMs).

GAP JUNCTIONS, TIGHT JUNCTIONS, AND DESMOSOMES

Gap junctions are channels for water and solutes (usually ions) that allow adjacent cells to communicate. They are composed of six proteins called connexins that are arranged into a hollow cylinder called a connexon. The connexon of one cell aligns with the connexon of an adjacent cell to form a gap junction. While gap junctions are found in nearly all cell types, they are especially important in cells specialized for conductivity, such as neurons and cardiac cells. **Tight junctions** are often described as leak-proof zippers that tightly seal one cell to another via branched networks of proteins called claudins. These junctions are common in epithelial tissues; particularly those of the digestive system where they help prevent the leakage of digestive enzymes. **Desmosomes** are button-like junctions that give strength and reinforcement to tissues that stretch. They are composed of proteins called cadherins that anchor to intermediate fibers of the cytoskeleton.

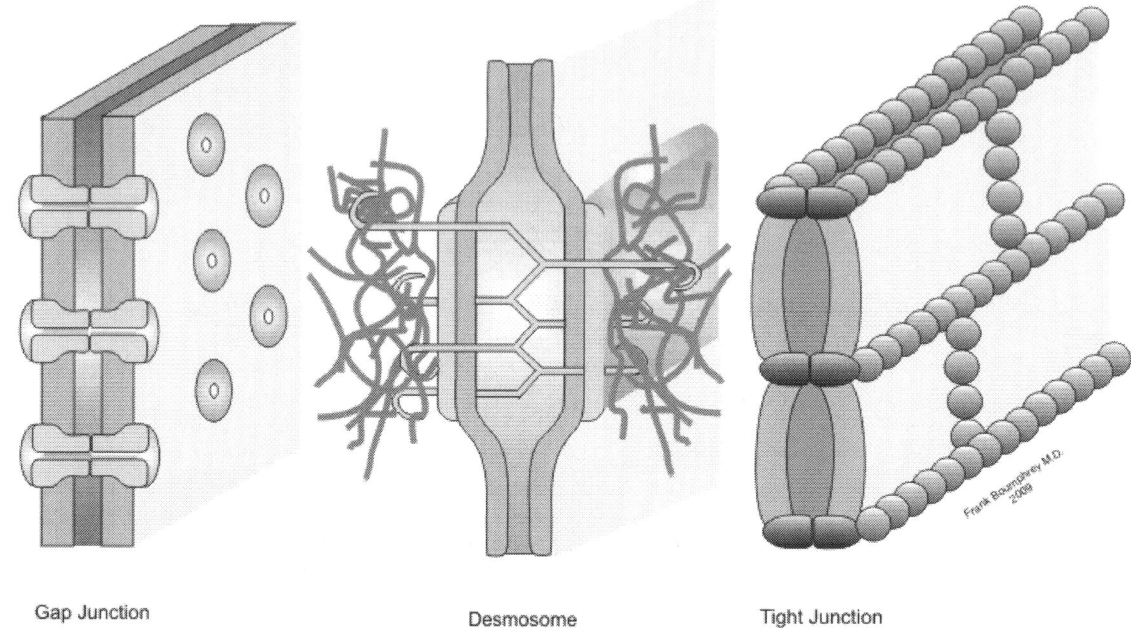

Gap Junction Desmosome Tight Junction

Membrane-Bound Organelles and Defining Characteristics of Eukaryotic Cells

Defining Characteristics of Eukaryotic Cells

Cells can be classified into two main groups based on the presence or absence of a nucleus. In fact, the terms **eukaryote** and **prokaryote** mean "true kernel" and "before the kernel," respectively. The nucleus is a membrane-bound structure that encloses nearly all the genetic material of a eukaryotic cell. Eukaryotic DNA molecules wrap around associated proteins to form linear chromosomes, and the genes within them are regulated by molecules within the nucleoplasm. For this reason, the nucleus is deemed the "control center" of the cell. Eukaryotic cells are also defined by the presence of other membrane-bound organelles, including mitochondria, endoplasmic reticulum, Golgi bodies, peroxisomes, and (in animal cells) lysosomes. Ribosomes and the cytoskeleton are not enclosed by membranes and are found in both prokaryotic and eukaryotic cells. These types of cells also differ in the way that they divide. While prokaryotes reproduce by a simple process called binary fission, eukaryotes undergo a more involved method of division called mitosis. During mitosis, duplicated chromosomes are lined up along the cell's equator and split at the centromere to form two identical daughter nuclei.

Review Video: Eukaryotic and Prokaryotic
Visit mometrix.com/academy and enter code: 231438

Nucleus

Compartmentalization, Storage of Genetic Information

The **nucleus** stores most of a cell's genetic information. (DNA is also found in mitochondria and chloroplasts.) Nuclear DNA is enclosed by the nuclear envelope: a double membrane that is perforated with pores. These pores are made of large protein complexes that regulate the passage of materials including RNA, ribosomal subunits, proteins, ions, and signaling molecules. Enclosed in the double membrane is the nucleoplasm (a semifluid), chromatin (DNA and associated histone proteins), and a non-membranous nucleolus which produces the ribosomal subunits. The inner nuclear membrane is covered by a mesh of protein filaments called the nuclear lamina which stabilizes the nucleus while regulating events such as DNA replication and cell division. The outer membrane is continuous with the endoplasmic reticulum.

The nucleus is responsible for the storage of DNA, and is also the site of DNA replication and transcription (the synthesis of RNA). Since gene expression is regulated largely at the level of transcription, the nucleus plays an important role in coordinating the activities of the cell.

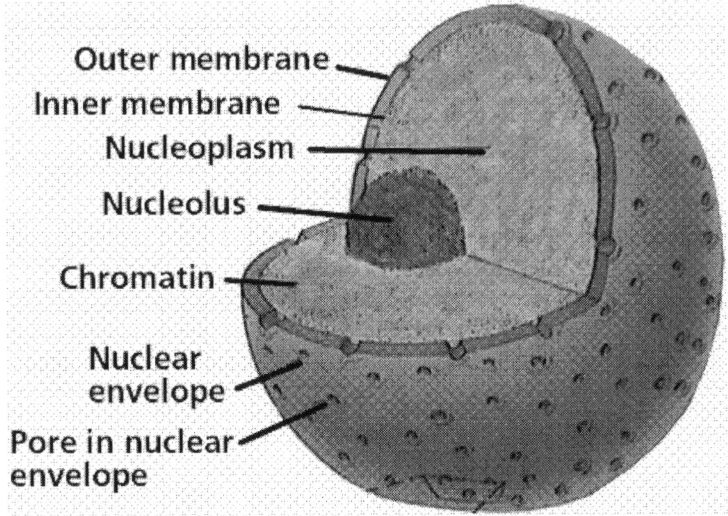

Nucleolus: Location and Function

The **nucleolus** is the largest structure inside the nucleus, and it is responsible for producing ribosomal subunits. It has no membrane, and is made of three regions: two thread-like fibrillar components and one granular component. The fibrillar center (FC) is where the ribosomal RNA genes are located and transcribed. The dense fibrillar center (DFC) processes the pre-rRNA, and the immature ribosomal subunits are assembled in the granular component (GC). All rRNA is synthesized in the nucleolus except the 5S-rRNA which is made in the nucleoplasm before being incorporated into ribosomal subunits. The subunits are exported from the nucleus through the nuclear pores.

The nucleolus disappears early in mitosis (prophase) and reappears in the final stage (telophase). However, it first appears as ten small units at various chromosome sites called nucleolus organizer regions (NORs) before aggregating into one structure.

Nuclear Envelope, Nuclear Pores

The **nuclear envelope** is the double membrane that encloses the nucleus, separating the nucleoplasm from the cytoplasm of the cell. There is a 20–40 nm gap between the two phospholipid bilayers called the perinuclear space, and the membranes are joined at the nuclear pores. Each pore is an octagonal aqueous channel made of hundreds of proteins called nucleoporins. These proteins interact with transporter proteins called karyopherins, which shuttle large molecules like RNA and certain proteins back and forth between the nucleus and the cytoplasm. Smaller molecules and ions are able to diffuse through the pore complex without the aid of a transporter. The pores are essential for the import of the enzymes and nucleotides that are required for DNA synthesis and transcription, and the export of mRNA, tRNA, and ribosomal subunits that are required for translation.

The outer membrane of the nuclear envelope is continuous with the endoplasmic reticulum (ER), and the lumen (inner space) of the ER is open to the perinuclear space. This allows for the easy exchange of materials between the two organelles. The nucleoplasmic side of the inner membrane is lined with a network of protein filaments called the nuclear lamina which supports the nucleus, while aiding in the organization of chromatin.

Mitochondria

Inner and Outer Membrane Structure

Mitochondria are described as the "powerhouses" of the cell because they produce most of a cell's ATP. They have two membranes: the outer membrane, which acts a selective barrier, and the inner membrane where most of the ATP is made. The inner membrane is folded into structures called cristae, and it is within these folds that the electron transport chain of aerobic respiration is located. Between the membranes is the intermembrane space where a proton motive force is used to drive **chemiosmosis**: the synthesis of ATP. The protons that are pumped across the intermembrane space during oxidative phosphorylation re-enter the mitochondrial matrix (the interior of the mitochondrion) through the protein ATP synthase, which is located in the inner membrane. The movement of the protons powers ATP synthase, allowing it to phosphorylate ADP. Inside the matrix are ribosomes and mitochondrial DNA. This DNA carries 37 genes (in humans) that are required for normal mitochondrion function. Mitochondria also play a role in apoptosis, or programmed cell death. Proteins associated with the inner mitochondrial membrane move into the cytoplasm in response to oxidative stress and activate other proteins that begin the degradation of the cell.

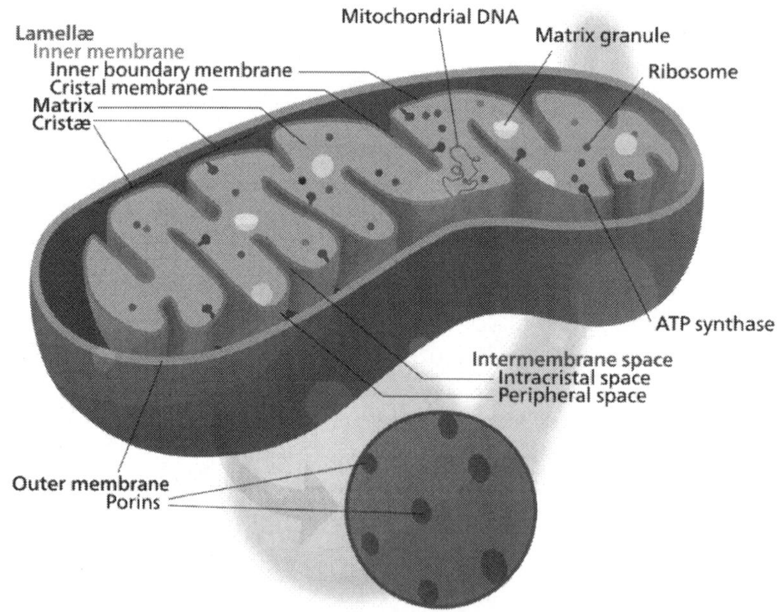

Review Video: Mitochondria
Visit mometrix.com/academy and enter code: 444287

Self-Replication

Mitochondria are described as semi-autonomous because each one has its own genome and ribosomes, and produces many of its own proteins. They also replicate in a manner similar to that of bacteria; they copy their circular DNA molecules before undergoing fission. However, mitochondria do rely on nuclear genes to produce many of the proteins required for DNA replication and other processes. These proteins are imported from the cytosol.

While the mitochondria are not fully autonomous, it is likely that they evolved from an autonomous heterotrophic prokaryote that established a symbiotic relationship with an ancestral host cell. It was probably engulfed by the host cell (hence the double membrane) and provided that cell with ATP. (This is known as the endosymbiont theory.) Its similarity to bacteria, both in structure and manner of reproduction, suggests that mitochondria were once free-living prokaryotes.

Lysosomes: Membrane-Bound Vesicles Containing Hydrolytic Enzymes

Lysosomes are organelles that function in the breakdown of various substances. They bud from the Golgi apparatus, and enclose hydrolytic enzymes that would damage the cell if not separated from the cytosol. These enzymes are active at a low pH of around 5, so hydrogen ions are pumped into the lysosome to maintain the acidic environment. Lysosomes play a vital role in cell homeostasis by dismantling various substrates and nonfunctioning intracellular components, and recycling them in a process called autophagy. Many of the substances destined for degradation are contained in a double-membrane vesicle called an autophagosome. Lysosomes can fuse with these (and with other vesicles created by endocytosis) releasing their enzymes and digesting the contents. Other substances can be transported into the lysosome directly by crossing the membrane. If enough lysosomes are damaged, the cell undergoes apoptosis, and in cases of severe damage, necrosis. Mutations of the hydrolases within the lysosomes are associated with a number of lysosomal storage diseases, including Tay Sachs.

Endoplasmic Reticulum

Rough and Smooth Components

Both the rough and smooth endoplasmic reticulum consist of a series of continuous membranes called cisternae, but each type of ER differs in both in structure and function.

The **rough ER** is continuous with the nuclear envelope, and its ribosome-studded cisternae have the appearance of flattened sacs. The ribosomes synthesize polypeptides which are then guided into the lumen of the rough ER before being modified, packaged in a vesicle, and sent to different regions within the cell, often the Golgi apparatus. The Golgi can then further modify the proteins and sort them based on their destinations. Many are shipped out of the cell via exocytosis.

The cisternae of the **smooth ER** are more tubular in shape than the rough ER, and they lack ribosomes. These membranes are continuous with the rough ER and the nucleus. Smooth ER is involved in many tasks, including the synthesis of lipids such as phospholipids and cholesterol. The smooth ER of liver cells detoxifies drugs, and the smooth ER of the muscles regulates and stores calcium ions.

Rough Endoplasmic Reticulum Site of Ribosomes

Secretory proteins (proteins destined to be exported from the cell) and proteins that are associated with the plasma membrane are synthesized on ribosomes that are bound to the cytoplasmic side of the rough endoplasmic reticulum. These ribosomes are not permanently fixed, and will bind to sites called translocons. Ribosomes that are free in the cytosol are very similar in structure to bound ribosomes, but the proteins they produce remain in the cytosol of the cell. As a polypeptide chain is growing out of a bound ribosome during translation, the chain is fed through a tiny pore into the lumen of the rough ER, where it folds into its proper conformation. Any proteins that do not fold properly into their native shape are recycled. Enzymes in the lumen may modify proteins by covalently bonding a carbohydrate to form a glycoprotein. (The Golgi continues the posttranslational modification of proteins.) Proteins that are shipped to other parts of the cell are first packaged into transport vesicles, and the vesicle will fuse with its target.

MEMBRANE STRUCTURE

The **endoplasmic reticulum** constitutes roughly half of all the plasma membrane in a cell. The membrane system of the rough ER is connected to the outer nuclear membrane, forming flattened sacs (cisternae) that connect to each other in a manner that resembles a multi-story parking garage. These helicoidal sheets are called **Terasaki ramps**. Newly synthesized proteins are packaged in transport vesicles that are coated with protein complexes that help direct each vesicle to its destination. (COPII coating proteins, for example, coat vesicles that fuse with the cis face of the Golgi apparatus.) These vesicles bud from a region of the ER known as transitional ER, where there are few ribosomes. The smooth ER lacks ribosomes altogether, and has a branched tubular structure. Some of these tubules fuse with one another.

ROLE IN MEMBRANE BIOSYNTHESIS

Both the smooth and rough endoplasmic reticulum are involved in membrane biosynthesis. Enzymes in the smooth ER (or SER) synthesize phospholipids by joining two fatty acid chains to a molecule of glycerol. This occurs on the cytoplasmic side of the membrane. The SER is also the site of another important membrane lipid, cholesterol, which serves as a membrane fluidity buffer. The rough ER is considered the "membrane factory" of the cell because it also produces phospholipids. These lipids are then inserted into the RER's own membrane so that vesicles can bud from it and eventually fuse with the plasma membrane and other parts of the endomembrane system. Ribosomes on the RER produce the integral proteins that are incorporated into the plasma membrane of the cell, or the membranes that enclose organelles.

ROLE IN BIOSYNTHESIS OF SECRETED PROTEINS

Proteins that are to be secreted from the cell, as well as integral membrane proteins, are produced by ribosomes that are bound to the rough ER, but initially these ribosomes are free-floating in the cytosol. They are directed to the RER before translation of the protein is complete. The growing polypeptide has a "signal sequence" of amino acids on the N-terminus of the chain. This sequence is recognized by a signal-recognition particle (SRP) which carries the polypeptide and ribosome to a receptor on the rough ER. The signal sequence contains a series of hydrophobic amino acids that helps the unfolded protein to pass through the RER membrane into the lumen. Once inside the lumen, the signal sequence is cleaved off, and the protein folds into its native shape. It is then packaged into a vesicle for shipment.

GOLGI APPARATUS: GENERAL STRUCTURE AND ROLE IN PACKAGING AND SECRETION

The **Golgi apparatus** consists of a series of curved, flattened sacs called cisternae. The cis face (the stack that is nearest to the ER) receives vesicles sent by the RER that contain immature proteins. The vesicles fuse with the membrane and release the proteins into the Golgi. The proteins then move from stack to stack, budding off a new vesicle which fuses with the next cisterna layer each time. During their travels, the proteins are modified by an assortment of Golgi enzymes. Proteins that were glycosylated in the ER may have some of their sugar residues removed, or more may be added. Sulfate and phosphate groups may be added as well. These "tags" influence the structure and function of the protein, and also aid in the sorting and delivery of these proteins to their destinations. The proteins are packaged into vesicles that bud from the trans face (or exit face) of the Golgi. Some of these proteins are secreted from the cell through exocytosis, while others become part of the cell membrane. Still others serve as hydrolytic enzymes inside lysosomes.

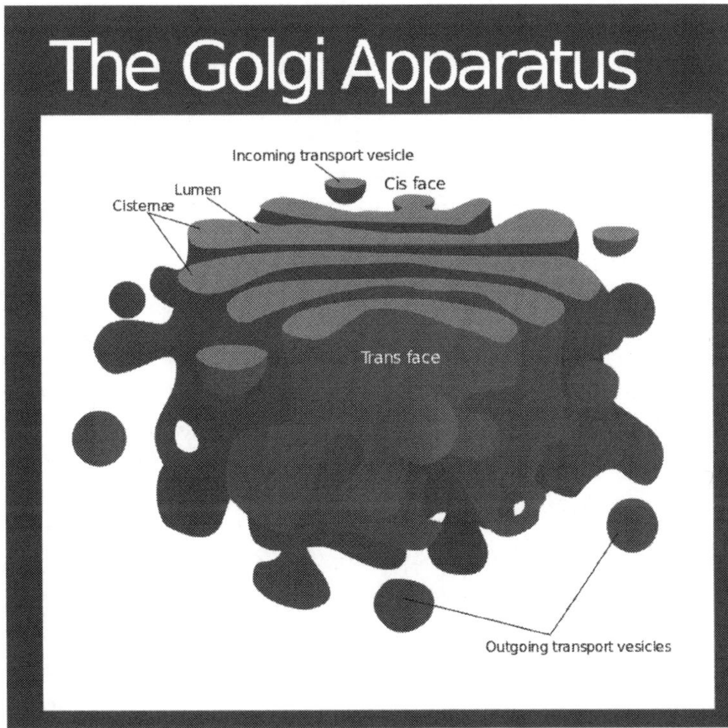

Peroxisomes: Organelles That Collect Peroxides

Peroxisomes are structurally similar to lysosomes; they are both membranous sacs filled with many types of enzymes. But unlike lysosomes, peroxisomes are found in all types of eukaryotic cells, and they can replicate independently using proteins that are imported from the cytosol. Their enzymes also function at a higher pH. Peroxisomes function in many metabolic processes, including biosynthesis of lipids, detoxification of alcohol, and the oxidation of amino acids and very long chain fatty acids. These oxidation reactions produce hydrogen peroxide (H_2O_2) as a byproduct, which is toxic to cells. Peroxisomes contain an enzyme called catalase that is able to break hydrogen peroxide down into water and oxygen gas. They also contain some of the enzymes involved in the pentose phosphate pathway, which produces NADPH to be used in reductive biosynthesis reactions.

Cytoskeleton

General Function in Cell Support and Movement

The **cytoskeleton** is a membraneless structure found in all cell types, and it is made of various types of protein fibers. In eukaryotes, the cytoskeleton has three major components: microfilaments, intermediate fibers, and microtubules. While the cytoskeleton is known for its role in cell shape and structure, it is also involved in the movement of materials within the cell, and movement of the cell itself. The cytoskeleton is dynamic and can extend and retract, allowing cells to maintain their shape, or change shape as needed. The network of protein fibers stabilizes most of the organelles, and also provides a "railway" for motor proteins to use to direct vesicles to their destinations. Components of the cytoskeleton help anchor the cell to neighboring cells, and in some cases, form extensions such as cilia and flagella that aid in cell movement. Cell division would be impossible without the cytoskeleton, as it is used to separate sister chromatids, and also pinches the cell into daughter cells during cytokinesis.

Microfilaments: Composition and Role in Cleavage and Contractility

Microfilaments are the thinnest components of the cytoskeleton, averaging about 6 to 8 nm in diameter. They are composed of protein molecules called actin that join together to form two rod-like polymers which twist around each other to form flexible tension-bearing filaments. These filaments organize into either bundles or networks, and they are involved in maintaining cell shape and events like cytokinesis, muscle contraction, and movement of the cell itself.

During cytokinesis, a cleavage furrow is formed through the contraction of microfilaments. These microfilaments are organized into a ring shape which decreases in size as they contract.

The cytoplasm is constricted until the original cell pinches into two daughter cells. Microfilaments are also involved in muscle contraction. The protein myosin binds to actin filaments forming myofibrils. The two components slide past each other as the cell contracts, and the muscle shortens. Microfilaments also aid in the gross movement of a cell by elongating the plus end (actin polymerization) while shortening the minus end (actin depolymerization).

Microtubules: Composition and Role in Support and Transport

Microtubules are the thickest components of the cytoskeleton (around 25 nm in diameter). They are made of a globular protein known as tubulin, which is a dimer made of α-tubulin and β-tubulin. These dimers stack upon each other to form linear rows called protofilaments, and 13 of these protofilaments arrange themselves in a ring to form a hollow tube. Microtubules can lengthen and shorten by polymerization and depolymerization of the tubulin dimers. They extend throughout the cell, helping the cell to resist compressional forces, while also providing a framework for motor proteins to travel on. Kinesins are motor proteins that tend to "walk" toward the plus end of the microtubule and dyneins travel toward the minus end. Many of these motor proteins carry vesicles to their destinations. Microtubules are also the major components of the mitotic spindle which segregates sister chromatids during mitosis. Cilia and flagella are also formed from microtubules which group together in nine pairs that surround a central pair.

Intermediate Filaments, Role in Support

Intermediate fibers are components of the cytoskeleton that are thinner than microtubules but thicker than microfilaments (about 10 nm in diameter). They are composed of over fifty types of proteins, and the types of proteins are specific to certain types of cells. For example, microfilaments made of keratin are found in epithelial cells, and microfilaments made of desmin are found in muscle cells. Lamins are proteins that form the microfilaments that line the inside portion of the nuclear envelope. Unlike their cytoskeletal counterparts, they are not polar, and they are not directly responsible for cell movement. They appear to only play a role in support. They help cells adhere to one another at cell junctions known as desmosomes, and also help to anchor the nucleus and other organelles. Intermediate filaments are specialized to withstand tensile forces, and thereby help to prevent cell distortion under mechanical stress. They do not polymerize and depolymerize the way that microtubules and microfilaments do.

Composition and Function of Cilia and Flagella

Both cilia and flagella are structures made of microtubules that extend from some types of cells. In eukaryotic cells, these microtubules are doubled up into pairs, and nine doublets form a ring around a central pair (the "9 + 2" arrangement). Each cilium and flagellum is about 0.25 μm in diameter, but flagella are usually much longer than cilia. Cilia are almost always found in high numbers, while cells rarely have more than a few flagella. Both structures are able to "wave" back and forth through the action of motor proteins called dyneins.

Some cells use cilia for locomotion while cells that are fixed within a tissue may use cilia to sweep materials along the surface. Ciliated cells of the respiratory tract move mucus out of the lungs, and cells of the female reproductive tract use cilia to mobilize the egg. Some cilia can even detect signals and transmit information to the inside of the cell. When cilia move, they do so in back-and-forth strokes, much like oars on a rowboat.

Flagella move differently; they are more whip-like with an undulating, beating pattern. Unlike cilia, they are only used for locomotion. Each human sperm uses a flagellum to move, and (like cilia) they can be found in many types of protists.

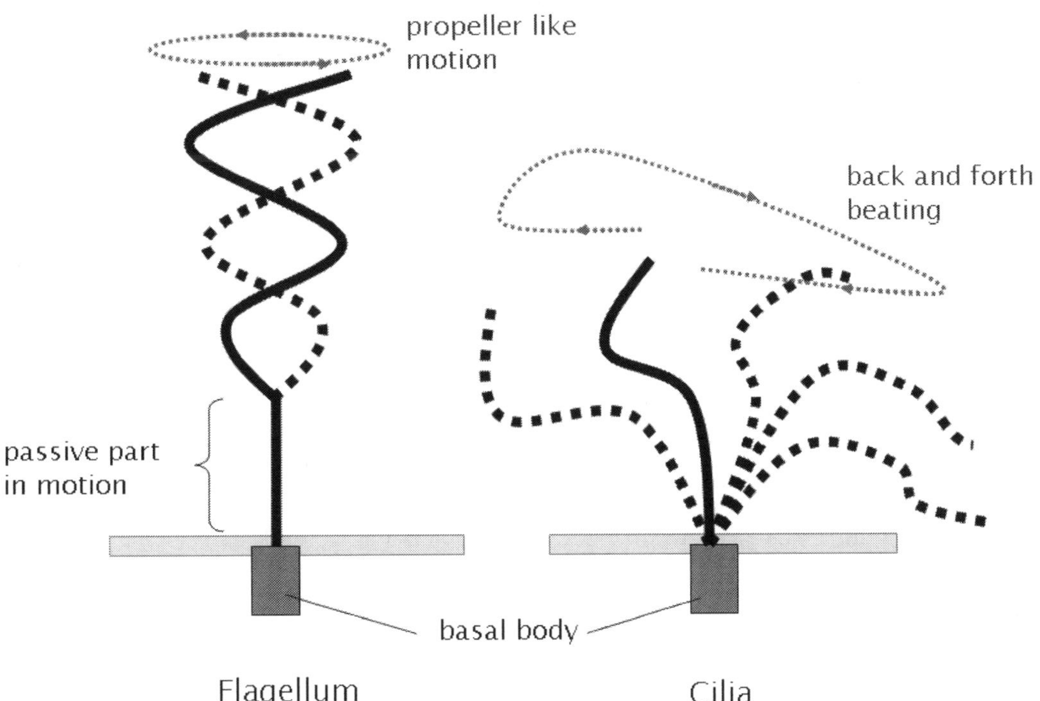

Centrioles, Microtubule Organizing Centers

Centrioles are cylindrical structures that are formed from nine triplets of microtubules arranged in a circle around a hollow center. In animal cells, two perpendicular centrioles form an organelle called a **centrosome**. Other types of eukaryotic cells have simple centrosomes, but only animal cells use centrioles to organize their microtubules. Centrosomes are typically found near the nucleus, but they migrate to opposite poles of the cell during cell division. Microtubules extend from the centrioles as the plus ends grow toward the metaphase plate, forming the spindle fibers of the mitotic spindle. Polar fibers extend from one centrosome to the other, while kinetochore fibers attach to the chromosomes, pulling the sister chromatids apart during anaphase.

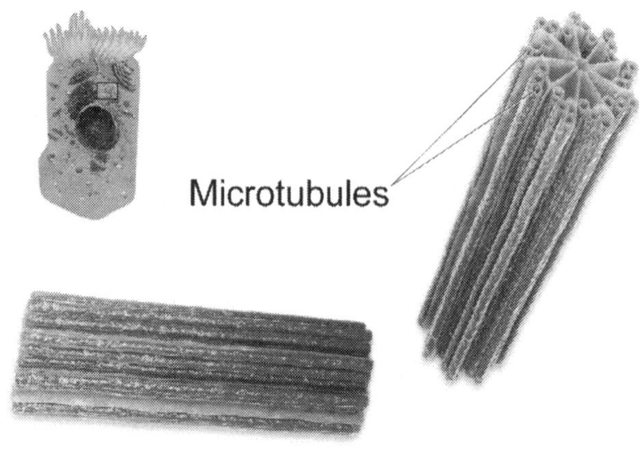

Centrioles

Tissues Formed from Eukaryotic Cells

Epithelial Cells

Epithelial cells come in a variety of shapes and functions, but they share the characteristic of being avascular. They are nourished by the diffusion of oxygen and nutrients from capillaries in the underlying layer of connective tissue called the basement membrane. Epithelial tissues are the lining and covering tissues of the body, and depending on their location may be involved in protection, absorption, secretion, and/or filtration. These tissues are classified according to the shape and arrangement of their cells:

Cell Shape	
flattened, scale-like	squamous
cube-shaped	Cuboidal
long, thin	Columnar
Arrangement	
single layer of cells	simple epithelia
appearance of multiple layers as a result of differences in cell shape and location	pseudostratified
multiple layers of cells	stratified epithelia

There are **many** types of epithelial tissues in the body. Stratified squamous epithelial tissues are found in locations that experience friction, such as the mouth, esophagus, and exterior skin. Simple columnar epithelia line the digestive tract, and harbor mucus-producing goblet cells. Simple squamous epithelia form membranes where filtration or diffusion occurs, such as the alveoli of the lungs. These are merely a few examples.

Connective Tissue Cells

Connective tissues are the most abundant tissues in the body. Most connective tissues are highly vascular, the exceptions being ligaments, tendons, and cartilage. In general, they support and protect the body, and are characterized by the presence of a nonliving matrix. This matrix is secreted by the cells of the connective tissue and it consists of ground substance (water, proteins, and carbohydrates) and protein fibers such as collagen, elastin, or reticular fibers. The consistency of these connective tissues varies greatly from one tissue type to another. Blood is a connective tissue made of blood cells and plasma, and it transports oxygen, carbon dioxide, nutrients, and wastes. Adipose tissue is made of fat cells that cushion and insulate the body. Osseous tissue, or bone, consists of osteocytes surrounded by a hard matrix of calcium salts and collagen. Cartilage, like bone, is a connective tissue that provides support, but it is made of cells called chondrocytes, and is more flexible. Ligaments and tendons are made of dense fibrous connective tissue, which is made mostly of collagen fibers.

The Structure, Growth, Physiology, and Genetics of Prokaryotes and Viruses

Cell Theory

History and Development and Impact on Biology

Before the invention of the microscope, it was unknown that living organisms were composed of cells. But the observations of Robert Hooke, Anton van Leeuwenhoek, Matthias Schleiden, Theodor Schwann, and Rudolph Virchow helped to form one of the most basic principles in biology: the cell theory. In 1665, Hooke constructed a primitive compound microscope and viewed, for the first time, what he termed "cells" in a sample of cork. Leeuwenhoek was the first to observe living cells (protists in pond water). Schleiden noted that plants were made entirely of cells (and cellular products) and Schwann expanded this observation to animals. At this time (1839) it was unclear how cells were formed. Virchow believed that cells did not form spontaneously, and rather came from the division of pre-existing cells. Together, these observations formed the cell theory:

- All living organisms are made of one or more cells
- The cell is the basic unit of life
- All cells arise from pre-existing cells

This theory has been modernized to include the fact that cells contain hereditary information, and pass it on during cell division. The cell theory forms the foundation of modern biology. It has helped scientists to understand how cells function, allowing for advances in biotechnology and medicine.

Classification and Structure of Prokaryotic Cells

Prokaryotic Domains

A three-domain system is used to classify all living organisms. These domains are Archaea, Bacteria, and Eukarya. The cell(s) of the organisms within the domain Eukarya are eukaryotic, and therefore have a nucleus and membrane-bound organelles. This domain includes the kingdoms Plantae, Animalia, Fungi, and Protista. The domains Archaea and Bacteria consist of single-celled organisms called prokaryotes. Prokaryotes share a common structure; they have a single circular chromosome that is *not* enclosed in a nucleus (it is concentrated in the nucleoid region), nor do they have membrane-bound organelles. They divide by binary fission, and do not have a mitotic spindle. They do have ribosomes (though they are smaller than eukaryotic ribosomes) and a plasma membrane, and are surrounded by a cell wall. They also have a primitive cytoskeleton. Prior to the 1970's, all prokaryotes were classified as a single kingdom (Monera) but research has shown that archaea and bacteria each have a distinct line of descent.

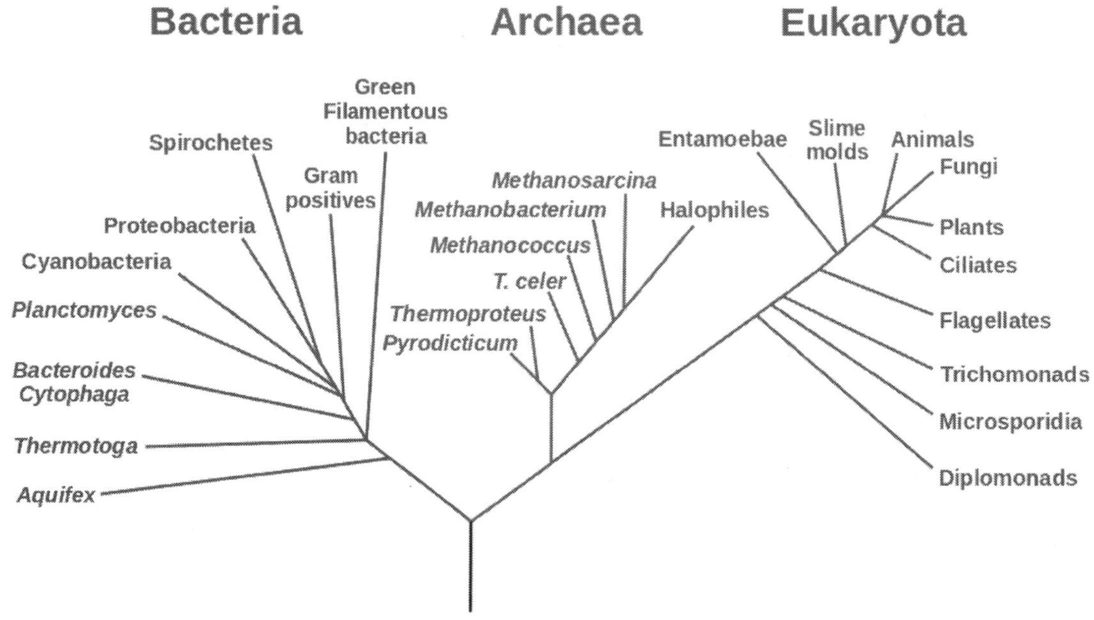

ARCHAEA VS. BACTERIA

Archaea and Bacteria both consist of unicellular prokaryotic organisms. They do not possess a nucleus or membrane-bound organelles, but they do have ribosomes, a single circular chromosome, a plasma membrane, and a cell wall. Despite these similarities, the two groups are quite different, hence the grouping into separate domains. Unlike that of bacteria, the hereditary material of archaea contains introns, and histone-like proteins are used to organize the DNA. The composition of ribosomal RNA and the cell wall is also different (only bacterial cells have peptidoglycan in their cell walls). Archaea are associated with extreme environments because many species have the ability to thrive in harsh conditions (high salt concentrations, extreme temperatures or pH, etc.). Many of them are chemosynthetic and can extract energy from inorganic sources. But archaea are not limited to extreme habitats. Some species even live in the human body, but pose no pathogenic threat. Bacteria can be beneficial to humans, but can also cause disease.

MAJOR CLASSIFICATIONS OF BACTERIA BY SHAPE

The three major classifications of bacteria by morphology are: bacilli, spirilla, and cocci.

Bacilli are rod-shaped bacteria, and may be gram-positive or gram-negative depending on the species. They can occur as a single bacillus, pairs called diplobacilli, or chains called streptobacilli. There are also oval-shaped bacilli called coccobacilli. Common examples of bacilli include *Listeria*, *Bacillus*, *Escherichia*, and *Salmonella*.

Spirilla are gram-negative, and have a spiral shape that may or may not be flexible depending on the type. Spirochetes are flexible, and have internal flagella. *Borrelia* are spirochetes that are responsible for Lyme disease. Spirilla, such as *Helicobacter*, are more rigid, and their flagella are external.

Cocci are spherical bacteria. They can be gram-positive or negative, and have many possible arrangements: pairs (diplococci), chains (streptococci), clusters of 4 (tetrads), cubes of 8 (sarcina), and irregular clusters (staphylococci). *Staphylococcus aureus* and *streptococcus pneumoniae* are cocci that are associated with infection.

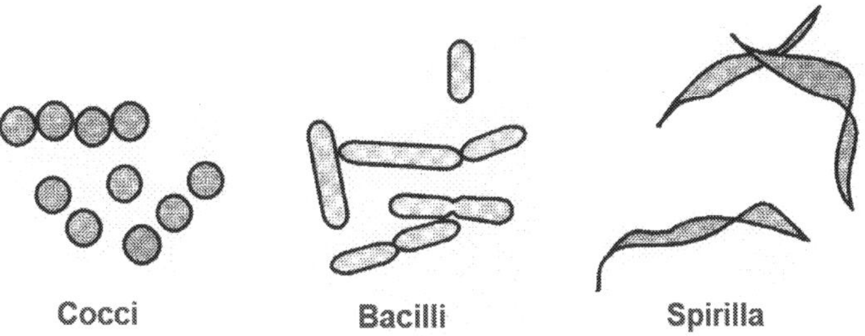

Presence of Cell Wall in Bacteria

The cells of plants, fungi, archaea, and bacteria have cell walls that vary in composition. The cell wall of a bacterium is made of a polymer of polysaccharides (glycosaminoglycan) and peptide chains called peptidoglycan (or murein). The thickness of this mesh differs between gram-positive and gram-negative bacteria. Gram-positive bacteria have up to 40 layers of peptidoglycan that surround a phospholipid bilayer (together these are called the **envelope**). The cell wall of gram-positive bacteria can be up to 100 nm thick. Gram-negative bacteria have far fewer layers, with a thickness of up to 10 nm. They also have an outer membrane that surrounds the cell wall, in addition to the inner membrane. The cell walls of gram-positive bacteria stain purple when stained with a Gram stain, and gram-negative bacteria stain pink. The cell wall gives strength and support to the cell, but is flexible enough to allow for growth and fission. It also helps to regulate the passage of materials by acting as a filter.

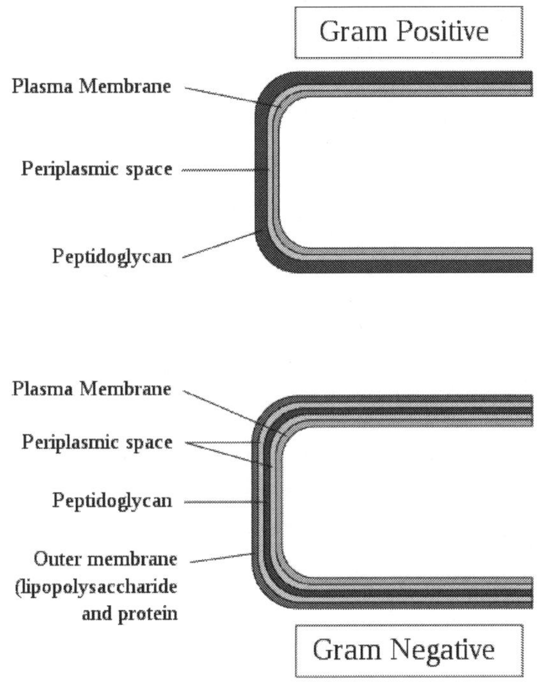

Flagellar Propulsion, Mechanism

A **flagellum** is a whip-like structure that many types of cells use for locomotion. A bacterial flagellum is made of a single filament (composed of the protein flagellin) with a diameter of about 20 nm, and a hollow central channel. A hook connects this filament to a complex structure called the **basal body**. The basal body is embedded in the plasma membrane and acts as a motor that can rotate clockwise or counterclockwise. The torque on the filament causes it to move. This process is powered by a proton motive force; the greater the concentration gradient, the greater the flow of hydrogen ions across the bacterial plasma membrane, and the faster it rotates. Bacteria can detect various chemicals and use flagellar propulsion to propel bacteria toward or away from the source of these chemicals. This is called **chemotaxis**.

The structure and mechanism for propulsion is different for bacteria than it is for archaea and eukaryotes. The flagella of archaea and eukaryotes are powered by ATP, not a proton motive force. Eukaryotic flagella are hollow and made of microtubules, while the flagella of archaea are solid, and made of many different types of proteins.

Growth and Physiology of Prokaryotic Cells

Reproduction by Fission

Bacteria reproduce asexually in a process known as **binary fission**. To prepare for this process, a bacterium must grow in volume and enlarge its membrane and cell wall. It replicates its circular chromosome, beginning at the origin of replication and continuing until the entire loop is copied. Each chromosome attaches to the membrane, and the cell wall and membrane grow inward at the middle to form a transverse septum with a replicated chromosome on each side. Other components such as ribosomes are randomly distributed to each daughter cell. Unlike in mitosis, there is no formation of a spindle apparatus. Each daughter cell is identical to the parent cell. Sometimes, cytokinesis is incomplete, and the cells remain attached to each other to form arrangements such as doublets, tetrads, and chains.

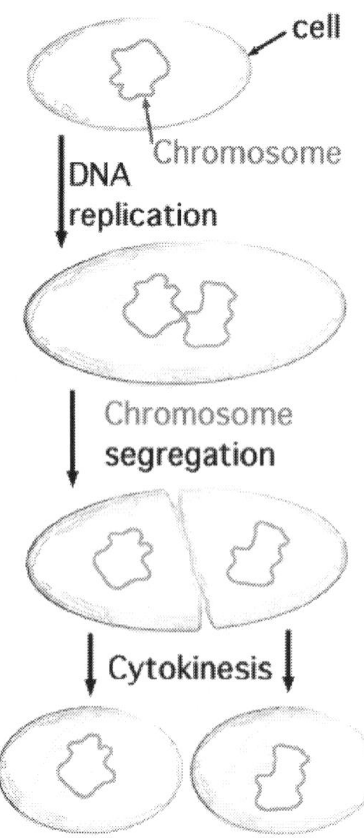

High Degree of Genetic Adaptability, Acquisition of Antibiotic Resistance

Bacteria, despite reproducing asexually, have a high degree of genetic adaptability. Random **mutations** in their DNA can give rise to genetically unique offspring. Depending on the location of that mutation, it could impart antibiotic resistance to the mutant. Bacteria can also exchange DNA with one another in a process called **conjugation**. The donor bacterium uses a narrow tube called a pilus to attach to the recipient bacterium before transferring a plasmid: a small piece of circular DNA. The plasmid often carries favorable genes, such as antibiotic resistance. Bacteria can also acquire new genes through **transformation**. In this process, the cells uptake fragments of DNA that are present in the surroundings (often left over from dead cells). The foreign DNA can be incorporated into the bacterial chromosome and expressed. Finally, **transduction**, or the injection of viral DNA from a bacteriophage, can also alter the bacterial genome.

Exponential Growth

The growth curve of a typical population of bacteria under favorable conditions has an exponential phase, but it usually begins with a lag phase. The **lag phase** occurs when the bacteria are introduced to a new environment. The population remains unchanged as they acclimate to the conditions, grow in size, metabolize nutrients, and perform normal functions. During the **exponential** (or log) **phase**, they divide regularly by binary fission. One cell produces two, then four, eight, sixteen, etc. This exponential growth can only continue until resources become limited and metabolic end products accumulate. This plateau in the growth curve is called the **stationary phase**. The **death phase** shows a decline in the population as the bacteria start to die off at a rate similar to the division rate in the exponential phase.

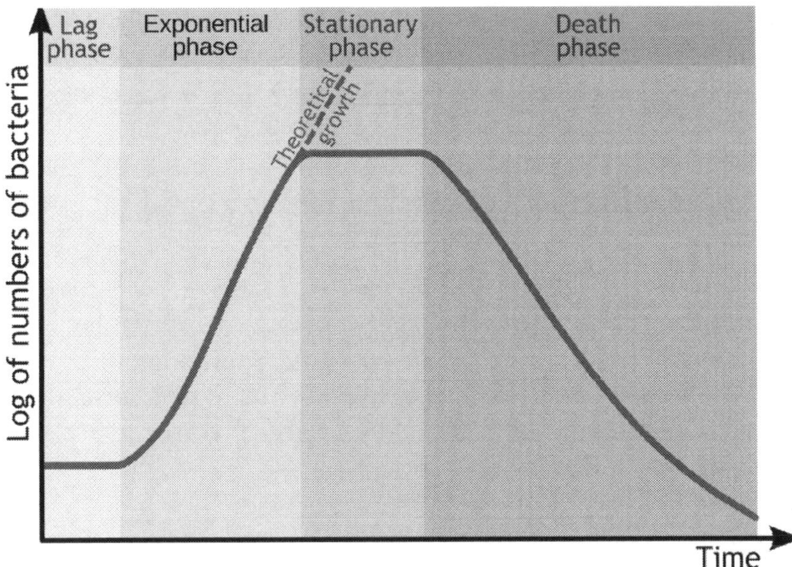

Existence of Anaerobic and Aerobic Variants

Bacteria can be classified into groups based on their response to oxygen. **Obligate aerobes** are bacteria that require oxygen for their metabolism. Like humans, they use glycolysis, the citric acid cycle, and oxidative phosphorylation to extract energy from organic compounds. **Obligate anaerobes**, on the other hand, cannot survive in the presence of oxygen because they lack the enzymes that protect them from oxidative damage, and must rely on either fermentation or anaerobic respiration to obtain energy. Anaerobic respiration, like aerobic respiration, involves glycolysis, the citric acid cycle, and an electron transport chain, but there is no oxidative phosphorylation. That is, oxygen is not reduced, but rather an alternative electron acceptor such as sulfate or nitrate is used. In fermentation, energy is extracted without the citric acid cycle or an electron transport chain. **Aerotolerant anaerobes** can tolerate oxygen, but do not use it in their metabolic processes. **Microaerophiles** do require oxygen, but can only survive in low concentrations. **Facultative anaerobes** can use aerobic respiration in the presence of oxygen, but can switch to fermentation or anaerobic respiration when oxygen is absent.

Parasitic and Symbiotic

Many species of bacteria can establish relationships that can benefit their host, but others can be harmful. Pathogenic bacteria grow at the expense of their host. They produce harmful toxins that result in diseases such as tetanus, tuberculosis, meningitis, and chlamydia. But far more common are mutualistic and commensal bacteria. Mutualistic bacteria benefit from their host, and the host is helped rather than harmed. For example, some bacteria in the human body keep the growth of harmful bacterial species in check. Other species in the digestive tract aid in digestion and synthesize B and K vitamins. There are also bacteria that exist in a commensalistic relationship and do not affect their host at all. *Streptococcus pyogenes* is a species that can thrive in certain body locations without causing harm, but a change in environment can lead to a variety of infections such as strep throat and impetigo.

Chemotaxis

Chemotaxis is the movement of an organism (often a bacterium) in response to a chemical stimulus. The direction, but not rate, of motion is determined by the concentration gradient of the chemical. In positive chemotaxis, a bacterium moves toward a favorable stimulus such as food, while in negative chemotaxis it moves away from an unfavorable stimulus such as a toxin. The direction of motion is controlled by signal transduction processes. Receptor proteins at one or both poles of the cell relay information about the chemical to the inside of the bacterium through a series of reactions. The end result is usually a change in the direction of flagellar rotation.

Genetics of Prokaryotic Cells

Existence of Plasmids, Extragenomic DNA

Many bacteria contain **extragenomic DNA**: DNA that is outside of their single chromosome. Plasmids, for example, are small circular strands of DNA that replicate independently and are passed onto daughter cells during cell division. (Some types of plasmids called episomes *can* get integrated into the bacterial chromosome.) While plasmids often contain genes that impart desirable traits such as antibiotic resistance or the ability to metabolize certain substances, they are rarely needed for survival under favorable conditions. A cell can contain anywhere from one to hundreds of copies of a plasmid. Sometimes, there are different types of plasmids within the same cell, assuming the plasmids are "compatible."

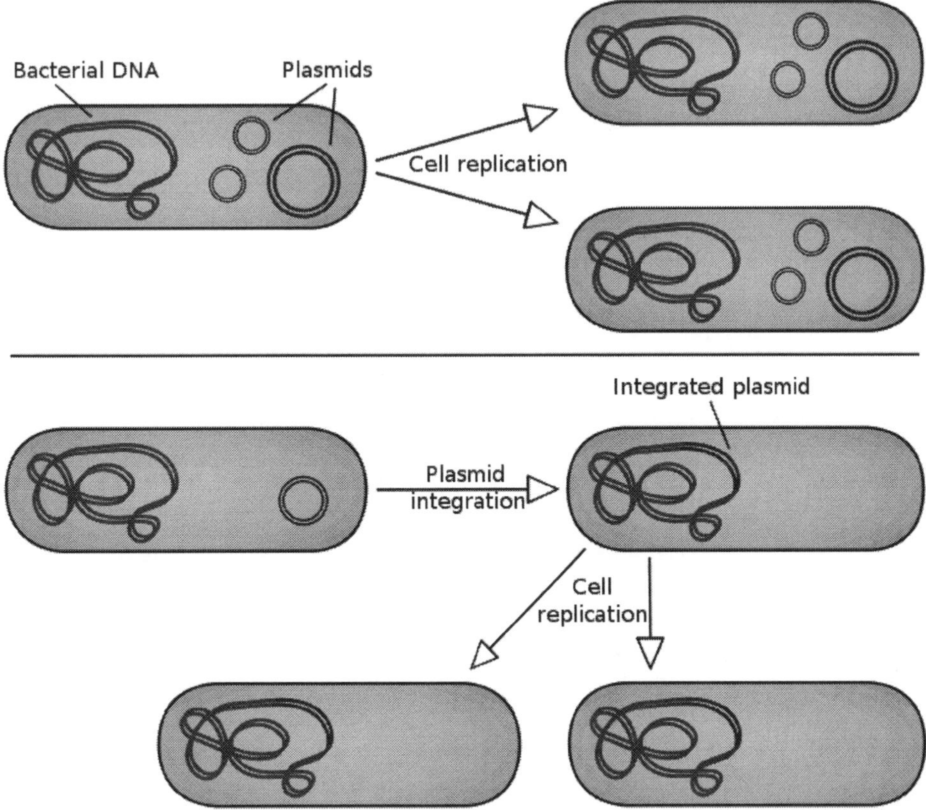

Transformation: Incorporation into Bacterial Genome of DNA Fragments from External Medium

When a bacterial cell dies, pieces of its DNA are released into the surrounding medium. These fragments can cross the envelope of surrounding bacteria if the cells are in a state of competence. Certain bacteria enter this state when nutrients are low, or if they are exposed to other stressful conditions. After the DNA is taken in, enzymes in the cell can either break down the fragments and use the nucleotides during DNA replication, or the fragments can be integrated into the bacterial chromosome. Any genes contained in the fragments can then be expressed by the bacterium. This is an example of horizontal gene transfer; DNA is passed between organisms, rather than from parent to offspring.

Conjugation

Conjugation is the process by which bacteria transfer DNA from one bacterium to another. Bacteria reproduce asexually, but conjugation is one mechanism for genetic recombination (the others being transformation and transduction). During conjugation, hereditary material is transferred in one direction from the donor to the recipient. For this to happen, the donor cell must have an F (fertility) plasmid which allows the donor "male" to form appendages called sex pili. The donor cell (also called the F^+ cell) uses a pilus to connect to the recipient female (or F^- cell). One nucleotide strand of the double stranded plasmid is given to the F^- cell, while the other strand remains in the F^+ cell. Once the complementary strand of each single strand is synthesized, the plasmids will be identical to each other. The recipient cell is now an F^+ cell, and can donate the plasmid to another F- cell. The F plasmid can be integrated into the bacterial chromosome or remain separate.

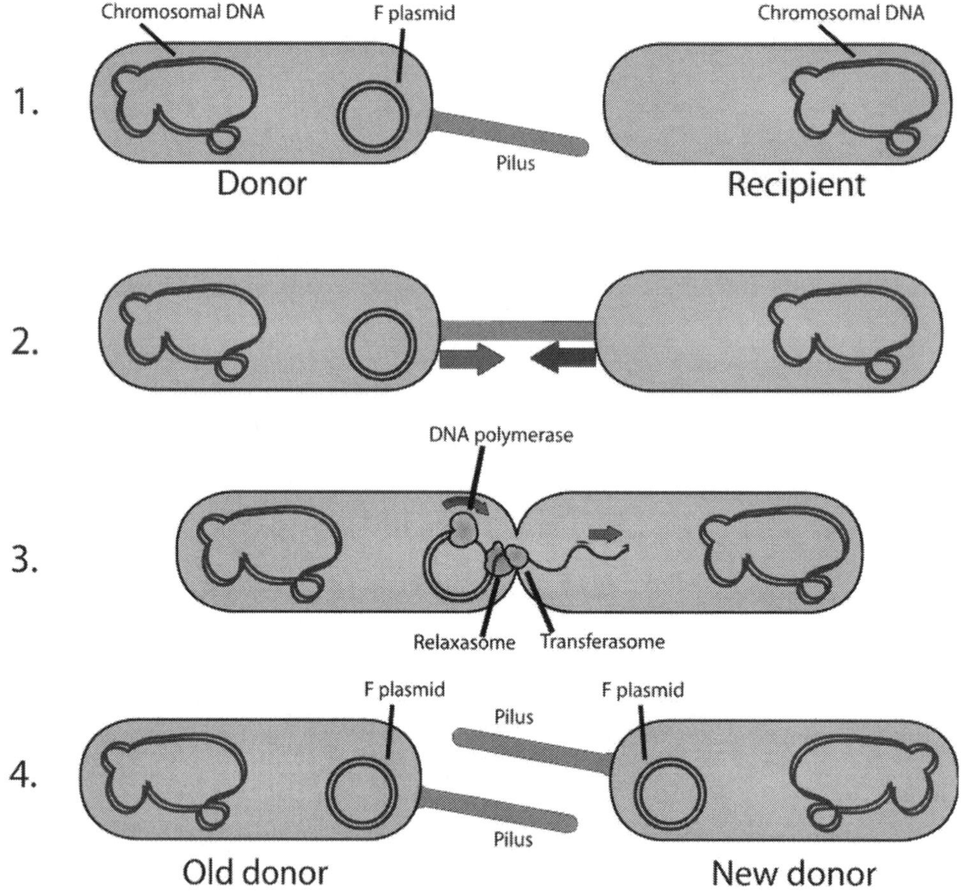

Transposons (Also Present in Eukaryotic Cells)

Transposons are segments of DNA that can move within the genome. They are found in both prokaryotic and eukaryotic cells. Transposons are sometimes called "jumping genes" because of their ability to translocate. They can cause mutations by interrupting gene sequences, but they can also carry their own genes. In bacteria, they often include an antibiotic resistance gene and can move back and forth between a plasmid and the chromosome.

There are two main classes of transposons: retrotransposons (class I) and DNA transposons (class II). Both encode the gene for the enzyme **transposase**, which facilitates the transfer of the genomic element from one location to another. Retrotransposons, however, are first transcribed into RNA, and then the enzyme **reverse transcriptase** synthesizes DNA from the RNA before it is inserted. DNA transposons are actually cut out of a genome before they are translocated.

Virus Structure

General Structural Characteristics (Nucleic Acid and Protein, Enveloped and Nonenveloped)

Viruses are particles that are classified somewhere between living and nonliving. They are made of proteins and nucleic acids, yet are acellular and entirely reliant on host cells to reproduce and to carry on metabolic processes. For this reason, viruses are described as obligate intracellular parasites. When they are outside of a host cell, they are referred to as **virions**.

Viruses share a common structure. They lack all of the organelles found in eukaryotic and prokaryotic cells, including ribosomes. They do have a protein coat called a capsid that is made of subunits called capsomeres. It encloses the viral genome, which may be DNA or RNA. The capsid comes in various shapes (such as rod and polyhedral) depending on the type of virus. Some viruses are surrounded by an envelope made of phospholipids and both bacterial and viral proteins.

Lack Organelles and Nucleus

Viruses contain DNA or RNA, but their genome is not enclosed in a nucleus. In fact, viruses do not have *any* organelles, and must rely on the ribosomes of the host cell to produce the proteins involved in the replication of their genome, as well as the proteins that form the capsid. It is not surprising that viruses are small, given that they are little more than a protein coat and genes. They must also be small enough to fit inside another cell so that they can replicate. They range from 20 to 400 nm in diameter, which is about 1/100 the size of a prokaryote, and 1/1000 the size of a typical eukaryotic cell.

Structural Aspects of Typical Bacteriophage

A **bacteriophage** (also called a "phage") is a virus that only infects prokaryotes, and therefore bacteriophages cannot infect humans. The name is appropriate because it means "bacteria eater", and these viruses destroy the cells that they infect. Most bacteriophages have a tail sheath that they use to inject their genome, and tail fibers that allow it to recognize and attach to a specific host. Like all viruses, the genome is encapsulated by a protein coat. This protein coat is left behind on the surface of the bacterium when the genome is injected.

Bacteriophages replicate in one of two ways: the lytic or lysogenic cycle. The method used is dependent on the type of virus and/or the environmental conditions. In the lytic cycle, the virus takes over the intracellular machinery of the host cell, producing progeny and lysing the cell. A virus in the lysogenic cycle does not typically cause symptoms because the genome is integrated into the host genome, without the production of more viruses. The genome is replicated when the host cell replicates, but no progeny are created unless a change in the environment causes it to leave the host genome and enter the lytic cycle.

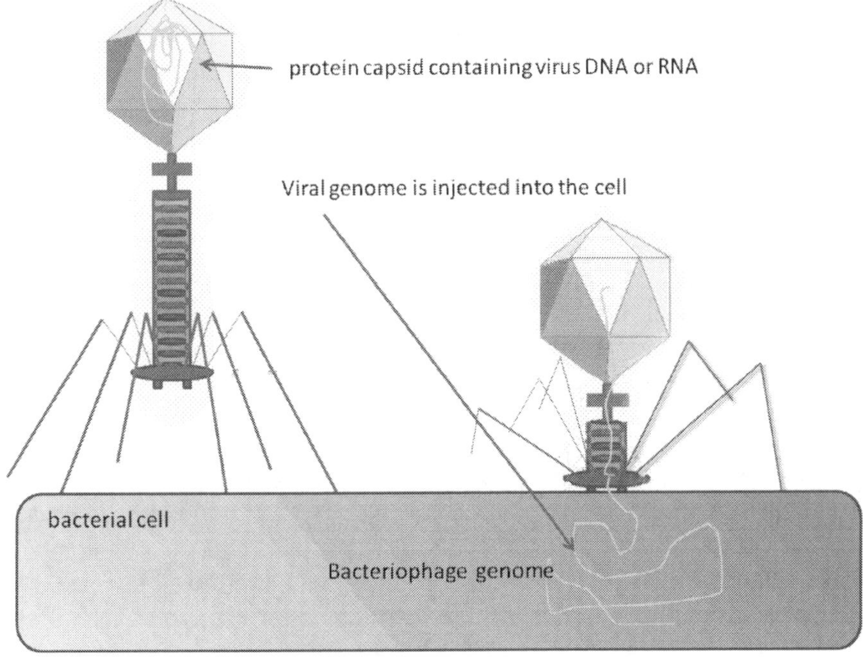

Genomic Content – RNA or DNA

All viruses encapsulate a genome. Viral genomes vary by size, and by the type of nucleic acid they contain. The average size of a viral genome is around 40 kilobase pairs, but there is a wide range from 1–2 kbp to a few hundred kbp. Most viruses contain RNA, but some have DNA, and each type of nucleic acids may be double or single stranded. Some single stranded (ss) RNA-containing viruses are "positive-sense," meaning their genes can be translated directly into proteins using the ribosomes of the host cell. Other RNA viruses are "negative-sense," and must synthesize a complementary transcript of the ssRNA. To do this, they use the enzyme RNA polymerase which they carry inside the capsid. The synthesized complementary strand is the "messenger RNA" used in translation. Some RNA viruses (called retroviruses) synthesize DNA from their ssRNA, and the DNA is integrated into the host DNA.

Viral Life Cycle

Self-Replicating Biological Units That Must Reproduce Within Specific Host Cell

Viruses cannot replicate outside of a host cell. To infect a cell, a virus must attach to specific receptors on the surface of a cell. If virus-specific receptors are not present, the cell cannot be penetrated. Once attached, the genome of the virus is either injected (typical of a bacteriophage), leaving the capsid behind, or the virus enters the cell intact (typical of a virus that infects eukaryotes). Once inside the host cell, the capsid (if present) is broken down, and the nucleic acid released. Many copies of the genome are produced, and the machinery of the host cell is used to make the proteins that are used in the assembly of new viruses. The genome and capsid proteins (capsomeres) spontaneously self-assemble into viral progeny. As progeny are produced, either they can bud off of the host cell (typical of enveloped viruses), or the cell may become so full of viruses that it bursts. The lysed cell dies, and virions are released to infect other cells. Cell damage and/or death, in combination with the body's immune response, account for the symptoms of a viral infection.

Generalized Phage and Animal Virus Life Cycles

Attachment to Host, Penetration of Cell Membrane or Cell Wall, and Entry of Viral Genetic Material

For a virus to attach to a host cell (a process called **adsorption**), it must bind to receptor proteins. The pathway for entry of the viral genome after adsorption varies according to the type of virus, and the type of host cell. Some viruses (particularly bacteriophages) use tail fibers to attach to the host cell's receptors before injecting their genome using the tail sheath. Viruses that infect eukaryotic cells tend to enter either by receptor-mediated endocytosis or by membrane fusion. In receptor-mediated endocytosis, attachment sites on the surface of the virus bind to cell surface receptors, and cell membrane invaginates around the virus, pinching off to forming a vacuole that enters the cytoplasm. Some cells mistake the virus for a desired resource, like nutrients. Enveloped viruses typically gain entry when proteins within their lipid envelope bind to receptor proteins on the cell membrane, and the envelope and membrane fuse. The virus enters, and the protein coat is degraded. If the cell does not have the specific receptor proteins used by a particular virus, then that cell cannot be infected.

Use of Host Synthetic Mechanism to Replicate Viral Components

Viruses depend on the biosynthetic machinery of the cell to replicate. They cannot copy their own genome, nor can they produce the proteins needed for the capsid. The host cell provides ATP, nucleotides, transfer RNA, amino acids, and most of the enzymes required for viral replication (though some viral genomes contain genes that are translated into enzymes). The cell's ribosomes are redirected to translate viral proteins that are used in the assembly of progeny. The cell can no longer perform its own functions, and has essentially become a virus factory.

Transduction: Transfer of Genetic Material by Viruses

Transduction is the transfer of DNA from one cell to another through the action of a virus, and is one way in which genetic recombination occurs in bacteria. When a bacteriophage infects a bacterium and replicates, the viral progeny may take parts of the bacterial genome with them when they exit the cell. The bacteriophages then inject the bacterial DNA (along with the viral genome) into new host cells. The bacterial DNA may simply be broken down by the new host cell, but if it matches up with a homologous sequence, crossover may occur, resulting in genetic recombination. There are two types of transduction. In **generalized transduction**, viruses can transfer any portion of the bacterial genome, whereas in **specialized transduction** only certain genes can be transferred.

Retrovirus Life Cycle: Integration into Host DNA, Reverse Transcriptase, HIV

Retroviruses are single-stranded RNA viruses that use the enzyme **reverse transcriptase** to transcribe their RNA into double-stranded DNA. The viral DNA becomes incorporated into the host cell's DNA with the help of the enzyme **integrase**. When the host cell replicates, it treats the viral DNA as its own and copies it, passing it on to each daughter cell. The viral genes within the host genome are transcribed and translated to produce the components of new viruses that bud from the cell to infect new ones. These types of viral infections are difficult to treat because once the viral DNA has been integrated into the host genome, the only way to kill it is to kill the cell itself. The human immunodeficiency virus (HIV) is an example of a retrovirus that infects white blood cells known as CD4 cells. As the number of CD4 cells declines, AIDS develops.

Prions and Viroids: Subviral Particles

Prions and viroids are tiny, non-living infectious particles that are much smaller than viruses. In fact, these pathogens are nothing more than proteins and RNA molecules, respectively.

Prions are misfolded variations of normal proteins that incubate for many years before symptoms of disease begin to show. They do not replicate, but rather prompt the misfolding of other proteins, though the mechanism is not well understood. The misfolded proteins group together, triggering the formation of even more prions. The cell cannot function normally under these conditions, and animal diseases such as mad cow disease and Creutzfeldt-Jakob disease result.

Viroids are short circular molecules (approximately 250–400 nucleobases) of ssRNA that are not translated into proteins, but replicate in host plant cells. Replication requires the enzyme RNA polymerase II, and occurs either in the nucleus or in chloroplasts. Viroids cause a number of plant diseases by silencing the normal RNA of the plant, and therefore interfering with gene expression. The human disease hepatitis D is caused by a viroid-like pathogen.

Processes of Cell Division, Differentiation, and Specialization

Mitosis

Mitotic Process: Prophase, Metaphase, Anaphase, Telophase, Interphase

Mitosis is the stage of the cell cycle in which the nucleus divides. It alternates with a much longer stage called interphase in which the cell performs its normal functions and prepares for division by copying organelles and duplicating chromosomes. If the cell passes the two major regulatory checkpoints of interphase, it proceeds through the four phases of mitosis, as summarized in the table below (though there will be one last checkpoint prior to anaphase). Mitosis is usually followed by cytokinesis, division of the cytoplasm, and results in two genetically identical daughter cells with the same number of chromosomes as the parent cell.

prophase	chromatin condenses into chromosomes the nucleolus and nuclear membrane break down the mitotic spindle begins to form
metaphase	the spindle aligns the chromosomes along the metaphase plate
anaphase	sister chromatids are split at the centromere and pulled toward opposite poles
telophase	chromosomes uncoil a nuclear membrane forms around each set of chromosomes a nucleolus forms in each new nucleus the mitotic spindle breaks down cytokinesis begins (it may also begin during anaphase)

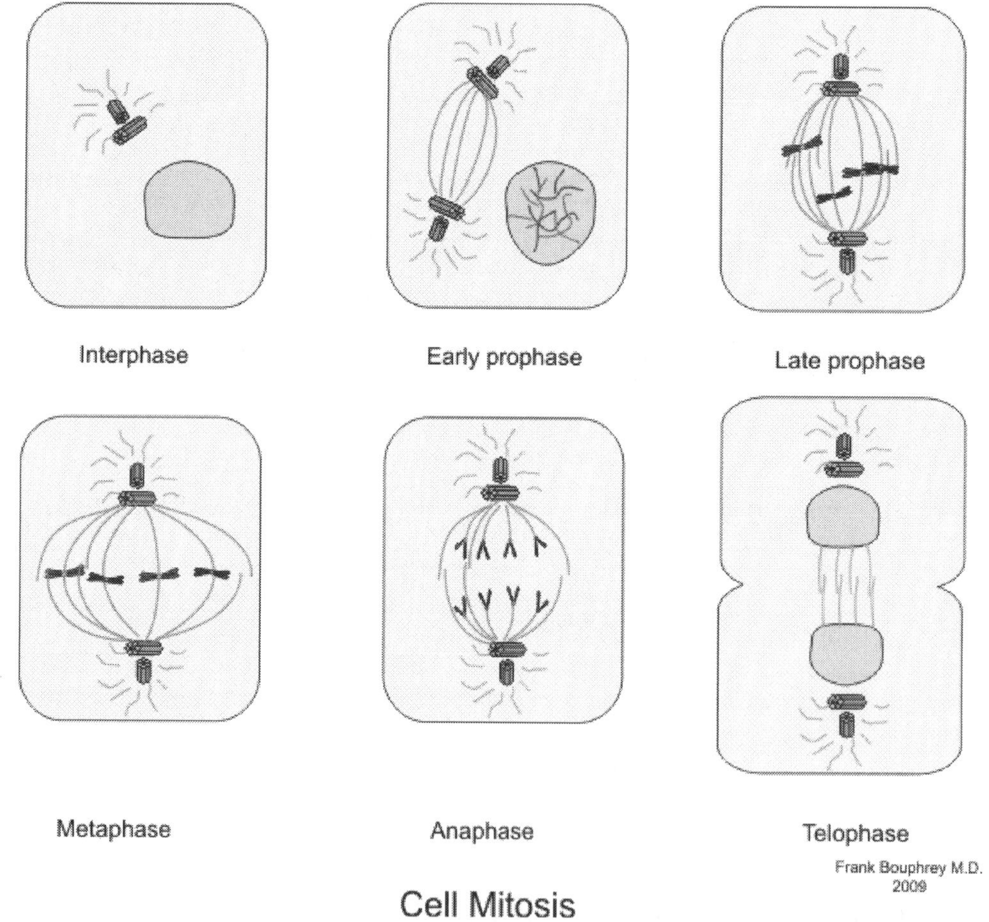

Cell Mitosis

Review Video: Mitosis
Visit mometrix.com/academy and enter code: 849894

At the onset of prophase, chromatin coils tightly into discrete chromosomes that are visible under a light microscope. The chromosomes resemble the shape of an "X", with identical DNA in each sister chromatid. The sister chromatids are bound together along their entire length by protein complexes called cohesins, but by metaphase all cohesins are broken down, except those found at the centromere. As the chromatin condenses, the nuclear envelope begins to disintegrate and the nucleolus disappears. Centrosomes, the microtubule organizing centers of the cell, migrate towards opposite poles of the cell as microtubules polymerize outward. This begins the formation of the mitotic spindle, which continues until metaphase. Protein-based structures called kinetochores form at the centromere to serve as an attachment point for the kinetochore fibers (microtubules) of the spindle. As the kinetochore microtubules attach to each chromosome at the centromere, other microtubules called polar fibers overlap at the center of the cell, never interacting with the chromosomes. By the end of prophase, the nuclear envelope has completely dissolved. This tends to be the longest stage of mitosis.

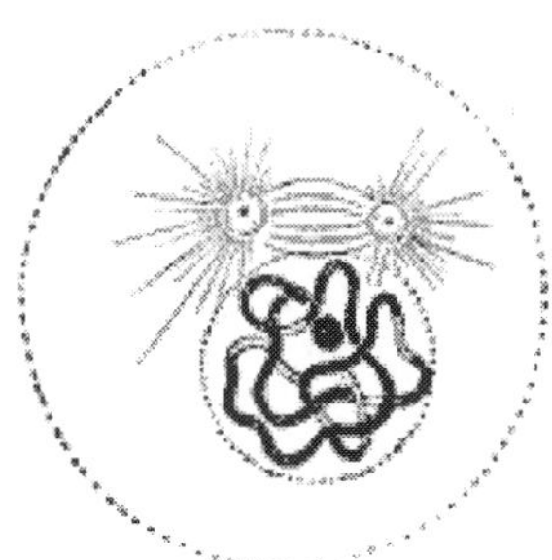

During metaphase, the centrosomes are at opposite poles of the cell, and chromosomes are positioned along an imaginary line between the two centrosomes known as the metaphase plate (sometimes called the spindle equator or equatorial plate). The kinetochore fibers lengthen or shorten as needed to line up the chromosomes, and the movement is assisted by forces exerted by motor proteins. Polar fibers continue to grow until they are sufficiently overlapped in preparation for the next stage of mitosis. Anaphase will only follow metaphase if the chromosomes are properly aligned, and every kinetochore on every sister chromatid is attached to a kinetochore fiber. Metaphase is usually shorter than prophase.

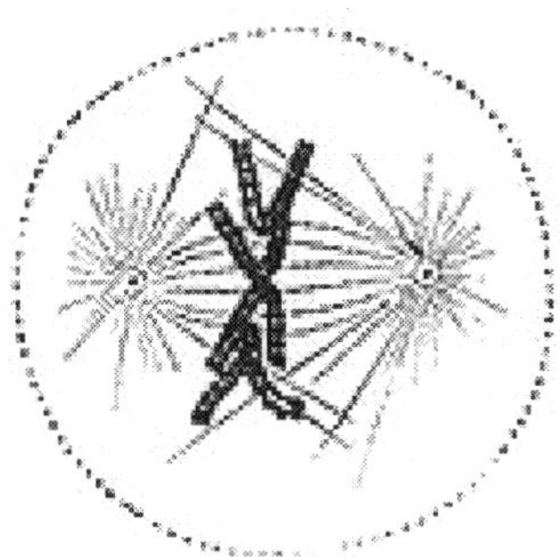

Chromosomes are at their most condensed form during anaphase. The stage begins when an enzyme known as separin cleaves the cohesins that hold sister chromatids together. The kinetochore fibers shorten as a result of depolymerization, splitting the centromeres and pulling the liberated chromosomes toward the centrosomes. As they are dragged through the cytosol, the linear chromosomes bend into a "V" shape as they trail behind the centromere. Meanwhile, the overlapping polar fibers push away from each other, causing the cell to elongate. There is now a complete set of chromosomes at each end of the cell.

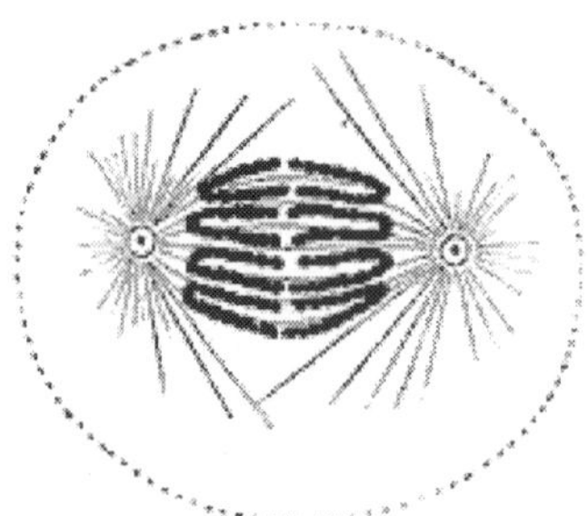

As liberated chromosomes arrive at the poles of the cell, a new nuclear membrane is formed around each group. The polar fibers continue to elongate the cell as the chromosomes uncoil and the nucleoli reform. The microtubules of the spindle are depolymerized and disappear. Cytokinesis begins during either telophase or late anaphase. A cleavage furrow forms near the site of the metaphase plate as a contractile ring of microfilaments beneath the plasma membrane begins to constrict the cell. This will continue after telophase, pinching the parent cell into two identical daughter cells.

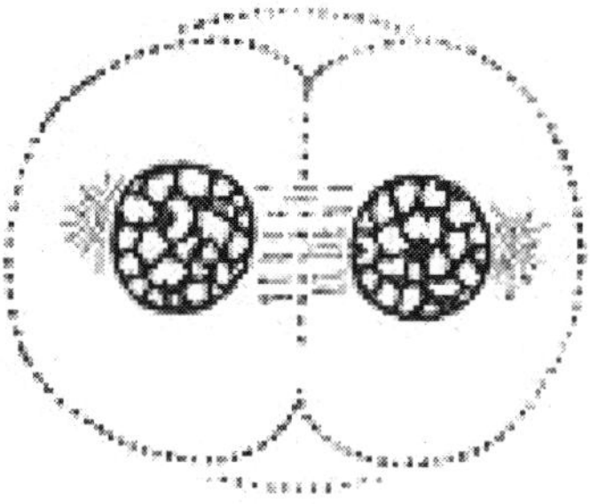

Mitotic Structures

Centrioles, Asters, Spindles

The mitotic spindle is responsible for segregating sister chromatids during mitosis. The assembly of the spindle begins with a structure called a **centrosome**, often described as the microtubule-organizing center of the cell. In animal cells, the microtubules are organized into structures called **centrioles**. Each centrosome is made of an amorphous matrix of proteins called pericentriolar material that encloses two centrioles that are oriented at right angles to each other. A centriole consists of nine triplets of microtubules arranged in a cylindrical shape. During the formation of the spindle, microtubules extend out from the centrioles to form spindle fibers. Some of these fibers attach to the chromosomes, and others overlap near the midline of the cell. A star-shaped array of shorter microtubules project from each centrosome to form an **aster**. Asters ensure the correct position of the mitotic spindle by anchoring the centrioles to the cell membrane at opposite poles of the cell.

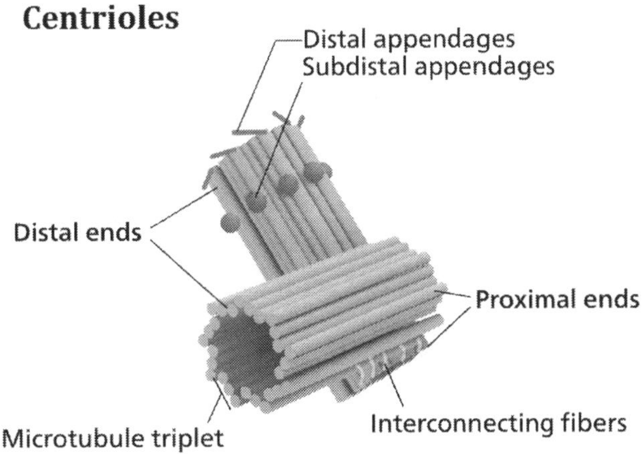

CHROMATIDS, CENTROMERES, KINETOCHORES

Chromosomes are duplicated during the S phase of the cell cycle so that a complete set of DNA can be distributed to each daughter cell during mitosis. Each "half" of a duplicated chromosome is called a **chromatid**, and they are attached to each other at the **centromere** by cohesin proteins. The centromere is characterized by repetitive sequences of DNA (centromeric DNA), and two protein complexes called **kinetochores** that form upon it. (Each chromatid has its own kinetochore.) The inner portion of a kinetochore associates with the centromeric DNA, and the outer portion provides an attachment point for the kinetochore microtubules of the mitotic spindle. When the microtubules contract, chromatids of a duplicated chromosome are separated at the centromere. They are no longer considered chromatids at this time, and are instead called chromosomes.

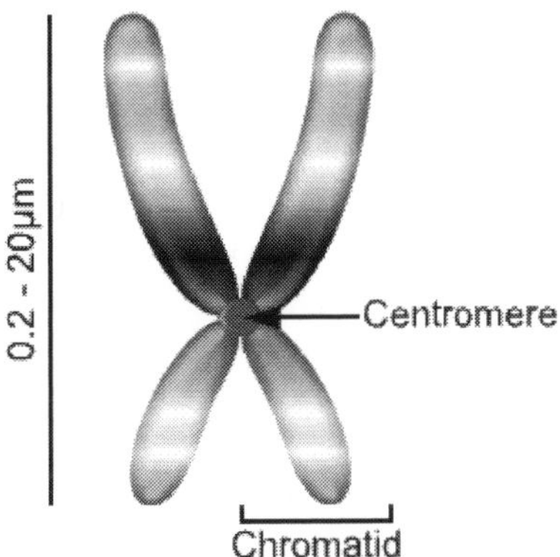

NUCLEAR MEMBRANE BREAKDOWN AND REORGANIZATION

In most eukaryotic cells, the nuclear membrane (also called the nuclear envelope, or NE) disappears during prophase so that the spindle fibers can access the duplicated chromosomes. It later reforms around each set of chromosomes during late anaphase or telophase. The disassembly of the NE is controlled by cyclin-dependent kinases. These enzymes phosphorylate proteins of the inner nuclear membrane, causing them to dissociate from the NE. This in turn causes the nuclear lamina (the structure that supports the nuclear envelope) to break down. Some elements from the disassembled NE diffuse into the cytosol, and others are incorporated into the endoplasmic reticulum. It is not entirely clear how the membrane reforms, but it is likely that inner membrane proteins are dephosphorylated, and parts of the endoplasmic reticulum are reorganized to form a new nuclear membrane.

MECHANISMS OF CHROMOSOME MOVEMENT

Chromosome movement is facilitated by the lengthening and shortening of microtubules, and is further aided by motor proteins. Microtubules are hollow structures made of protein dimer subunits called alpha and beta tubulin. During prophase, these dynamic structures radiate from the centrosome by adding tubulin at the plus end, while the minus end remains fixed at the centrosome. Eventually, the kinetochores of every chromosome will be "captured" by a microtubule. The chromosomes are then pushed and pulled by polymerization or depolymerization of the microtubules until they are positioned along an imaginary midline called the metaphase plate. This movement is mediated by ATP-driven motor proteins called kinesins that "walk" along the microtubules toward the plus end. When the chromosomes are aligned, the microtubules that are attached to the chromosome depolymerize by the removal of tubulin from the plus end. As the kinetochore fibers shorten, the chromosomes separate at the centromere. Meanwhile, the polar microtubules that overlap in the center of the cell lengthen and push against each other. The combined effect of the elongating polar microtubules and shortening kinetochore microtubules moves the chromosomes towards the poles of the cell.

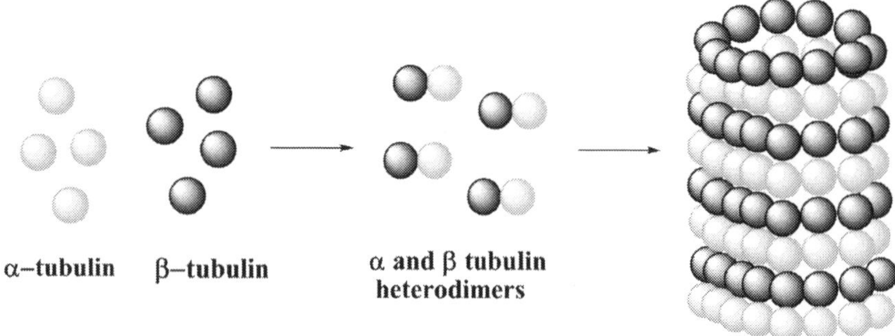

Section of a Microtubule

Review Video: Chromosomes
Visit mometrix.com/academy and enter code: 132083

PHASES OF CELL CYCLE: G0, G1, S, G2, M

The **cell cycle** can be described as the life of a cell, beginning with the formation of the cell, and ending with its own division. The phases of the cycle are G_1 (first gap), S (synthesis), G_2 (second gap) and M (the mitotic phase). Many cells, however, enter a non-growing G_0 state in which the cell performs its job but does not divide. This may happen for a number of reasons, and it is not always reversible. Cells that are deficient in nutrients or growth factors may be blocked from proceeding to the S phase, and only called back to the cycle when favorable conditions are restored. Mature liver cells and many adult stem cells exist in a reversible **quiescent** state, and only divide in response to stimuli such as tissue damage. Some cells leave the cell cycle permanently. A cell with damaged DNA, for example, is likely to enter an irreversible state of **senescence**, meaning that it will cease to divide and grow. This allows the cell to avoid apoptosis (programmed cell death), but it will remain in G_0 indefinitely. Other highly differentiated cells such as nerve and cardiac muscle cells permanently leave the cell cycle because they are genetically programmed to do so.

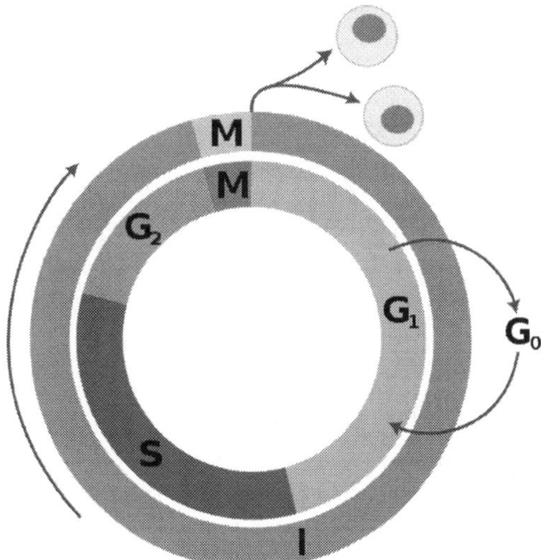

The G_1 (first gap) phase of the cell cycle is the first part of interphase, and it begins immediately after cell division. During this stage, the volume of the cell increases, and the metabolic activities that were inhibited during mitosis are accelerated. The cell begins the task of copying its organelles, synthesizing mRNA, tRNA, and rRNA, and producing the enzymes required for DNA replication, all while continuing to perform its given function. The time duration of this phase varies greatly, but it tends to be the longest phase of the cell cycle, averaging 6-12 hours. Some cells remain in this phase for years. Before the cell is allowed to proceed to the S phase, it is inspected at the G_1 checkpoint. It "passes" if it has grown enough and has sufficient nutrients and growth factors, and the DNA is not damaged. If it "fails" it enters the G_0 phase.

The S (synthesis) phase of the cell cycle falls between G_1 and G_2 of interphase. During this time (which averages 6–8 hours) each molecule of DNA is replicated, doubling the genetic content from 2n to 4n. Note that this does *not* change the ploidy of the cell; the chromosome number remains at 46. Helicases separate the two complementary strands of DNA at multiple sites along each molecule, and DNA polymerases add nucleotides at a rate of about 50 nucleotides per second. By the end of the S phase, there is an identical copy of each DNA molecule, ensuring that each daughter cell that is created during the M phase will have a complete genome. Centrosomes are duplicated during this stage as well, while transcription and protein synthesis are inhibited.

The G_2 (second gap) phase follows DNA replication, and is the final part of interphase. It is characterized by roughly 3–4 hours of cell growth, continued replication of organelles, and protein synthesis. The centrosomes that were duplicated during the S phase begin to mature, as microtubules become more organized and the centrioles elongate. As it prepares for mitosis, the cell performs its usual metabolic functions-but before the cell is allowed to divide, it must pass inspection at the G_2 checkpoint. If any errors are detected in the duplicated chromosomes, the cell cycle is arrested until the DNA can be repaired. Cells that are significantly and irreparably damaged will either enter a state of senescence, or be eliminated through programmed cell death.

Mitosis (nuclear division) and cytokinesis (cytoplasmic division) together make up the M phase of the cell cycle. There is no growth during this phase, and normal metabolic functioning is inhibited to devote the cell's resources to the division process. During mitosis, the chromosomes condense (prophase), align along the metaphase plate (metaphase), split at the centromere and segregate (anaphase), and uncoil as a new nuclear membrane is built around each full set (telophase). Cytokinesis overlaps with the final stages of mitosis.

In animal cells, cytokinesis results from the formation of a contractile ring of actin and non-muscle myosin II filaments. This ring forms around the equator of the cell, directly beneath the plasma membrane, and parallel to the metaphase plate. Myosin is a motor protein that uses ATP to move the actin filaments, causing the ring to contract like a drawstring. As this is happening, vesicles from inside the cell fuse along the cleavage furrow to form a plasma membrane. The two cells become physically separated in a process called abscission. The M phase is the shortest phase of the cell cycle, averaging 1–2 hours.

Growth Arrest

Cell growth can be halted in response to signals from both inside and outside the cell. For example, most cells require anchorage to neighboring cells or substrates to proliferate. Cells that exhibit anchorage dependence usually exhibit density-dependent inhibition as well. As they become crowded, the physical constraints may stop the cells from growing. Crowding may also activate signal transduction pathways that arrest cells at certain points in the cell cycle. Growth arrest may also occur in conditions of oxidative stress, infection, or depleted levels of nutrients and/or growth factors. (Growth factors are proteins that stimulate cell growth.) Finally, any cells with damaged or incompletely replicated DNA, or chromosomes that are not properly aligned along the midline of the cell during mitosis, are arrested before they divide by checkpoint proteins. If the problem can be corrected, the cell will be allowed to progress. Cells that are too damaged will either remain in an arrested state permanently, or undergo apoptosis.

Control of Cell Cycle

There are three significant checkpoints that control the cell cycle: G_1, G_2, and M. These regulation points can be compared to traffic lights. If a cell fails inspection, then its progression to the next stage is halted. Checkpoints respond to signals from both inside the cell (such as incomplete DNA replication) and outside the cell (such as overcrowding, or a deficiency in growth factors).

Checkpoint	Assesses the cell for the following conditions:
G_1 (G_1 / S transition)	Sufficient cell growth Presence of adequate growth factors Sufficient energy reserves / nutrients DNA integrity (no damage) Side note: This checkpoint is called the "restriction point." Once the cell has passed it, the cell is committed to division.
G_2 (G_2 / M transition)	Completely replicated chromosomes following S phase DNA integrity (no damage)
M (metaphase of mitosis)	Chromosomes are aligned along the metaphase plate during metaphase Every kinetochore is anchored to a spindle fiber

Checkpoints are controlled by proteins, namely cyclins and cyclin-dependent kinases (CDKs) that respond to intracellular and extracellular cues. Cyclins belong to a family of proteins that activate CDKs by binding to them to form cyclin-dependent kinase complexes (CDKCs). Concentrations of cyclins fluctuate throughout the cycle to control the timing of each phase. Once a CDKC becomes enzymatically active, it can phosphorylate target proteins (such as transcription factors) within the cell cycle. Phosphorylation may increase or decrease the activity of the target, which in turn affects the progression of the cell cycle. A well-known CDKC is MPF, or maturation-promoting factor. It phosphorylates proteins in the nuclear membrane, causing it to break down at the onset of mitosis. Later, it activates APC/C. or anaphase-promoting complex, in order to initiate its own destruction and move the cell from the M phase to the G_1 phase.

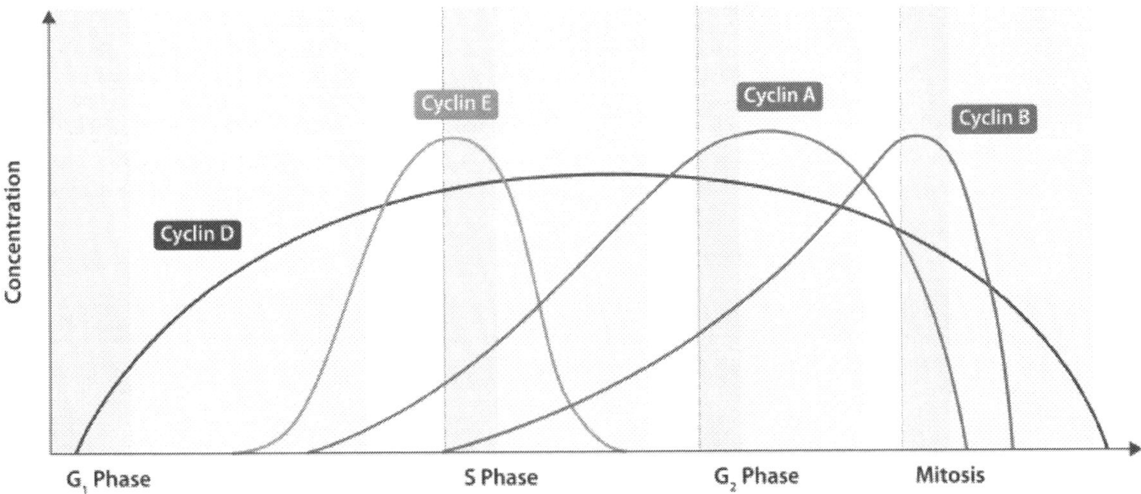

Loss of Cell Cycle Controls in Cancer Cells

Cancer cells do not respond to signals that control the cell cycle. They bypass checkpoints and proliferate in conditions that should trigger senescence or apoptosis. This can happen as a result of mutations in the genes that produce either positive or negative regulatory proteins. For example, there are tumor suppressor genes, including the RB (retinoblastoma), BRCA, and p53 genes that control the production of proteins that *inhibit* the cell cycle in unfavorable conditions. P53 is nicknamed the "guardian of the genome" because when DNA is damaged, the p53 protein (a transcription factor) triggers the synthesis of the p21 protein, which forms a complex with CDK, arresting the cell cycle before the S phase. Many incidences of cancers are associated with a p53 mutation.

Mutations can also arise in genes called proto-oncogenes that synthesize proteins that *stimulate* the cycle. For example, a mutation could transform a proto-oncogene into an oncogene that allows a CDK to function without partnering with a cyclin. In short, a mutation in any of the proteins that play a role in the cell cycle can lead to uncontrolled cell division.

Biosignaling

Oncogenes, Apoptosis

Biosignaling is a messaging system that cells use to coordinate their activities. It involves the use of receptor proteins and the signal molecules that they bind from outside the cell. Proto-oncogenes encode the information for growth factors and their receptors, and are therefore important players in the signaling pathways that regulate the cell cycle. When proto-oncogenes are over-expressed or mutated, they can accelerate the signaling pathways that promote cell division. The RAS oncogene is one of many genes commonly associated with cancer. The RAS protein is a GTPase that regulates the cell cycle by toggling back and forth between an active and inactive state. But when it is mutated, it remains in its active form, signaling the cell to divide even in the absence of growth factors. Oncogenes can also inhibit apoptosis, a natural process that eliminates damaged or unhealthy cells. When a cell is targeted to die, enzymes are released from the mitochondria which activate caspases in the cytosol, and the caspases digest the intracellular components. Oncogenes can both prevent the release of the mitochondria enzymes and directly inactivate the caspases.

REPRODUCTIVE SYSTEM

GAMETOGENESIS BY MEIOSIS

Gametogenesis is the process by which diploid germ cells give rise to haploid gametes (sex cells). Germ cells are produced in the early stages of embryogenesis, and migrate from the primitive streak to the gonads where they later undergo meiosis. Germ cells are distinguished from somatic cells because they can undergo both mitosis and meiosis. All other cells are restricted to mitosis, and have no potential to produce gametes. Mitosis is a single division that results in two identical cells, each with the same number of chromosomes as the parent cell. In meiosis, a germ cell undergoes two rounds of cell division (meiosis I and meiosis II). During meiosis I, homologous pairs of chromosomes exchange portions of their DNA before they are separated and distributed independently to daughter cells. These events ensure that the daughter cells are genetically unique, and the chromosome number is cut in half. The steps of meiosis II are similar to those of mitosis, and result in four haploid cells. These cells differentiate to give rise to the mature gametes that fuse during fertilization, restoring the diploid number. The production of ova and sperm is more specifically called oogenesis and spermatogenesis, respectively.

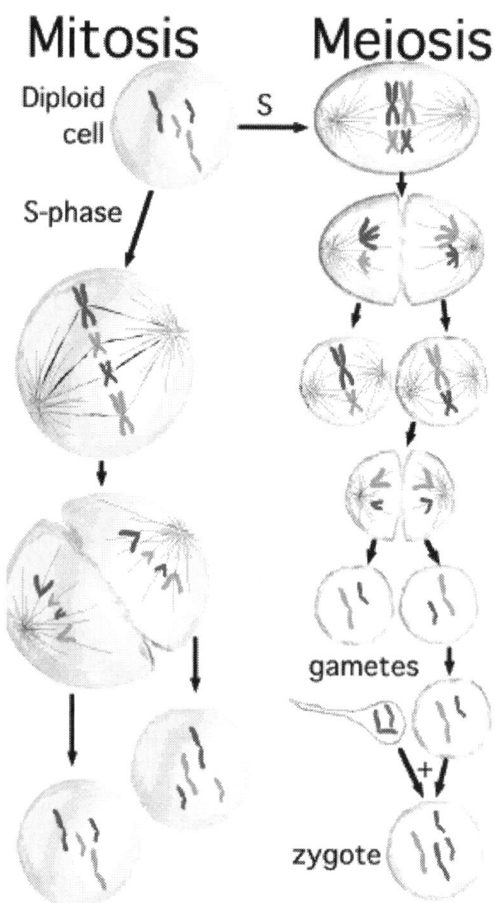

Ovum and Sperm

Ova and sperm are reproductive cells that are produced during the processes of oogenesis and spermatogenesis, respectively. Both types of gametes are haploid (human eggs and sperm each have 23 chromosomes while somatic cells contain 46), and they originate from a diploid primordial germ cell (PGC). The development from a PGC to a mature gamete can be summarized as follows:

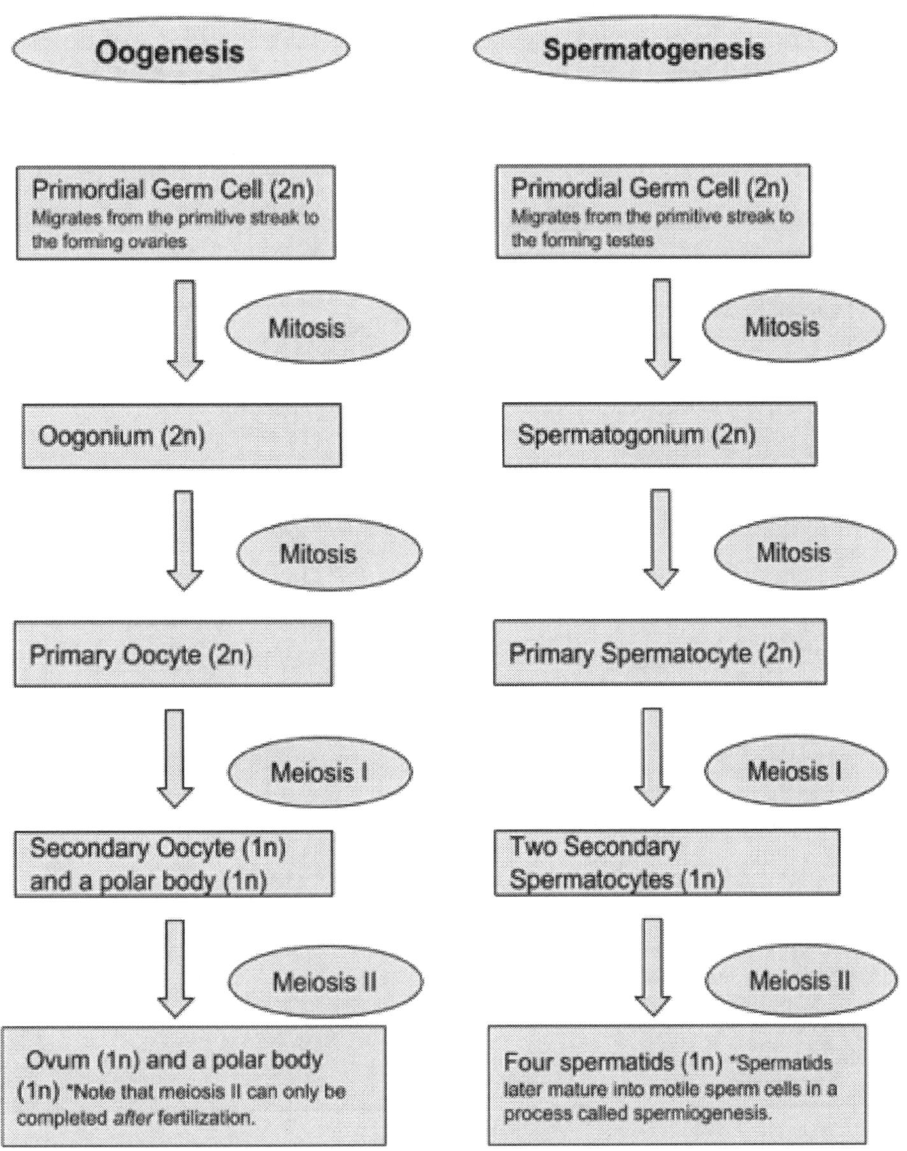

Differences in Formation

Both oogenesis and spermatogenesis begin with diploid germ cells. These diploid cells give rise to gametogonia (via mitosis), which develop into primary gametocytes (mitosis), then into secondary gametocytes (meiosis I), and then gametes (meiosis II). The differences between the processes are summarized as follows:

Oogenesis	Spermatogenesis
Nearly the entire process occurs in the ovaries; completion occurs in the oviduct	Occurs entirely in the testes
Only some oogonia develop into oocytes	All spermatogonia become spermatocytes
Oogonia give rise to a finite number of primary oocytes during fetal development	Spermatogonia continually give rise to primary spermatocytes at the onset of puberty (millions per day)
Nucleus does not condense; it is much larger than the nucleus of a sperm cell	Nucleus condenses to help streamline the cell
Meiosis is arrested at prophase I (resumes monthly between puberty and menopause) and arrested again at metaphase II (resumes only if sperm penetrates the secondary oocyte)	Meiosis is continuous
Cells divide unequally to produce one ovum and two or three polar bodies (polar bodies are not viable and break down)	Cells divide equally to produce four spermatids
No gametes released after menopause	Gamete production continues throughout life

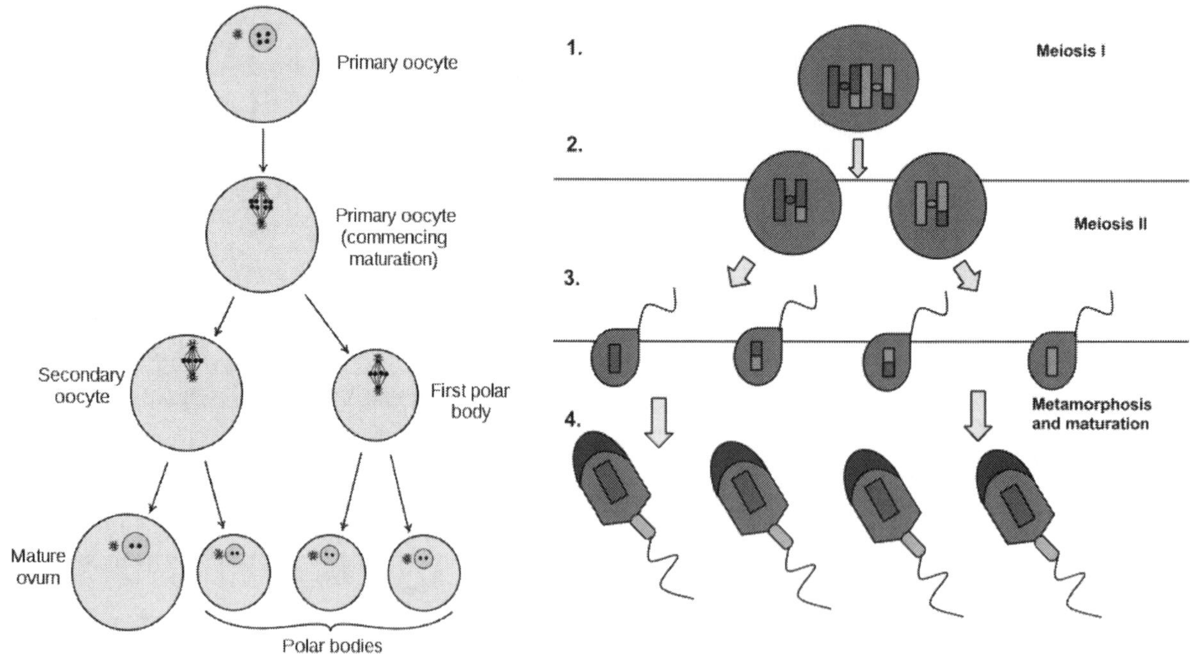

Differences in Morphology

An ovum is one of the largest human cells. At around 0.1 mm in diameter, it is visible to the naked eye. It is commonly confused with the follicle, a larger structure that houses an oocyte as it matures. The ovum itself is a spherical cell full of nutritional reserves for a developing embryo. The cytoplasm, nucleus, and nucleolus of the ovum are more precisely known as the **ooplasm** (or yolk), **germinal vesicle**, and **germinal spot**, respectively. **Cortical granules** near the plasma membrane help to prevent fertilization by more than one sperm. The ovum is coated in a jelly-like layer of glycoproteins called the **zona pellucida**, which plays a vital role in fertilization by triggering the reactions within a sperm cell that allow it to penetrate the ovum. This protein layer is produced by secretions from both the egg and the surrounding granulosa cells of the follicle known as the **corona radiata**. As the egg matures, the follicle enlarges until it is ejected from the ovary during ovulation.

In the Image Below:

- *FC* = follicle cells of the corona radiata
- *Y* = yolk (ooplasm)
- *B* = sperm cells
- *Memb* = plasma membrane and zona pellucida
- *N* = nucleus (germinal vesicle)

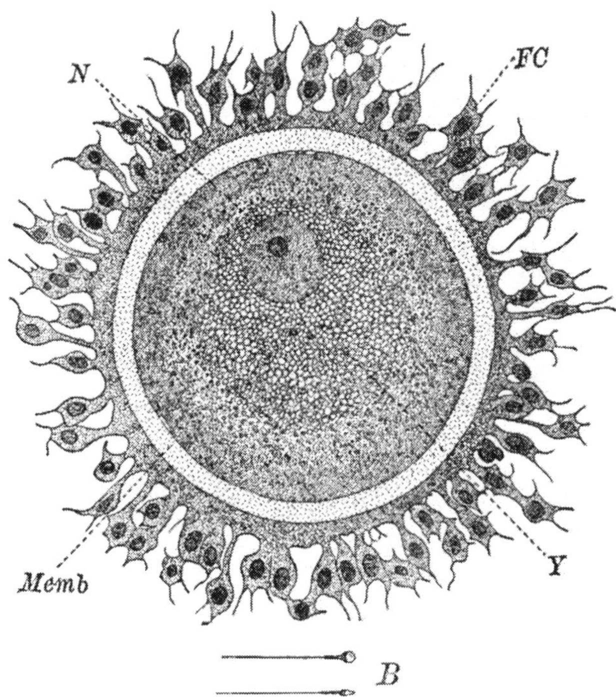

A sperm cell is the smallest of human cells, measuring about 0.05 mm in length. It has three distinct sections: the head, midpiece, and tail; its streamlined form is well suited to its function. The head contains centrioles and a compacted nucleus with tightly coiled DNA. The anterior surface of the head is capped with the **acrosome,** *a* Golgi-derived structure that is packed with enzymes that assist in the penetration of the zona pellucida, and is therefore essential for fertilization. Between 50 and 100 mitochondria spiral around the midpiece, which is the only part of the sperm that contains any mitochondria. The ATP produced by the mitochondria powers the sliding motion of the microtubules within the tail, or **flagellum**, of the sperm, which in turn causes it to undulate. The microtubule-based core of the flagellum is called the **axoneme**, and consists of nine doublets of microtubules arranged around a central pair.

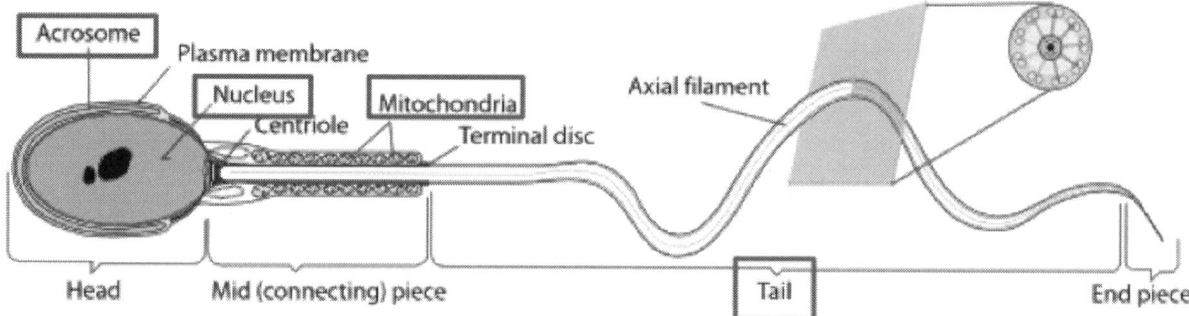

RELATIVE CONTRIBUTION TO NEXT GENERATION

When an oocyte undergoes meiosis and cytokinesis, the cytoplasm divides unequally to produce one large viable ovum. This ensures that nearly all of the resources that are required for the survival of a zygote are present. The ooplasm of the egg contains an abundance of nutrients that will sustain the zygote, and later the daughter cells (blastomeres) that are produced by mitosis. All of the molecules (enzymes, RNA) needed for protein synthesis are present as well. It also contains the organelles, with the exception of the centrioles, which are degraded during oogenesis. These structures are instead donated by the sperm cell. Sperm cells do contain mitochondria, but they are left behind when the midpiece and tail are released from the head during fertilization. Any paternal mitochondria that manage to enter the egg are quickly destroyed, leaving only maternal mitochondria. Each gamete contributes 22 autosomes (non-sex chromosomes) and one sex chromosome to the zygote. The egg always contributes an X chromosome, and the sperm contributes either an X or a Y chromosome.

REPRODUCTIVE SEQUENCE: FERTILIZATION; IMPLANTATION; DEVELOPMENT; BIRTH

Fertilization usually occurs in the fallopian tube within 24 hours of ovulation. Of the hundreds of millions of sperm that are ejaculated, an average of 200 reach the secondary oocyte. When a sperm makes contact with the oocyte, it burrows through the corona radiata and binds to receptor proteins in the zona pellucida. The acrosome releases enzymes that allow the sperm to pass through the zona pellucida to the membrane of the oocyte. Here, actin filaments extend from the sperm to form a tubular structure called the acrosomal apparatus through which its pronucleus is passed. (The midpiece and tail are left behind.) Entry of the pronucleus stimulates the cortical reaction; enzymes from cortical granules beneath the membrane of the oocyte diffuse into the zona pellucida, causing it to harden, and preventing fertilization by more than one sperm. Another block to polyspermy is the depolarization of the oocyte membrane that occurs in response to calcium ions that are released when the sperm meets the membrane. The oocyte then divides unequally by meiosis II to produce an ovum and a nonviable polar body. The pronucleus of the sperm fuses with the pronucleus of the ovum, and a zygote (fertilized egg) is formed.

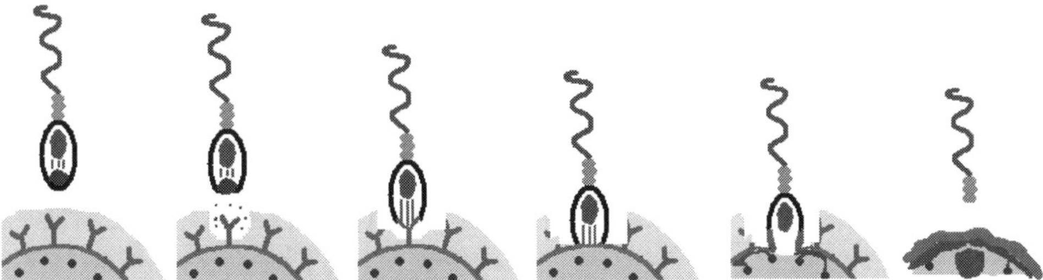

After fertilization, the zygote develops into a cluster of cells called a **morula**. The morula is pushed from the fallopian tube to the uterine cavity by peristalsis (muscle contractions) and the wave-like motions of cilia. It floats freely in the uterus for around 3 days, using uterine secretions as nourishment. The cells of the morula begin to differentiate and give rise to a blastocyst with a fluid-filled cavity and two types of cells. The inner cell mass will give rise to the embryo, and the outer trophoblasts develop into the placenta. Degeneration of the zona pellucida, followed by "zona hatching", occurs around six days after fertilization in preparation for implantation. As this transformation happens, the blastocyst secretes human chorionic gonadotropin (hCG) which stimulates the production of other hormones. These hormones help to maintain the corpus luteum (preventing menses) and prepare the endometrium for implantation. About one week after ovulation, the blastocyst (now over 200 cells) attaches to the endometrium, and outer cells of the trophoblast fuse to form large multinucleated syncytiotrophoblasts that extend like fingers (called chorionic villi) into the endometrium. Fetal blood vessels form inside these villi. About two weeks after fertilization, the blastocyst is fully implanted, and the endometrium is now called the decidua (the maternal contribution to the placenta).

During the pre-embryonic stage of development, the zygote undergoes **cleavage**, dividing mitotically to form a morula. The morula continues to divide and differentiate into a fluid-filled blastocyst. The blastocyst implants in the uterine wall, and the embryonic stage of development commences. During **gastrulation**, the cells of the embryo are reorganized to form the embryonic germ layers (ectoderm, mesoderm, and endoderm) that will produce the tissues and organs of the embryo. A neural plate derived from the ectoderm invades the mesoderm to form the neural tube in a process called **neurulation**. **Organogenesis** continues with the development of a rudimentary heart that beats at around the third week. The digestive system and other internal organs form, as well as the placenta and umbilical cord. By the end of eight weeks, the organ systems have formed and the embryo is now a fetus. During the fetal stage, development continues with the differentiation of the reproductive organs, coordinated movements of limbs, ossification of bones, and an increase of subcutaneous fat. Birth normally occurs around 40 weeks post fertilization.

The fetus must adapt quickly as it transitions from an intrauterine environment to an extrauterine environment. This transition is facilitated by hormones, notably cortisol and catecholamines. Before birth, the neonate relies on oxygen from the mother's blood, and its lungs are collapsed and fluid-filled. As labor approaches, the secretion of fluid from the fetal lungs decreases, while reabsorption increases. At birth, the lungs fill with air and the rest of the fluid leaves the lungs. This first breath triggers critical circulatory changes. Pulmonary resistance decreases, pulmonary blood flow increases, and the shunts that cause the blood to bypass the lungs and liver close or constrict. (The **foramen ovale** that bypasses the lungs closes at first breath. The **ductus arteriosus**, which also bypasses the lungs, and the **ductus venosus** that bypasses the liver, both constrict at birth and close soon after.) The neonate will no longer receive nourishment from the placenta, and will rely on mother's milk and stores of glycogen in the liver. The neonate must also expend energy to keep warm, and so increases its metabolic rate through muscle movements and the burning of brown fat.

EMBRYOGENESIS

STAGES OF EARLY DEVELOPMENT

FERTILIZATION AND CLEAVAGE

Fertilization is the fusion of a sperm and egg to create a zygote. The zygote prepares for the first mitotic division by replicating the maternal and paternal chromosomes, but does not increase in volume. Approximately thirty hours after fertilization, the zygote splits to form a two-celled embryo. These cells are called blastocysts. The cleavage process is holoblastic, meaning the division is complete (as opposed to meroblastic, or partial cleavage). These cells continue to divide rapidly. Initially, all cells divide simultaneously, but after several divisions they begin to divide independently. There is little time for growth between divisions. In fact, the G_1 and G_2 phases of the cell cycle are nearly non-existent, and the mulberry-shaped morula is the same size as the original zygote. As this period of rapid division called **cleavage** continues, the blastomeres differentiate and compact to form an inner mass surrounded by the cells of the trophoblast. By day 5, the morula has developed into a blastocyst, which implants in the uterus.

BLASTULA FORMATION

Blastulation is the development of a blastula from a morula. In mammals, a blastula is known as a **blastocyst**. Around three days after fertilization, the cells of the morula begin to compact and differentiate. These pluripotent cells are called **embryoblasts**. As they compact into an inner cell mass, a fluid-filled cavity called a **blastocoel** is formed. An outer ring of cells called the **trophoblast** creates a boundary between the blastocoel and the extracellular environment. As the blastocyst develops, the zona pellucida that once protected the egg and aided in fertilization is broken down, and the trophoblasts divide and differentiate. The inner trophoblast cells, called **cytotrophoblasts**, fuse to give rise to an outer layer of **syncytiotrophoblasts**, which form the outer portion of the **placenta**. The embryoblasts continue to differentiate as they separate from the trophoblast to form a disc of tissue that separates the blastocoel from the newly formed amniotic cavity. This **bilaminar disc** consists of two layers: the **epiblast** that is exposed to the amniotic cavity, and the **hypoblast** that is exposed to the blastocoel. The epiblasts migrate, lining the amniotic cavity to begin the formation of the amnion. The hypoblasts migrate as well, lining the blastocoel, which becomes a primitive yolk sac. The yolk sac provides nourishment to the embryo until the placenta takes over.

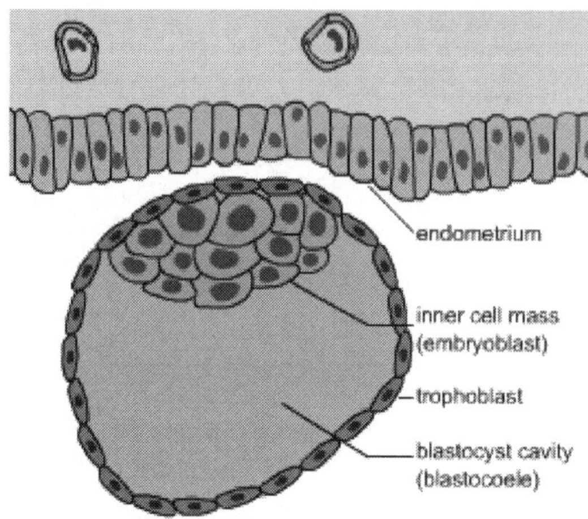

Gastrulation: First Cell Movements

Gastrulation is the process by which the cells of an embryo are reorganized into a multi-layered gastrula. Most animals form three germ layers during gastrulation: the endoderm, mesoderm, and ectoderm. The coordinated movements of cells are under the control of signaling pathways, and the timing and pattern varies from species to species. Some common types of cell movements include:

- **Invagination** - the folding of a sheet of cells to form a pouch
- **Ingression** - the breaking away and migration of cells
- **involution** - the rolling of a sheet of cells to form another layer
- **epiboly** - the spreading out of cells to form a thinner layer
- **delamination** - the splitting of one sheet of cells into two separate populations
- **intercalation** - the rearrangement of cells from different layers to form a single layer

Gastrulation: Formation of Primary Germ Layers (Endoderm, Mesoderm, Ectoderm)

In humans, three distinct germ layers are established in the third week of development, and it begins with the formation of the **primitive streak** on day 15. Signaling pathways trigger the coordinated movements of cells along the midline of the epiblast, defining the left and right parts of the embryo. A furrow called the **primitive groove** appears as the epiblast cells divide rapidly - more rapidly than the hypoblast cells. This causes the epiblast layer of the bilaminar disc to invaginate, and the cells begin to detach and migrate into the hypoblast. At day 16, nearly all the cells of the hypoblast layer are displaced, and there is now a layer of cells between the epiblast and hypoblast layer called the **mesoderm**. The remaining cells of the epiblast gives rise to the **ectoderm**, and the hypoblast cells give rise to the **endoderm**, forming a trilaminar embryo. The rearrangement and migration of cells also drives the formation of four extraembryonic membranes: the amnion, chorion, yolk sac, and allantois.

Neurulation

Neurulation describes the early stages of the formation of the nervous system. It begins in the third week of development with the differentiation of cells within the mesoderm. These cells form a rod-like structure called a **notochord** that runs along the length of the embryo within the mesoderm layer. This flexible structure induces a change in the ectoderm, causing it thicken into a **neural plate**, which invaginates into the mesoderm layer. This **neural groove** deepens until the ridges on each side (**neural folds**) make contact with each other and form a cylindrical structure called the **neural tube**. This tube will later develop into the central nervous system (brain and spinal cord). **Neural crest cells** that were once at the "crest" of each neural fold break away, and will develop into the peripheral nervous system, as well as other important tissues. Neurulation (and early embryogenesis) is finished when the entire length of the neural tube is closed. Failure of the neural tube to close completely results in a disease called spina bifida.

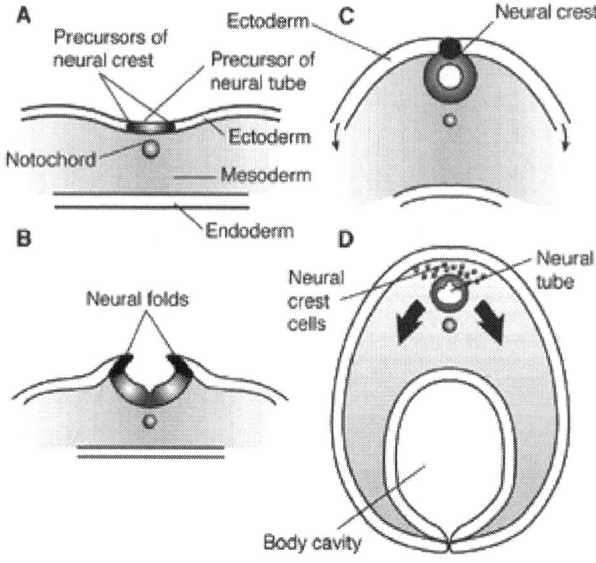

Major Structures Arising out of Primary Germ Layers

Each germ layer that forms during gastrulation contributes to specific structures and systems within the body, as described in the table below:

Primary Germ Layer	Important Derivatives
Endoderm (innermost layer)	epithelial lining of the digestive system, liver, and pancreas (excluding mouth and anus) epithelial lining of the respiratory system (excluding nasal passageways) thymus, thyroid, and parathyroid glands of the endocrine system bladder and distal urinary tract of the urinary system
Mesoderm (middle layer)	the muscular system the cardiovascular system the lymphatic system the skeletal system connective tissues of the digestive and respiratory tract dermis gonads adrenal cortex
Ectoderm (outermost layer)	central and peripheral nervous system epidermis and its appendages (hair, hair follicles, sweat glands, sebaceous glands) epithelial lining of the mouth, salivary glands, nasal passageways, and anus tooth enamel and dentin some skeletal elements of the jaw pituitary gland, and adrenal medulla

Neural Crest

Neural crest cells develop along the crests of the neural folds that arise during neurulation. When the neural tube closes, they can be found along the border of the ectoderm and neural plate (dorsal aspect). The non-neural ectoderm, neural plate, and mesoderm collectively induce the formation of these cells through a variety of signaling pathways. An important characteristic of neural crest cells is their capacity to migrate to distant locations in the body. Despite their origins in the ectoderm, these multipotent cells are sometimes called the fourth germ layer because of the many structures that they form. Neural crest cells give rise to the peripheral nervous system, including sensory ganglia, sympathetic and parasympathetic ganglia, and Schwann cells. They also contribute to other organ systems-producing the adrenal medulla, calcitonin-secreting thyroid cells, melanocytes, dentin of the tooth, smooth muscle cells, facial cartilage and bones, and a variety of other connective tissues.

Environment–Gene Interaction in Development

The development of an embryo results from complex interactions between genes and the environment. Embryogenesis is a period of accelerated gene expression that mediates the differentiation of cells, and the formation of the organ systems. Cell-cell communication, activation of transcription factors, methylation of DNA, and acetylation of histone proteins all play a role in development, and any errors in these processes can have serious consequences. Teratogens are agents that cause developmental aberrations, often by altering gene expression, which in turn may induce apoptosis or block the migration of cells. For example, high doses of vitamin A are known to interfere with the Hox genes that control the basic body plan, which disrupts the migration of neural crest cells. Other teratogenic agents include radiation, alcohol, drugs, chemicals, viruses, and bacteria.

Mechanisms of Development

Cell Specialization

Cell specialization is the process by which an immature cell develops into a cell with a specific form and function. The fate of a cell is determined largely by cues from surrounding tissues, and these cues drive gene expression. Cells destined to be a part of the same tissue coordinate their activities and give rise to properties not seen at the cellular level. Specialization consists of two main phases: determination and differentiation. A **determined** cell has no detectable morphological differences as compared to its derivative, but it is irreversibly committed to becoming a certain type of cell. A **differentiated** cell has specific structural characteristics (such as size and shape) and functional characteristics (such as responsiveness to signals, membrane potential, and metabolic activities). Such specialization arises not from modifications in the genome, but from selective gene expression.

Determination

Cell determination is the irreversible commitment of a cell to follow a specialized course of development. It is preceded by a less restrictive phase called specification. A **specified** cell can still be influenced by its surroundings, and its fate reversed or changed. **Determined** cells will not stray from their fates, even when placed in a foreign region of the embryo.

Determination can occur as a result of the asymmetric distribution of cytoplasmic molecules that mediate gene expression (such as transcription factors and the mRNA molecules that code for them) during cleavage. One of the daughter cells remains a stem cell, while the cell with the cytoplasmic determinants becomes committed to a specific lineage. Determination can also be caused by an external influence. Inductive signaling molecules called morphogens are secreted by nearby cells, and create a gradient as they diffuse across the tissues of the embryo. The response elicited by the cells that they act on is dependent on the concentration of the morphogen. Cells exposed to a high concentration will have a different fate than those exposed to a lower concentration. Only after a cell is determined will it begin the process of differentiation.

Differentiation

Differentiation refers to the biochemical, structural, and functional changes that a cell undergoes as it matures into a cell with a clearly defined role. This transition from a determined cell to a specialized cell occurs as a result of differential gene expression, which in turn is driven by transcription factors. The least differentiated cells are referred to as **totipotent**, and they have the capacity to differentiate into any type of cell, including cells of the embryo and placenta. The only human totipotent cells are the zygote itself and the cells that arise in the first few divisions. Cells that give rise to the primary germ layers are **pluripotent**, because they have the capacity to form all cell types except the trophoblasts that give rise to placental structures. **Multipotent** cells are more specialized. They can still differentiate, but have limited options. Umbilical cord stem cells and the hematopoietic stem cells that give rise to blood cells are multipotent. **Oligopotent** cells are even more restricted, and finally **unipotent** cells can only produce one type of cell. It is uncertain if true unipotent cells exist.

Tissue Types

Differentiation of the inner cell mass of the blastocyst produces the primary germ layers that ultimately give rise to four main tissue types: epithelial, connective, muscle, and nervous. Tissues are organized groups of cells that coordinate their activities to accomplish a specific function. The role of a tissue is mainly determined by the types of cells it contains, the arrangement and orientation of those cells, and the regulation of cell division and apoptosis.

Epithelial tissues consist of tightly packed cells that cover and line surfaces such as the skin and body cavities. These tissues are specialized for protection, secretion, absorption, and filtration. **Connective** tissues are characterized by an acellular matrix that surrounds the cells. They are the most abundant tissues in the human body, and function to support, protect, and connect body parts. Examples include bone, cartilage, adipose, and blood tissue. **Muscle** tissues, which include smooth, cardiac, and skeletal, contract to produce movement. **Nervous** tissue receives and responds to stimuli. It is composed of neurons that generate and conduct electrical impulses, and the glial cells that support them.

Cell–Cell Communication in Development

Cell-cell communication is crucial for the proper development of an embryo. When cells are "competent" they are able to receive signals from adjacent or nearby cells, inducing them to become a certain type of cell. (Competence is not a permanent state, and may change during the course of development.) A developing cell may also secrete inducing factors of its own. Cells that secrete signal molecules are called **inducers**, and cells that differentiate in response to those signals are called **responders**. Most of these signals are growth factors that only act on cells of a specific tissue. **Autocrine** signals are self-generated; they act on the same cell that secreted them. **Paracrine** signals diffuse to cells in close proximity. **Endocrine** signals enter the blood and travel to distant tissues. **Juxtacrine** signals require direct contact between cells. When the contact is made, signals from one cell bind to the receptors of another. Sometimes, two different tissues respond to each other's signals, promoting differentiation in each other. This is called reciprocal induction.

Cell Migration

Cell migration is required for normal embryonic development; it begins during gastrulation and continues throughout life. Any errors in the migration pathway can lead to malformations, diseases, or even demise of the embryo. Migration is initiated by signaling molecules that trigger the detachment of cells from their substrate. The cell polarizes to define a leading edge, while actin filaments of the cytoskeleton polymerize to push the cell forward in a crawling motion. Rearrangement of the cytoskeleton forms flat, sheet-like projections called **lamellipodia** at the leading edge. Sometimes, finger-like projections called **filopodia** extend beyond the lamellipodia in the direction of motion. Contraction of the cell occurs when actin interacts with myosin. Chemical messengers continually influence the direction and rate of motion, ensuring that cells reach the intended site in the body at the right time. Some cells migrate individually, while others (such as epithelial and mesenchymal cells) migrate collectively.

Pluripotency: Stem Cells

Potency describes the ability of a cell to differentiate. Only totipotent cells (the zygote and cells that arise after the first few divisions) have complete potency, but pluripotent stem cells still have great differentiation potential. They can develop into any cell type, with the exception of placental cells. As the zygote and subsequent blastomeres undergo cleavage, the once totipotent cells give rise to two lineages: the cells of the trophoblast, and the embryonic stem cells that give rise to the primary germ layers (the ectoderm, mesoderm, and endoderm). All of the hundreds of types of human cells stem from these germ layers—however, pluripotent cells cannot form an entire organism because they can't produce the needed placental tissues.

Because of the malleability of pluripotent cells, they can used therapeutically in the treatment of various diseases. Researchers have identified ways to reprogram somatic cells in a way that reverses the differentiation process. These induced pluripotent stem cells, or iPS cells, provide an alternative to the harvesting of stem cells from an embryo.

Gene Regulation in Development

Differential gene expression is the mechanism for cell specialization and ultimately the development of an organism. Many factors collectively determine which genes are expressed and *when* they are expressed. In cell-cell communication, target cells detect and respond to signals (such as growth factors) released by other cells. When a signaling molecule binds to a membrane receptor, it causes a conformational change in the receptor. The signal transduction pathway continues with the phosphorylation of cytoplasmic proteins, which leads to the activation of transcription factors. Transcription factors bind to DNA and either promote or suppress gene expression.

Other strategies exist to regulate gene expression as well. **Epigenetic regulation** involves the methylation of DNA and modification of the histone proteins that it wraps around. These heritable modifications alter the structure of the chromosome. (Regions of DNA that are more condensed are less accessible to RNA polymerase.)

Regulation continues beyond the level of transcription. For example, coding regions (exons) of messenger RNA can be spliced together in different orders to produce different proteins from the same transcript. The proteins that are produced during translation may also require activation at a later time.

Programmed Cell Death

Programmed cell death, or apoptosis, is an important part of embryonic development. It is induced by signals that activate proteases called caspases. Caspases cleave certain cytoplasmic proteins, setting a series of events in motion. The cell shrinks and loses its anchorage to adjacent cells. Chromatin condenses as the cell membrane bulges out into protrusions called blebs. The DNA and organelles are broken down into fragments, and the blebs break free of the cell, taking a portion of the cytoplasm with them. The blebs, now called apoptotic bodies, are engulfed and digested by phagocytic cells. No intracellular components leak out during this process (unlike necrosis, in which an injured cell releases its contents into the surroundings).

This regulated process is used to eliminate abnormal, mispositioned, or misplaced cells. It also helps to sculpt certain structures. For example, many of the precursors to neural cells are eliminated in order to create a more direct pathway for electrical impulses. Apoptosis also helps to shape the hands and feet. If the process is incomplete, toes or fingers may be fused in a condition known as syndactyly. Sometimes, apoptosis occurs as a result of teratogenic agents, leading to malformations or fetal death.

Existence of Regenerative Capacity in Various Species

Regenerative capacity describes the ability to regrow damaged or lost tissues. There are different mechanisms by which this can happen. **Somatic cell proliferation** occurs when differentiated cells produce more of their own kind. This is used by complex organisms as a way to heal, and rarely used to grow a complex structure such as a limb. Another means of regeneration is the **differentiation** of adult stem cells. The hematopoietic stem cells that reside in the bone marrow, for example, can give rise to any type of blood cell. **Dedifferentiation** describes the ability of specialized cells to revert back to a less differentiated state. They then proceed through a similar migration pattern as seen during development to restore the injured or missing structure. Complex structures can be regenerated this way—for example, the regrowth of a salamander limb. **Transdifferentiation** is the direct differentiation of a somatic cell into a cell of a different lineage without dedifferentiation. Pancreatic cells can transdifferentiate into liver cells.

Regeneration is used by all species to varying degrees. The hydra can regenerate its entire body from just a small fragment. Many amphibians can regenerate complex structures like limbs and tails. Birds and mammals have a much narrower range of regenerative capabilities. The human liver can quickly replace lost tissue, but the heart cannot.

Senescence and Aging

Senescence is a progressive decline in function as a result of biological aging. The term can be used to describe an organism as a whole, or the irreversible state of a cell that can no longer divide but remains physiologically active. Senescence can be brought on by the activation of an oncogene or the deactivation of a tumor suppressor gene, as a way to reduce the threat of cancer. This non-proliferative state can also be induced by oxidative stress, DNA damage, and telomere shortening. **Telomeres** are repetitive non-coding sequences of DNA found at the ends of chromosomes that protect the coding sequences. Every time a cell divides, the chromosomes shorten because DNA polymerase cannot replicate the end portion. Eventually the telomeres are lost and the cell must enter a state of senescence to prevent damage to important genes. An enzyme called telomerase *can* add nucleotides to these problematic end portions, but it is only found in certain types of cells, such as embryonic stem cells, germ cells, cancerous cells, and even adult stem cells (in low amounts). The proportion of senescent cells tends to increase with age, but evidence shows that senescence is also a strategy used during embryonic development to halt the growth of certain tissues, thereby helping to shape the embryo.

Structure and Functions of the Nervous and Endocrine Systems and Ways in Which These Systems Coordinate the Organ Systems

Nervous System: Structure and Function

Major Functions

The nervous system is responsible for coordinating and controlling all of the activities of the body. It is composed of a complex network of neurons and the neuroglial cells that support them. Neurons are responsible for carrying out the **sensory**, **integrative**, and **motor** functions of the nervous system. Sensory receptors detect changes in the internal and external environment, such as pain, pressure, light, or temperature. During integration, the information is brought to the central nervous system where it is processed and interpreted. The motor function refers to the voluntary or involuntary response that is carried out by effectors, such as the contraction of a muscle, or the secretion of products by gland cells. These rapid responses are essential for the maintenance of homeostasis, heart rate, breathing, regulation of temperature, movement, sensations, memory, emotion, language, and more.

Review Video: The Nervous System
Visit mometrix.com/academy and enter code: 708428

High Level Control and Integration of Body Systems

The nervous system is responsible for the integration of body systems. The central nervous system (CNS) consists of the brain and spinal cord. It is considered the control/integration center because it combines sensory information from various sources. It communicates with the rest of the body via the peripheral nervous system (PNS). The **afferent** division of the PNS brings information *to* the CNS, and the **efferent** division delivers messages *from* the CNS to muscles or glands.

The nervous system works particularly closely with the endocrine system. Nerve impulses send information about the condition of the body to the hypothalamus, which regulates the release of hormones from the pituitary. The pituitary, or "master gland," controls other glands of the endocrine system. All body systems ultimately require direction from the nervous system to function properly and maintain homeostasis. Heart rate, digestion, body temperature, movement, and higher functions such as cognitive ability, memory, emotion, and fine motor skills are under the control of the nervous system.

Adaptive Capability to External Influences

The nervous system is the first body system to respond to changes in the environment. The receptors of afferent neurons (sensory neurons) are specialized to detect certain types of stimuli, and these neurons transmit action potentials to the CNS where a motor response may be called for. Sensory receptors are found nearly everywhere in the body. They can be classified by location, morphology (free vs. encapsulated nerve endings), the nature of the stimuli they detect (pressure, chemicals, light, temperature), and rate of adaptation.

Sensory adaptation refers to the change in sensitivity that occurs when receptors are exposed to a prolonged stimulus. Adaptation rates vary greatly across the different types of receptors, but they can be classified into two main groups. **Phasic** receptors quickly adapt to a constant stimulus, meaning that action potentials decrease over time and eventually stop. This explains the loss of sensation of clothes against the skin, or how an odor seems to disappear when the source is still present. Most tactile and chemoreceptors are phasic. **Tonic** receptors adapt slowly, constantly alerting the CNS of the stimulus with action potentials. Proprioceptors (receptors that provide feedback about position and movement of the body) are tonic receptors, as are photoreceptors (light-detecting receptors) and nociceptors (pain receptors).

Organization of Vertebrate Nervous System

The nervous system is divided into two main parts: the central nervous system (CNS), which consists of the brain and spinal cord, and the peripheral nervous system (PNS), which consists of nervous tissues (nerves, ganglia) that are outside the CNS. The CNS integrates sensory information, and the PNS sends information to and from the CNS, allowing it to communicate with the rest of the body. Afferent neurons of the PNS transmit impulses to the CNS, and efferent neurons transmit impulses to effectors.

The PNS is further divided into the autonomic system (ANS) and somatic nervous system (SNS). The SNS controls voluntary movements, such as the contraction of skeletal muscles. The ANS controls involuntary movements, such as the contraction of smooth and cardiac muscles, and glandular secretions. The ANS has two subdivisions that tend to work antagonistically (though there are exceptions). The sympathetic division activates the "fight or flight" response, preparing the body for action by increasing heart rate, dilating pupils and bronchial tubes, and suppressing functions that are not required for immediate survival. The parasympathetic division activates the "rest and digest" functions by decreasing heart rate, constricting pupils and bronchial tubes, and promoting digestion.

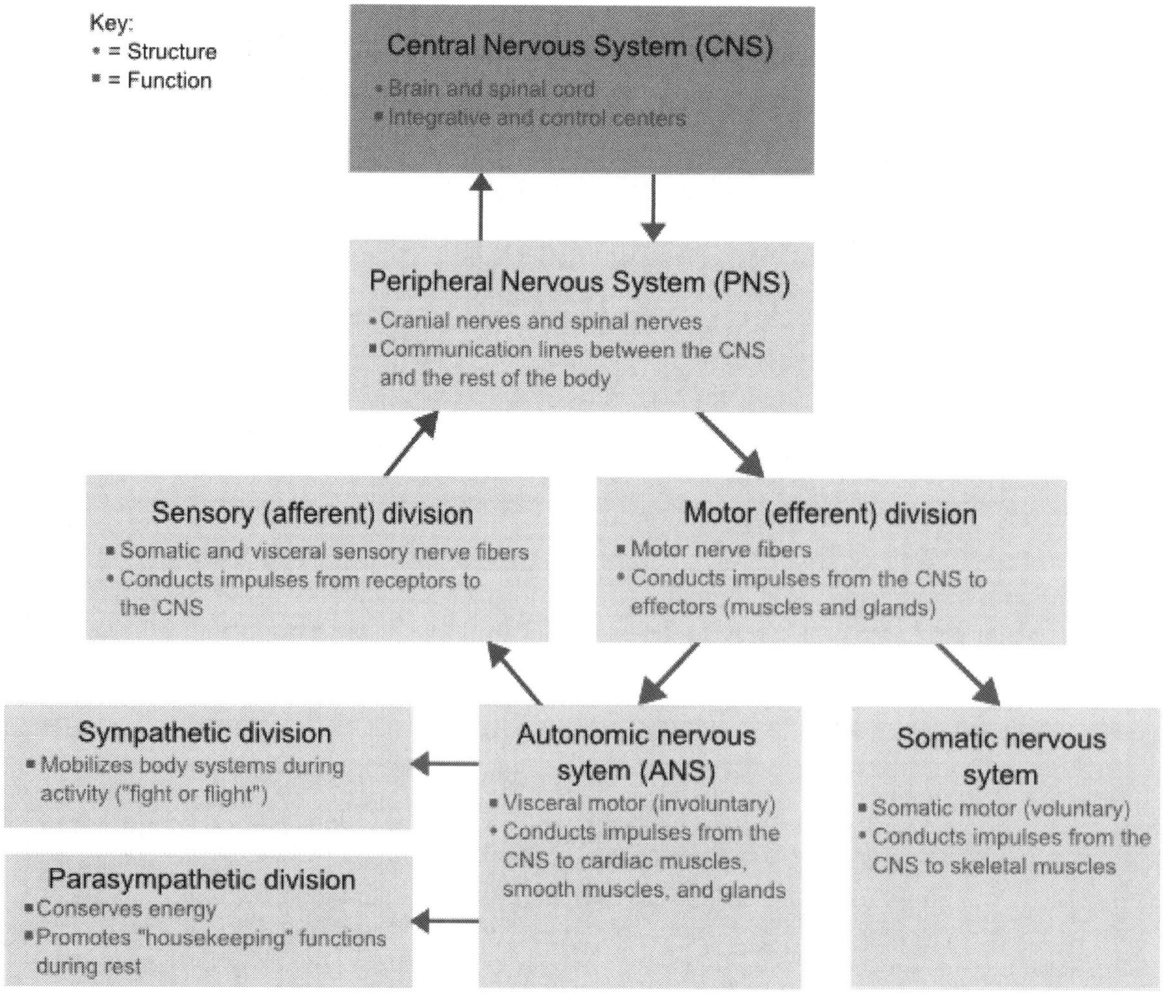

Key:
• = Structure
▪ = Function

Central Nervous System (CNS)
• Brain and spinal cord
▪ Integrative and control centers

Peripheral Nervous System (PNS)
• Cranial nerves and spinal nerves
▪ Communication lines between the CNS and the rest of the body

Sensory (afferent) division
▪ Somatic and visceral sensory nerve fibers
• Conducts impulses from receptors to the CNS

Motor (efferent) division
▪ Motor nerve fibers
• Conducts impulses from the CNS to effectors (muscles and glands)

Sympathetic division
▪ Mobilizes body systems during activity ("fight or flight")

Parasympathetic division
▪ Conserves energy
▪ Promotes "housekeeping" functions during rest

Autonomic nervous sytem (ANS)
▪ Visceral motor (involuntary)
• Conducts impulses from the CNS to cardiac muscles, smooth muscles, and glands

Somatic nervous sytem
▪ Somatic motor (voluntary)
• Conducts impulses from the CNS to skeletal muscles

Sensor and Effector Neurons

Sensory neurons are the afferent neurons that deliver impulses to the CNS. They are sometimes classified by the type of stimulus that they respond to. **Mechanoreceptors** respond to changes in pressure or tension. Cutaneous touch receptors such as Meissner's corpuscles, Merkel's disks, Pacinian corpuscles, and Ruffini endings are all mechanoreceptors, as are the muscle spindles that detect stretching of skeletal muscle and the receptors of the inner ear that detect vibrations. **Chemoreceptors** such as olfactory and taste receptors detect the presence of chemicals. **Photoreceptors** such as the rod and cone cells of the eye respond to light. **Thermoreceptors** sense both absolute temperature, and changes in temperature. **Nociceptors** detect pain.

Sensory neurons can also be categorized by location. **Exteroceptors** near the body surface transmit information about the external environment. **Proprioceptors** within the inner ear, skeletal muscles, and joints provide information about movement, position, and equilibrium. **Interoceptors** of visceral organs and blood vessels provide information about internal stimuli.

Once the sensory information has been processed, **effector neurons** (motor neurons) transmit the impulse away from the CNS to activate muscles and glands. All motor neurons of the somatic division run directly from the CNS to the effector without synapsing with another neuron. The autonomic division uses two-neuron pathways.

Sympathetic and Parasympathetic Nervous Systems: Antagonistic Control

The autonomic nervous system has two divisions, sympathetic and parasympathetic, and they tend to have antagonistic effects when they both innervate the same organ. Both divisions use a two-neuron pathway, consisting of a preganglionic neuron which runs from the CNS to a ganglion, and a postganglionic neuron which innervates the effector.

The sympathetic nervous division is responsible for triggering the "fight or flight" response. Preganglionic neurons of the sympathetic nervous system release acetylcholine (ACh), which is the stimulus for the release of norepinephrine from postganglionic neurons. Norepinephrine acts on target tissues, prompting a rapid and unified response. The heart rate increases, respiration rate increases, blood flow to the heart and skeletal muscle increases, pupils dilate, and glycogen is broken down.

The parasympathetic nervous division is responsible for the "rest and digest" response. *Both* pre- and postganglionic neurons of the parasympathetic nervous system release acetylcholine. The parasympathetic nervous system stimulates events that are slower-paced, and less essential for immediate survival. The heart rate and respiration rate decrease, blood flow is directed to digestive organs, peristalsis is promoted, pupils constrict, and glycogen is synthesized.

Reflexes

A **reflex** is a nearly instantaneous, unconscious, and involuntary response to a stimulus. The stimulus (for example, the sensation of heat when one touches a hot stove) is detected by the receptors of afferent neurons, and sensory information is sent to interneurons in the spinal cord. (Interneurons are entirely restricted to the central nervous system, and act as bridges between sensory and motor neurons.) From here, the signal travels along motor neurons to the effectors (the muscles of the arm and hand). Before the signal for pain has reached the brain, the hand has already been withdrawn. While reflexes do not require conscious thought, some have pathways that involve the brain. The brain can sometimes override reflex actions—for example, trying not to blink during an eye exam. Sometimes, a reflex involves a direct link between the sensory and motor neuron—for example, the patellar reflex, or knee-jerk reaction. This is referred to as a monosynaptic reflex. Polysynaptic reflexes are more complex because they involve interneurons.

FEEDBACK LOOP, REFLEX ARC

A reflex arc describes a neural pathway that triggers a reflex action. It begins with a **receptor**—the site or organ that receives the stimulus. A **sensory neuron** carries the impulse along the afferent pathway to the **integration center** within the central nervous system. Interneurons process the information and pass the impulse to a **motor neuron**. The impulse travels along the efferent pathway to the **effector**—the responding muscle or gland.

Most reflexes attempt to maintain homeostasis by inhibiting a change in condition; this is called negative feedback. The maintenance of body temperature is one of many examples. As body temperature changes, thermoreceptors send information to the hypothalamus. If body temperature is too high, a command is sent to dilate blood vessels and release sweat. If the temperature is too low, the body shivers and blood vessels constrict. Positive feedback loops are less common, and sometimes harmful because they enhance the stimuli rather than inhibit them. A beneficial form of positive feedback occurs during childbirth. When the cervix is stretched by the descending fetus, impulses are sent to the pituitary, which sends a command to increase uterine contractions. The more the fetus is pushed, the more the cervix stretches. This positive feedback loop continues until birth.

ROLE OF SPINAL CORD AND SUPRASPINAL CIRCUITS

The spinal cord is a major reflex center that connects the afferent and efferent pathways. It is made of an exterior layer of white matter that surrounds an interior core of grey matter. The white matter consists of glial cells and myelinated bundles of axons that form tracts to and from the brain. There are no cell bodies or dendrites in white matter. Grey matter consists mostly of interneurons, but also contains motor neurons and glial cells. (The axons are mostly unmyelinated, giving the tissue its grey appearance.) The cell bodies of afferent neurons reside in dorsal root ganglia, just outside the spinal cord. Afferent fibers enter into the posterior/dorsal aspect of the spinal cord (a region called the posterior grey horn) through the anterior root, while efferent fibers exit on the anterior/ventral aspect (the anterior grey horn) through the posterior root. Spinal neurons usually innervate structures that are inferior to the neck.

Not all reflexes are mediated by spinal neurons. Supraspinal circuits require input from the brain or brainstem, and are involved in actions such as the blinking and gagging reflexes.

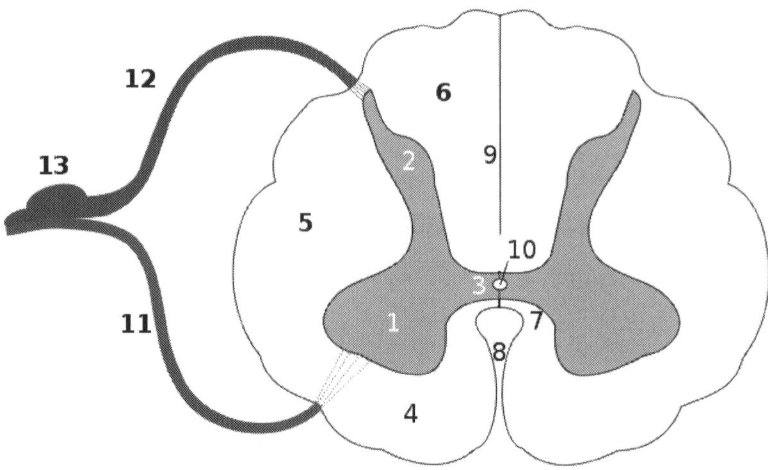

Cross section of a spinal cord		
Gray matter	**White matter**	**Other structures**
1. Anterior horn	4. Anterior funiculus	10. Central canal
2. Posterior horn	5. Lateral funiculus	11. Anterior root
3. Grey commissure	6. Posterior funiculus	12. Posterior root
	7. Anterior commissure	13. Dorsal root ganglion
	8. Anterior median fissure	
	9. Posterior median sulcus	

Integration with Endocrine System: Feedback Control

The nervous system is closely integrated with the endocrine system. Both systems control the body—the nervous system through electrical impulses, and the endocrine system though slower-acting, but longer-lasting hormones. The two systems are linked via the hypothalamus, a region in the brain that controls the autonomic nervous system as well as the pituitary gland. In fact, neurons within the hypothalamus have axons that extend through the infundibulum and terminate in the posterior pituitary. The hypothalamus produces oxytocin and antidiuretic hormone (ADH), but these hormones are stored in and secreted by the posterior pituitary. The release of other important hormones from the anterior pituitary is also regulated by the hypothalamus. Pituitary hormones go on to control other endocrine glands and body functions. Hormones travel through the bloodstream to target tissues, eliciting responses that are important for growth, development, metabolism, and the maintenance of homeostasis. An example of the interaction between the two systems can be seen in the letdown of milk during nursing. As a baby begins to nurse, the stimulus sends an impulse to the hypothalamus, causing the pituitary to release oxytocin into the blood. The hormone targets the mammary gland, inducing it to release milk.

Nerve Cell

Cell Body: Site of Nucleus, Organelles

The cell body, or soma, of a neuron contains the organelles that are responsible for the metabolic activities of the neuron. The interior of the cell body contains a nucleus with a prominent nucleolus. The DNA within the nucleus encodes the information for the many proteins that are needed for the neuron to function. The neuronal cytoplasm contains most of the organelles that are characteristic of animal cells (cytoskeleton, rough and smooth endoplasmic reticulum, Golgi bodies, lysosomes, peroxisomes, and mitochondria). There are relatively high numbers of mitochondria to support the high metabolic needs of the neuron. Granular Nissl bodies (made of rough ER and clusters of free ribosomes) synthesize proteins for use within the cell. Notably absent in mature neurons are centrioles, as differentiated neurons have lost their ability to divide. Various projections (dendrites and/or an axon) extend from the cell body, and neurons can be classified according to these structural differences.

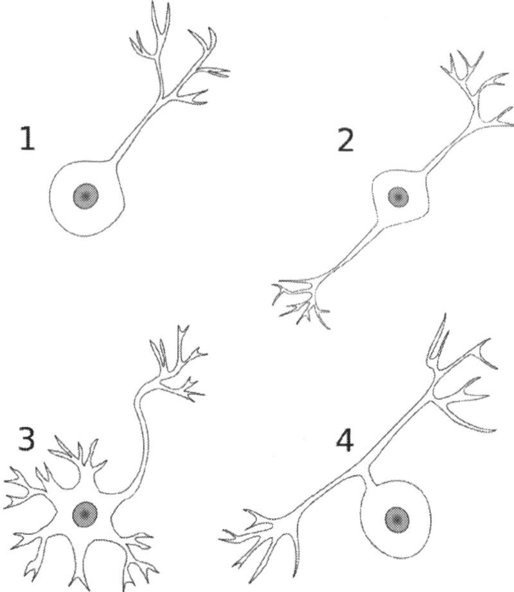

- 1: unipolar (many sensory neurons are unipolar)
- 2: bipolar (rare—associated with retina of the eyes, and inner ear)
- 3: multipolar (most common type—interneurons and motor neurons)
- 4: pseudounipolar (sensory neurons)

Dendrites: Branched Extensions of Cell Body

Dendrites are relatively short, branched extensions of the cell body that receive incoming chemical signals (neurotransmitters) from the other neurons. These tree-like projections taper with every branch, maximizing the surface area for synaptic inputs. Many dendrites have tiny protrusions called dendritic spines that synapse with a single axon. The cytoplasm within the dendrites contains the same organelles as the cell body, with the exception of the nucleus.

The neurotransmitters that are released from axon terminals of the presynaptic cell cross the synaptic cleft, where they bind to receptor sites on the dendrites of the postsynaptic cells. These signals may be excitatory or inhibitory, and the net effect of these signals determines whether the neuron is inhibited or triggered to fire (in which case the chemical message will be converted to an electrical impulse that travels down the axon).

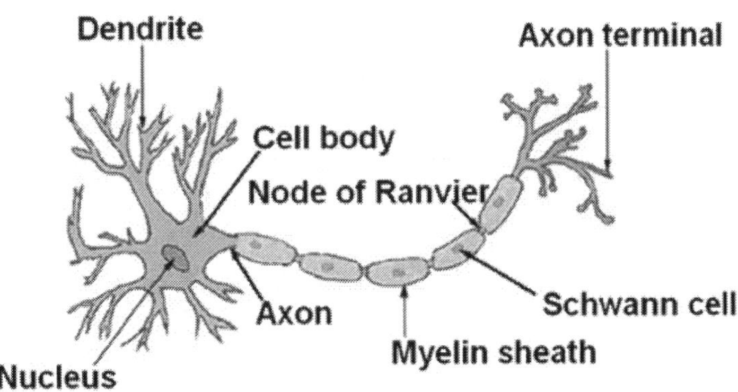

Axon: Structure and Function

An axon is a smooth, cable-like nerve fiber that is specialized to conduct electrical impulses away from the soma. Most neurons have one long axon, but the axon's length can vary, and some neurons have no axon at all. The axon emerges from a slightly elevated structure called the **axon hillock** that connects the soma to the axon. The cytoplasm of the axon is called **axoplasm**, and it lacks the Golgi bodies, Nissl bodies, and ribosomes found in dendritic cytoplasm. Since there is little to no translation, proteins must be imported from the soma. The axon often splits into **collaterals** that allow one neuron to interact with more than one cell. At the end of each axon are highly branched structures called **axon terminals**. These club-shaped endings contain synaptic vesicles filled with neurotransmitters. When an action potential is generated at the axon hillock, it propagates along the axon. When it reaches the axon terminals, the neurotransmitters are released to a target cell.

Myelin Sheath, Schwann Cells, Insulation of Axon

The axons of many neurons are sheathed in a lipid-based coating called **myelin**. Myelin insulates the axon much like the coating on electrical wire. It also increases the rate at which an impulse can travel. There are intermittent gaps in the sheath called nodes of Ranvier that allow the impulse to jump quickly from one node to the next.

Neurons of the peripheral nervous system are myelinated by **Schwann cells**. These glial cells curve around the axon, wrapping their plasma membranes around it like a bandage to form multiple lipid-rich layers. The nucleus and cytoplasm remain outside the myelin sheath, but are encased in the outer **neurilemmal** sheath of the Schwann cell. Axons of very small diameter may be supported by Schwann cells, but are not myelinated by them. These are called non-myelinating Schwann cells. **Oligodendrocytes** are responsible for sheathing the neurons of the central nervous system. Unlike Schwann cells, a single oligodendrocyte can myelinate dozens of axons by extending its membrane in multiple directions and wrapping around the axons. White matter of the CNS is made mostly of myelinated axons, while the axons associated with grey matter are unmyelinated.

Multiple sclerosis, the leukodystrophies, and many other diseases result from damaged myelin. Without the proper insulation, the neurons of affected individuals cannot effectively conduct an impulse.

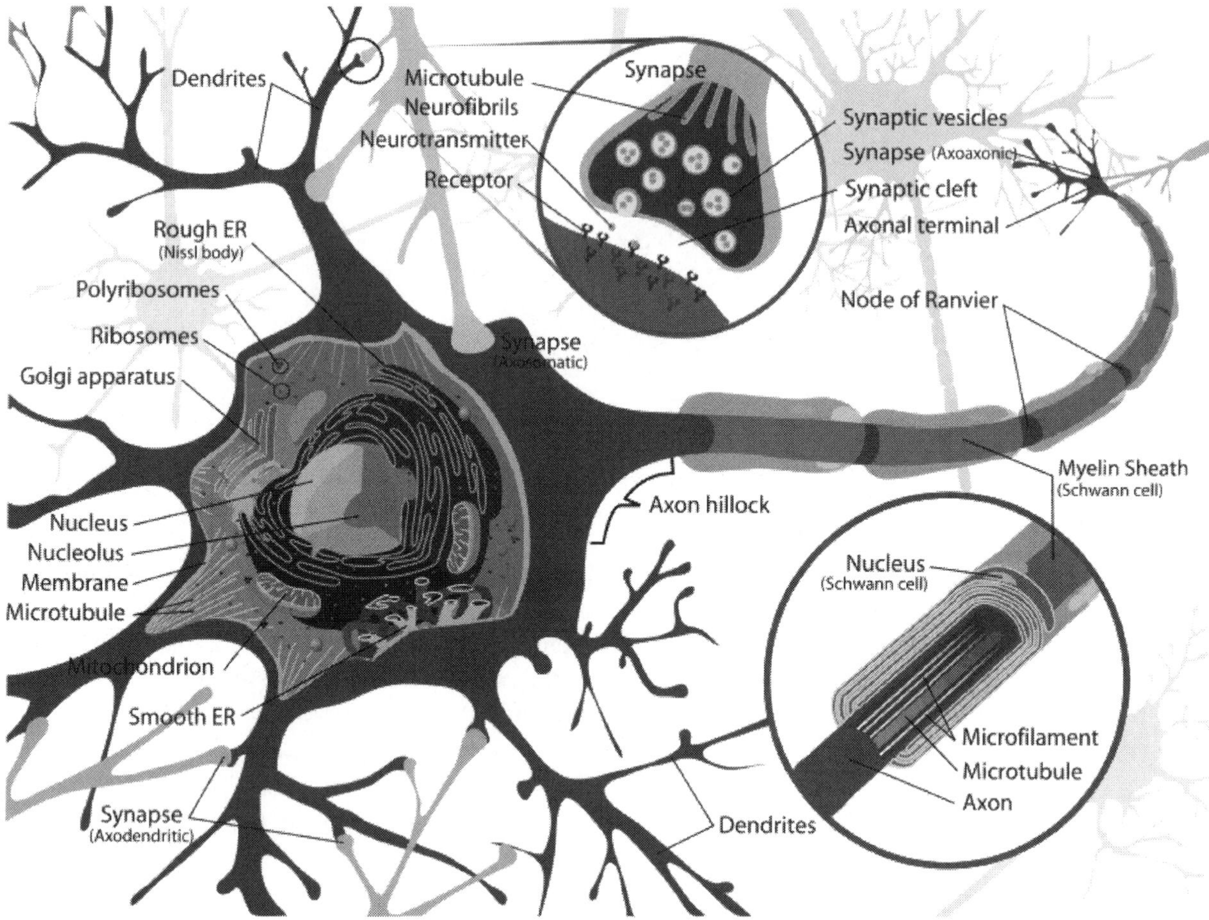

Nodes of Ranvier: Propagation of Nerve Impulse Along Axon

Nodes of Ranvier are uninsulated gaps between myelinated portions of the axon that increase the rate of conduction. These exposed portions are about 1 μm in length, and they contain a high density of voltage gated sodium and potassium channels. The channels open to allow the passage of these ions, depolarizing the membrane. Since ions are unable to diffuse through the myelin, the action potential must jump to the next node. This is called **saltatory propagation**. This type of conduction is faster and more efficient than the continuous conduction that is seen along the entire length of an unsheathed axon. Large-diameter myelinated axons conduct impulses much faster (80–120 m/s) than thin unmyelinated axons (0.5–10 m/s). While rapid conduction has its benefits, myelinated axons have less neuroplasticity than unmyelinated axons; that is, they are more limited in their ability to form new connections with other neurons.

Synapse: Site of Impulse Propagation Between Cells

A **synapse** is a communicating junction between two neurons, or between a neuron and an effector (muscle or gland). The synapse consists of a presynaptic element, a tiny gap called the synaptic cleft, and a postsynaptic element. Impulses are transmitted across the synaptic cleft through the action of neurotransmitters. Synapses can be classified according to the nature of the postsynaptic element. **Axodendritic** synapses terminate on the dendrites of a postsynaptic neuron. **Axosomatic** synapses terminate on a postsynaptic soma. **Axoaxonic** synapses are rare, terminating on a postsynaptic axon.

They can also be classified by the mode in which the impulse is transmitted. Most synapses are unidirectional **chemical** junctions, using neurotransmitters to send messages to the postsynaptic cell. When the impulse reaches the axon terminals, the vesicles that store the neurotransmitters fuse with the plasma membrane, releasing the signals into the synaptic cleft before they bind to receptors on the postsynaptic target. At this point, the postsynaptic membrane will either be excited (depolarized) or inhibited (hyperpolarized). Bidirectional **electrical** synaptic junctions do not use neurotransmitters. They are linked by gap junctions that allow the flow of ions between cells. Electrical synapses are faster, always excitatory, and rarer.

Generic Neurotransmitter System

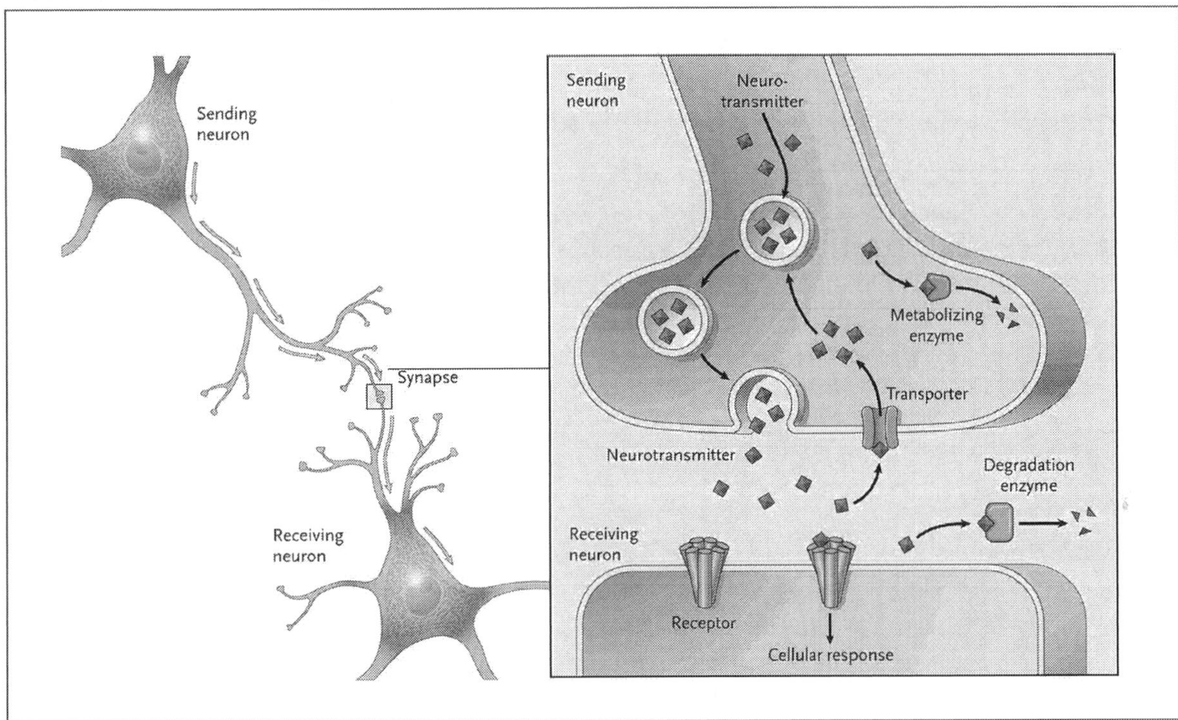

SYNAPTIC ACTIVITY: TRANSMITTER MOLECULES

When an action potential reaches the axon terminal, voltage-gated calcium channels open in response to the depolarization of the membrane. Calcium ions enter, triggering the release of neurotransmitters by exocytosis. The neurotransmitters diffuse across the synaptic cleft, binding to receptors in the target cell and eliciting either an excitatory or an inhibitory response. The neurotransmitters are then recycled back to the presynaptic cell, are degraded by enzymes, or diffuse away from the synaptic cleft to prevent overstimulation.

Common neurotransmitters and their actions are summarized below:

Neurotransmitter	Action
Acetylcholine (ACh)	Stimulates skeletal muscle
Norepinephrine (NE)	Influences mood and sleep patterns
Dopamine	Associated with mood, attention, reward system, and movement
Histamine	Works with the hypothalamus, promotes wakefulness
Serotonin	Many roles–mostly inhibitory. Influences sleep, mood, hunger, and arousal
GABA	The major inhibitory neurotransmitter
Glutamate	The major excitatory neurotransmitter

Resting Potential: Electrochemical Gradient

The resting potential describes the voltage across a non-signaling neuron's membrane. It averages −70 millivolts due to an excess of negative charge in the cytoplasm as compared to the extracellular fluid. In this resting state, most of the voltage-gated sodium and potassium channels are closed. There are, however, many ungated potassium channels that allow the leakage of potassium ions (K^+) out of the cell (down the concentration gradient). There are far fewer leak channels for the sodium ions (Na^+) that are more concentrated on the outside of the cell. This differential permeability is an important factor in the establishment of the resting potential membrane. As potassium ions diffuse out of the cell, they leave behind negatively charged organic ions in the cytoplasm. Eventually their diffusion is opposed by electrical forces, and the ions are pulled back into the cell. (This combination of forces is called an electrochemical gradient.) For the difference in electric potential to be maintained, the concentration gradients of potassium and sodium must also be maintained. An ATP-powered enzyme called the sodium/potassium pump transports 3 Na^+ out of the cell for every 2 K^+ that it takes in. This counteracts the leakage of ions, maintaining a resting potential of −70 mV.

Action Potential

An **action potential** is the rapid change in membrane potential that occurs when an impulse is generated. At rest, the voltage-gated sodium channels of a neuron are closed, but a stimulus can cause some of them to open. The entry of Na^+ **depolarizes** the membrane; the membrane potential becomes more positive. If the stimulus meets or exceeds the threshold, more sodium channels open. The Na^+ that was concentrated outside the cell diffuses in, completely depolarizing the membrane, peaking at around +30 mV. The gates close quickly, but not before triggering nearby channels to open. A chain reaction takes the action potential down the axon.

The membrane potential is restored during **repolarization**. Voltage-gated potassium ions open as the sodium channels close, and K^+ leaves the cell, causing the inside to become negatively charged again. The membrane becomes momentarily **hyperpolarized** (around −80 mV) as more K^+ leave the cell than is necessary to establish resting potential. During the **refractory period**, the neuron either requires a greater than normal stimulus to respond (relative refractory period) or does not respond at all (absolute refractory period). The sodium-potassium pump establishes the original concentration gradients of Na^+ and K^+ by pumping sodium out and potassium in, and the neuron can fire again.

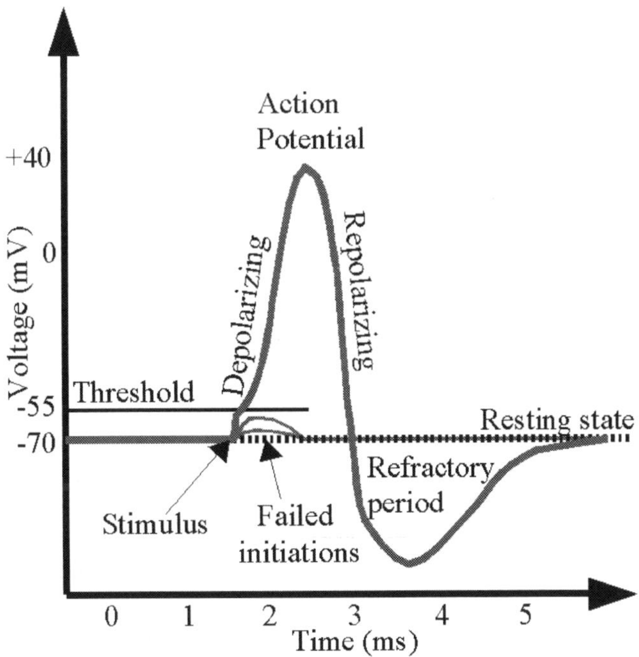

Threshold, All-or-None

The threshold potential is the level of depolarization that is required to trigger an action potential. The average threshold value is about −55 mV. When neurotransmitters bind to the postsynaptic neuron, their effects may be excitatory or inhibitory. Whether or not the neuron fires depends on the sum of these effects. If the excitatory signals outweigh the inhibitory signals enough to reach the critical threshold, an action potential will be generated (usually at the axon hillock), sending an impulse down the neuron.

The threshold potential follows an "all-or-nothing" principle. If the stimulus is too weak to depolarize the membrane to −55 mV, then the neuron will not fire. As soon as the threshold potential is reached, the neuron will fire, and it will always fire with the same intensity - even if it overshoots the threshold. There are no "weak" or "strong" action potentials, but the neuron *can* fire more frequently as the strength of a stimulus increases.

Sodium/Potassium Pump

The potential difference (or voltage) across a membrane is determined by the relative concentrations of ions on each side of the membrane. Potassium ions are more concentrated inside the cytoplasm of a neuron, and sodium ions are more concentrated on the outside. These ions diffuse down their concentration gradients through leak channels, though the membrane is far less permeable to sodium. Without some mechanism to restore the concentration gradients, the membrane would depolarize. A transmembrane protein called the sodium/potassium pump solves this problem by using active transport to pump 3 Na^+ out of the cell for every 2 K^+ that are pumped inside. Before it is phosphorylated by ATP, this electrogenic pump has an affinity for the sodium ions inside the cell. Once it is phosphorylated, it changes shape, exporting 3 Na^+. In this conformation, the pump now has an affinity for the potassium ions that are outside the cell. The phosphate group is released, and 2 K^+ enter. The imbalance of ion shuttling maintains the polarity of the membrane.

Excitatory and Inhibitory Nerve Fibers: Summation, Frequency of Firing

A single neuron can have thousands of synapses with presynaptic neurons. Some of these synapses will have excitatory effects–increasing the probability that an action potential will be generated—, and others will have inhibitory effects—decreasing the probability that an action potential will be generated. The neurotransmitters released by an **inhibitory** nerve fiber will open potassium channels in the postsynaptic cell, allowing the *outflow* of K^+. This leads to localized *hyperpolarization* known as an inhibitory postsynaptic potential (IPSP). The neurotransmitters released by an **excitatory** nerve fiber will open sodium channels in the postsynaptic cell, allowing the *inflow* of Na^+. This leads to localized *depolarization* known as an excitatory postsynaptic potential (EPSP). The summation of these IPSPs and EPSPs determines whether or not the neuron will fire. **Temporal summation** is the integration of repeated signals from a single neuron over a short time, while **spatial summation** is the integration of simultaneous signals from two or more neurons. If the membrane depolarizes to threshold level, an action potential will result. The strength of the EPSP has a direct effect on the frequency of action potentials, but not on the intensity of the action potentials. For this reason, the nervous system is said to be "frequency modulated" as opposed to "amplitude modulated."

Glial Cells, Neuroglia

Glial cells, also called neuroglia, support and protect neurons within the central and peripheral nervous system. Despite their inability to conduct impulses, there are many more glial cells than neurons within nervous tissue. Glia also have the ability to divide, and so nearly all brain tumors arise from them.

CNS Glial Cell	**Structure / Characteristics**	**Function**
Astrocytes	Star-shaped The most abundant cells found in neural tissue	Anchor neurons Facilitate the exchange of materials between capillaries and neurons Uptake excess ions and neurotransmitters
Microglia	Spider-shaped—relatively few extensions	Phagocytic—immune defense, digest dead neurons and debris
Oligodendrocytes	Structurally similar to an astrocyte, but fewer extensions Extensions wrap around axons of CNS neurons	Produce the myelin sheaths that insulate CNS neurons Speed up neurotransmission
Ependyma	Ciliated cells that form the epithelial lining of the ventricles and central canal of the spinal cord Columnar or cuboidal	Circulate cerebrospinal fluid (CSF) Facilitate the exchange of materials between the CSF and interstitial fluid of brain and spinal cord

PNS Glial Cell	**Structure / Characteristics**	**Function**
Schwann cells	Extensive lipid membranes wrap around PNS axons to form layers	Produce the myelin sheaths that insulate PNS neurons Speed up neurotransmission
Satellite cells	Flattened cells that surround the soma of neurons within PNS ganglia	Protect and cushion PNS neurons

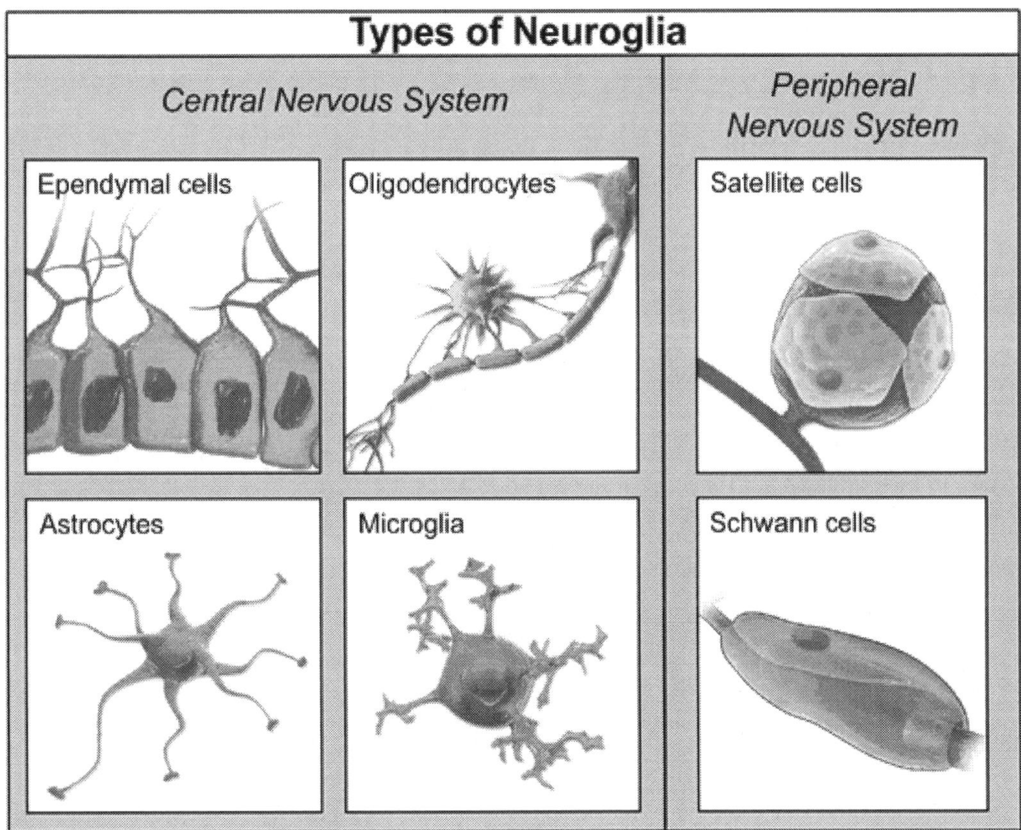

ELECTROCHEMISTRY

CONCENTRATION CELL: DIRECTION OF ELECTRON FLOW, NERNST EQUATION

The cell membrane of a neuron can be compared to a type of a galvanic cell known as a concentration cell. The difference in concentration of ions on each side of the cell membrane sets up a voltage, much like the two half-cells of a concentration cell (each half differs only in concentration, not material). The Nernst equation relates the voltage (or Nernst potential) to the concentration gradient and charge of the ion in question (only one species of ion can be considered in the calculation.) As can be seen in the equation, if there is no difference in concentration across the membrane, then there will be no voltage, since the natural log of 1 is zero. The equation below examines potassium (K^+) but any ion can be substituted in for K.

$$V = \frac{RT}{zF}\ln\frac{[K^+]_o}{[K^+]_i}$$

- V (or E) = membrane potential
- R = ideal gas constant (8.314 JK−1 mol−1)
- T = temperature (Kelvins)
- z = charge on the ion
- F = Faraday's constant (96485 C mol−1)
- ln = natural log
- $[K^+]_o$ = potassium concentration outside the cell
- $[K^+]_i$ = potassium concentration inside the cell

Biosignaling

Gated Ion Channels

Voltage Gated

Voltage-gated ion channels are transmembrane proteins that open and close in response to a change in membrane potential. Typically, these channels are highly selective, only allowing the passage of one type of ion. When an electrically excitable cell like a neuron is at its resting potential, voltage-gated channels are closed. But as a membrane depolarizes, the new electric field causes the proteins to change conformation.

Voltage-gated sodium channels have two gates: the activation gate (**gate m**) and the deactivation gate (**gate h**). These gates allow a sodium channel to shift between three conformations: closed, open, and inactivated. In the closed state (resting potential), gate m is closed, and gate h is open. Gate m opens in response to a stimulus and sodium ions diffuse into the cell, further depolarizing the membrane. At the peak of depolarization, gate h closes to block the inflow of sodium ions, and the channel is in an inactive state.

Voltage-gated potassium channels only have one gate: **gate n**. Gate n opens immediately before the sodium channels are inactivated. As potassium ions flow out of the cell, the membrane repolarizes. The potassium channel closes relatively slowly, allowing an excess of potassium ions to exit the cell.

Ligand Gated

Ligand-gated ion channels (LGICs, or ionotropic receptors) are receptor proteins that are commonly found in electrically excitable cells because they can respond very quickly to a stimulus. These transmembrane proteins undergo a rapid change in conformation in response to the binding of a particular substance, often a neurotransmitter. In a postsynaptic neuron, LGICs receive the neurotransmitters that are released from the presynaptic axon terminals. When the ligands bind, they trigger the opening of a channel within the protein that allows the flow of certain ions down their concentration gradients. These channels tend to be less specific than voltage-gated ion channels, and sometimes allow the passage of more than one type of ion. The ligand itself, however, is very specific to its receptor—fitting into it like a lock and key. As ions cross the membrane, the voltage changes, and the chemical message is translated into an electrical message. GABA, for example, is the primary inhibitory neurotransmitter in the nervous system. When it binds to its ionotropic receptor, the channel opens to allow chloride ions (Cl^-) into the cell. The cell becomes hyperpolarized and therefore less likely to fire.

Receptor Enzymes

Receptor enzymes are transmembrane proteins that act as catalysts in response to the binding of a ligand. These proteins share a common structure; they have an extracellular **ligand-binding domain**, an intracellular **enzymatic domain**, and a transmembrane domain that connects them. When a signal molecule from outside the cell binds to the ligand-binding domain, the protein undergoes a conformational change which activates the catalytic function of the enzymatic domain. This in turn triggers a signaling cascade inside the cell.

The most common class of receptor enzymes are **receptor tyrosine kinases** (RTKs). When activated by ligands (often growth factors), they phosphorylate tyrosine residues on a variety of proteins within the cytosol. These physiological changes promote differential gene expression, and help to regulate the growth and development of a cell. Neurotrophins, for example, are ligands that bind to the Trk family of RTKs. They play a critical role in the survival and proper functioning of neurons.

G Protein-Coupled Receptors

G protein-coupled receptors (GPCRs) are a large class of receptor proteins that respond to a wide array of signals, including neurotransmitters, ions, light, hormones, and odor molecules. There are roughly 1,000 types of GPCRs in humans, and all share the same general structure regardless of the specific ligand that they interact with. The α-helices of the protein span the membrane seven times, with the ligand-binding site on the extracellular side. When a ligand binds, the conformation of the protein changes, activating the G protein to which it is coupled. G proteins are heterotrimeric (they consist of an alpha, beta, and gamma subunit) and are capable of binding to guanosine triphosphate (GTP) and guanosine diphosphate (GDP). When the G protein is activated, the α-subunit replaces the bound GDP with GTP. This causes the α-subunit (along with the bound GTP) to dissociate from the β- and γ-subunits, while remaining within the membrane. The G protein, depending on the type, will then go on to either stimulate or inhibit certain biosignaling pathways. G proteins are typically responsible for increasing or decreasing amounts of cyclic AMP or triggering the flow of calcium ions into the cell.

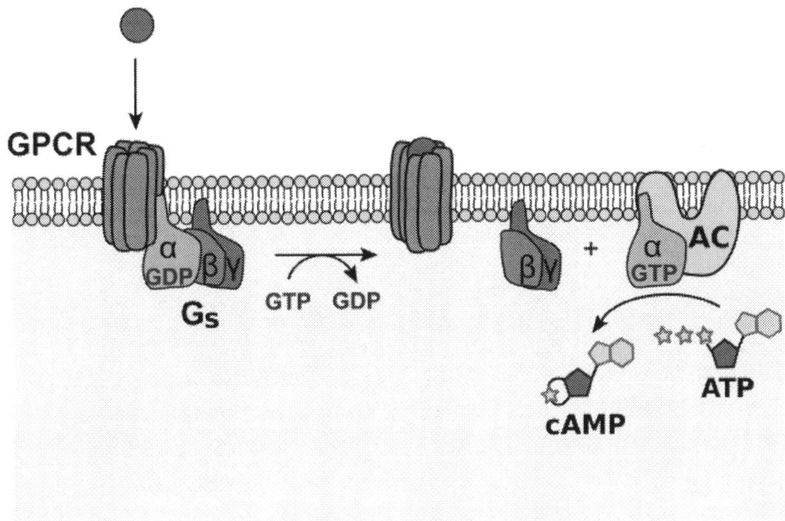

Lipids

Description; Structure

Lipids are a class of structurally and functionally diverse biomolecules that are characterized by their hydrophobic properties; they do not dissolve in water but do mix well with nonpolar substances. They can be classified according to structure into two main groups: saponifiable and non-saponifiable. Saponifiable lipids, such as triacylglycerols and phospholipids, contain fatty acid chains with ester linkages that can be easily hydrolyzed. Non-saponifiable lipids, such as steroids and terpenes, are non-ester lipids that lack fatty acids.

Lipids are involved in a variety of functions. Triacylglycerols can be metabolized for energy, and serve as energy storage. Phospholipids are the major structural components of cell membranes, and a type of glycolipid known as galactocerebroside forms the myelin sheaths that insulate neurons. Lipids play active roles as well, including biosignaling. Steroid hormones such as glucocorticoids, mineralocorticoids, and the sex hormones travel through the blood, diffuse into target cells, and bind to receptors that directly regulate gene expression.

Review Video: Lipids
Visit mometrix.com/academy and enter code: 269746

Steroids

Steroids consist of four fused cycloalkane rings (three hexanes and one pentane). Cholesterol is a **sterol** (a steroid alcohol) that acts as a fluidity buffer in cell membranes. It is also the precursor to bile acids, vitamin D, and steroid hormones.

Steroid hormones include the sex hormones and corticosteroids. Sex hormones are responsible for secondary sex characteristics. They are secreted primarily by the gonads and placenta, but are also produced in small amounts by the adrenal cortex. The "female" sex hormones are the estrogens (such as estradiol), and the "male" hormones are the androgens (such as testosterone). Progesterone is produced by the corpus luteum and the placenta, and is important for the preparation and maintenance of pregnancy.

The adrenal cortex secretes glucocorticoids and mineralocorticoids. These corticosteroids help to control inflammation, electrolyte and water balance, stress responses, immune responses, and metabolism. A common glucocorticoid is the stress hormone cortisol, which acts as an anti-inflammatory. Aldosterone is a mineralocorticoid that regulates the levels of sodium and potassium in the blood, helping to maintain blood pressure.

Since these hormones are insoluble in water, they rely on plasma proteins to transport them in the bloodstream. Once released from these proteins, the hormones can diffuse through the cell membrane, bind to intracellular receptors, and directly regulate gene expression.

Terpenes and Terpenoids

Terpenes are plant-made, generally odiferous lipids that can be built up into many other biological molecules, including steroids. Terpenes arise from the polymerization of **isoprene**: a hydrocarbon with the general formula C_5H_8. The formula for a terpene follows the C5 rule; it will always be a multiple of C_5H_8—or $(C_5H_8)_n$ where n = the number of linked isoprene units. Monoterpenes have two isoprene units, diterpenes have four, triterpenes have six, tetraterpenes have eight, and so on. **Squalene** ($C_{30}H_{48}$) is a triterpene that undergoes cyclization to give rise to cholesterol, which is the precursor to steroid hormones. **Terpenoids** are simply terpenes that have been modified by the addition of oxygen or the shifting or removal of methyl groups. There are over 20,000 distinct types of terpenes and terpenoids.

Isoprene:

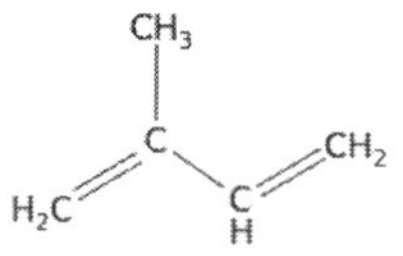

Squalene:

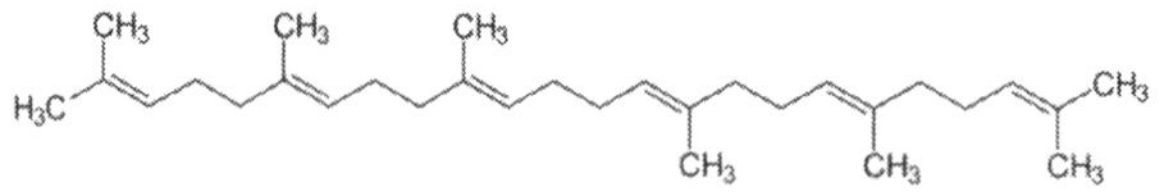

Cholesterol:

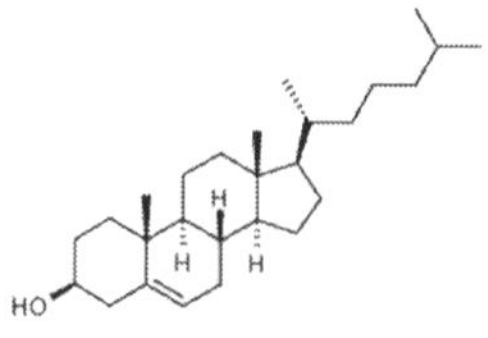

Endocrine System: Hormones and Their Sources

Function of Endocrine System: Specific Chemical Control at Cell, Tissue, and Organ Level

The endocrine system consists of all the glands and tissues that secrete chemical messengers called hormones. The endocrine system works closely with the faster-acting nervous system to coordinate and regulate important processes including growth, development, metabolism, immune function, reproduction, response to stress, and water and electrolyte balance. In short, the endocrine system is essential for the maintenance of homeostasis in the body. When hormones are secreted into the extracellular fluid, they diffuse into the bloodstream and are carried throughout the body. Only cells with receptors that are specific to the secreted hormones are affected. This specificity allows hormones to control targeted tissues and organs—often other endocrine glands (these are called tropic hormones). Major glands of the endocrine system include the hypothalamus, pineal gland, pituitary gland, thyroid, parathyroid glands, thymus, adrenal glands, gonads, and pancreas. Certain cells within the heart, kidneys, gastrointestinal tract, and placenta also have endocrine functions.

Definitions of Endocrine Gland, Hormone

An **endocrine gland** produces hormones and secretes them directly into the blood without the use of a duct. (*Endo* = within, *crine* = separate or secretion.) When the hormones are first released by the gland, they enter the interstitial fluid before diffusing into nearby capillaries. The circulatory system then delivers the hormones to target organs. By contrast, **exocrine glands** release non-hormone products such as sweat, oil, tears, and bile through ducts to their target locations—usually a cavity or epithelial surface inside or outside the body. Unlike hormones, exocrine products do not bind to receptors.

Hormones are molecules that bind to receptors and deliver regulatory messages. Many of these signaling molecules are steroids derived from cholesterol. These include the sex hormones and corticosteroids. The rest are non-steroids, and include amines, peptides, and proteins.

There are also signaling molecules called eicosanoids (ex: prostaglandins) that are sometimes referred to as "local hormones," and while they do bind to receptors, they are not secreted by endocrine glands, and do not travel through the bloodstream. Paracrine signals act on target cells that are near the secreting cell, and autocrine signals target the same cell that secreted them.

Major Endocrine Glands: Names, Locations, Products

The **hypothalamus** is the link between the nervous system and the endocrine system. It is located in the brain, superior to the pituitary and inferior to the thalamus. The hypothalamus communicates with the pituitary by secreting "releasing hormones" (RH) and "inhibiting hormones" (IH). Hormones of the hypothalamus include:

Hormone	Action
GnRH - gonadotropin RH	Stimulates anterior pituitary to release LH and FSH
GHRH - growth hormone RH	Stimulates anterior pituitary to release GH
GHIH - growth hormone IH (somatostatin)	Inhibits the release of GH from the anterior pituitary
TRH - thyrotropin RH	Stimulates anterior pituitary to release thyrotropin (TSH)
PRH - prolactin RH	Stimulates anterior pituitary to release prolactin
PIH - prolactin IH (dopamine)	Inhibits the release of prolactin from the anterior pituitary
CRH - corticotropin RH	Stimulates anterior pituitary to release ACTH

Hormone	Action
Oxytocin	Targets the uterus - stimulates contractions. Targets the mammary glands - milk secretion
ADH - antidiuretic hormone (vasopressin)	Targets the kidneys and blood vessels - increases water retention

The **pituitary** is nicknamed the "master gland" because many of the hormones it secretes act on other endocrine glands. It is located within the sella turcica of the sphenoid bone, beneath the hypothalamus. This pea-sized gland hangs from a thin stalk called the infundibulum, and it consists of an anterior and posterior lobe - each with a different function.

Source	Hormone	Action
Pituitary gland (anterior)	TSH - thyroid stimulating hormone (thyrotropin)	Targets the thyroid - stimulates the secretion of thyroid hormones
	ACTH - adrenocorticotropic hormone	Targets the adrenal cortex - stimulates the release of glucocorticoids and mineralocorticoids
	GH - growth hormone	Targets muscle and bone - stimulates growth
	FSH - follicle stimulating hormone	Targets the gonads - stimulates the maturation of sperm cells and ovarian follicles
	LH - luteinizing hormone	Targets the gonads - stimulates the production of sex hormones; surge stimulates ovulation in females
	PRL - prolactin	Targets the mammary glands - stimulates production of milk
Pituitary gland (posterior)	Oxytocin (produced in hypothalamus; stored and released by posterior pituitary)	Targets the uterus - stimulates contractions Targets the mammary glands - stimulates milk secretion
	ADH - antidiuretic hormone (vasopressin) (produced in hypothalamus; stored and released by posterior pituitary)	Targets the kidneys and blood vessels - increases water retention

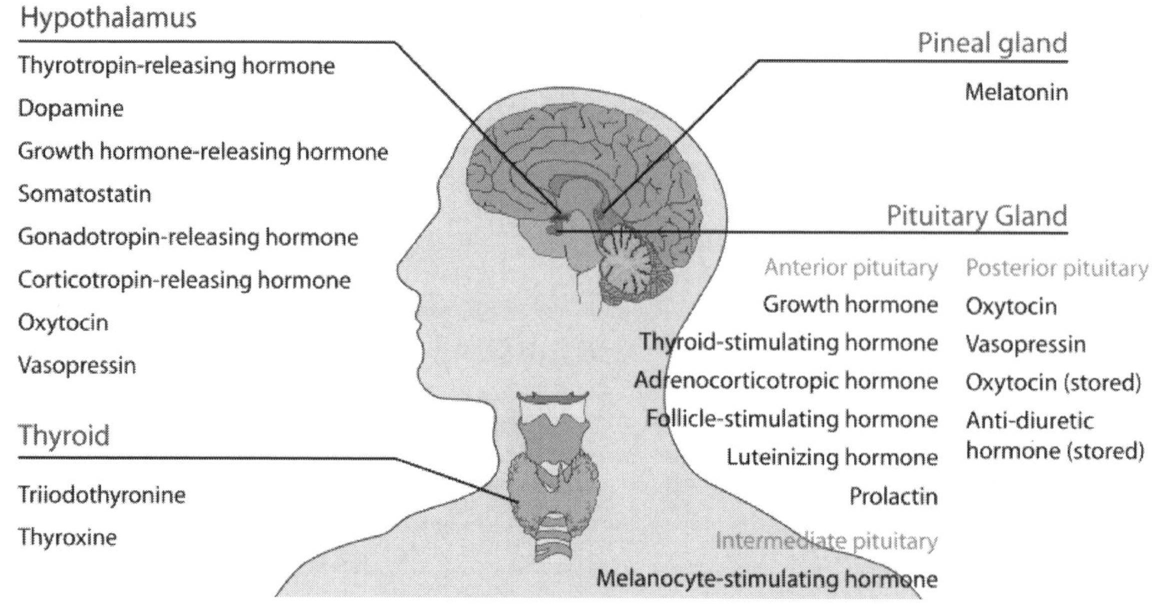

Source/Description	Hormone	Action
Pineal gland Situated between the two hemispheres of the brain where the two halves of the thalamus join.	Melatonin	Targets the brain - regulates daily rhythm (wake and sleep)
Thyroid gland Butterfly-shaped gland; the point of attachment between the two lobes is called the isthmus. The isthmus is on the anterior portion of the trachea, with the lobes wrapping partially around the trachea.	T_3 - triiodothyronine	Targets most cells - stimulates cellular metabolism
	T_4 - thyroxine	Targets most cells - stimulates cellular metabolism
	Calcitonin	Targets bone and kidneys - lowers blood calcium
Parathyroid gland Four small glands that are embedded in the posterior aspect of the thyroid.	PTH - Parathyroid hormone	Targets bone and kidneys - raises blood calcium

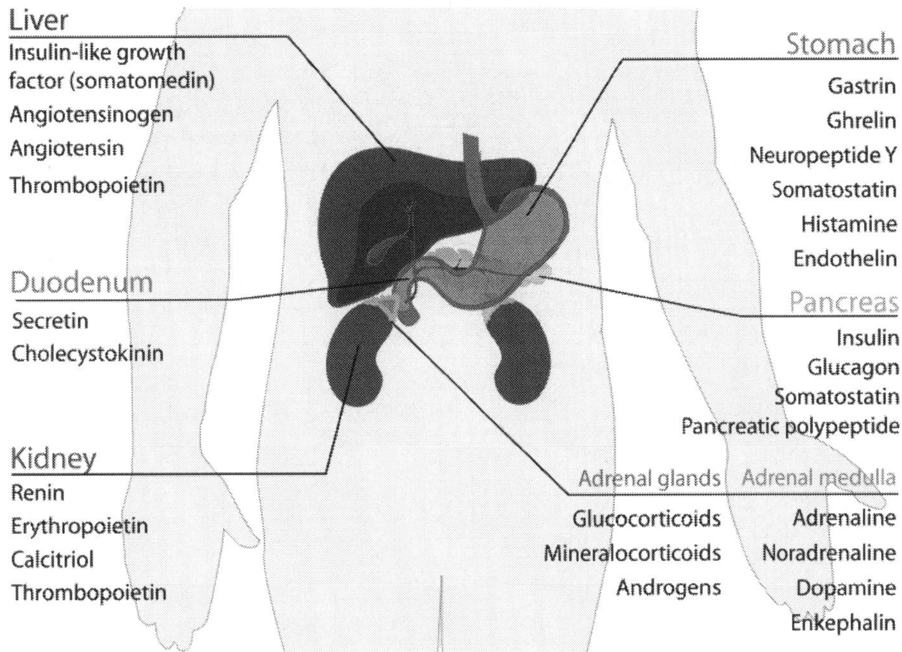

Source/Description	Hormone	Action
Thymus gland Located between the sternum and the heart, embedded in the mediastinum. It slowly decreases in size after puberty.	Thymosin	Targets lymphatic tissues - stimulates the production of T-cells
Pancreas The head of the pancreas is situated in the curve of the duodenum and the tail points toward the left side of the body. The pancreas is mostly posterior to the stomach.	Insulin	Targets the liver, muscle, and adipose tissue - decreases blood glucose
	Glucagon	Targets the liver - increases blood glucose
	GHIH - growth hormone IH (somatostatin)	Inhibits the secretion of insulin and glucagon

Source/Description	Hormone	Action
Adrenal medulla Located on top of the kidneys. The adrenal medulla is the inner part of the gland.	Epinephrine and norepinephrine	Target heart, blood vessels, liver, and lungs - increase heart rate, increase blood sugar (fight or flight response)
Adrenal cortex The adrenal cortex is the outer portion of the adrenal gland.	Mineralocorticoids (aldosterone)	Target the kidneys - increase the retention of Na^+ and excretion of K^+
	Glucocorticoids	Target most tissues - released in response to long-term stressors, increase blood glucose (but not as quickly as glucagon)
	Androgens	Target most tissues - stimulate development of secondary sex characteristics
GI tract	Gastrin	Targets the stomach - stimulates the release of HCl
	Secretin	Targets the pancreas and liver - stimulates the release of digestive enzymes and bile
	CCK - cholecystokinin	Targets the pancreas and liver - stimulates the release of digestive enzymes and bile
Kidneys	Erythropoietin	Targets the bone marrow - stimulates the production of red blood cells
	Calcitriol	Targets the intestines - increases the reabsorption of Ca^{2+}
Heart	ANP - atrial natriuretic peptide	Targets the kidneys and adrenal cortex - reduces reabsorption of Na^+, lowers blood pressure
Adipose Tissue	Leptin	Targets the brain - suppresses appetite

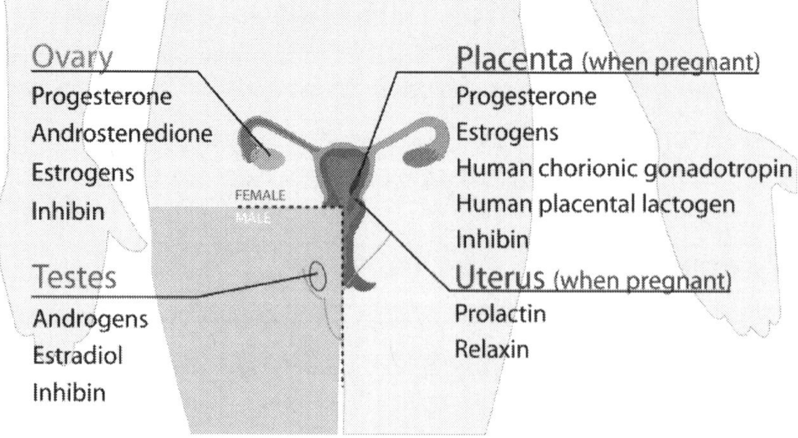

Source/Description	Hormone	Action
Ovaries The ovaries rest in depressions in the pelvic cavity on each side of the uterus. (Note that ovaries produce testosterone in small amounts.)	Estrogen	Target the uterus, ovaries, mammary glands, brain, and other tissues - stimulate uterine lining growth, regulate menstrual cycle, facilitate the development of secondary sex characteristics
	Progesterone	Targets mainly the uterus and mammary glands - stimulates uterine lining growth, regulates menstrual cycle, required for maintenance of pregnancy
	Inhibin	Targets the anterior pituitary - inhibits the release of FSH
Placenta Attached to the wall of the uterus during pregnancy	Estrogen, progesterone, and inhibin	(See above)
	Human chorionic gonadotropin (hCG)	Targets the ovaries - stimulates the production of estrogen and progesterone
Testes Located within the scrotum, behind the penis.	Testosterone	Targets the testes and many other tissues - promotes spermatogenesis, secondary sex characteristics
	Inhibin	(See above)

Major Types of Hormones

Hormones can be broadly classified into lipid-soluble hormones (steroids) and water-soluble hormones (non-steroids). Steroid hormones are derived from cholesterol, and their base structure consists of four fused carbon rings. They are released by the adrenal cortex, testes, ovaries, and the placenta. Major types of steroid hormones include the **sex hormones** (estrogens, androgens, progesterone) and the **corticosteroids** (glucocorticoids and mineralocorticoids). Since these hormones are lipid-soluble, they can diffuse through the cell membrane and bind to the nuclear receptors that regulate transcription.

Non-steroid hormones tend to elicit faster responses than steroid hormones. They cannot diffuse into the cell, and instead bind to receptors on the cell membrane, activating second-messenger systems. These hormones are classified into amines, peptides, and proteins. **Amines** are derivatives of the amino acids tyrosine or tryptophan, and include epinephrine, norepinephrine, thyroxine, and melatonin. **Peptide hormones** are short chains of amino acids. Common examples include oxytocin, somatostatin, and antidiuretic hormone. **Protein hormones** such as insulin, growth hormone, and parathyroid hormone consist of longer chains—generally over 100 amino acids. Hormones can also be **glycoproteins**. Follicle-stimulating hormone, thyroid-stimulating hormone, and luteinizing hormone all have carbohydrate attachments.

Neuroendocrinology – Relation Between Neurons and Hormonal Systems

Neuroendocrinology is the study of the interplay between the nervous system and endocrine system. The nervous system uses neurotransmitters to communicate, while the endocrine system uses slower-acting hormones (though the effects are longer-lasting). Hormones can trigger the firing of neurons, and neurons can stimulate the release of hormones. Both systems work together to maintain homeostasis. The physical bridge between these two systems is an almond-sized region of the brain called the hypothalamus. A slender stalk called the infundibulum extends down from the hypothalamus and connects to the pituitary gland. The hypothalamus communicates with the anterior lobe (adenohypophysis) of the pituitary through a network of capillaries, controlling the release of the six anterior pituitary hormones. The posterior lobe (neurohypophysis) is connected to the hypothalamus via neurons. It stores and releases oxytocin and ADH, which are produced by the hypothalamus. When changes in homeostasis are detected, the hypothalamus directs the pituitary to act.

Endocrine System: Mechanisms of Hormone Action

Cellular Mechanisms of Hormone Action

When hormones are released in response to a stimulus, they enter the bloodstream and are exposed to nearly all the cells in the body. Only cells with receptors specific to those hormones are affected. The mechanism of hormone action depends largely on the chemical nature of the hormone.

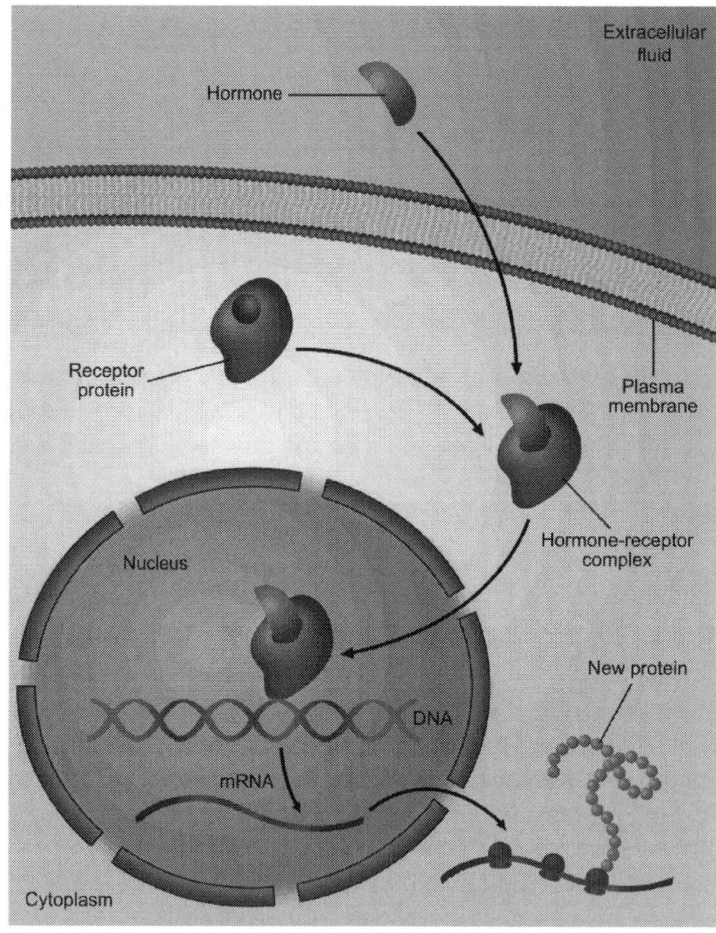

Steroid hormones are lipid-soluble, and can diffuse through the cell membrane of target cells. The hormones bind to intracellular receptors, which are usually in the nucleus but can also be in the cytoplasm. The hormone-receptor complex undergoes a conformational change, allowing it to bind to a region within the promoter sequence of DNA called the hormone-response element (HRE). This action directly controls gene activity by initiating or blocking transcription. The proteins that are translated may stimulate or inhibit certain metabolic pathways. The greater the number of hormone-receptor complexes that are formed, the greater the response from the target cell.

Non-steroid hormones are water-soluble, and (with the exception of thyroid hormones) cannot diffuse into cells. Instead, they act as first messengers by binding to receptors on the outer surface of the plasma membrane. This action activates a second messenger, which initiates a signaling cascade, ultimately changing the metabolic activities of the cell.

A common second messenger is cyclic AMP (cAMP). When the hormone binds to the receptor, it activates a G protein within the membrane. The G protein then activates the enzyme adenylate cyclase which forms cAMP from ATP. cAMP activates protein kinases, which go on to phosphorylate cytoplasmic proteins, altering their function.

Inositol triphosphate (IP3) and diacylglycerol (DAG) are also used as second messengers. When the G protein is activated by the binding of a hormone, it activates the enzyme phospholipase C, which cleaves IP3 off of a membrane phospholipid (PIP_2), and the remaining DAG is left within the membrane. IP3 diffuses to the endoplasmic reticulum and triggers the release of calcium ions from the lumen. These ions activate enzymes involved in various metabolic pathways. DAG plays a role in biosignaling by activating protein kinases.

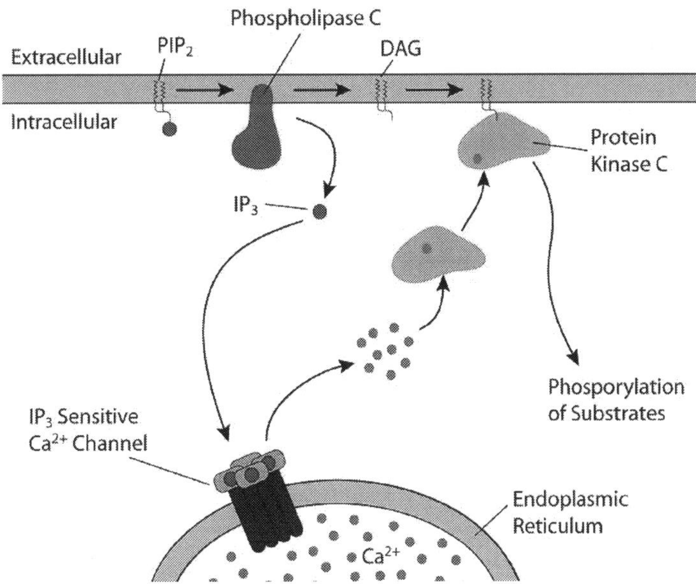

TRANSPORT OF HORMONES: BLOOD SUPPLY

Hormones are secreted from endocrine cells into in the interstitial fluid, usually through the process of exocytosis. This may occur in response to humoral stimuli (changes in the composition of extracellular fluids / blood), neural stimuli, or hormonal stimuli. The hormones diffuse into nearby capillaries and are transported to distant locations using the bloodstream. Some water-soluble hormones (most amines, peptides, and proteins) can dissolve in the blood and circulate freely, but lipid-soluble hormones (steroids and thyroid hormones) cannot. They bind loosely to carrier proteins such as albumin or globulins during transportation, and are inactive in this state. They dissociate from the carrier proteins, often in response to low hormone concentration, before binding to receptors on the target cells.

SPECIFICITY OF HORMONES: TARGET TISSUE

Hormones are able to enter systemic circulation while only affecting target tissues. Such specificity is dependent on the types of protein receptors present on or within target cells. A portion of the hormone has a shape that is nearly complementary to the binding domain of the receptor, though the receptor will flex to create a more perfect fit. Cells without the required receptors are invisible to the hormone.

The number of receptors on a target cell can change. As the number of receptors increases, the effect of the hormone increases proportionally. If the concentration of hormones in the blood is low, more receptors can be synthesized to increase the sensitivity to the hormone. This is called **up-regulation**. A prolonged increase in hormone concentration triggers a loss of receptors, desensitizing the cell to the hormone. This is called **down-regulation**.

Integration with Nervous System: Feedback Control

The endocrine system is regulated primarily by negative feedback mechanisms. When the concentration of hormones in the blood is high, the release of hormones and/or production of their receptors decreases. Conversely, when concentrations are low, the hormones and/or receptors can be upregulated. Various types of stimuli can trigger the release of hormones. **Humoral** stimuli refer to changes in chemical concentrations in the blood, such as ions or glucose. **Neural** stimuli (signaling from neurons) can also cause the secretion of hormones, as seen in the fight-or-flight response. Lastly, tropic hormones can stimulate endocrine glands (**hormonal** stimuli).

When the hypothalamus detects changes in homeostasis, it signals the pituitary gland to secrete hormones into the bloodstream where they travel to their target organ. As blood concentrations increase, feedback is sent to the hypothalamus and pituitary to inhibit further signaling to the target. The nervous system has the ability to adjust the "normal" levels of a hormone for a given situation—for example, in response to stress.

Structure and Integrative Functions of the Main Organ Systems

Respiratory System

General Function

The respiratory system includes the nose, mouth, nasal cavity, sinuses, pharynx, larynx, trachea, bronchial tree, and lungs. These organs facilitate the delivery of oxygen to the cells of the body for use in cellular respiration. The **conductive zone** brings inhaled air to the **respiratory zone** where gas exchange occurs. As oxygen is loaded into the blood, carbon dioxide is removed. Essential to this process are the diaphragm and intercostal muscles which are used to enlarge the chest cavity during pulmonary respiration (breathing). External respiration is the exchange of gas between the lungs and the blood. Internal respiration is the exchange of gas between the blood and tissues. Secondary functions of the respiratory system include pH regulation of the blood, thermoregulation, odor detection, and the production of speech.

Review Video: Respiratory System
Visit mometrix.com/academy and enter code: 783075

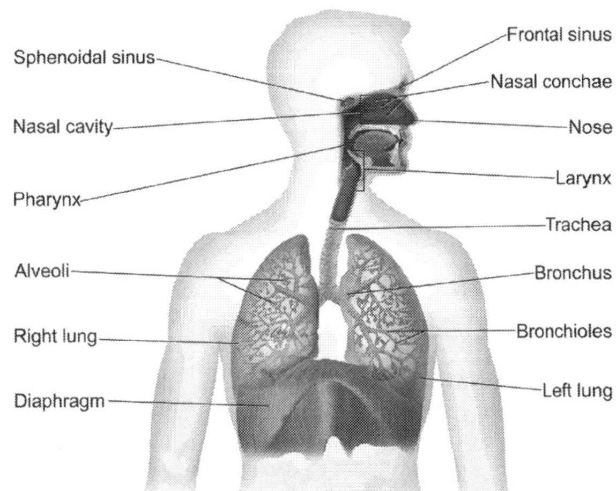

The Respiratory System

GAS EXCHANGE, THERMOREGULATION

Gas exchange is the loading of oxygen into pulmonary blood, and the removal of carbon dioxide. Inhaled air moves from through the mouth or nose to the pharynx, larynx, trachea, right / left main bronchi, and bronchioles, and then the alveoli. It is here that gases diffuse down their partial pressure gradients across a shared membrane between the capillaries and alveoli called the respiratory membrane. Oxygen diffuses into the blood where it is delivered to tissues throughout the body, and carbon dioxide diffuses out of the blood as a waste product of cellular respiration.

The respiratory system is also involved in **thermoregulation**: the regulation of body temperature. Capillaries within the respiratory tract, particularly the nasal passages and trachea, can constrict to conserve heat and dilate to release heat. The exhalation of warm, moistened air also helps to cool the body.

PROTECTION AGAINST DISEASE: PARTICULATE MATTER

A secondary role of the respiratory system is protection against disease and filtration of particulate matter. Some particles are filtered by nostril hairs and others get caught in mucus. Lysozymes within the mucus help to break down the trapped debris, and the cilia that line the respiratory tract then sweep it away. Immunoglobulin A (IgA) is also produced in the mucosal lining, and these antibodies aid in immune defenses by neutralizing pathogens. Mast cells within the respiratory tract release inflammatory chemicals that increase blood flow to the region, and alert the immune system to a threat. Large phagocytic cells called macrophages can also help to protect the lungs by engulfing small cells and particulates.

STRUCTURE OF LUNGS AND ALVEOLI

The lungs are spongy, porous organs that occupy most of the thoracic cavity. A serous membrane called the pleura lines the thoracic cavity (**parietal pleura**) as well as the surface of the lungs (**visceral pleura**). The three-lobed right lung is separated from the two-lobed left lung by the **mediastinum**. The trachea forks into primary bronchi which enter the left and right lung (along with blood and lymphatic vessels) at a region called the **hilum**. Each primary bronchus splits repeatedly into secondary bronchi, tertiary bronchi, and bronchioles to form the bronchial tree. The terminal bronchioles further divide into respiratory bronchioles, which are characterized by the presence of some alveoli. The respiratory bronchioles lead into alveolar ducts, which terminate in alveolar sacs.

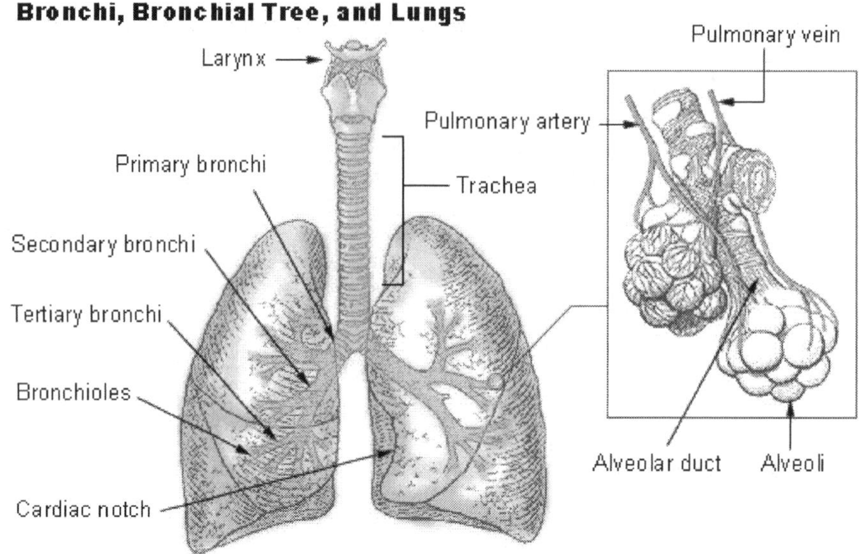

Within the alveolar sacs of the bronchi are clusters of **alveoli**: microscopic pouches where gas exchange occurs. The lungs contain hundreds of millions of these sacs, with a combined surface area that averages 70 m^2. The wall of each alveolus consists of a single layer of epithelial cells, most of which are type I cells. These squamous cells are involved in gas exchange. Type II cells are cuboidal cells that secrete surfactant to prevent the alveoli from collapsing. The alveolar walls are perforated by pores that connect adjacent alveoli, providing an alternate route for the passage of air in case of blocked ducts. The outer surfaces are covered with a network of capillaries. The basement membrane of a capillary fuses with the alveolar basement membrane to form the **respiratory membrane** (which also includes the capillary and alveolar epithelial cells).

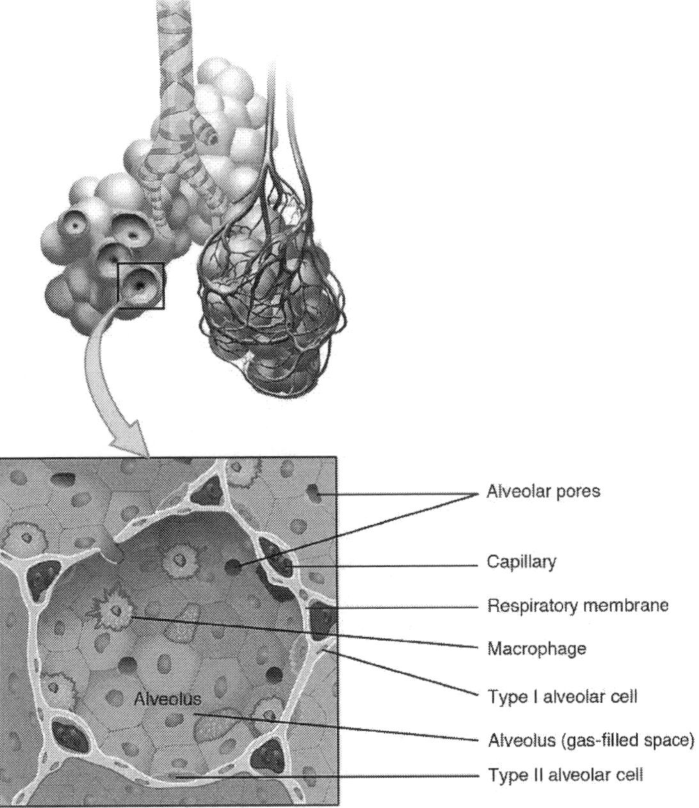

Breathing Mechanisms

Diaphragm, Rib Cage, Differential Pressure

The diaphragm is a thin, dome-shaped muscle that separates the abdominal cavity from the thoracic cavity. This muscle, along with the external and internal intercostal muscles of the rib cage, are responsible for changing the volume, and therefore the pressure, of air in the lungs. This mechanism of breathing follows **Boyle's law**: the pressure and volume of a gas have an inverse relationship, assuming the temperature is constant.

When the diaphragm and external intercostals contract, the volume of the thoracic cavity increases, and the rib cage and sternum elevate and expand outward. The increase in volume results in a decrease in intrapleural pressure, and air enters the lungs in a process called **inspiration**. This is called **negative-pressure breathing** because the pressure in the lungs is lower than atmospheric pressure (and gases move down the pressure gradient). **Expiration** is usually a more passive process, and it is achieved by simply relaxing the same muscles that facilitated inhalation. As the volume of the thoracic cavity decreases, intrapleural pressure increases, and air leaves the lungs.

Air can be forcibly pushed out through the contraction of the internal intercostals and abdominal muscles.

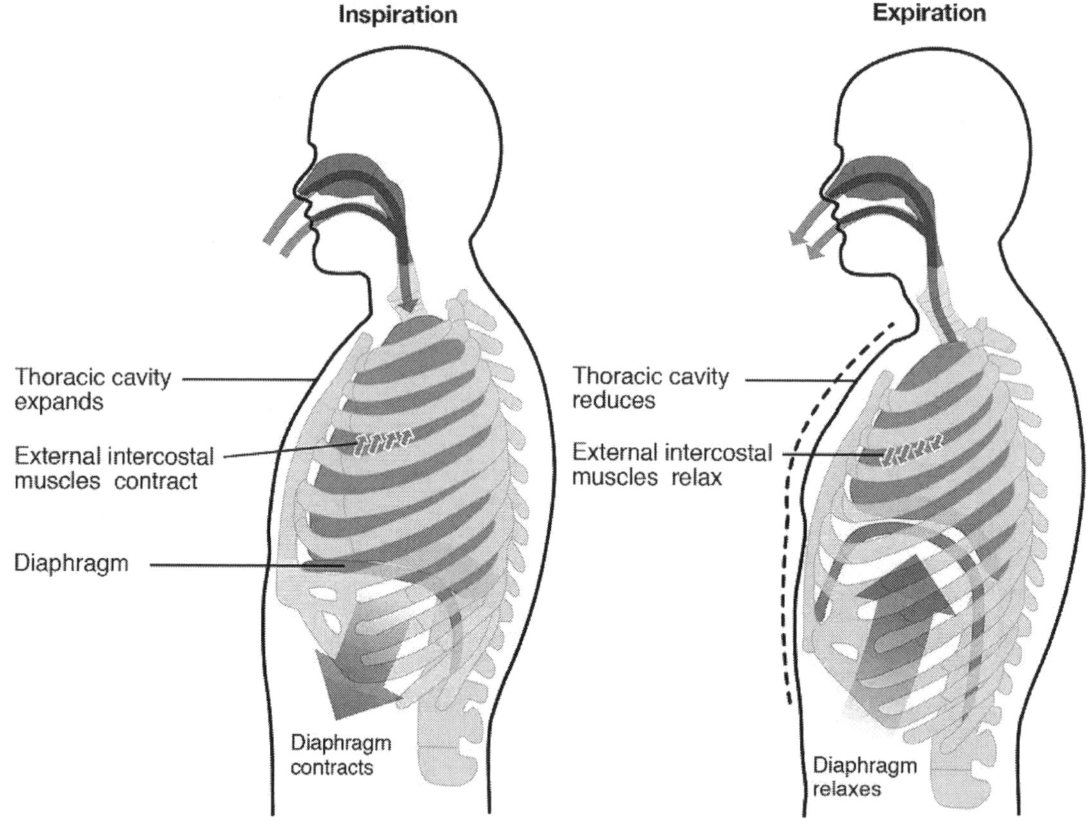

Resiliency and Surface Tension Effects

The connective tissues of the lungs contain elastin, allowing them to bounce back after each inhalation. The greater the ability of the lung to stretch, the greater its **compliance**. Elasticity, combined with the forces of surface tension, would cause the lungs to collapse without a corrective mechanism.

The inner surface of each alveolus is coated with film of fluid. The polar water molecules at the fluid's surface are attracted to one another, and as a result of this surface tension, the volume of the alveoli is reduced. By extension, the pressure in each alveolus increases. According to the **Law of Laplace**, pressure is directly proportional to surface tension and inversely proportional to the radius ($P = \frac{2T}{r}$). Since surface tension is a constant regardless of the radius, smaller alveoli have greater pressure. Type II alveolar cells solve this problem by secreting a **surfactant**: a substance that reduces surface tension when dissolved in a liquid. The surfactant, made mostly of amphipathic lipoproteins, counteracts the cohesive forces between water molecules, making them easier to inflate. And since the surfactant has proportionally greater effects in smaller alveoli, the pressure from one alveolus to the next is somewhat uniform. Surfactant also increases the compliance of the lungs and reduces the likelihood of alveolar collapse.

Thermoregulation: Nasal and Tracheal Capillary Beds; Evaporation, Panting

A secondary role of the respiratory system is thermoregulation. In humans, body temperature is regulated mainly by vasodilation / vasoconstriction, sweating, and shivering, but breathing plays a role as well. When air is inhaled, it is exposed to the mucosa of the conducting zone, and quickly equilibrates to the temperature of the blood. Most heat exchange occurs at the highly vascular nasal and tracheal epithelial lining. By the time it reaches the lungs, the air has already been warmed and moistened. During exercise, heavy breathing not only delivers more oxygen to the blood, but is also a mechanism for cooling the body. As respiratory rate increases, so does moisture evaporation along the epithelial lining. Animals that pant rely on this cooling mechanism more than non-panting species because they have little to no ability to sweat.

Particulate Filtration: Nasal Hairs, Mucus/Cilia System in Lungs

On average, humans inhale about 20,000 liters of air per day. This air contains particulates such as dust, pollen, mold spores, bacteria, and viruses that must be filtered and broken down. Filtration begins in the nose, where nasal hairs prevent larger particles from proceeding through the respiratory tract. The next line of defense is the mucus that lines the airways, trapping particles that were not filtered by the nose hairs. The conducting passageways of the respiratory tract are also lined with ciliated epithelial cells, and the cilia beat in a direction that pushes trapped debris and pathogens toward the throat where it is either swallowed, spat out, or expelled through the nostrils. The alveoli, however, are not coated in mucus or cilia, and they depend on white blood cells called macrophages to engulf potentially harmful particles and digest them. They also send signals to other cells of the immune system to alert them to a possible threat.

Alveolar Gas Exchange

Diffusion, Differential Partial Pressure

Exchange of gas between the air and blood occurs along the respiratory membrane of the alveoli. The blood that is brought to the alveoli via pulmonary arterioles is deoxygenated, with a concentration of carbon dioxide that is greater than that of the air. Each gas moves down its partial pressure gradient by simple diffusion. Oxygenated blood is then taken toward the heart via pulmonary venules.

Partial pressure is the pressure that one type of gas within a mixture would exert if it were to occupy the same volume as the total mixture. The partial pressure of carbon dioxide (P_{CO_2}) in the blood that enters the pulmonary capillaries is 45 mmHg, but the P_{CO_2} in the alveolar air is only 40 mmHg. Therefore, CO_2 diffuses out of the blood and into the air. The oxygen in the blood entering the capillaries has a partial pressure of 40 mmHg, but the P_{O_2} in the alveolar space is 104 mmHg. Therefore, O_2 diffuses into the blood down its partial pressure gradient. The blood that leaves the capillaries has the same partial pressures of oxygen and carbon dioxide as the air in the alveolar space.

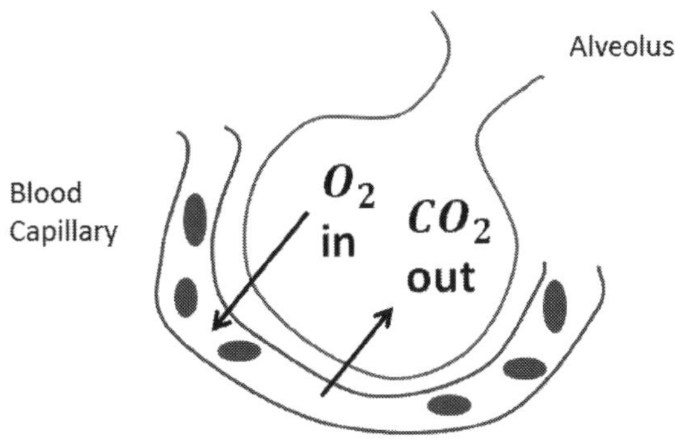

Henry's Law

According to Henry's Law, the concentration of dissolved gas in a liquid is directly proportional to the solubility and partial pressure of that gas. That is, the greater the partial pressure of a gas, the greater the rate of diffusion of that gas into a liquid.

Henry's Law:

$$c = kP$$

- c = concentration of dissolved gas
- k = Henry's law constant; unique to each gas, depends on solubility
- P = partial pressure of the gas

This relationship can be used to predict the behavior of a gas (such as oxygen or carbon dioxide) when it is exposed to a liquid (such as blood). Gases move from areas of high pressure to low pressure, and the steeper the gradient, the greater the rate of diffusion. Solubility is also a factor. Carbon dioxide is more soluble in blood than oxygen, but oxygen has a steeper pressure gradient so the rates of diffusion balance out. Nitrogen has the highest partial pressure of all the atmospheric gases, but its blood concentration is very low due to its poor solubility.

pH Control

The normal pH of blood ranges from 7.35 to 7.45. The lungs and kidneys each play a role in controlling these levels, as even minor disturbances can lead to serious consequences. A pH level below the normal range is called **acidemia**, and a value above the normal range is called **alkalemia**. The respiratory system uses the **bicarbonate buffer system** to balance the pH of the blood. When carbon dioxide combines with water, a weak acid (carbonic acid: H_2CO_3) is formed, before dissociating into its conjugate base (a bicarbonate ion: HCO_3^-) and a hydrogen ion (H^+) as seen in the following equation: $CO2 + H2O \leftrightarrow H2CO3 \leftrightarrow HCO3- + H+$. If the pH of the blood is low (as caused by excess hydrogen ions), then the rate of respiration increases, and the reaction shifts to the left. Excess hydrogen ions are accepted by the bicarbonate ions, and the pH increases. If the pH is high, then breathing slows, the reaction shifts to the right, the concentration of hydrogen ions increases, and pH decreases. The kidneys also help to monitor blood pH, but the response is slower and longer-lasting.

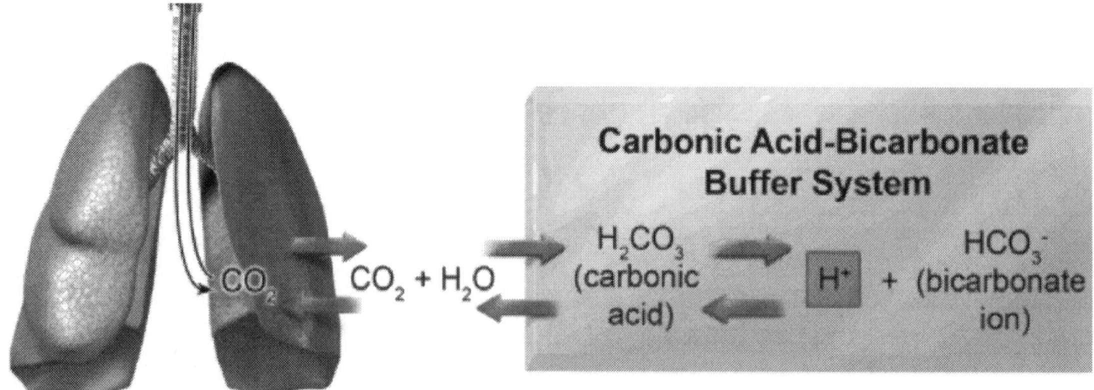

Regulation by Nervous Control

CO_2 Sensitivity

The rate and depth of breathing are controlled by the nervous system, which responds to changes in the chemical composition of the blood. Carbon dioxide has the greatest effect on the rate of respiration. Chemoreceptors in the brain, specifically the medulla oblongata and pons, indirectly respond to CO_2 concentration. As levels in the blood increase, CO_2 diffuses into the cerebrospinal fluid of the brain, and reacts with water to form carbonic acid. The acid quickly ionizes to form its conjugate base and hydrogen ions. It is the hydrogen ions that stimulate the chemoreceptors of the central nervous system. The respiratory centers of the brain respond by increasing the rate of respiration, and more CO_2 is exhaled. The greater the stimulus, the greater the response.

Chemoreceptors of the peripheral nervous system, located in the aortic and carotid bodies, also regulate respiratory rate. These receptors are sensitive to CO_2, hydrogen ions, and to a lesser degree oxygen. Only when oxygen levels are critically low do receptors signal the brain to increase the rate of respiration.

Circulatory System

Functions

The circulatory system is primarily associated with the transport of oxygen, nutrients, hormones, ions, and fluids throughout the body, as well as the removal of metabolic wastes.

Oxygen moves down its partial pressure gradient from the air into the blood of the alveolar capillaries, where most of it binds to hemoglobin molecules in the red blood cells. A small amount dissolves in the blood. Without oxygen, cells would be unable to transfer the energy in glucose to ATP during cellular respiration.

The carbon dioxide that is produced during cellular respiration is transported away from tissues and diffuses out of the alveolar capillaries. Like oxygen, carbon dioxide can dissolve in blood or bind to hemoglobin, but most travels in the form of bicarbonate ions. Other metabolic waste products such as urea are brought to the kidneys to be filtered. The kidneys also help to regulate the levels of fluids and ions in the blood.

Digested nutrients such as glucose, amino acids, and fats are circulated to target cells where they are absorbed. Hormones released by endocrine glands also reach their target cells in this way. Lipid-soluble molecules require the use of a carrier protein to be transported in blood.

Role in Thermoregulation

The circulatory system plays an important role in thermoregulation. The human body maintains an average temperature of around 98.6 °F (37 °C), which is optimal for metabolic processes and defense against pathogens. Heat exchange occurs at the surface of the skin, where blood vessels can dilate or constrict in response to signals from the brain.

Sensory neurons called thermoreceptors detect changes in temperature and send impulses to the hypothalamus, which then sends signals to the effectors—the smooth muscles that surround cutaneous arterioles. If the body temperature is too warm, the smooth muscle relaxes, and the arterioles dilate. Vasodilation allows more blood to flow through the capillary beds near the surface of the skin, and more heat is lost to the surroundings. If the temperature is too cool, the smooth muscle contracts, and the arterioles constrict. Vasoconstriction reduces the volume of blood that flows near the body's surface, which minimizes heat loss to the surroundings. Sweating and shivering also help to control body temperature.

Four-Chambered Heart: Structure and Function

The wall of the heart is a composed of three layers of tissue. The outer layer is the **epicardium**, which protects the heart and secretes lubricating serous fluid. The middle layer is the muscular **myocardium**, which contracts to pump blood. The innermost layer is the **endocardium**, which lines the chambers and valves.

The heart is a four-chambered organ. The superior "receiving" chambers are the atria. The **right atrium** receives blood from the vena cava, and the **left atrium** receives blood from the pulmonary veins. The muscular "discharging" chambers are the ventricles. The **right ventricle** pumps blood into the pulmonary trunk, and the **left ventricle** pumps blood into the aorta.

The **tricuspid valve** (also called the right atrioventricular valve, or right AV valve) prevents backflow into the atrium when the ventricle contracts. The **pulmonary semilunar valve** prevents the return of blood into the right ventricle. The **bicuspid valve** (also called the left AV valve, or mitral valve) prevents blood from entering the left atrium when the ventricle contracts. The **aortic semilunar valve** stops the backflow of blood into the right ventricle as it leaves through the aorta.

The path of blood through the heart is traced in the diagram below:

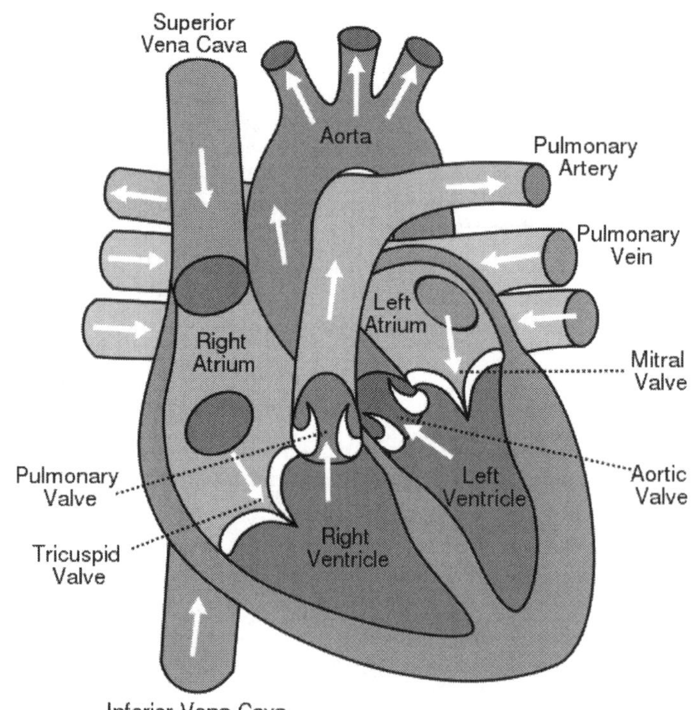

Review Video: The Heart
Visit mometrix.com/academy and enter code: 451399

Endothelial Cells

The thin inner lining of blood vessels (and the lymphatic vessels) is called the **endothelium**. This tissue lines the entire circulatory system, including the interior of the heart. It is composed of a single layer of squamous endothelial cells that are connected by tight junctions and adherens junctions. This allows the endothelium to act as a selectively permeable barrier between the blood and the surrounding tissue, though some vessels have pores and gaps that allow the passage of larger molecules. The smoothness of the endothelium reduces friction between the blood and the vessel wall. Endothelial cells also play a role in vasoconstriction by releasing peptides called endothelins that cause the smooth muscle within the vessel walls to contract. They also secrete chemicals that inhibit the coagulation of blood, but if the endothelium is damaged, they release different chemicals required for clot formation.

Systolic and Diastolic Pressure

Blood pressure is the force per unit area that is exerted by the blood on the walls of the vessels. Unless otherwise indicated, blood pressure refers specifically to the pressure within the major arteries, since arterioles, capillaries, venules, and veins have progressively less pressure. Blood pressure is often expressed as two numbers, and in units of millimeters of mercury (mmHg). The first number refers to the **systolic pressure**, or the maximum pressure that is exerted during **systole**. During this time, the ventricles contract, forcing blood into the aorta and pulmonary trunk. As the blood enters the arteries, the elastic walls stretch to accommodate the increased volume, and then return to their normal diameter during **diastole**. Diastole is the period in which the ventricles relax and blood pressure is at its lowest point. The normal average blood pressure for an adult at rest is 120/80 mmHg, where 120 is the systolic bp, and 80 is the diastolic bp. High blood pressure can damage the walls of the blood vessels and increase the risk of heart disease, heart failure, and stroke. Low blood pressure is only concerning if it occurs suddenly, or if it causes noticeable symptoms such as lightheadedness or fainting.

Pulmonary and Systemic Circulation

The **pulmonary circuit** is the part of the circulatory system that carries blood from the heart to the lungs and back to the heart. When deoxygenated blood is expelled from the right ventricle, it moves through the pulmonary trunk, which bifurcates into the right and left pulmonary arteries. Each branch extends into the lungs, eventually giving rise to arterioles and then the capillaries where gas exchange occurs by diffusion. Oxygenated blood leaves the capillaries through venules which fuse into veins, finally merging into four pulmonary veins that return blood to the left atrium. Note that in the pulmonary circuit, the arteries have *less* oxygen than the veins. Low blood oxygen in the pulmonary circuit triggers vasoconstriction, which redirects blood to better ventilated parts of the lung.

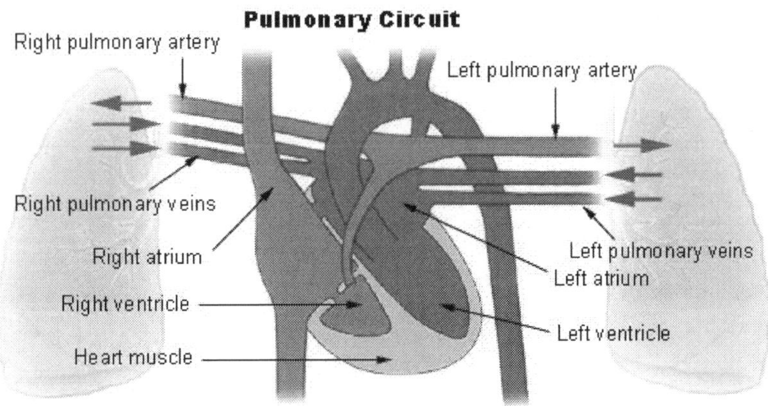

The **systemic circuit** carries blood from the muscular left ventricle of the heart to the aorta, which gives rise to the arteries that eventually branch into arterioles and then the capillary beds within the tissues of the body. Oxygen and nutrients enter the tissues, and carbon dioxide and other wastes enter the blood. Deoxygenated blood leaves the capillary beds through venules, which merge into larger veins. The blood then enters the right atrium through the superior and inferior vena cava. Because this circuit is much longer than the pulmonary circuit, blood pressure is *higher.* Unlike the pulmonary circuit, blood in the arteries carries *more* oxygen than blood in the veins. When oxygen levels are low, vessels dilate to promote blood flow to tissues that need it.

Systemic Circuit

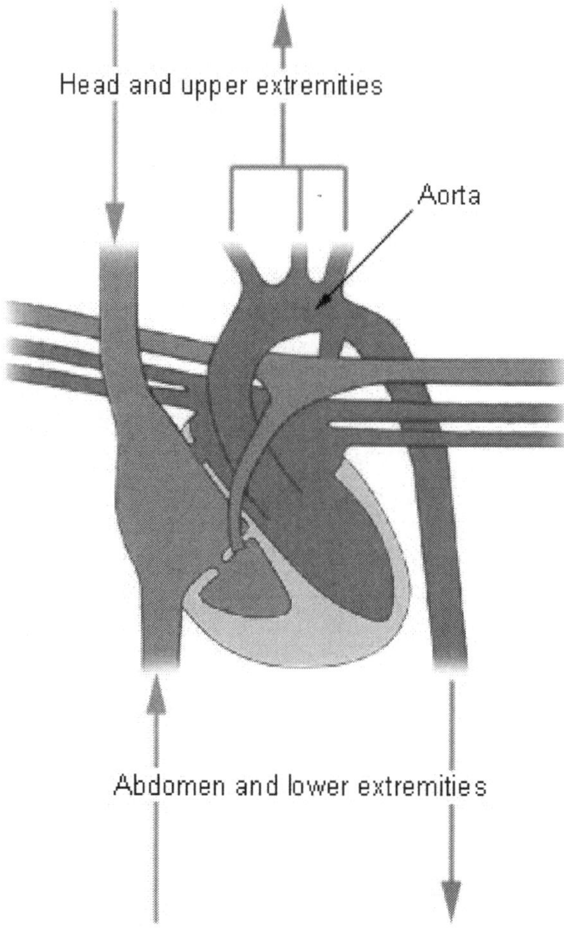

ARTERIAL AND VENOUS SYSTEMS (ARTERIES, ARTERIOLES, VENULES, VEINS)

STRUCTURAL AND FUNCTIONAL DIFFERENCES

The walls of all blood vessels (except the capillaries) consist of three layers: the innermost **tunica intima**, the **tunica media** consisting of smooth muscle cells and elastic fibers, and the outer **tunica adventitia**.

Arterial System:	**Elastic arteries**	**Muscular arteries**	**Arterioles**
Structure	Includes the aorta and major branches Tunica media has more elastin than any other vessels Largest vessels in the arterial system	Includes the arteries that branch off of the elastic arteries Tunica media has a higher proportion of smooth muscle cells, and fewer elastic fibers as compared to elastic arteries	Tiny vessels that lead to the capillary beds Tunica media is thin, but composed almost entirely smooth muscle cells
Function	Stretch when blood is forced out of the heart, and recoil under low pressure	Regulate blood flow by vasoconstriction / vasodilation	Primary vessels involved in vasoconstriction / vasodilation Control blood flow to capillaries

Venous System:	**Venules**	**Veins**
Structure	Tiny vessels that exit the capillary beds Thin, porous walls; few muscle cells and elastic fibers	Thin tunica media and tunica intima Wide lumen Valves prevent backflow of blood
Function	Empty blood into larger veins	Carry blood back to the heart

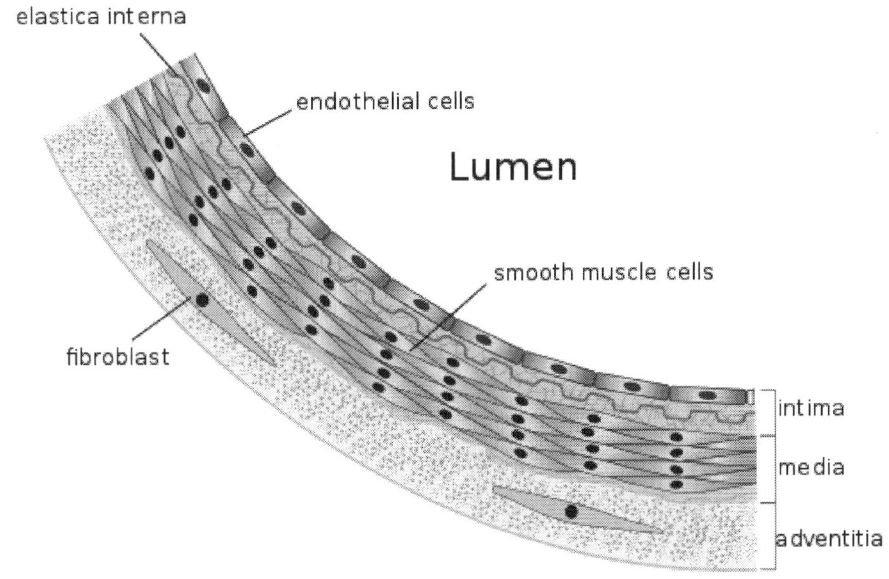

PRESSURE AND FLOW CHARACTERISTICS

Blood pressure is highest in the main arteries of the systemic circuit, particularly the aorta. The pressure decreases progressively as blood flows through the arterioles, capillaries, venules, and veins. The blood pressure is lowest in the vena cava. The steepest *drop* in blood pressure (as opposed to absolute pressure) occurs at the arterioles. The large reduction in diameter from artery to arteriole results in an increase in resistance as blood moves against the vessel wall. This slows down the flow of blood, and decreases the pressure.

Blood flow can be described as turbulent or laminar. Turbulence is an unsteady, swirling flow of blood that can occur during periods of high velocity, when the blood encounters an obstruction, or when the vessels take a sharp turn or narrow suddenly. Turbulent flow usually produces sounds, while laminar flow is silent. Laminar flow is the steady, streamlined flow of blood that occurs throughout most of the circulatory system.

CAPILLARY BEDS

MECHANISMS OF GAS AND SOLUTE EXCHANGE

Capillaries have only a single layer of endothelial cells that rest on a basement membrane. Capillary beds are groups of interconnected capillaries that facilitate the exchange of gas and solutes between the blood and interstitial fluid. Nutrients and oxygen enter the interstitial fluid, and carbon dioxide and other wastes enter the capillary blood. Gases and lipid-soluble substances can cross the endothelial cell membranes by simple diffusion, but ions and large particles often require the help of transport proteins or vesicular transport. Sometimes materials move through **intercellular clefts**: channels between adjacent endothelial cells. Capillaries with a nonporous continuous endothelium are called **continuous capillaries**. These are the most common types of capillaries in the body, and also the most impermeable. **Fenestrated capillaries** have pores that increase their permeability and are found in the kidneys and small intestine. **Sinusoidal capillaries** have a discontinuous endothelium that permits the passage of large particles and even blood cells. They are the most permeable of the capillaries.

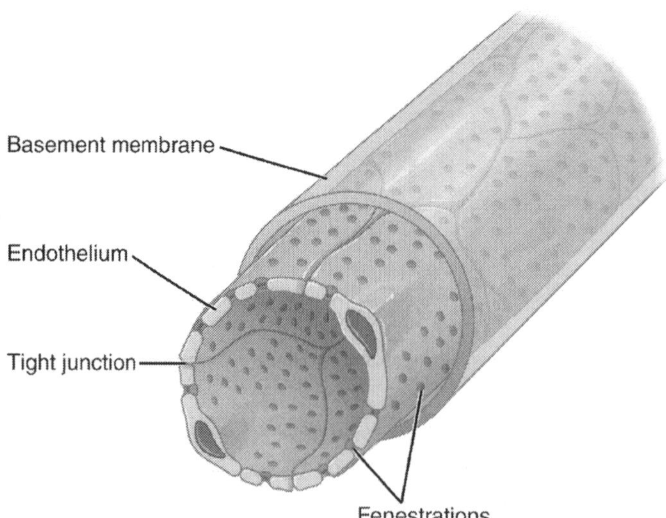

SOURCE OF PERIPHERAL RESISTANCE

Peripheral resistance is the resistance of the vessels to the flow of blood as a result of friction. As resistance increases, the rate of blood flow decreases. The main factors that affect peripheral resistance are diameter and length of the vessel, and volume and viscosity of the blood.

Resistance is most affected by changes in the *diameter* of the vessel. The relationship is inverse; as radius decreases, the resistance increases proportionally to the fourth power of the radius. For example, if the radius of a blood vessel is cut in half due to the buildup of plaque, resistance increases by a factor of 16. As such, vasoconstriction and vasodilation are critical to maintaining the appropriate level of resistance and flow. As *length* of the vessel increases, the resistance increases proportionally due to the increased surface area. As a person gains weight, the new blood vessels that nourish the new adipose tissue cause the total resistance of the system to increase. Blood volume and blood viscosity are usually not subject to sudden changes, but the effects of such changes are fairly intuitive. A decrease in either of these factors results in a decrease in resistance and an increase in flow rate.

Composition of Blood

Plasma, Chemicals, Blood Cells

Blood is a mixture of plasma, chemicals, and blood cells. The clear, straw-colored liquid portion that makes up 55% of the blood is called **plasma**, and the remaining 45% consists of **formed elements**: the red and white blood cells and platelets.

Plasma is a solution of water, plasma proteins (albumin, antibodies, clotting proteins), carbohydrates, amino acids, lipids, vitamins, salts, gases, hormones, and waste products. About 92% of plasma is water.

Most of the cells in the blood are **red blood cells** (RBCs, or erythrocytes). These biconcave cells lack organelles, leaving room for hemoglobin - a protein to which oxygen and carbon dioxide can bind. The percentage of red blood cells by volume is called **hematocrit**, and averages about 42% for women and 46% for men. Less than 1% of blood consists of white blood cells and platelets. White blood cells (WBCs, or leukocytes) are the only blood cells with nuclei. Unlike RBCs, they are not confined to the blood and can move in and out of vessels. There are many types of WBCs, and all are specialized to fight pathogens in different ways. **Platelets** (thrombocytes) are cell fragments that initiate clotting, and they outnumber WBCs about 40:1.

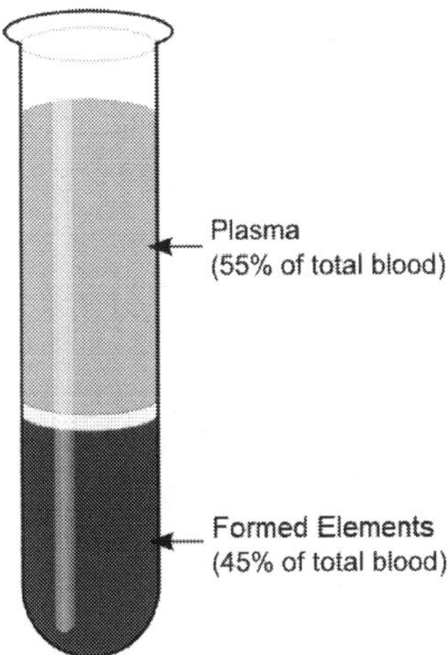

Erythrocyte Production and Destruction; Spleen, Bone Marrow

Erythropoiesis (the production of red blood cells) occurs in the red bone marrow. When oxygen levels are low, the hormone **erythropoietin** (produced by the kidneys and liver) targets the marrow, stimulating **myeloid stem cells** to differentiate into **erythroblasts**. These immature RBCs divide many times, filling up with newly synthesized hemoglobin. The nuclei condense, and are ejected along with other organelles until only some endoplasmic reticulum remains. These cells are called **reticulocytes**, and they are released into the blood. After 1-2 days, the rest of the endoplasmic reticulum is lost, and mature **erythrocytes** are formed. Note that these cells are incapable of division.

After about 120 days, old and damaged RBCs are recognized and engulfed by phagocytes that are concentrated in the liver, spleen, and bone marrow. Hemoglobin is broken down into its four globin polypeptide chains and heme groups. Amino acids are released from the chains and enter the blood. The iron within the heme groups is either stored as ferritin in the liver or returned to the marrow to make more hemoglobin. The rest of the heme group is degraded to bilirubin and excreted in the bile.

Regulation of Plasma Volume

Plasma volume is influenced by hydrostatic pressure and osmotic pressure. The pressure within the vessels and capillaries tends to be higher than the pressure of the interstitial fluid. This difference in pressure drives fluid out of the blood and into the surrounding fluid in a process called filtration. When water crosses the walls of the vessels, many solutes including plasma proteins are left behind, and the osmolarity (concentration) of the blood increases. When the osmolarity of the blood is high, water diffuses from the interstitial fluid into the blood, increasing plasma volume and decreasing osmolarity. This osmotic pressure helps to counteract the leakage of water from the capillaries.

Plasma volume is also regulated by the nervous and endocrine systems. Osmoreceptors detect changes in blood osmolarity, and baroreceptors detect changes in pressure. If solute concentration of the blood increases and/or blood volume decreases, the pituitary gland releases ADH to promote the reabsorption of water in the kidneys, rather than excreting it in urine. The adrenal cortex plays a role as well by releasing aldosterone. Aldosterone promotes the reabsorption of salt, which leads to an increase in water reabsorption, increasing the plasma volume.

Coagulation, Clotting Mechanisms

When a blood vessel is damaged, the smooth muscle constricts at the site of injury and platelets adhere to the exposed collagen of the vessel wall. The platelets develop spine-like projections, and release chemicals to attract other platelets and promote further vasoconstriction. A plug is formed as platelets aggregate, but this is rarely a sufficient fix without the coagulation of the blood.

There are two clotting mechanisms: extrinsic and intrinsic. In the extrinsic clotting mechanism, damaged tissue releases thromboplastin, which triggers a cascade of reactions that results in the production of an enzyme called prothrombin activator. Prothrombin activator is also produced by the slower-acting *intrinsic* clotting mechanism. When blood encounters a foreign substance or tissue, the Hageman factor (also called coagulation factor XII) is activated, leading to the production of prothrombin activator. From here, the clotting pathways are the same. Prothrombin activator converts prothrombin to thrombin using calcium as a cofactor. Thrombin splits fibrinogen to form fibrin, but also stimulates its own production (a positive feedback loop). Fibrin is a fibrous protein that forms a mesh-like network that traps more platelets and red blood cells. This forms a clot that seals the injured region of the blood vessel.

Oxygen Transport by Blood

Hemoglobin, Hematocrit and Oxygen Content

Almost all oxygen is transported by molecules of **hemoglobin** (Hb) that are found within erythrocytes, though 1.5% of blood oxygen is dissolved in the plasma. Hemoglobin has a protein component and a heme component. The protein component consists of four polypeptide chains known as globin (two alpha chains and two beta chains). Associated with each chain is a heme group that gives blood its red color. The heme group consists of a single iron atom surrounded by a complex organic ring called **protoporphyrin**. When blood passes through the capillaries of the lungs, it picks up oxygen. Each iron atom binds a molecule of oxygen—so one hemoglobin can bind up to four molecules of oxygen, and each erythrocyte carries around 250 million molecules of hemoglobin. The oxygenated form of hemoglobin is called **oxyhemoglobin**.

Hemoglobin can also transport up to four carbon dioxide molecules, though CO_2 binds to amino acids within the globin, not iron. Only about 23% of carbon dioxide is transported in this form, known as **carbaminohemoglobin**. Roughly 70% travels in the form of bicarbonate ions (as seen in the bicarbonate buffer system), and the rest is dissolved in the plasma.

Oxygen Affinity

As the partial pressure of oxygen increases, so does the saturation level of hemoglobin. When the first oxygen molecule binds, the conformation of hemoglobin changes, making it easier for the second and third oxygen molecules to bind. The fourth and last oxygen molecule does not bind as easily, as seen in the S-shaped dissociation curve below.

Other factors can cause the curve to shift to the left (increasing affinity) or right (decreasing affinity). An increase in pH (as caused by a decrease in carbon dioxide) will also increase the affinity of hemoglobin for oxygen. Conversely, a decrease in pH (as caused by an increase in carbon dioxide) reduces affinity. This is known as the **Bohr effect**. Other factors that affect affinity include temperature, BPG, and carbon monoxide. As temperature increases, the affinity for oxygen decreases, and vice versa. BPG (2,3-bisphosphoglycerate, also called DPG) is a byproduct of glycolysis that decreases affinity for oxygen. Hemoglobin has a much higher affinity for carbon monoxide than for oxygen, and as such CO easily displaces O_2.

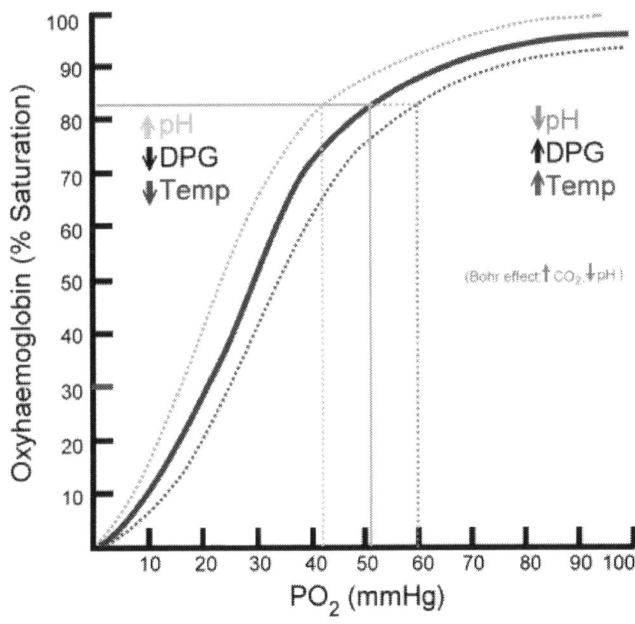

Nervous and Endocrine Control

Heart rate and blood pressure are greatly influenced by the nervous and endocrine systems. The sympathetic division of the autonomic nervous system increases the heart rate by releasing norepinephrine (NE), which acts on the SA node of the heart. The parasympathetic division has the opposite effect. The vagus nerves that innervate the heart release acetylcholine (ACh), which slows the heart rate. Central and peripheral chemoreceptors also help to regulate heart rate by monitoring levels of pH, carbon dioxide, and oxygen.

Blood pressure is regulated by baroreceptors in the aortic arch and carotid arteries (both of which detect high blood pressure) and also the venae cavae, pulmonary veins, and atrial walls (all of which detect low blood pressure). When high blood pressure is detected, the blood vessels dilate and heart rate decreases to restore homeostasis. Blood pressure is also regulated by hormones of the endocrine system. When blood pressure drops, the kidneys secrete a hormone called renin which initiates a series of reactions that ultimately cause the release of aldosterone from the adrenal glands. Aldosterone promotes the reabsorption of water, increasing the plasma volume.

Lymphatic System

Structure of Lymphatic System

The lymphatic system includes the thymus, bone marrow, tonsils, spleen, lymphatic vessels, lymph nodes, and lymph. Lymph is a clear liquid similar in composition to plasma. It is transported in one direction (toward the neck) where it is emptied into the subclavian veins. Lymph consists of white blood cells and the fluid that leaks out of the blood capillaries. Lymphatic vessels are similar in structure to veins; they have thin walls, and also have valves to prevent backflow. Their walls are more porous, however, allowing the lymph to drain into them for circulation. Lymph is moved by contractions of both smooth and skeletal muscle. Lymphatic vessels are found nearly everywhere in the body except the central nervous system and avascular tissues. The vessels are interrupted by oval-shaped masses of tissue called lymph nodes that contain lymphocytes and filter out foreign substances. The primary organs of the lymphatic system (bone marrow and thymus) produce mature lymphocytes. There are also secondary organs (such as the spleen and tonsils) that house lymphocytes. These specialized white blood cells destroy disease-causing microorganisms.

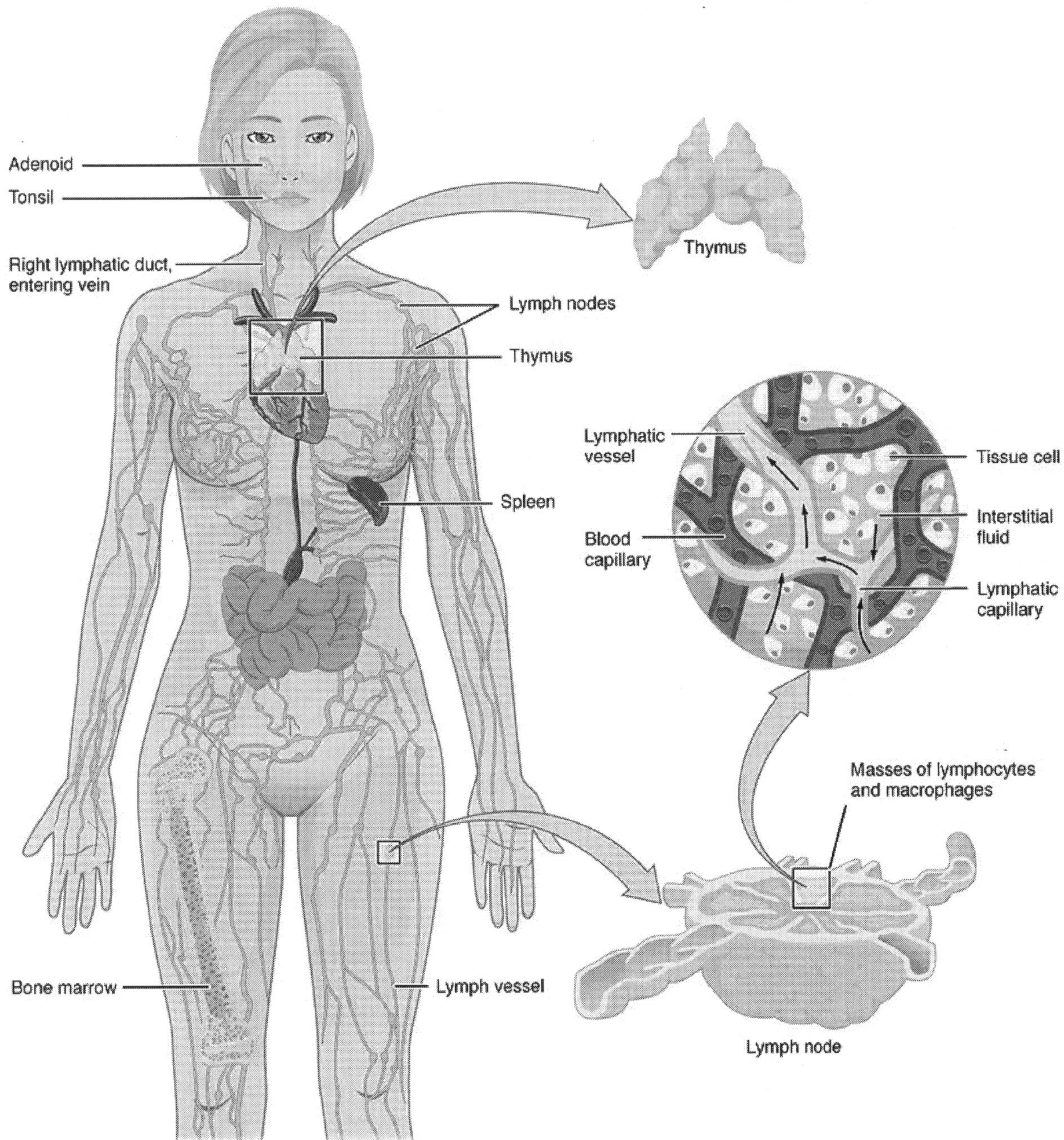

MAJOR FUNCTIONS

EQUALIZATION OF FLUID DISTRIBUTION AND TRANSPORT OF PROTEINS AND LARGE GLYCERIDES

One key function of the immune system is the equalization of fluid between the blood and tissues. Greater hydrostatic pressure in the blood vessels (as compared to the interstitial fluid) causes fluid to leak out of the vessels into the surrounding tissues. Porous lymphatic capillaries collect excess interstitial fluid (now called lymph) for delivery to the right and left subclavian veins. As it travels through the lymphatic system, the lymph passes through lymph nodes where it is filtered and cleansed. Eventually, it reaches either the right lymphatic duct (which drains into the right subclavian vein) or the thoracic duct (which drains into the left subclavian vein), returning fluid back into the blood. If pressure is too great in the lymphatic vessels, edema will occur as fluid leaks back into the tissues.

The lymphatic system also helps to transport certain biomolecules. The villi of the small intestine harbor specialized lymph capillaries called **lacteals** that absorb fats. These fats are transported in the form of **chylomicrons**, which give the lymph (called **chyle**) a whitish appearance. The lymphatic system is also used to return plasma proteins or cells that leaked out of the blood vessels back into the bloodstream.

Production of Lymphocytes Involved in Immune Reactions

The bone marrow and thymus are the "primary" lymphatic organs because they are the sites of lymphocyte production. Stem cells in the red bone marrow called **hemocytoblasts** give rise to immature lymphocytes. Lymphocytes that stay in the bone marrow differentiate into **B cells** and **natural killer (NK) cells**, and other immature lymphocytes migrate to the thymus where they differentiate into **T cells**. Lymphocytes use the bloodstream to migrate from these primary lymphatic organs to "secondary" lymphatic organs, such as the lymph nodes, spleen, and tonsils. When they make contact with antigens, the lymphocytes are activated and mature into effector cells that can participate in immune reactions.

Immune System

Innate (Non-Specific) vs. Adaptive (Specific) Immunity

Innate immunity refers to the nonspecific first line of defense against pathogens that is present at birth. There is no potential for this system to "learn" from previous pathogens or adapt to new threats. The first barriers to infection include mechanical barriers such as the skin and mucous membranes. Chemical barriers include the low pH of gastric juice, interferons that block viral replication, lysozyme in tears, and other antimicrobial proteins such as defensins, collectins, and complements. Pathogens can also be engulfed by phagocytes, or by the destruction of the infected cell by natural killer cells. Fever and inflammation can offer nonspecific protection as well. **Adaptive immunity** develops over time. It may be slow to act initially, but the "memory" of the first encounter with an **antigen** (a toxin or a molecule on the surface of a pathogen that triggers an immune response) allows for faster responses in subsequent exposures to that same antigen. The antigen is recognized as foreign, and the appropriate type of cell is selected to combat the pathogen with which it is associated. These cells are primarily lymphocytes. Depending on the type of lymphocyte, they respond to infection by producing antibodies, killing infected cells, or directing other immune responses.

Review Video: Immune System
Visit mometrix.com/academy and enter code: 622899

Adaptive Immune System Cells

T-Lymphocytes and B-Lymphocytes

There are two main types of lymphocytes that are involved in adaptive immune responses: T-lymphocytes (T cells) and B-lymphocytes (B cells).

T cells mature in the thymus, and are involved in cell-mediated immunity. The initial activation of T cells occurs when they encounter their specific antigen on the surface of an antigen-presenting cell (or APC). When they bind to these APCs, they proliferate and differentiate into various types of T cells. **Cytotoxic T cells** are specialized to kill infected or abnormal cells. Some cytotoxic T cells produce **memory T cells** that respond to subsequent infections. **Helper T cells** secrete cytokines that stimulate the division of T and B cells, while alerting other types of WBCs. **Regulatory (suppressor) T cells** inhibit T and B cells to stop the immune response.

B cells mature in the bone marrow, and are involved in humoral-mediated immunity. The initial activation of B cells occurs when they encounter freely circulating antigens. (Many B cells require co-stimulation by a helper T cell.) After binding to specific antigens, B cells differentiate into plasma cells and memory B cells. **Plasma cells** secrete antibodies that bind to antigens. **Memory B cells** also produce antibodies, but only during a subsequent infection.

Innate Immune System Cells

Macrophages and Phagocytes

There are various types of cells involved in innate immunity, many of which are phagocytes. **Neutrophils** account for most of the white blood cells in the bloodstream. These phagocytes are usually the first to arrive at the site of infection and they chase pathogens using chemotaxis. **Eosinophils** regulate inflammatory responses and release chemicals that kill foreign invaders—often parasitic worms. **Mast cells** (found in connective tissues) and **basophils** (which circulate in the blood before entering tissues) both release histamine to promote inflammation and heparin to inhibit clotting. **Macrophages** (derived from monocytes, the largest leukocytes) are large WBCs that engulf debris and pathogenic microorganisms, and function as antigen presenters to effector T cells. **Dendritic cells** function in much the same way, except they activate "naive" T cells (T cells that have not yet encountered their antigen). **Natural killer cells** are not phagocytes; they destroy cells that have been infected with a pathogen by binding to them and releasing granzymes that trigger apoptosis.

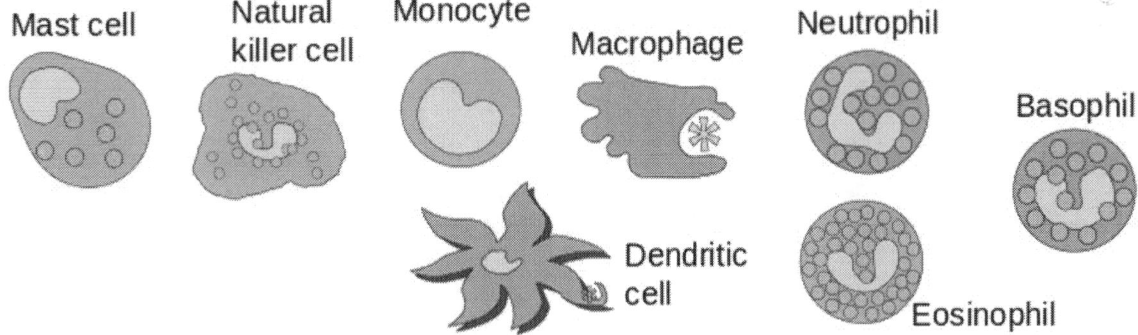

Tissues

The functions of the major tissues and organs that play a role in the immune system:

Tissue of the Immune System	Function
Bone Marrow	Produces hematopoietic stem cells that give rise to all types of blood cells, including lymphocytes Site of B cell differentiation
Thymus	Site of T cell differentiation
Spleen	Splenic cords of the red pulp contain an abundance of macrophages and lymphocytes that help to filter aged blood cells, pathogens, and debris from the blood The white pulp is a lymphatic tissue that consists almost entirely of B and T cells, and provides a place for these lymphocytes to proliferate
Lymph nodes	Provide a place for lymphocytes and other WBCs to proliferate (cortex contains B cells and macrophages, medulla contains T cells) Filter the lymph of microorganisms, toxins, and wastes B cells produce antibodies that assist in the immune response
MALT	Mucosa-associated lymphoid tissue refers to the small clusters of lymphatic cells that are found in the tonsils, appendix, and Peyer's patches of the small intestine. T cells, B cells, and macrophages provide protection against pathogens

Concept of Antigen and Antibody

An **antigen** is a substance that elicits a response from the immune system. Antigens are usually large biomolecules (often proteins) that are identified as foreign or non-self. They can be found on the surfaces of antigenic substances such as viruses, bacteria, fungi, and pollen grains. **Foreign antigens** originate outside the body, and include the examples listed above. **Self-antigens** are produced by the body and rarely initiate an immune response. They often trigger a response in other people, as seen in the rejection of transplanted tissues or organs.

Antibodies (also called immunoglobulins) are products of B cells that bind to specific antigens. The binding of an antibody to an antigen can disarm the pathogen in a variety of ways. In some cases, the pathogens **agglutinate** (clump together) before being destroyed. Antibodies can also **neutralize** the antigen by blocking its ability to attach to cells, or cause it to become insoluble and **precipitate** out of solution. Sometimes, they activate **complement**—a system of proteins that enhances the effectiveness of the immune response. Other cells of the immune system can be called to action, and phagocytosis can be enhanced in a process called **opsonization**. Antibodies also promote **inflammation** to help slow the spread of infection.

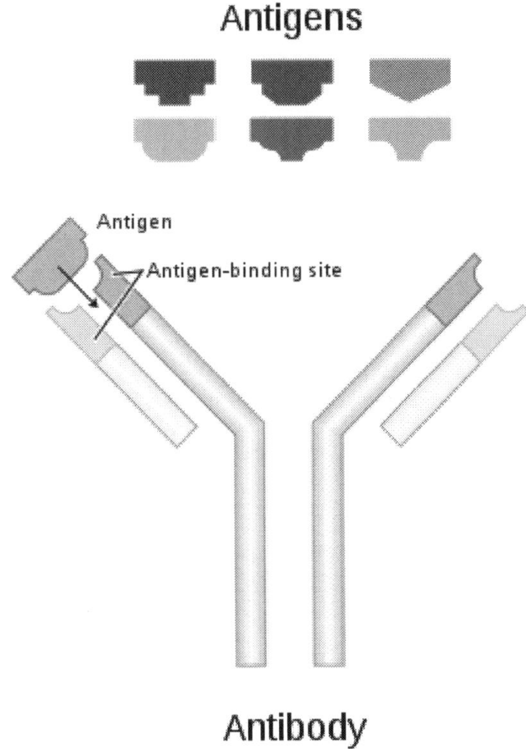

ANTIGEN PRESENTATION

T cells do not recognize free antigens, and so antigens must be presented to them by other cells. The mechanism of presentation depends on the source of the antigen.

Extracellular (exogenous) antigens are engulfed by an antigen-presenting cell, such as a macrophage or dendritic cell. Lysosomal enzymes digest the antigen into small peptides which are brought to the cell surface to be displayed. The antigen pieces are presented on glycoproteins known as **major histocompatibility complexes (MHC) class II**. Only when a helper T cell encounters an antigen presented in this manner will it activate B cells and cytotoxic T cells.

Intracellular (endogenous) antigens, such as viral proteins, are produced inside of a cell. They are digested into small peptides by proteases and then displayed on **MHC class I** molecules. These antigens are recognized by cytotoxic T cells, which go on to destroy infected or cancerous cells.

CLONAL SELECTION

Within the body is a large pool of lymphocytes that differ according to the antigen receptors that they possess. This varied population allows the body to be ready to defend against any antigen it may encounter. But in order to mount an effective response, the cell that is "selected" by the antigen (as determined by its capability to bind to B cell receptors [BCRs] or T cell receptors [TCRs]) must undergo clonal expansion. The selected cell divides rapidly to give rise to a large population of cells that are all equipped with the proper receptors. The clones that are produced will either be effector cells that combat the infection (such as plasma cells or cytotoxic cells), or memory cells that are prepared for a secondary response. This process occurs mainly in the lymph nodes.

Structure of Antibody Molecule

Antibodies are Y-shaped proteins that consists of four polypeptide chains (two identical heavy chains, and two identical light chains) linked together by disulfide bonds. At each tip of the "Y" is a variable region of amino acids that is specific to the **epitope**: the part of the antigen to which the antibody binds. The rest of the antibody is called the **constant region**. (There are five major types of antibodies [IgG, IgM, IgA, IgE, and IgD] that differ according to the constant portion of the heavy chain.)

The variable region of the antibody has a unique conformation that is complementary to the shape of a specific antigen. These specialized regions are called **antigen binding sites**. When the epitope (also called the antigenic determinant site) binds, an antigen-antibody complex is formed.

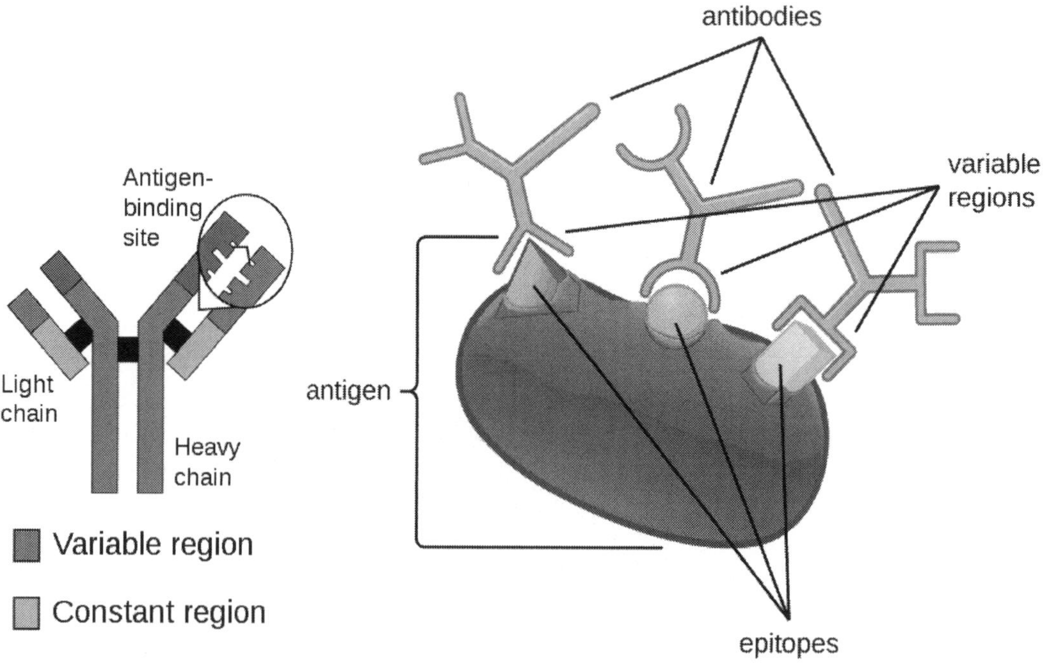

Recognition of Self vs. Non-Self, Autoimmune Diseases

Self-antigens are present on all body cells, and it is important for the immune system to distinguish these antigens from foreign, or non-self, antigens. The antigen receptors on immature lymphocytes are generated randomly, and some are likely to respond to the self-antigens present in the environment. Any B cells in the bone marrow, or T cells in the thymus, that respond to self-antigens are killed in a process called negative selection. A backup mechanism is in place for any cells that escape this process, as can be seen in B cell activation. When a B cell presents an antigen on its surface, it must be activated by a helper T cell that is bound to an identical antigen. It is unlikely that the T cell will have responded to the same self-antigen, and the B cell remains inactive. Failure of this two-step verification process can result in an attack on self-cells. B cells produce antibodies and T cells act against the cells of the body. Conditions that result from such attacks are known as autoimmune diseases. Common examples include rheumatoid arthritis, psoriasis, and multiple sclerosis.

Major Histocompatibility Complex

Nearly all body cells are tagged with glycoproteins known as major histocompatibility complexes, or MHCs. These MHCs are different for each person (which explains the rejection of transplanted organs or tissues.) Alterations of these MHCs mark the cells as non-self.

MHC-I (MHC class I molecules) are found on nucleated cells (nearly all cells except red blood cells). Antigens produced within the cell (endogenous) are degraded, and portions of them combine with MHC-I before being displayed on the cell surface. T cells will be activated when their receptors bind to MHC-I / antigen complexes, and the antigen-presenting cell is destroyed.

MHC-II (MHC class II molecules) are found on antigen-presenting cells, such as dendritic cells, B cells, and macrophages. Antigens from extracellular pathogens (exogenous) are engulfed and broken down and the fragments combined with MHC-II before being displayed on the cell surface. This presentation alerts other immune system cells to the antigen.

DIGESTIVE SYSTEM

INGESTION

SALIVA AS LUBRICATION AND SOURCE OF ENZYMES

When food is ingested, it is immediately moistened by saliva. This lubricating fluid is secreted by hundreds of minor salivary glands that are scattered throughout the oral cavity, and three pairs of major salivary glands: the parotid, submandibular, and sublingual glands.

Saliva contains a variety of solutes, many of which are enzymes. **Salivary amylase** begins the chemical breakdown of polysaccharides into simpler sugars, and **lingual lipase** begins the breakdown of fats. The effects of salivary enzymes are minimal, however, compared to the digestion that occurs later in the stomach and small intestine. Saliva contains antimicrobial agents as well. **Lysozyme** is an enzyme that works together with immunoglobulin A to break down the cell walls of many bacteria. Other components of saliva include bicarbonate ions that help the saliva to maintain a pH that is optimal for salivary enzymes, as well as other ions. **Mucin** is a protein that helps to form a gel-like coating that lubricates the bolus of food.

Review Video: Gastrointestinal System
Visit mometrix.com/academy and enter code: 378740

INGESTION; ESOPHAGUS, TRANSPORT FUNCTION

The esophagus is a 25-cm tube extending from the pharynx to the stomach that functions as a passageway for food. It is not involved in digestion or absorption of nutrients, but it does secrete mucus to lubricate the esophagus and aid in the transport of food. The esophagus (and the alimentary canal that follows) has a wall that consists of four layers: the mucosa, submucosa, muscularis externa, and adventitia. Most of the digestive tract has a muscularis externa made of smooth muscle tissue, but the upper third of the esophagus is composed of skeletal muscle, and is under voluntary control. The middle portion is a mixture of both skeletal and smooth muscle, and the lower third is entirely smooth muscle. Food does not simply "fall" into the stomach; it is pushed along by **peristalsis**: an involuntary process in which the muscles in the wall of the digestive organ rhythmically contract and relax. The upper esophageal sphincter at the superior end of the esophagus and the lower esophageal sphincter at the inferior end control the passage of food by contracting and relaxing.

STOMACH

STORAGE AND CHURNING OF FOOD

The stomach is a muscular organ that can stretch to accommodate a high volume of food. While some chemical digestion does occur, the primary role of the stomach is the storage and mechanical breakdown of food. The inner surface (mucosa) is folded into a series of ridges called rugae that allow the stomach to expand as it fills with food. The stomach holds about 1 liter after a typical meal, but can stretch to accommodate nearly four times that amount. It churns and pummels food for an average of three to four hours with the help of a third muscle layer in the muscularis externa that is unique to the stomach. As the food is mixed with gastric juices, it turns into a creamy paste called chyme. A valve called the pyloric sphincter regulates the passage of chyme into the small intestine.

PRODUCTION OF DIGESTIVE ENZYMES, SITE OF DIGESTION

The mucosa of the stomach contains gastric glands which open into numerous gastric pits. There are four types of cells in these glands: mucous cells, parietal cells, chief cells, and endocrine cells. **Endocrine cells** (G cells) release hormones such as gastrin into the blood, and do not contribute to gastric juices. The rest of the glands are exocrine, and secrete their products into the stomach.

Parietal cells secrete intrinsic factor, which is required for the absorption of vitamin B_{12} in the small intestine. They also release hydrochloric acid (HCl), which lowers the pH of gastric juice to an average range of 1 to 3. This acidic environment is required for the activation of pepsinogen, which is secreted by the **chief cells**. The active form of pepsinogen is called pepsin—a digestive enzyme that breaks down proteins into smaller peptide chains. Chief cells also secrete gastric lipase, which continues the digestion of fats (though most fat and protein digestion occurs in the small intestine). The **mucous cells** secrete bicarbonate-containing mucus to protect the stomach from the acidity and digestive enzymes.

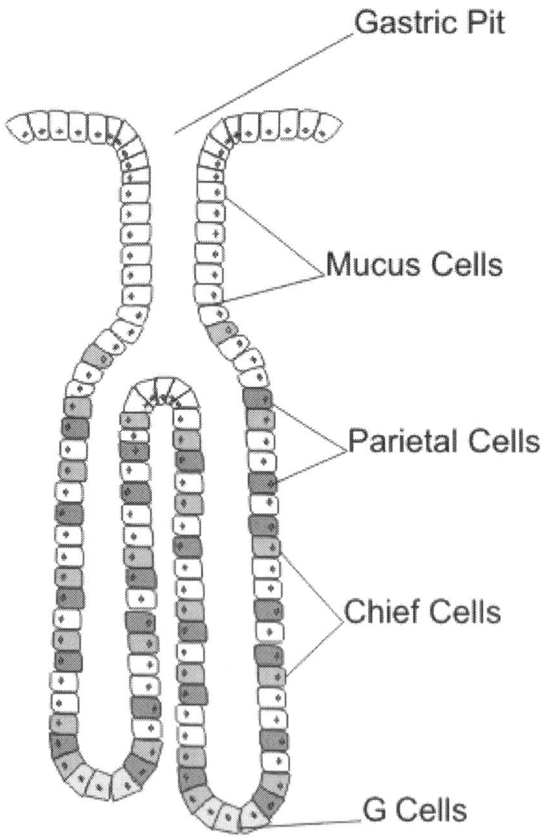

STRUCTURE (GROSS)

The stomach is a muscular organ located in the left superior region of the abdomen. The gastroesophageal sphincter (also called the lower esophageal or cardioesophageal sphincter) found at the junction between the esophagus and stomach helps to prevent the reflux of acidic contents. The stomach itself can be divided into four main parts: the cardiac region, the fundus, the body, and the pylorus. The **cardiac region** is the area where food is emptied into the stomach. The **fundus** is the most superior region of the stomach, and the **body** is the largest, most central region. The body curves toward the right to form a "J" shape, with a lesser curvature and a greater curvature. It then narrows into a funnel-shaped region called the **pylorus**. The wider end of the pylorus is called the pyloric antrum and the narrow portion is the pyloric canal. The pyloric sphincter is the valve that regulates the release of small amounts of chyme into the small intestine. Other features of the stomach include the gastric folds (rugae) of the mucosa that allow the stomach to stretch and expand. The stomach is also characterized by an inner oblique layer of smooth muscle that is not seen in the rest of the alimentary canal.

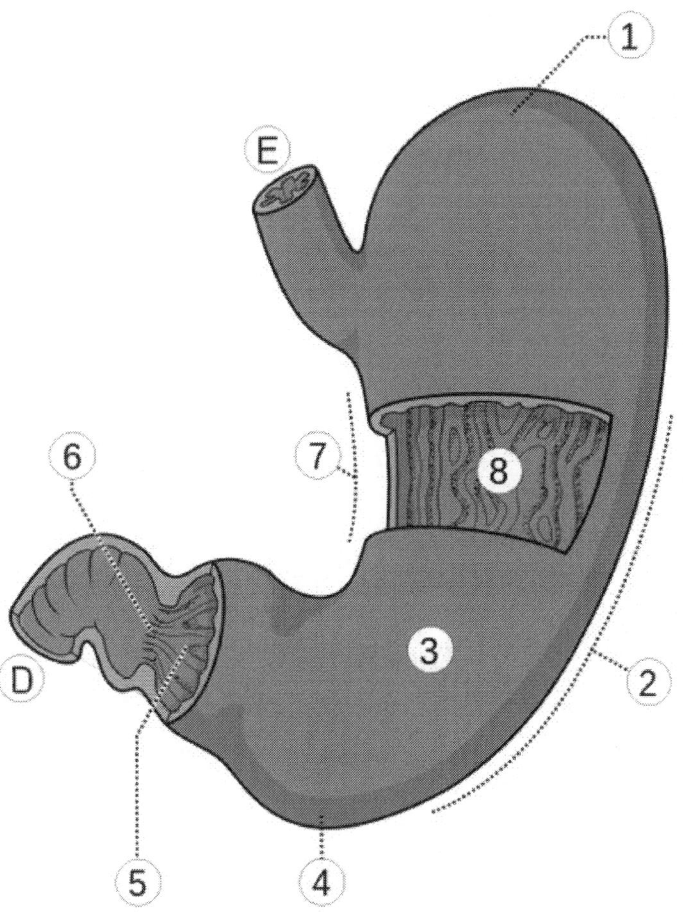

- 1. Fundus
- 2. Greater curvature
- 3. Body
- 4. Pyloric region
- 5. Pyloric antrum
- 6. Pyloric canal
- 7. Lesser curvature
- 8. Rugae
- E. Esophagus
- D. Duodenum of small intestine

LIVER

STRUCTURAL RELATIONSHIP OF LIVER WITHIN GASTROINTESTINAL SYSTEM AND THE PRODUCTION OF BILE

The liver is an essential component of the gastrointestinal system, but is not a part of the alimentary canal. This large, four-lobed organ acts as an accessory organ by performing many functions such as the production of bile, nutrient metabolism, and detoxification.

The primary digestive function of the liver is the synthesis of bile. Bile is a yellow-green solution of bile salts, pigments (mainly bilirubin from the breakdown of hemoglobin), cholesterol, and electrolytes. Only the bile salts play a role in digestion, and they do so mechanically (not enzymatically) by emulsifying fats into smaller globules called micelles that can be acted on by lipases in the small intestine. Bile also enhances the absorption of the fat-soluble vitamins A, D, E, and K. Liver cells synthesize bile salts from cholesterol.

Bile is stored and concentrated in the gallbladder. When food enters the small intestine, a hormone called cholecystokinin (CCK) signals the gallbladder to contact, and the bile is squeezed into the common bile duct. This duct joins with the pancreatic duct at the hepatopancreatic ampulla (ampulla of Vater) and bile spills into the duodenum via the duodenal papilla. Bile can also flow directly from the liver to the duodenum.

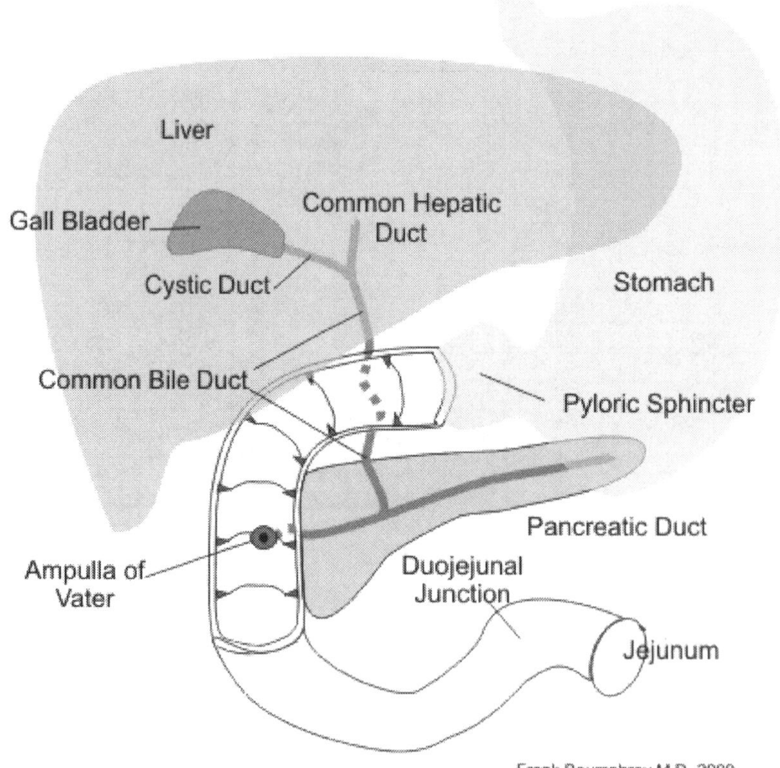

ROLE IN BLOOD GLUCOSE REGULATION, DETOXIFICATION

The liver performs many metabolic functions, including the regulation of blood glucose concentration (which averages 100 mg/dl). Blood from the digestive tract enters the liver through the hepatic portal vein. If the blood sugar is too high, the liver polymerizes glucose to form glycogen in a process called **glycogenesis**. If blood sugar is too low, liver cells break down stored glycogen and release glucose monomers in a process called **glycogenolysis**. In cases of prolonged fasting, the liver can produce glucose from non-carbohydrate sources such as proteins and fats. This is called **gluconeogenesis**.

The liver also has a vital role in detoxification. Ammonia (a toxic waste product of the metabolism of amino acids) is converted to urea in the liver and excreted by the kidneys. Hormones that are circulating in the blood are inactivated by the liver and eliminated by the kidneys as well. The liver also breaks down exogenous compounds, such as drugs and alcohol.

Pancreas

Production of Enzymes and Transport of Enzymes to Small Intestine

The **pancreas** is a triangular-shaped organ with both endocrine and exocrine functions. (As an endocrine gland, it releases insulin, glucagon, and somatostatin into the blood.) It is located below the stomach, and extends from the duodenum to the spleen. Its role in digestion is the production and secretion of digestive juices. When chyme reaches the duodenum, enteroendocrine cells secrete cholecystokinin (CCK), which stimulates the acinar cells of the pancreas to release enzyme-rich juices. Secretin is secreted as well, which stimulates the duct cells to release a bicarbonate-rich solution that raises the pH. This provides the optimal environment for enzymes released by the pancreas. Pancreatic amylase digests starch, and pancreatic lipase digests fats. Proteases are released in their inactive form, but are activated in the small intestine. These activated protein-digesting enzymes include trypsin, carboxypeptidases A and B, and chymotrypsin. Nucleases digest nucleic acids. Pancreatic juice is emptied into the main pancreatic duct, which merges with the common bile duct at the hepatopancreatic ampulla. Juices enter the duodenum at the duodenal papilla. There is also an accessory pancreatic duct that empties directly into the duodenum at the minor papilla.

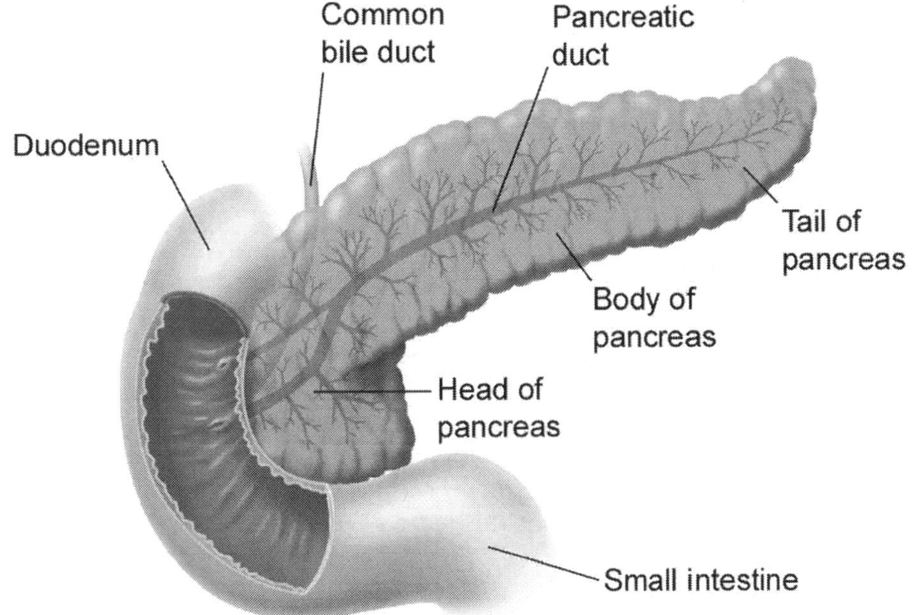

National Cancer Institute

Small Intestine

The small intestine is a long tube that extends from the pyloric sphincter to the ileocecal valve. Pancreatic enzymes and enzymes of the small intestine continue the digestion of food so the nutrients are small enough to be absorbed. These enzymes (called brush border enzymes) are embedded in the **microvilli**: tiny folds of the apical cell membrane that increase surface area. The core of each microvillus consists of actin filaments that extend out from the cytoplasm. Finger-like projections of the mucosa (villi) and deep circular folds of the mucosa and submucosa (plicae circulares) also increase the surface area available for absorption.

Absorption of water and food molecules occurs mostly in the jejunum and ileum of the small intestine. Amino acids and most sugars are taken into the intestinal cells using cotransport with sodium ions (secondary active transport). Lipid components and water are absorbed into the cells by simple diffusion. Short-chain fatty acids, sugars, amino acids, water, and electrolytes enter the bloodstream by diffusing into capillaries within the villi and traveling to the liver.

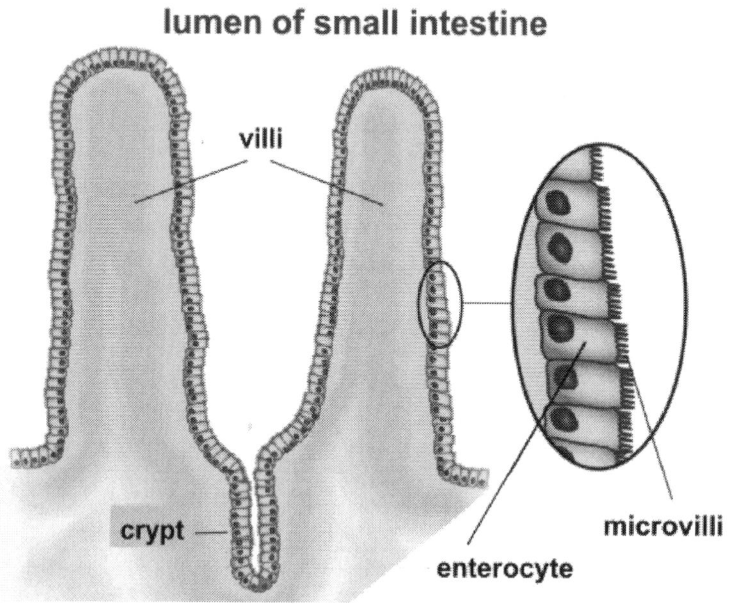

Production of Enzymes, Site of Digestion and Neutralization of Stomach Acid

Most of the chemical digestion of food occurs in the small intestine. Brush border enzymes of the microvilli (as well as pancreatic enzymes) break down carbohydrates, fats, proteins, and nucleic acids into smaller components which are then absorbed. Some mechanical digestion occurs in the small intestine as well. Peristalsis moves chyme toward the small intestine, while segmentation pushes it back and forth to help mix enzymes into the chyme. Brunner's glands in the duodenum secrete bicarbonate-containing fluid that (with the help of alkaline pancreatic juice) neutralizes the acidic chyme, providing the optimal pH for enzyme activity.

Brush border enzymes and the substrates that they break down are summarized in the table below.

Brush border enzyme	Substrate
Dextrinase	Oligosaccharides
Glucoamylase	Oligosaccharides
Maltase	Maltose (disaccharide)
Lactase	Lactose (disaccharide)
Sucrase	Sucrose (disaccharide)
Aminopeptidase	Peptides
Dipeptidase	Dipeptides

Nucleosidase	Nucleotides
Phosphatase	Nucleotides

STRUCTURE (ANATOMIC SUBDIVISIONS)

The small intestine is subdivided into three regions: the duodenum, jejunum, and ileum. At about 25 cm, the C-shaped **duodenum** is the shortest segment, but it has the widest diameter. It receives chyme from the stomach and neutralizing digestive juices from the pancreas. Most of the chemical digestion of food occurs here. It does not play a large role in absorption, with the exception of iron. The **jejunum** is the main site of absorption. It averages 2.5 meters in length, and is characterized by prominent plicae circulares, long villi, and dense microvilli. The longest segment of the small intestine is the **ileum**. It averages 3.5 meters in length, but is the most narrow in diameter. Small aggregates of lymphatic cells called Peyer's patches are common in this segment, but they can be found throughout the small intestine. The primary role of the ileum is to absorb vitamin B_{12}, bile salts, and any nutrients that were not absorbed by the jejunum. It has few circular folds, and they disappear altogether in the distal region. It terminates at the ileocecal valve, which controls the movement of chyme into the large intestine.

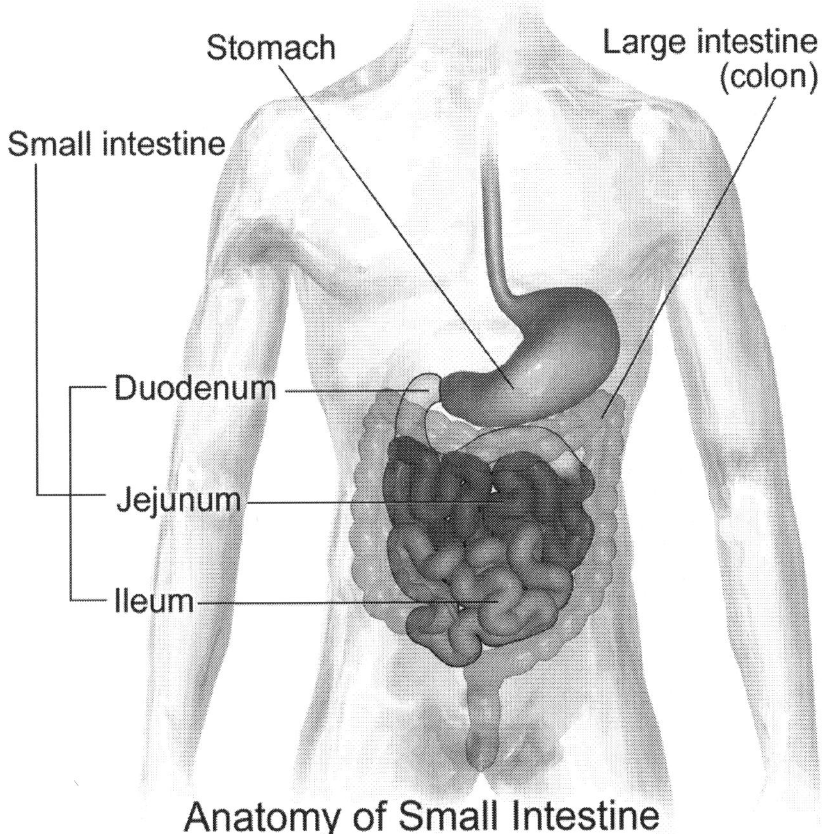

Anatomy of Small Intestine

LARGE INTESTINE

ABSORPTION OF WATER

The large intestine specializes in the absorption of vitamin K, biotin, sodium ions, chloride ions, and water. By the time chyme reaches the large intestine, most of the water (approximately 80%) has already been absorbed by the small intestine. As the chyme is pushed through the colon 90% of the remaining liquid is absorbed, leaving a mass of indigestible food, water, and bacteria. If the feces are excreted before enough water is absorbed, they leave as diarrhea. Constipation results when too much water is absorbed.

Bacterial Flora

The large intestine does not secrete digestive enzymes, but there are hundreds of species of resident bacteria that can digest certain materials left in chyme. These beneficial microbes are nourished by small amounts of cellulose and other carbohydrates, and they release gases such as carbon dioxide and methane as waste products of fermentation. The bacteria also release vitamin K, biotin, thiamin, riboflavin, and vitamin B_{12}. Vitamin K (required for the synthesis of clotting proteins) and biotin (a cofactor for many enzymes) are absorbed for use in the body. Resident gut flora also help to keep populations of pathogenic bacteria in check. The appendix *may* serve as a reservoir for beneficial species of bacteria, though it is often infected with harmful microbes.

Structure (Gross)

The large intestine is the portion of the alimentary canal that begins at the **ileocecal valve** and terminates at the anus. It is larger in diameter than the small intestine, but much shorter in length - averaging 1.5 meters. The first portion of the large intestine is a pouch called the **cecum**, and it receives chyme from the small intestine. It is also the site of a blind-ended tube called the **appendix**. The middle portion of the large intestine is the **colon**, which can be further subdivided into the ascending colon (right side of the body), transverse colon (extends across the abdominal cavity), descending colon (left side of the body), and sigmoid colon. The sigmoid colon lies in the pelvic cavity and becomes the **rectum**, which opens to the anus. There are no villi in the large intestine, but there are pouch-like sacculations called **haustra** that are separated by folds called plicae semilunares. These pouches are formed by the contraction of smooth muscle within the muscularis layer. The walls of the large intestine are lubricated by mucus, which is secreted by goblet cells.

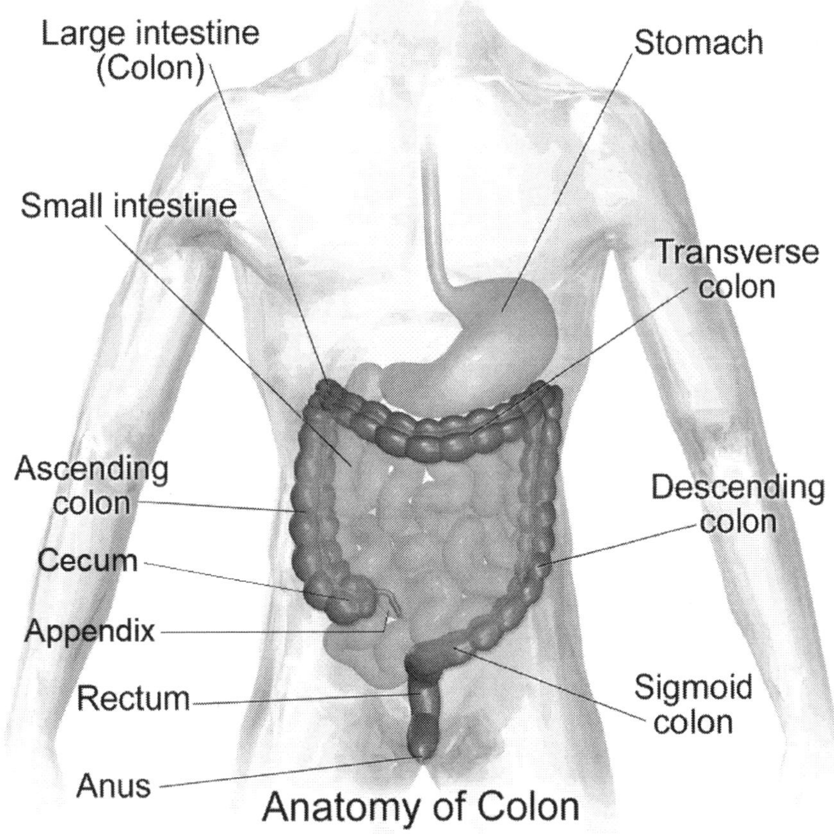

Anatomy of Colon

RECTUM: STORAGE AND ELIMINATION OF WASTE, FECES

The final 12 to 15 cm of the large intestine is called the rectum. In humans, it curves to conform to the shape of the sacrum and coccyx bone. The **anal canal** is the last portion of the rectum, and it ends with an involuntary internal sphincter and a voluntary external sphincter. A dilated region (superior to the anal canal) called the **rectal ampulla** functions as a storage area for feces before they are eliminated in the process of defecation. Feces consist of bacteria, water, undigested material, epithelial cells, and bile (which accounts for the brown coloration). As this material accumulates, the walls of the rectum expand and stretch receptors send signals that cause the rectal muscles to contract, the internal sphincter to relax, and the external sphincter to contract. At this point, the decision can be made to eliminate or delay elimination.

MUSCULAR CONTROL

PERISTALSIS

Mechanical digestion begins in the mouth with the voluntary act of chewing (mastication). Skeletal muscles of the mouth and pharynx aid in swallowing (deglutition), which consists of three phases: the voluntary buccal phase and the involuntary pharyngeal and esophageal phases. The muscularis externa of the digestive tract consists of two layers of muscle tissue (three in the stomach) that contract radially and then relax to squeeze food in one direction. This involuntary propulsive process is called **peristalsis**. Peristalsis moves food from the pharynx to the esophagus to the stomach where an extra muscle layer helps to churn and mix the food. Another involuntary process called **segmentation** occurs in the intestines, in addition to peristalsis. In segmentation, non-adjacent portions of the digestive tract contract and relax to move the chyme, partly digested food, back and forth. Haustral contractions in the large intestine are a form of segmentation that moves chyme from one haustrum to the next. Mass peristalsis describes the movements that occur two to four times a day to push large amounts of chyme toward the rectum. Movement along the digestive tract is also controlled by the gastroesophageal sphincter, pyloric sphincter, and anal sphincters.

Endocrine Control

Hormones and Target Tissues

Hormones associated with the GI tract	
Hormone	**Target / Action**
Gastrin	Targets the parietal cells of the stomach—stimulates the release of HCl from G cells Stimulates smooth muscle contraction in the stomach and intestines, promoting motility Promotes relaxation of pyloric sphincter
CCK—cholecystokinin	Targets the pancreas and liver—stimulates the release of digestive enzymes and bile into the duodenum - stimulates gallbladder contraction - relaxes the hepatopancreatic sphincter Promotes the contraction of the pyloric sphincter (inhibits gastric emptying)
Secretin	Targets the pancreas and liver—augments the effects of CCK Stimulates the release of bicarbonate from the pancreas
GIP—Gastric Inhibitory Peptide	Inhibits gastric motility and secretions
Motilin	Targets the esophagus and intestines—promotes peristalsis between meals
VIP—Vasoactive intestinal peptide	Promotes relaxation of smooth muscle (particularly the sphincters) Vasodilator

Nervous Control: The Enteric Nervous System

The network of neurons buried in the lining of the gastrointestinal tract that controls the function of the digestive system is called the **enteric nervous system** (ENS). The ENS can operate independently of the brain and spinal cord, and communicates with the CNS through the parasympathetic and sympathetic nervous systems. The parasympathetic nervous system stimulates digestive activities, while the sympathetic nervous system inhibits them.

The ENS is divided into two main parts: the submucosal and myenteric plexuses. The **submucosal plexus** is embedded in the connective tissue of the submucosa. It functions in regulating local secretions, absorption, contraction of submucosal muscle, and blood flow. The **myenteric plexus** is located between the circular and longitudinal layers of the muscularis externa. This network exerts control over the motility of the GI tract. It increases the tone, as well as the rate, intensity, and velocity of contractions.

EXCRETORY SYSTEM

ROLES IN HOMEOSTASIS

BLOOD PRESSURE

When osmoreceptors detect an increase in blood osmolality, or when baroreceptors detect a decrease in blood pressure, the pituitary gland secretes **antidiuretic hormone** (ADH). ADH stimulates the reabsorption of water in the kidney so that less water is excreted in the urine. This increases the volume and pressure of the blood.

The **renin-angiotensin-aldosterone system** (RAAS) is another mechanism by which blood pressure is regulated. When granular juxtaglomerular cells of the afferent arterioles of the kidneys detect a drop in blood pressure, they secrete an enzyme called **renin**. Renin interacts with a plasma protein called **angiotensinogen**, producing **angiotensin I**. As angiotensin I enters the capillaries of the lungs, it is acted on by another enzyme that converts it to **angiotensin II**. This hormone raises blood pressure by promoting vasoconstriction and stimulating the adrenal cortex to release **aldosterone**. Aldosterone increases the reabsorption of sodium, which increases water reabsorption, causing the blood volume and pressure to increase.

OSMOREGULATION

Osmoregulation describes the regulation of water and solute concentrations of body fluids. The primary organ involved in this process is the kidney. Dehydration or excessive salt intake will raise the osmolality of the blood. (Plasma osmolality is determined mainly by the concentrations of electrolytes, such as Na^+, Cl^-, and K^+.) When osmoreceptors in the hypothalamus detect an increase in osmolality, signals are sent to the pituitary gland to release ADH. ADH causes the collecting ducts in the kidneys to be more permeable to water, and water crosses the epithelium from the urine into the interstitium where it is returned to the blood. As a result, the blood osmolality decreases, and urine osmolality increases.

Aldosterone also plays a role in osmoregulation. When blood pressure is low, this hormone is secreted by the adrenal cortex. Aldosterone increases sodium reabsorption, which causes more water to leave the collecting tubule, thus raising blood osmolality. It also regulates the concentrations of other ions, such as potassium and chloride.

ACID–BASE BALANCE

The kidneys are key players in the maintenance of blood pH, which must be kept within a narrow range of 7.35 and 7.45. This is achieved by regulating the ratio of hydrogen ions to bicarbonate ions. (The higher the concentration of H^+ ions, the lower the pH.) Buffer systems in the body such as the phosphate, protein, and bicarbonate systems are in place to resist changes in H^+ concentration. Recall that the respiratory system helps to control pH through the bicarbonate buffer system. When carbon dioxide combines with water, carbonic acid (H_2CO_3) is formed, before dissociating into bicarbonate ions (HCO_3^-) and H^+. (Reaction: $CO_2 + H_2O \leftrightarrow H_2CO_3 \leftrightarrow HCO_3^- + H^+$.) Increasing the rate of respiration decreases the concentration of H^+, which increases pH. The reverse is true when the rate of respiration decreases. The response from the *kidneys* is slower, but lasts longer. As blood pH decreases, H^+ ions are excreted by the renal tubules via urine (which is now more acidic) and bicarbonate ions are retained. The intercalated cells of the late distal tubule and collecting duct can also generate new bicarbonate ions. The kidneys lower pH by reabsorbing H^+ ions and secreting bicarbonate ions.

Removal of Soluble Nitrogenous Waste

Nitrogen-containing wastes such as ammonia, urea, uric acid, and creatinine are excreted in urine. **Ammonia** is a toxic base that is formed during the breakdown of amino acids. Enzymes in the liver convert it to a less toxic form called **urea**. There is a high concentration of urea in the medulla because the collecting ducts are permeable to it. Much of the urea enters the interstitium, and it is then reabsorbed into the descending loop of Henle. Urea is the most abundant nitrogenous waste product in the urine, but since most of it is recycled, only a small amount is eliminated in urine. The high concentration of urea in the interstitium is helpful because it promotes the reabsorption of water. **Uric acid** is another nitrogenous waste that is excreted in the urine. It is formed as a byproduct of the catabolism of purine nucleotides, and most of it is reabsorbed in the proximal tubule by active transport. Like urea, only a small percentage is excreted. **Creatinine** is produced in the muscles as byproduct of the metabolism of creatine phosphate. It is filtered by the kidneys and excreted. Unlike urea and uric acid, creatinine is not reabsorbed by the tubules.

Kidney Structure

The kidneys are bean-shaped organs located in the lumbar region of the body that function in the filtering of blood and the excretion of wastes. Each kidney is surrounded by three protective layers of connective tissue: the **renal fascia**, the **adipose capsule**, and the innermost **renal capsule**. The capsule surrounds the outer region of the kidney called the **renal cortex**. The cortex contains many filtration units called **nephrons**, which have tubules that dip into the interior region called the **medulla**. The tubules in the medulla run parallel to each other and form striped cone-shaped masses of tissue called **medullary pyramids**. A cavity called the **renal sinus** contains the basin-like **renal pelvis**, which funnels the urine into the ureter. The **hilum** is the concave region of the kidney where the blood vessels and nerves enter and leave. Blood enters the kidney through the renal artery, which branches into smaller and smaller arteries until the blood reaches a tuft of capillaries called the **glomerulus**. Here, the blood is filtered before leaving the kidney through a network of veins that merge into the renal vein.

Frontal section through the Kidney

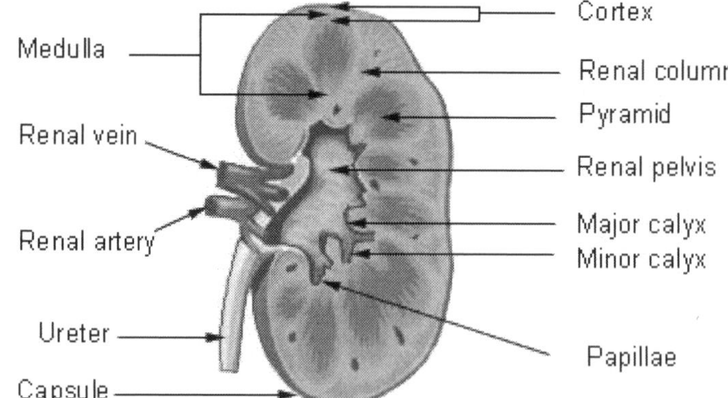

Cortex

The renal cortex is the outer portion of the kidney, and it is the site of **ultrafiltration**: the nonspecific filtration of blood under high pressure. It is also responsible for the majority of reabsorption of water. The cortex is very vascular, and has a granular appearance due to the presence of nephrons. The renal corpuscles and the convoluted tubules of the nephrons are within the cortex (forming the **cortical labyrinth**), but the loops of Henle extend into the adjacent region known as the renal medulla. The thick, straight portions of the proximal and distal tubules, as well as the collecting ducts, form **medullary rays** that begin in the cortex and run perpendicular to the capsule. About 85% of nephrons (cortical nephrons) have short loops of Henle that extend only slightly into the medulla. The remaining 15% (juxtamedullary nephrons) have longer loops that extend deeper. Extensions of the cortex called **renal columns** dip down in between the renal pyramids of the medulla.

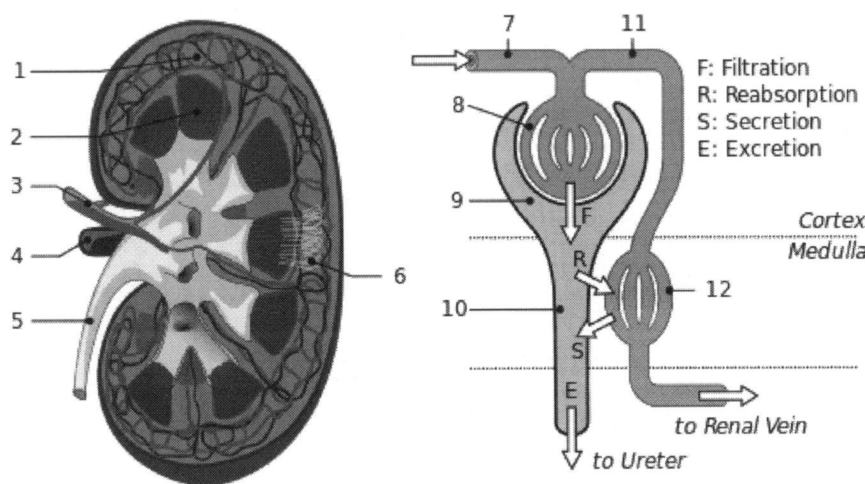

1: Renal cortex. 2: Medulla. 3: Renal artery. 4: Renal vein. 5: Ureter. 6: Nephrons. 7: Afferent arteriole. 8: Glomerulus. 9: Bowman's capsule. 10: Renal tubule. 11: Efferent arteriole. 12: Peritubular capillaries.

MEDULLA

The adrenal medulla is the inner part of the kidney, and it continues the reabsorption of water and salts that began in the cortex. These substances enter the peritubular capillaries that are associated with the nephrons. Any filtrate that is not reclaimed by the circulatory system will leave as urine.

The medulla contains cone-shaped regions of tissue called **renal pyramids** that are separated by **renal columns**. The tips of the pyramids are oriented toward the pelvis of the kidney, and the bases face the cortex. The renal pyramids contain tubules that transport renal filtrate from the renal cortex to the apex of the pyramids. At the apex is a structure called the **renal papilla** that contains ducts that allow the processed filtrate (now called urine) to pass out of the medulla to collecting chambers called **calyces**. From here the urine passes through the renal pelvis, through the ureter, and finally into the bladder.

NEPHRON STRUCTURE

The nephron is the functional unit of the kidney. Each kidney has over a million of these microscopic structures, and each one consists of two main parts: the **renal corpuscle** (which filters the blood) and the **renal tubule** (which collects and concentrates the filtrate). The renal corpuscle consists of a cup-shaped structure called **Bowman's capsule** that wraps partially around a cluster of capillaries called the **glomerulus**. The renal tubule is a looping canal that is continuous with Bowman's capsule. It consists of different regions that differ in structure and function. The **proximal convoluted tubule** begins at Bowman's capsule and then plunges into the medulla, forming a u-shape called the **loop of Henle**. It then becomes the **distal convoluted tubule**, which is continuous with the **collecting duct**. The collecting duct is typically considered as a separate structure, and not part of the nephron.

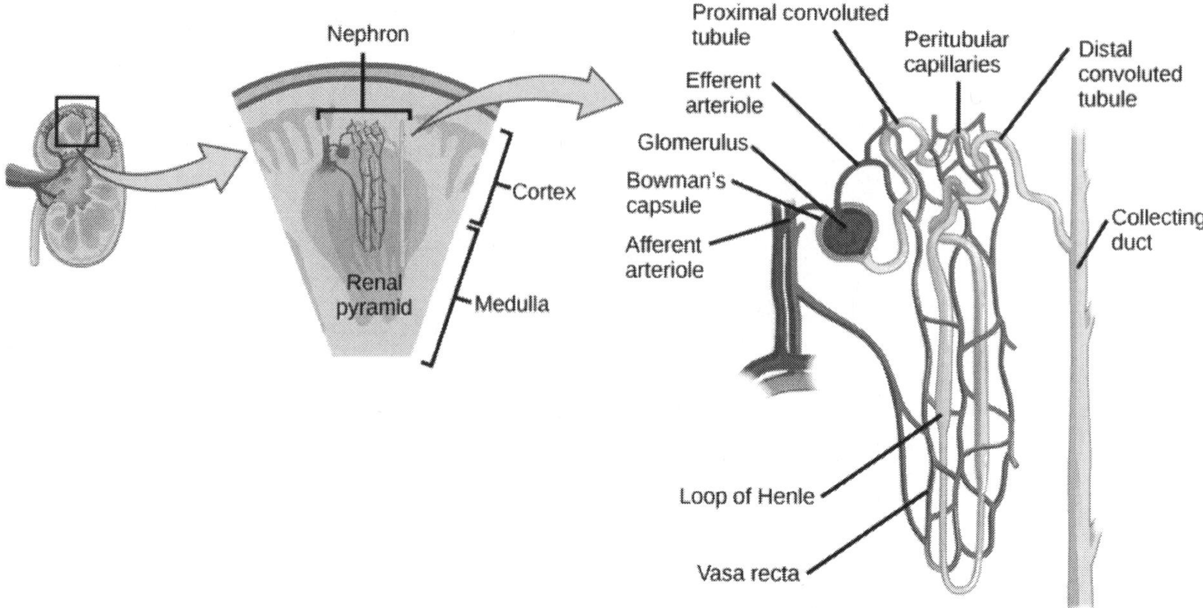

Glomerulus and Bowman's Capsule

Each renal corpuscle consists of a **glomerulus** and a **Bowman's capsule**. The glomerulus is a tangled network of blood capillaries that occupies Bowman's capsule. These fenestrated capillaries are lined with a thin layer of epithelial cells. An **afferent arteriole** takes blood to the glomerulus and an **efferent arteriole** takes it away. The smaller diameter of the efferent arteriole increases the pressure within the glomerulus, which is required for ultrafiltration. **Mesangial cells** contract to regulate blood flow, and also support the capillary network.

Bowman's capsule is a cup-like structure at the closed end of the renal tubule that encloses the glomerulus. It has an outer layer of epithelial cells that form the parietal layer, and a visceral layer of **podocytes** with processes called **pedicels** that wrap around the capillaries. Gaps between the pedicels (filtration slits) allow the passage of tiny molecules and ions. Together, the endothelial cells of the capillaries, the basement membrane, and the pedicels make up the **filtration membrane**. Fluid from the blood leaves the fenestrated capillaries and passes through the filtration membrane and collects in **Bowman's space** (the cavity between the two layers of Bowman's capsule). From here, the filtrate enters the renal tubule.

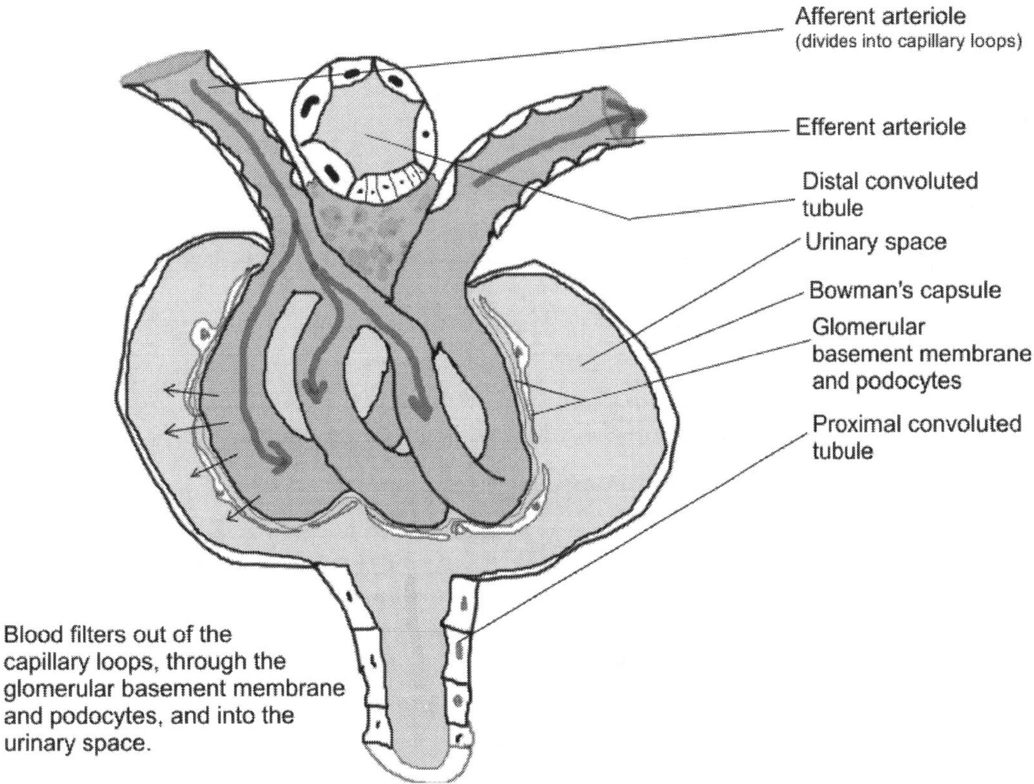

Proximal Tubule, Loop of Henle, and Distal Tubule

The renal tubule is divided into three continuous regions: the proximal convoluted tubule, the loop of Henle, and the distal convoluted tubule. The **proximal convoluted tubule** extends from Bowman's capsule, and this coiled tube is characterized by cuboidal cells with dense microvilli that aid in reabsorption and secretion. There are only sparse microvilli in the rest of the tubule. The middle, hairpin-shaped portion of the renal tubule is called the **loop of Henle**, and it maintains a relatively high solute concentration in the medulla, which in turn assists in the reabsorption of water. The loop consists of a descending limb (which reabsorbs water) that plunges into the medulla, a U-turn that curves back toward the cortex, and an ascending limb (which reabsorbs ions). The ascending limb widens into a thick portion composed of larger epithelial cells. The loop is lined with simple squamous epithelial cells, with the exception of the thick ascending limb which is lined with simple cuboidal cells. This limb becomes the **distal convoluted tubule** (also lined with cuboidal cells), which is involved in absorption and secretion, but not to the extent of the proximal convoluted tubule. It is also shorter in length.

Collecting Duct

The collecting duct is the final site of reabsorption in the kidney, and it is shared by multiple nephrons. The distal tubule empties filtrate into the collecting tubule, which merges with other collecting tubules to form the collecting duct. Collecting tubules are lined with simple cuboidal epithelium, but these cells elongate to form columnar cells as they get closer to the duct. Some of these cells are **principal cells**, which reabsorb sodium ions and water (under ADH and aldosterone control). Other cells are **intercalated cells**, and they play an important role in acid-base balance and the reabsorption of sodium ions. Both these types of cells can also be found toward the end part of the distal tubule, but there are fewer microvilli than in the collecting duct. The filtrate that passes through the collecting duct enters the minor calyces at the apex of a medullary pyramid.

Formation of Urine

Glomerular Filtration

The formation of urine begins with glomerular filtration. This nonspecific filtration is driven by the hydrostatic pressure of the blood. This pressure is higher than in other capillaries because the efferent arterioles that exit the glomerulus have a smaller diameter than the afferent arterioles that enter. Water and small solutes from the blood are forced through fenestrations in the capillaries, leaving behind larger particles. The fluid must pass through the 3-layered filtration membrane before entering Bowman's space as renal filtrate. The first layer is the endothelial lining of the capillaries. Fenestrations in the capillaries prevent the passage of blood cells. The second layer is the basement membrane, which excludes plasma proteins such as albumin. The third layer is the visceral lining of Bowman's capsule. Small filtration slits between the podocytes allow only the smallest of particles to pass. The concentration of a solute in the glomerular filtrate is the same as the concentration in the blood. On average, about 1/5 of the blood is filtered, but this varies depending on the pressure.

Secretion and Reabsorption of Solutes

Secretion removes solutes from the blood and adds them to the filtrate, while reabsorption removes solutes from the filtrate and returns them to the blood. Solutes are moved by either primary active transport, secondary active transport, or diffusion, and water is reabsorbed by osmosis. The functions of each region of the renal tubule and collecting duct are summarized in the table below:

Region	Role in Secretion
Proximal convoluted tubule	H^+, creatinine, NH_4^+, drugs, toxins—active transport
Loop of Henle—Descending limb	Urea
Distal convoluted tubule	K^+, H^+
Collecting duct	K^+, H^+

Region	Role in Reabsorption
Proximal convoluted tubule	Main site of reabsorption in the kidney; 60–70% of the volume of filtrate is reclaimed in the PCT. Glucose, amino acids, vitamins, Na^+, Cl^-, K^+, Ca^{2+}, Mg^{2+}, bicarbonate, phosphate, water, urea
Loop of Henle—Descending limb	Water
Loop of Henle—Ascending limb	Na^+, Cl^-, K^+, Mg^{2+}, Ca^{2+}
Distal convoluted tubule	Cl^-, Ca^{2+} Na^+, Water (variable permeability—opening of Na^+ channels is dependent on aldosterone)
Collecting duct	Urea, bicarbonate Na^+, Water (variable permeability—dependent on aldosterone and ADH)

Concentration of Urine

The concentration of urine is influenced by the high solute concentration of the medulla, and the hormones that control the permeability of the distal convoluted tubule and collecting duct.

The **countercurrent mechanism** describes the use of active transport to move solutes out of the ascending loop of Henle (which is impermeable to water) into the medullary interstitium. The osmotic gradient that is created causes water diffuse out of the descending limb (which *is* permeable to water), concentrating the filtrate. The recycling of urea also helps to maintain a high medullary osmolarity. The descending loop of Henle and the collecting duct are both permeable to urea, but the descending limb and the distal tubule are not. Urea enters the descending loop from the interstitium, and travels through the renal tubule to the collecting duct, where it reenters the interstitium.

The concentration of urine is also regulated by hormones. The permeability of the distal convoluted tubule to sodium is dependent on aldosterone. Aldosterone promotes the reabsorption of Na^+, and since water follows the sodium, the urine becomes more concentrated. The permeability of the collecting duct is dependent on both aldosterone and ADH. ADH increases the duct's permeability by water by inserting aquaporins that allow the passage of water.

Counter-Current Multiplier Mechanism

A countercurrent system in the loop of Henle is responsible for the generation of an osmotic gradient in the medulla that promotes the reabsorption of water. The descending limb is permeable to water, but not solutes. The ascending limb is permeable to solutes, but not water. Na^+, Cl^-, and other ions are actively transported from the ascending limb into the medullary interstitium. The concentration gradient causes water to leave the descending limb by osmosis, which increases the concentration of the filtrate in the descending limb. As the filtrate moves up the ascending limb, ions are actively absorbed, raising the solute concentration in the medulla. This positive feedback loop is known as the countercurrent *multiplier* mechanism because it multiplies the concentration of the interstitial fluid as a result of the functional differences between the two limbs.

The countercurrent multiplier system is distinguished from the countercurrent *exchange* system, in which the hypertonicity of the medulla is *maintained* (not generated) by the countercurrent flow of blood in the vasa recta. As blood in the *descending* part of the vasa recta passes the *ascending* limb, it picks up ions that left the filtrate. As blood in the *ascending* vasa recta passes the *descending* limb, most of the ions diffuse back into the medulla.

Countercurrent Multiplier Mechanism:

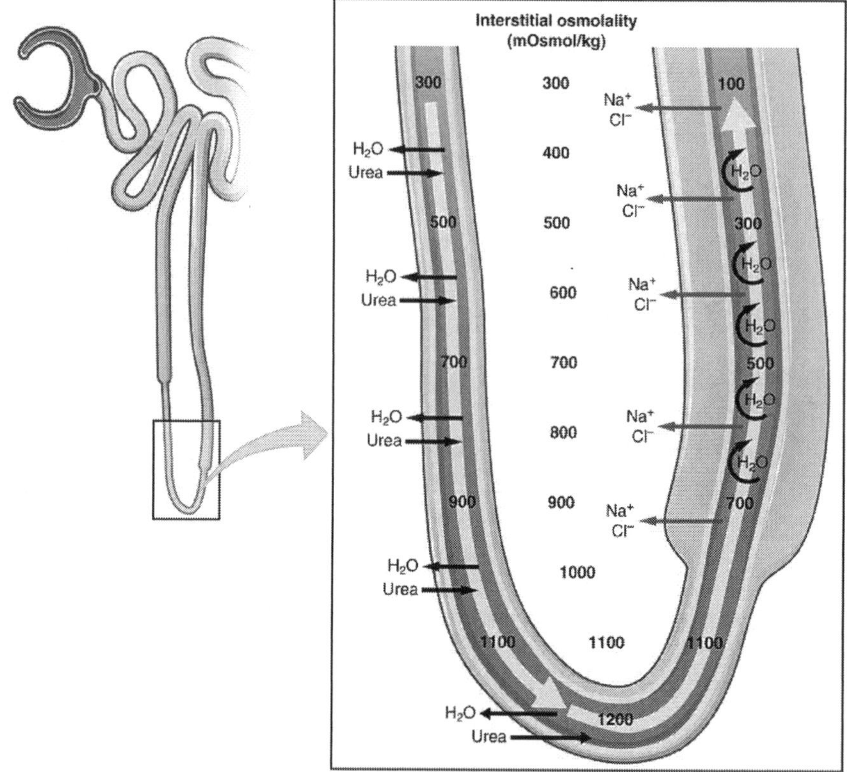

STORAGE AND ELIMINATION: URETER, BLADDER, URETHRA

A **ureter** is a tubular organ that delivers urine from the kidney to the bladder for storage. The collecting ducts (the final sites of reabsorption) empty urine into the ureter, and both gravity and peristalsis move the urine into the bladder. The bladder is a bag-like organ that can store up to 600 ml of urine (though the desire to urinate begins at around 150 ml). The ureters, bladder, and superior portion of the urethra are lined with transitional epithelial tissue that allows expansion. When the organ becomes distended, the stretched epithelium appears to have fewer cell layers.

Urine is stored in the bladder until contraction of the **detrusor muscle** (the smooth muscle within the bladder wall) forces urine into the urethra. Contraction of the bladder is controlled by the parasympathetic nervous system. Stretch receptors in the bladder send impulses to the sacral region of the spinal cord. Impulses are then sent along efferent neurons to the bladder, telling it to contract. A circular smooth muscle called the internal urethral sphincter relaxes, and (if the timing is appropriate) the voluntary external urethral sphincter relaxes as well. Urine flows from the bladder, through the urethra, and out of the body in a process called micturition.

MUSCULAR CONTROL: SPHINCTER MUSCLE

There are two sphincters of the urethra that delay the emptying of the bladder. The **internal urethral sphincter** (IUS) is found between the bladder and the urethra. It consists of smooth muscle and is continuous with the smooth muscle of the bladder (the detrusor muscle). The sympathetic nervous system keeps the IUS contracted until the micturition reflex is triggered. The IUS relaxes as a result of sympathetic inhibition, allowing urine to pass through. The second sphincter that controls the elimination of urine is the **external urethral sphincter** (EUS), which is made of skeletal muscle, and under the control of the somatic nervous system. A conscious decision can be made to relax the EUS under appropriate circumstances. Involuntary contraction of the detrusor forces urine out of the body, and the voluntary contraction of abdominal muscles can increase the rate of flow by compressing the bladder.

Reproductive System

Male and Female Reproductive Structures and Their Functions

Gonads

The gonads are the components of the reproductive system that produce gametes (sex cells) and secrete hormones. The male gonads are the **testes**. These structures are housed in the scrotum and encapsulated by a fibrous layer of connective tissue called the **tunica albuginea**. Thin layers of tissue extend from the tunica albuginea and divide the testes into 250 to 300 compartments called **lobules**. Each lobule contains -one to four **seminiferous tubules**—the sites of spermatogenesis. The epithelial lining of these tubules consists of the **spermatogenic cells** that give rise to sperm, as well the cells that nourish them (**sustentacular cells**, also called **Sertoli cells**). **Interstitial cells** (**Leydig cells**) around the seminiferous tubules produce testosterone, which stimulates the production of sperm. The seminiferous tubules join together to form a network of channels called the **rete testis** that bring maturing sperm cells to the **efferent ducts** where they exit the testes and enter the **epididymis**.

The female gonads are the **ovaries**. Ovaries are oval-shaped structures that rest in slight depressions on either side of the uterus known as the **ovarian fossae**, and they are held in position by several peritoneal ligaments. Each ovary is covered by two types of tissue: a layer of simple cuboidal epithelium known as the **germinal epithelium**, and the underlying **tunica albuginea**. The ovary is subdivided into the outer cortex and the inner medulla. The **cortex** has a granular appearance due to the presence of thousands of nourishing **follicles** in various stages of development. Each of these saclike follicles contains an oocyte. Initially, the oocyte is surrounded by a single layer of **follicular cells**, but as the follicle matures, the cells give rise to a multi-layer of estrogen-producing **granulosa cells**. After ovulation, a gland called the **corpus luteum** forms, and it secretes progesterone and small amounts of estrogen. This gland disappears unless pregnancy occurs. The interior of the ovary, or **medulla**, is made of loose areolar connective tissue, and contains many blood vessels, lymphatic vessels, and nerves that enter and leave through the **hilum**.

Genitalia

The internal male genitalia include the epididymides, vasa deferentia, and accessory glands including the seminal vesicles, prostate gland, and Cowper's glands (the bulbourethral glands). The **epididymis** is a convoluted tube attached to the outside of a testicle that nourishes sperm as they finish maturing, and stores them until ejaculation. From here the sperm pass through the **vas deferens** (sperm duct), **ejaculatory duct**, and **urethra**, and exit through the penis. The **seminal vesicles** secrete fluid into the ejaculatory duct that makes up roughly 60% of the volume of semen. The contents of this mildly alkaline fluid include fructose, prostaglandins, and proteins. Secretions of the **prostate gland** (about 30% of semen volume) nourish the sperm and increase their motility. **Cowper's glands** secrete a lubricating fluid that makes up 2–5% of semen volume.

The external male genitalia include the penis and scrotum. The **penis** is the erectile organ responsible for delivering sperm to the female. It consists of three cylinders of spongy tissue: a pair of **corpora cavernosa** and the **corpus spongiosum** that surrounds the urethra. The **scrotum** is the sac that protects the sperm-producing testes and keeps them at the proper temperature.

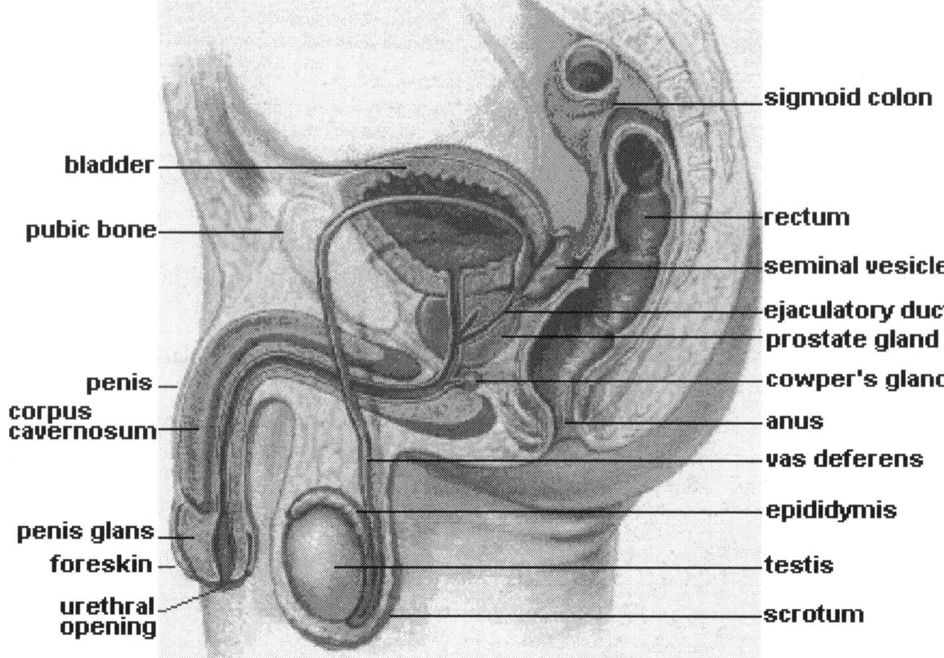

The internal female genitalia include the ovaries, the fallopian tubes, the uterus, and the vagina. The **ovaries** produce oocytes, and also secrete sex hormones. When an oocyte is released during ovulation, it is "captured" by the **fallopian tube**, also known as the uterine tube or oviduct, which is not directly connected to the ovaries. Fertilization typically occurs in the fallopian tube, and implantation of the fertilized egg usually occurs in the endometrium of the uterus. The **uterus** is a muscular, pear-shaped organ that nourishes and protects the developing embryo. The neck of the uterus that opens to the vagina is called the **cervix**. The **vagina** is a muscular canal that receives the penis during intercourse. During childbirth, the baby passes through the vagina—also called the birth canal.

The external female genitalia include the structures of the **vulva**. These include the mons pubis, the labia majora and labia minora, Bartholin's glands, and the clitoris. The **mons pubis** is a mound of fatty tissue that lies over the pubic bone. The skin folds that form the **labia** help to protect the more delicate tissues beneath. **Bartholin's glands** produce a fluid that lubricates the vagina. The **clitoris** consists of erectile tissue full of nerve endings that contribute to sexual arousal.

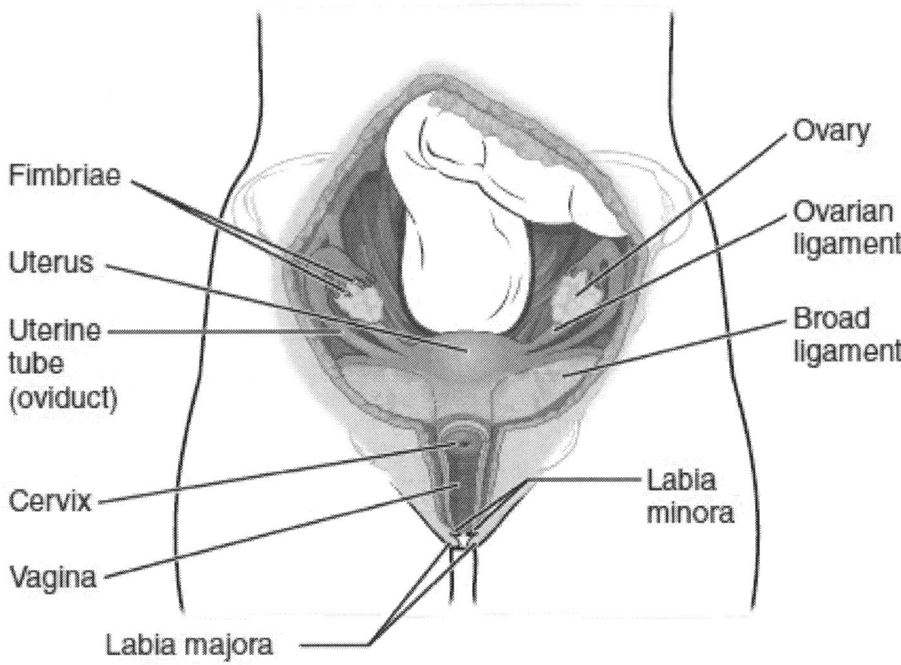

DIFFERENCES BETWEEN MALE AND FEMALE STRUCTURES

Many of the structures within the male and female reproductive are "homologous" to each other because they share a common developmental pathway. But these structures become specialized for different roles in reproduction.

The male reproductive system is designed to produce sperm and deliver it to the female for fertilization. Most of the male reproductive structures are external, which helps to keep the sperm at the optimal temperature. The testes produce much higher levels of testosterone than female gonads, and they produce millions of gametes per day after puberty. The male urethra is a common passageway for both urine and semen.

In contrast, the female reproductive system is designed to nurture a developing embryo. The reproductive structures are housed internally. The ovaries produce much higher levels of estrogen than male gonads. They contain all of the oocytes that they will ever have before birth, and only one is released per month during ovulation. The female urethra is not connected to the reproductive system.

HORMONAL CONTROL OF REPRODUCTION

Ovaries	
Hormone	**Action**
Estrogens (secreted by granulosa cells and corpus luteum)	Target the uterus, ovaries, mammary glands, brain, and other tissues—stimulate uterine lining growth, regulate menstrual cycle, facilitate the development of secondary sex characteristics
Progesterone (secreted by corpus luteum)	Targets mainly the uterus and mammary glands—stimulates uterine lining growth, regulates menstrual cycle, required for maintenance of pregnancy Inhibits GnRH
Inhibin (secreted by granulosa cells)	Targets the anterior pituitary—inhibits the release of FSH
Placenta	
Estrogen and progesterone	(See above)
Inhibin	(See above)
Human chorionic gonadotropin (hCG)	Targets the ovaries—stimulates the production of estrogen and progesterone
Anterior Pituitary	
Follicle-Stimulating Hormone (FSH)	Targets the granulosa cells of the ovarian follicles—stimulates the maturation of the follicle Targets the Sertoli cells of the testes—stimulates spermatogenesis
Luteinizing Hormone (LH)	Targets the ovary—stimulates ovulation and development of the corpus luteum Targets the Leydig cells of the testes—stimulates the production of testosterone
Hypothalamus	
GnRH—gonadotropin releasing hormone	Stimulates anterior pituitary to release LH and FSH
Testes	
Testosterone (secreted by Leydig cells)	Targets the testes and many other tissues—promotes spermatogenesis, secondary sex characteristics
Inhibin (secreted by Sertoli cells)	(See above)

MALE AND FEMALE SEXUAL DEVELOPMENT

Sex determination occurs at birth; two X chromosomes will give rise to a female, and XY gives rise to a male. The SRY gene on the Y chromosomes is responsible for the development of the male reproductive organs and the repression of female reproductive organs. In the absence of the Y chromosome, the embryo will be female. **Wolffian ducts** give rise to male internal reproductive structures, and **Mullerian ducts** give rise to female internal reproductive structures. As one system develops, the other is broken down. Seven weeks after conception, the differences in external genitalia become evident. At puberty, there is a surge in development as the hypothalamus releases gonadotropin releasing hormone (GnRH). This triggers the secretion of luteinizing hormone (LH) and follicle stimulating hormone (FSH) from the anterior pituitary gland. These gonadotropins increase the production of sex hormones, which allow the male and female reproductive organs to mature. Spermatogenesis begins in males, and ovulation and menstruation begin in females. Secondary sex characteristics emerge as well. Males develop facial, axillary, and pubic hair, and the voice deepens as the larynx grows. Females develop pubic hair and begin to ovulate and menstruate, and the hips become wider.

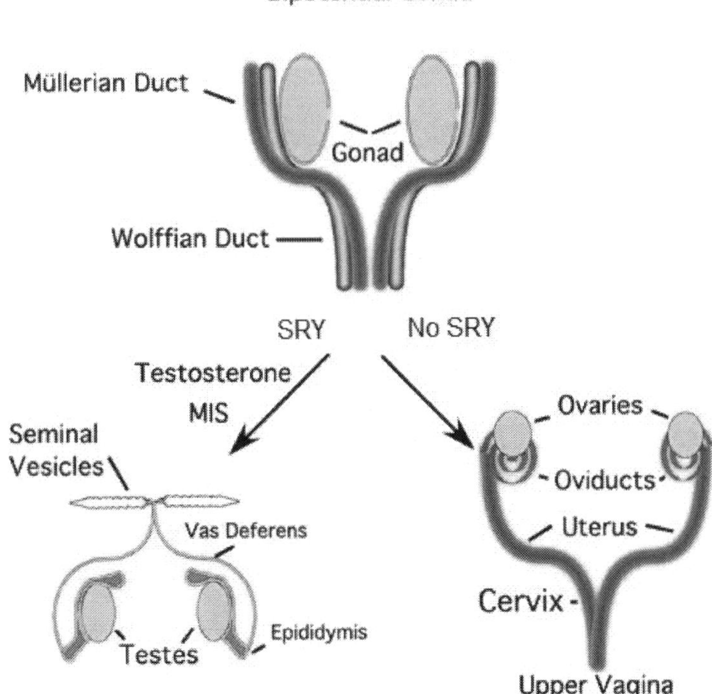

FEMALE REPRODUCTIVE CYCLE

The female reproductive cycle is characterized by changes in both the ovaries and the uterine lining (endometrium).

The ovarian cycle has three phases: the follicular phase, ovulation, and the luteal phase. During the **follicular phase**, FSH stimulates the maturation of the follicle, which then secretes estrogen. Estrogen helps to regenerate the uterine lining that was shed during menstruation. **Ovulation**, the release of a secondary oocyte from the ovary, is induced by a surge in LH. The **luteal phase** begins with the formation of the corpus luteum from the remnants of the follicle. The corpus luteum secretes progesterone and estrogen, which inhibit FSH and LH. Progesterone also maintains the thickness of the endometrium. Without the implantation of a fertilized egg, the corpus luteum begins to regress, and the levels of estrogen and progesterone drop. FSH and LH are no longer inhibited, and the cycle renews.

The uterine cycle also consists of three phases: the proliferative phase, secretory phase, and menstrual phase. The **proliferative phase** is characterized by the regeneration of the uterine lining. During the **secretory phase**, the endometrium becomes increasingly vascular, and nutrients are secreted to prepare for implantation. Without implantation, the endometrium is shed during **menstruation**.

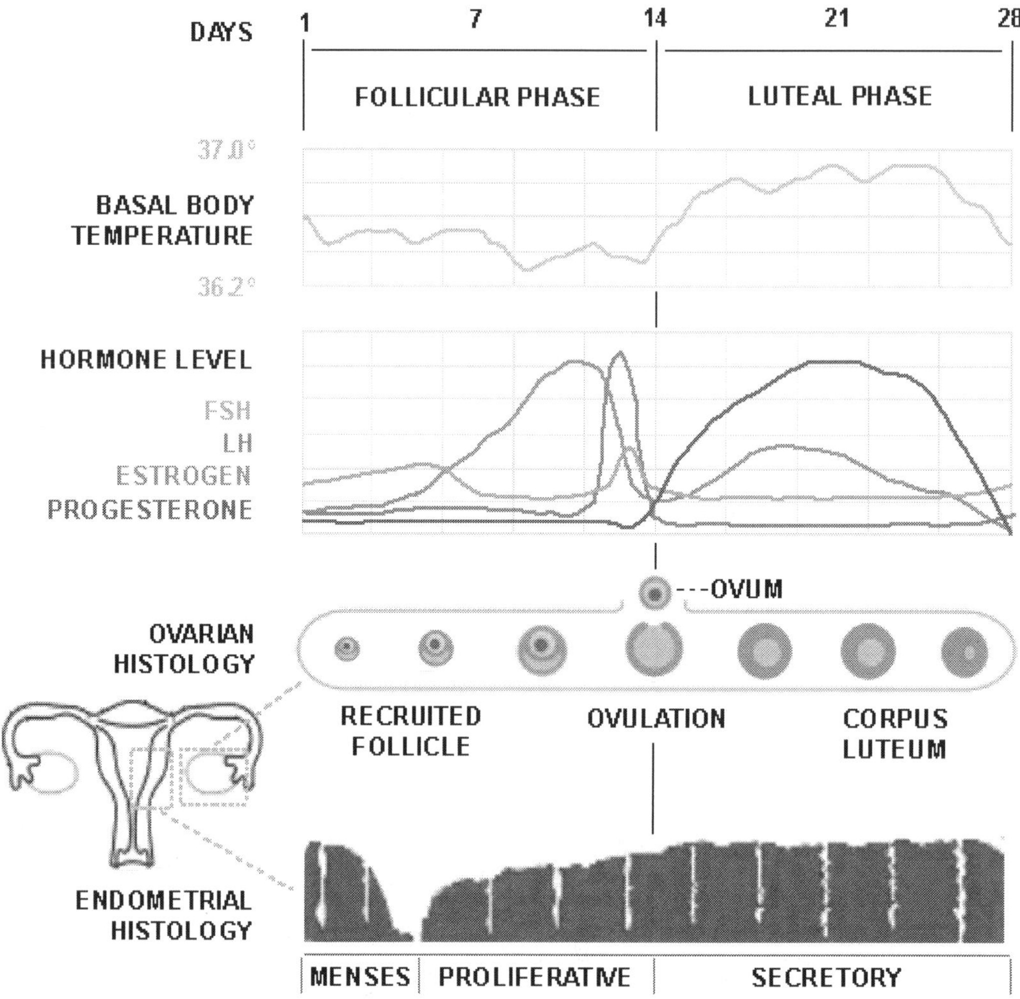

Pregnancy, Parturition, Lactation

Pregnancy: When a blastocyst implants in the uterine lining, it releases hCG. This hormone prevents the corpus luteum from degrading, and it continues to produce estrogen and progesterone. These hormones are necessary to maintain the uterine lining. By the second trimester, the placenta secretes enough of its own estrogen and progesterone to sustain pregnancy and the levels continue to increase throughout pregnancy, while hCG hormone levels decrease.

Parturition: The precise mechanism for the initiation of parturition (birth) is unclear. Birth is preceded by increased levels of fetal glucocorticoids, which act on the placenta to increase estrogen and decrease progesterone. Stretching of the cervix stimulates the release of oxytocin from the posterior pituitary gland. Oxytocin and estrogen stimulate the release of prostaglandins, and prostaglandins and oxytocin increase uterine contractions. This positive feedback mechanism results in the birth of the fetus.

Lactation: During pregnancy, levels of the hormone prolactin increase, but its effect on the mammary glands is inhibited by estrogen and progesterone. After parturition, the levels of these hormones decrease, and prolactin is able to stimulate the production of milk. Suckling stimulates the release of oxytocin, which results in the ejection of milk.

Integration with Nervous Control

Communication between the nervous system and reproductive system is required for sexual development, the female reproductive cycle, sexual behavior, and pregnancy and childbirth. The hypothalamus of the central nervous system exerts control over the endocrine system, which is responsible for producing the hormones that allow the body to coordinate such functions. The hypothalamus produces GnRH in response to various stimuli, and GnRH stimulates the anterior pituitary to release FSH and LH. These gonadotropins have a stimulatory effect on the gonads. As levels of sex hormones increase, the hypothalamus (and GnRH production) is inhibited by negative feedback. Positive feedback mechanisms also play a role in the reproductive system. The LH surge that induces ovulation occurs when high levels of estrogen actually *stimulate* the hypothalamus to secrete GnRH, which in turn causes the pituitary to secrete more LH. Another example of positive feedback occurs during childbirth. Stretching of the uterus sends nerve impulses to the hypothalamus, which signals the release of oxytocin. Oxytocin promotes uterine contractions, which increases the stretching of the uterus. These are but a few examples of how the nervous system exerts control over the reproductive system.

Muscle System

Important Functions

Support: Mobility

The muscle system is made up of skeletal, smooth, and cardiac muscles that contract to produce nearly all body movements. Skeletal muscles are used for voluntary actions. Walking, jumping, smiling, eye movements, and the maintenance of posture are all under the control of the somatic nervous system. The muscles that coordinate voluntary movements are attached to bone by tendons, and the bone is moved when the muscle shortens. Skeletal muscles also work with the tendons, ligaments, and bone to support and stabilize the joints.

Contraction of smooth muscle is involuntary, and therefore under autonomic control. Smooth muscle in the gastrointestinal tract contracts rhythmically to propel food along the gastrointestinal tract. This is called peristalsis. Blood pressure is regulated by contraction and relaxation of the smooth muscle within the vessel wall. Vasoconstriction increases blood pressure and decreases blood flow, while vasodilation decreases blood pressure and increases blood flow. Cardiac muscle of the heart contracts to pump blood throughout the body.

Peripheral Circulatory Assistance

The return of blood to the heart is assisted by a system called the **skeletal muscle pump**. Large peripheral veins in the legs and arms have valves that prevent the backflow of blood. When the skeletal muscles around these deep veins contract, the vessel is compressed, and blood is forced through the valves in the direction of the heart. Exercising these muscle groups increases the rate of blood flow.

The **thoracic pump** also facilitates venous return. During inspiration, contraction of the diaphragm and intercostal muscles expands the thoracic cavity. The increased volume results in a decrease in pressure, which is transmitted to the right atrium. This drop in pressure helps the blood to return to the heart. Also, when the pressure in the thoracic cavity decreases, the pressure in the abdominal cavity increases, squeezing the blood in the inferior vena cava toward the heart.

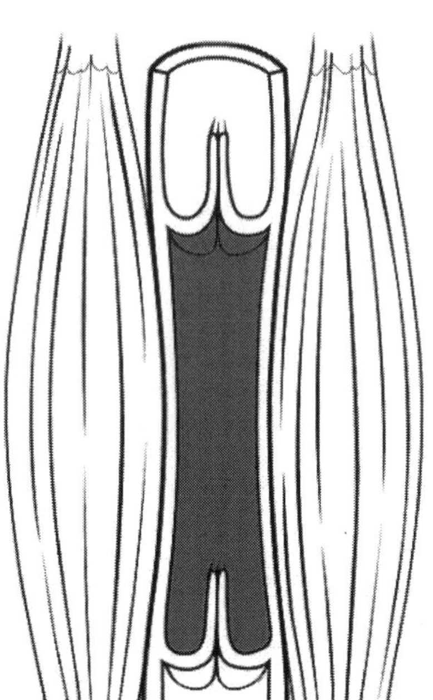

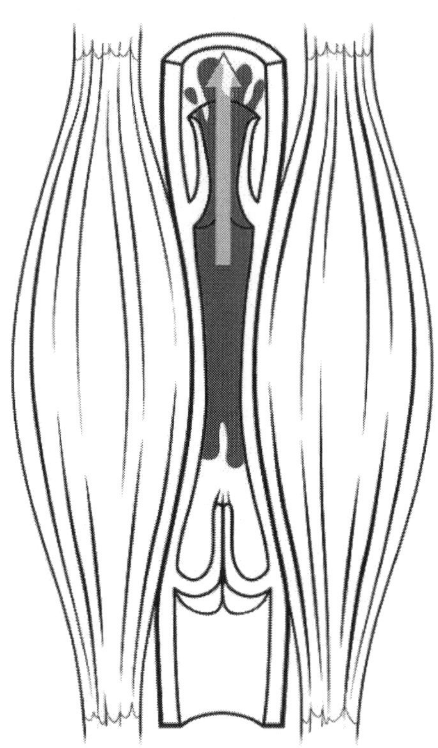

THERMOREGULATION (SHIVERING REFLEX)

When thermoreceptors detect a drop in temperature, impulses are sent to the posterior hypothalamus, which then sends signals to the effectors. Smooth muscles in the walls of the cutaneous arterioles contract involuntarily to reduce the blood flow near the surface of the skin. This minimizes heat loss to the environment. Arrector pili muscles also contract, causing hairs to stand on end in an attempt to trap warm air. If the core body temperature drops, the shivering reflex is triggered by the posterior hypothalamus. Shivering is involuntary shuddering, caused by the rapid contracting and relaxing of skeletal muscles. Contraction of these muscles requires the hydrolysis of ATP, and this exothermic reaction releases energy in the form of heat. Some heat is also generated as a result of friction between the sliding filaments of the muscle.

When thermoreceptors detect a rise in temperature, the anterior hypothalamus tells the smooth muscles that surround cutaneous arterioles to relax. Vasodilation allows more blood to flow near the surface of the skin, and heat is lost to the environment.

STRUCTURE OF THREE BASIC MUSCLE TYPES: STRIATED, SMOOTH, CARDIAC

Skeletal muscle is under somatic (voluntary) control and does not display myogenic activity. (Skeletal muscles require external stimulation to contract.) They are involved in the movement of bone, support, thermoregulation, and venous return to the heart. These muscles are **striated**; the muscle fibers have alternating regions of light and dark bands. A single skeletal myocyte is cylinder-shaped and has many nuclei.

Smooth muscle is under autonomic (involuntary) control and is capable of using myogenic mechanisms to contract (independent of nervous stimulation). Smooth muscle tissue is found in the walls of hollow organs and vessels, and aids in the movement of substances such as food and blood. The cells are spindle-shaped, non-striated, and uninucleated.

Like smooth muscle, cardiac muscle is under autonomic control and exhibits myogenic activity. Cardiac muscle tissue is found in the walls of the heart, and is required for the pumping of blood. The cells are branched, striated, and usually uninucleate (but may have two nuclei). They are connected to each other by intercalated discs with gap junctions that allow the cells to communicate.

Muscle Structure and Control of Contraction

T-Tubule System

Transverse tubules, or **T-tubules**, are tunnel-like invaginations of the **sarcolemma**—the plasma membrane of striated muscle cells. The membranes of this system contain a high concentration of ion channels, allowing them to play an important role in muscle contraction. When an action potential propagates along the sarcolemma, the T-tubules help to depolarize the cell by carrying the impulse to the **sarcoplasmic reticulum** (SR) that surrounds the **myofibrils** in a muscle cell. The SR is a form of smooth endoplasmic reticulum that is specialized to store and release calcium ions. The t-tubules are sandwiched between two enlarged chambers of the SR called **terminal cisternae**. This "sandwich" makes up a structure called the **triad**. When the impulse reaches the SR, the calcium channels in the SR membrane open, releasing calcium ions that ultimately cause contraction of the muscle. ATP-powered calcium pumps within the SR membrane pump Ca^{2+} back into the SR to relax the muscle.

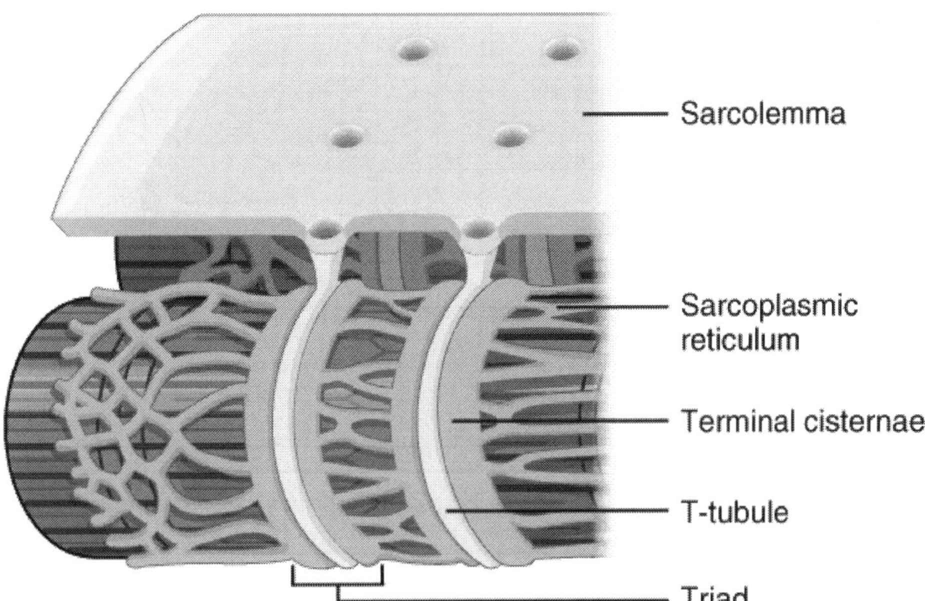

Contractile Apparatus

The **contractile apparatus** describes a unit within muscle tissue that is specialized for contraction. The structure of the contractile apparatus is similar among striated muscle tissues, and consists of a repeating unit called a **sarcomere**. Tens of thousands of these sarcomeres lie end to end to form a **myofibril**. One sarcomere is separated from another by a boundary called the **Z line**, where a network of proteins serves as a point of anchorage for **actin** (thin filaments). Six thin filaments surround a single thick myosin filament. The filaments themselves do not change length during contraction; their arrangement allows them to slide over each other when myosin heads pull on the thin filaments, causing the sarcomeres to shorten, and the muscle to contract. Note that while smooth muscle cells do contain actin and myosin, the filaments are disorganized, and no sarcomeres are present.

Contractile Velocity of Different Muscle Types

There are three main types of skeletal muscle fibers: slow-twitch oxidative (SO—type I), fast-twitch oxidative-glycolytic (FOG—type IIa), and fast-twitch glycolytic (FG—type IIb). Most muscles consist of an even blend of these fibers, but the proportions vary in certain muscles, depending on function. For example, muscles associated with maintaining posture will have a high percentage of slow-twitch fibers, while muscles in the lower legs of a sprinter will have a high percentage of fast-twitch fibers.

The characteristics of each type of fiber are summarized in the following table:

	Slow Twitch, Type I	**Fast Twitch, Type IIa**	**Fast Twitch, Type IIb**
Fiber Diameter	Smaller	Intermediate	Larger
Capillary density	High	Moderate	Low
Myoglobin Concentration / Color	High / Red	Moderate / Red-Pink	Low / White
Metabolism	High aerobic capacity, low anaerobic capacity	Both aerobic and anaerobic capabilities	Low aerobic capacity, high anaerobic capacity
Concentration of Mitochondria	High	Moderate	Low
Resistance to Fatigue	High	Moderate	Low
Contractile Velocity	Slow	Rapid	Rapid
Force Production	Low	Moderate	High
General Use	Prolonged, low-intensity aerobic activities / maintenance of posture	Moderate intensity activities, such as running	Short bursts of activity, such as sprinting or heavy lifting

Regulation of Cardiac Muscle Contraction

Cardiac muscle demonstrates myogenic activity. The pacemaker cells of the sinoatrial (SA) node of the heart generate their own action potential, which then travels to the atrioventricular (AV) node (the secondary pacemaker), the bundle of His, the bundle branches, and finally the Purkinje fibers. Gap junctions between adjacent cardiac cells facilitate the transmission of the action potential from one cell to the next. As the impulse travels through the sarcolemma of a cardiac muscle cell, voltage-gated calcium ion channels open, allowing the entry of extracellular Ca^{2+}. The inflow of Ca^{2+} triggers the release of even more Ca^{2+} from the sarcoplasmic reticulum. Calcium ions cause the cardiac muscle to contract in a similar manner to skeletal muscle cells (the sliding filament mechanism). Note that skeletal muscle cells do not generate their own action potential, and the action potential is more prolonged in cardiac cells.

While the heart is autorhythmic, the muscle contraction is further regulated by the autonomic nervous system. Sympathetic stimulation increases heart rate, while parasympathetic stimulation (the vagus nerve) decreases heart rate. The endocrine system influences heart rate as well. Epinephrine secreted from the adrenal medulla and thyroxine from the thyroid gland both increase heart rate.

Oxygen Debt: Fatigue

Oxygen debt is the amount of oxygen required to restore metabolic conditions to resting levels. Muscle activity is powered by the hydrolysis of ATP. In a resting state, aerobic respiration provides enough ATP for muscles to function. Stored ATP is quickly used up during intense exercise, and a molecule called **creatine phosphate** phosphorylates ADP to produce ATP. Anaerobic respiration also supplies ATP relatively quickly, but only for a short amount of time. If oxygen is available, aerobic respiration synthesizes ATP. When oxygen levels become depleted, **lactic acid** (a byproduct of anaerobic respiration) begins to accumulate. The buildup of lactic acid, along with the depletion of ATP and oxygen, causes muscle fatigue. Lactic acid that does not remain in the muscles is brought to the liver, where it is converted into glucose. The amount of oxygen required to accomplish this task, and to replenish the levels of ATP and creatine phosphate, is called oxygen debt.

Nervous Control

Motor Neurons, Neuromuscular Junction, Motor End Plates

The stimulus for skeletal muscle cell contraction comes from motor neurons, and the synapse between the neuron and muscle cell is called the **neuromuscular junction**. A single motor neuron can form synapses with multiple muscle cells. The neuron and the muscle cells that it innervates are collectively called a **motor unit**. This arrangement allows a large group of cells to contract together. All the motor neurons that innervate the same muscle make up a **motor pool**.

When an action potential reaches an axon terminal, voltage-gated calcium ions in the membrane are opened, and Ca^{2+} enters. These ions bind to synaptic vesicles that store acetylcholine (ACh), causing them to fuse with the membrane and release ACh into the synaptic cleft. ACh binds to nicotinic receptors on a folded portion of the sarcolemma known as the motor end plate. The permeability of the muscle cell changes, and the cell depolarizes. The action potential is taken into the muscle cell via T-tubules, causing calcium channels in the sarcoplasmic reticulum to open. The release of calcium into the sarcoplasm causes the muscle to contract.

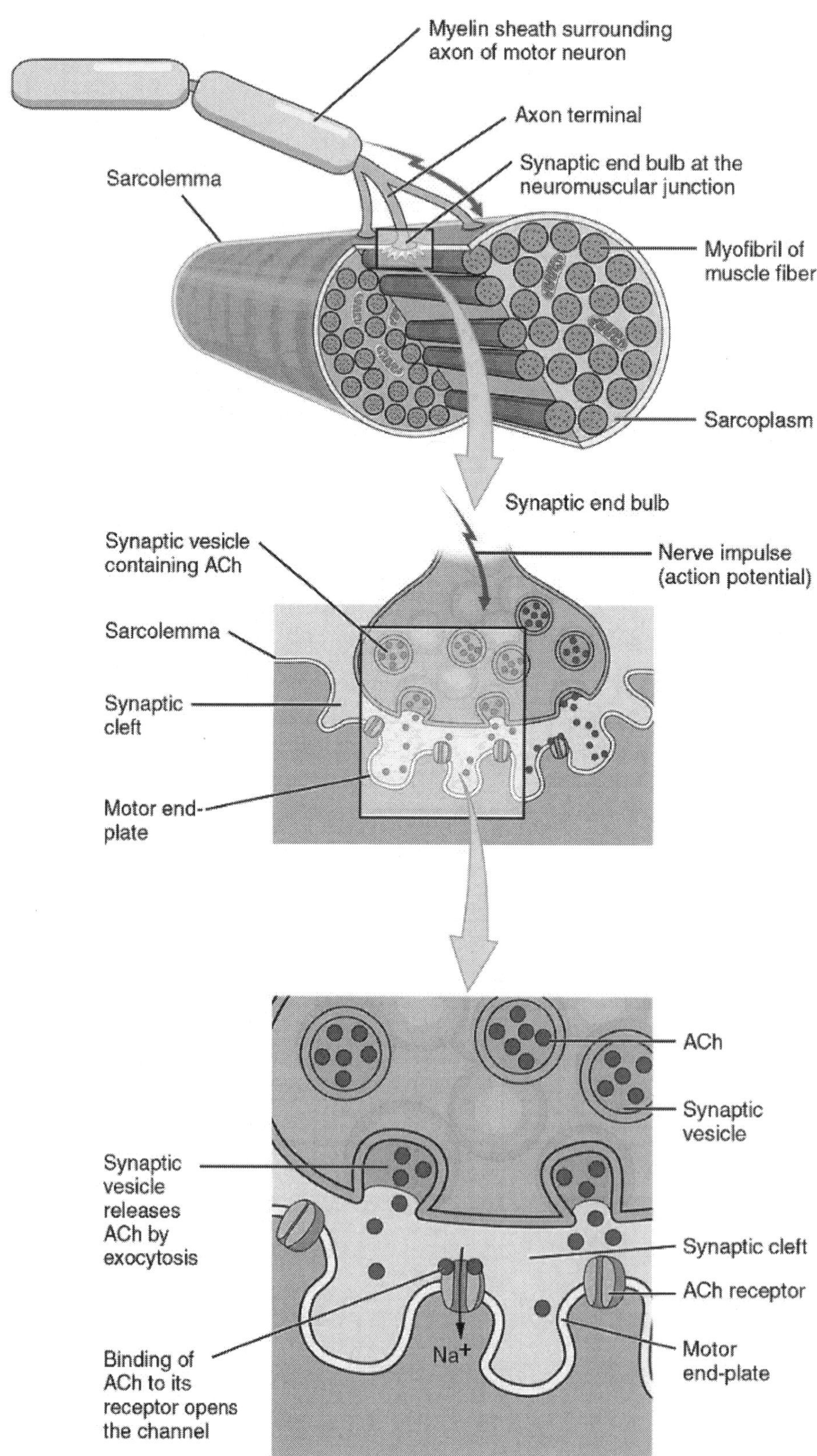

SYMPATHETIC AND PARASYMPATHETIC INNERVATION

Involuntary muscle tissues (smooth, cardiac) are innervated by motor neurons of the sympathetic and parasympathetic divisions of the autonomic nervous system. Motor pathways of the ANS consist of *two* neurons: a preganglionic and a postganglionic neuron. The cell body of a preganglionic neuron resides in the central nervous system and synapses with the cell body of one or more postganglionic neurons within an autonomic ganglion. Postganglionic nerve fibers are shorter than presynaptic fibers, and they extend to the effectors. *Pre*ganglionic neurons of both the sympathetic and parasympathetic systems release acetylcholine (ACh). *Post*ganglionic neurons of the parasympathetic division release ACh, but those of the sympathetic division release norepinephrine (NE).

In general, the sympathetic and parasympathetic systems tend to have antagonistic effects on the muscles (and glands) they innervate. The sympathetic division induces a fight or flight response, which causes the heart rate and blood pressure to increase, and blood to be diverted away from the digestive system. The parasympathetic division induces a rest and digest response, which causes the heart rate and blood pressure to decrease, and promotes digestion.

VOLUNTARY AND INVOLUNTARY MUSCLES

The peripheral nervous system is divided into the somatic and autonomic nervous systems. Voluntary muscles are composed of skeletal muscle tissue and are under the control of the somatic nervous system. Most voluntary muscles are connected to bone. These muscles usually contract in response to a conscious thought process, but they are also involved in certain involuntary reflexes, such as the knee jerk reflex. The motor cortex of the brain is responsible for generating most of the nerve impulses that initiate voluntary movements.

Involuntary muscles are innervated by motor neurons of the autonomic nervous system. These muscles include the smooth muscles found in the walls of hollow organs such as the intestines and blood vessels, as well as the cardiac muscle of the heart. The lower part of the brainstem called the medulla oblongata sends signals to involuntary muscles that play a role in digestion, vasodilation/vasoconstriction, heart rate, respiratory rate, and other visceral functions.

SPECIALIZED CELL - MUSCLE CELL

ABUNDANT MITOCHONDRIA IN RED MUSCLE CELLS: ATP SOURCE

Red muscle fibers are specialized for endurance activities of low intensity such as walking, light lifting, or the maintenance of posture. They are relatively slow to contract, but are resistant to fatigue and have abundant mitochondria. Mitochondria are the sites of oxidative phosphorylation. When levels of blood oxygen are insufficient, a protein called myoglobin supplies oxygen that is used in the synthesis of ATP. (Myoglobin is similar to hemoglobin, but it found in muscle tissue, has a higher affinity for oxygen, and can only carry one oxygen molecule per molecule of myoglobin.) The red coloration of these slow-twitch fibers comes from the extensive capillary network that surrounds them and the high myoglobin content. In contrast, white muscle fibers are specialized for high intensity activities, contain low amounts of mitochondria and myoglobin, and fatigue quickly.

ORGANIZATION OF CONTRACTILE ELEMENTS: ACTIN AND MYOSIN FILAMENTS, CROSS BRIDGES, SLIDING FILAMENT MODEL

The interior of a skeletal muscle cell consists of elongated structures called **myofibrils** that run in parallel columns along the length of the cell. Myofibrils are polymers of repeating contractile units called **sarcomeres**. Within each myofibril are two types of filaments: **thin filaments** and **thick filaments**. Thin filaments are made mostly of **actin** molecules arranged in a helical configuration. Other proteins called **troponin** and **tropomyosin** can be found along the length of the filament, and they help to regulate the access of myosin to actin. **Myosin** proteins make up the thick filaments. These golf-club shaped molecules twist together, with the heads protruding out of the filament. The myosin heads form **cross bridges** when they bind to active sites on the actin filaments. The myosin changes shape, pulling the actin filament toward the middle of the sarcomere in a process called the **power stroke**. This causes the sarcomere to shorten via the **sliding filament mechanism**. ATP is required to revert the myosin heads to their original position. Cardiac muscle cells have a similar arrangement of actin and myosin, but the filaments of smooth muscle cells are less organized.

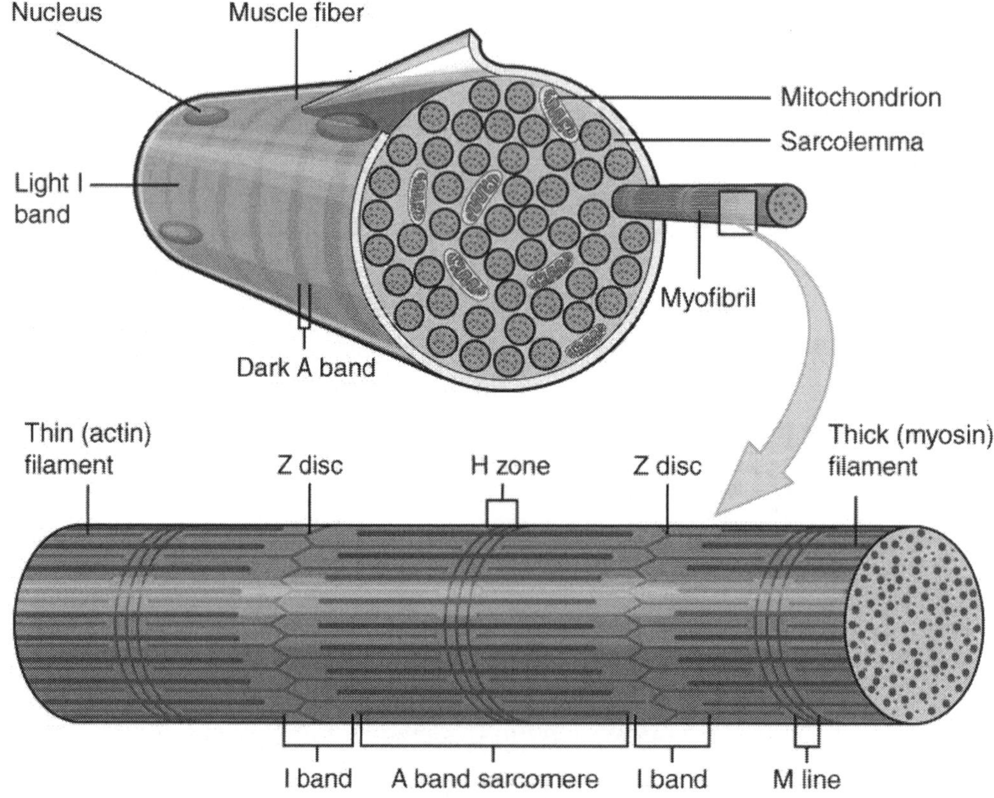

Sarcomeres: "I" and "A" Bands, "M" and "Z" Lines, "H" Zone

A sarcomere is the smallest contractile unit of striated muscle that is capable of contracting. A myofibril consists of tens of thousands of sarcomeres lined up end-to-end, each one divided into various bands, lines, and zones that account for the striated appearance. The **Z-line** is made of a protein network that anchors the thin actin filaments and forms the boundary of each sarcomere. It can be seen within a light region known as the isotropic band (**I-band**) which consists only of actin filaments. An anisotropic band (**A-band**) consists of the entire length of the thick myosin filaments, including areas of overlap with the thin filaments. In the center of the A-band is the **H-zone**, made only of myosin filaments. Within the H-zone (and at the center of the sarcomere) is the **M-line**, where proteins of the cytoskeleton attach to myosin filaments. When a sarcomere is fully contracted, the ends of the actin filaments overlap, the I-bands narrow, and the H bands disappear. The lengths of the A-bands remain the same.

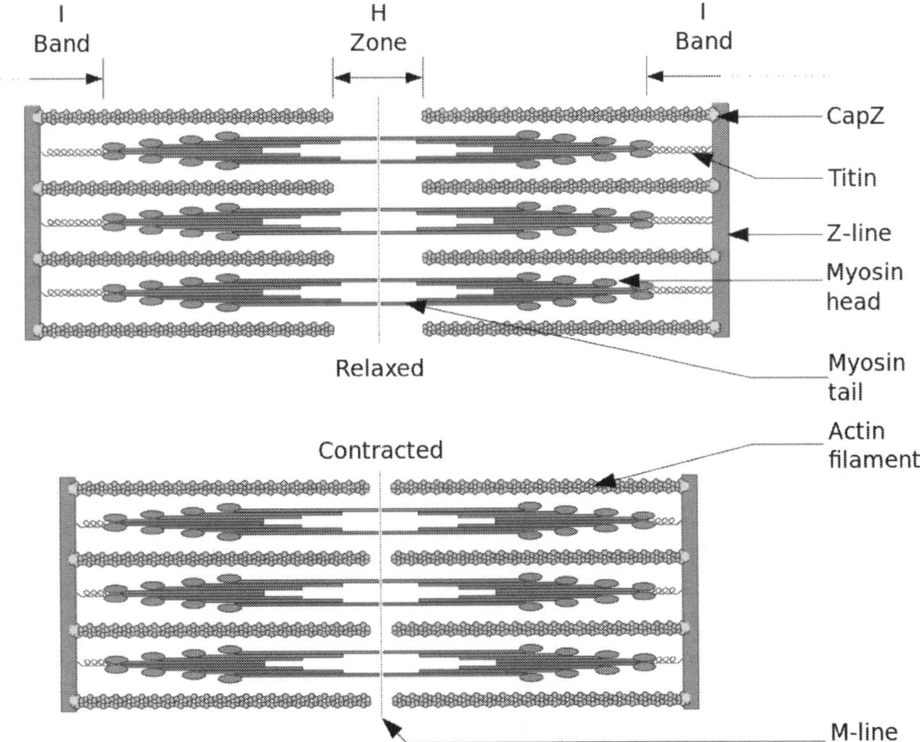

Presence of Troponin and Tropomyosin

Troponin and tropomyosin are regulatory proteins that initiate the contraction of striated muscles when calcium levels are high, and inhibit contraction when calcium levels drop. **Troponin** is a globular protein complex that consists of three subunits: troponin I, T, and C. **Troponin I** binds to actin filaments and inhibits the binding of myosin. **Troponin T** is bound to the protein **tropomyosin**—a fibrous, rope-like protein that winds around actin and blocks the sites where myosin heads attach to the actin filaments. **Troponin C** has a high affinity for the calcium ions that regulate muscle contraction. When calcium binds to troponin C, a series of conformational changes occur that ultimately causes tropomyosin to slip out of place, allowing myosin to form cross bridges with actin and contract the sarcomere.

Note that smooth muscles lack troponin C. Instead, calcium binds to **calmodulin**, which leads to the phosphorylation of myosin and contraction of the muscle.

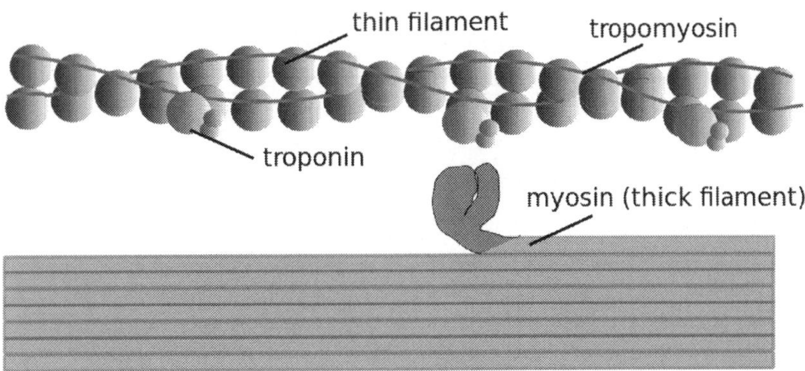

Calcium Regulation of Contraction

Muscle contraction is directly tied to the concentration of calcium ions in the sarcomere. When an action potential travels from a motor neuron to a muscle cell, the sarcolemma depolarizes, and the action potential is brought into the cell by the T-tubules. Ca^{2+} is released from the sarcoplasmic reticulum (SR) at all points that come in contact with the T-tubules. Calcium ions flow into the cytoplasm of the cell (the sarcoplasm) and bind to troponin, which causes tropomyosin to reveal the myosin-binding sites on actin. When myosin binds to actin, cross bridges are formed between the myosin heads and the actin filaments. The myosin heads change shape, causing the thin actin filaments to slide past the thick myosin filaments, and the muscle fiber contracts. When the action potential is terminated, ATP-powered calcium pumps in the membrane of the sarcoplasmic reticulum pump calcium back into the SR. As the concentration of calcium ions in the sarcoplasm decreases, the sarcomeres relax.

Skeletal System

Functions

Structural Rigidity and Support

The skeletal system provides a framework for the body that consists of bones, ligaments, tendons, cartilage, and other tissues. This system is essential in the support and physical protection of the body. Bones support the weight of the body, give shape to body parts, and help to keep internal organs in place. Bones also serve as attachment points for muscles, allowing for body movement. Skeletal muscles connect to bones via tendons, and bones attach to each other via ligaments. Cartilage is more flexible, and supports body parts such as the ear, the nose, the trachea, and various joints. The skeletal system also protects vital organs. The skull encloses the brain, the vertebrae surround the spinal cord, the thoracic cage protects the heart and lungs, and the pelvic girdle protects the inferior portion of the digestive system, the bladder, and the internal reproductive organs. Delicate bone marrow is also protected within the hollow spaces of certain bones.

Review Video: Skeletal System
Visit mometrix.com/academy and enter code: 256447

Calcium Storage

Bone is a reservoir for calcium. The bone cells produce a hard acellular **matrix** composed of about 35% collagen and 65% inorganic material. Most of the inorganic matter is a type of **calcium phosphate** known as **hydroxyapatite**. Calcium is required for a number of processes, including the contraction of muscles, the conduction of a nerve impulse, and the clotting of blood. The body takes in calcium in the diet, and about 99% of absorbed calcium is stored in bones and teeth. When calcium levels are high, bone-forming cells called **osteoblasts** remove calcium from the blood and deposit it into the bone along with other components of the matrix. Eventually, these cells become surrounded by the hard, calcium-rich secretion and differentiate into mature bone cells called **osteocytes**. If blood calcium is low, cells called **osteoclasts** can break down bone and put calcium back into the blood. In a healthy individual, there is a balance between the amount of calcium deposited and the amount removed. Homeostatic imbalances result in hypercalcemia or hypocalcemia.

Skeletal Structure

Specialization of Bone Types, Structures

Bones can be classified as long, short, flat, irregular, and sesamoid. **Long bones** function primarily in movement and supporting body weight. They are rod shaped, and are longer than they are wide. The extremities of a long bone (**epiphyses**) are covered in articular cartilage, and they are wider than the shaft (**diaphysis**). Most of the bones of the upper and lower limbs are long bones, as are the collar bones. **Short bones** are roundish or cube-shaped. They have little to no role in movement, and instead function in support and stability. Examples of short bones include the carpals and tarsals of the wrist and ankle, respectively. **Flat bones** are flattened, thin bones that are usually curved. Their broad shape is suited for protection, as well as muscle attachment. The scapulae, sternum, ribs, ilia of the pelvic girdle, and certain cranial bones are all flat bones. **Irregular bones** have complex shapes that do not fit the classifications above, and their form is suited to their function. Examples of irregular bones include the vertebrae and many facial bones. **Sesamoid bones**, such as the kneecap, are found embedded in tendons where there is considerable mechanical stress.

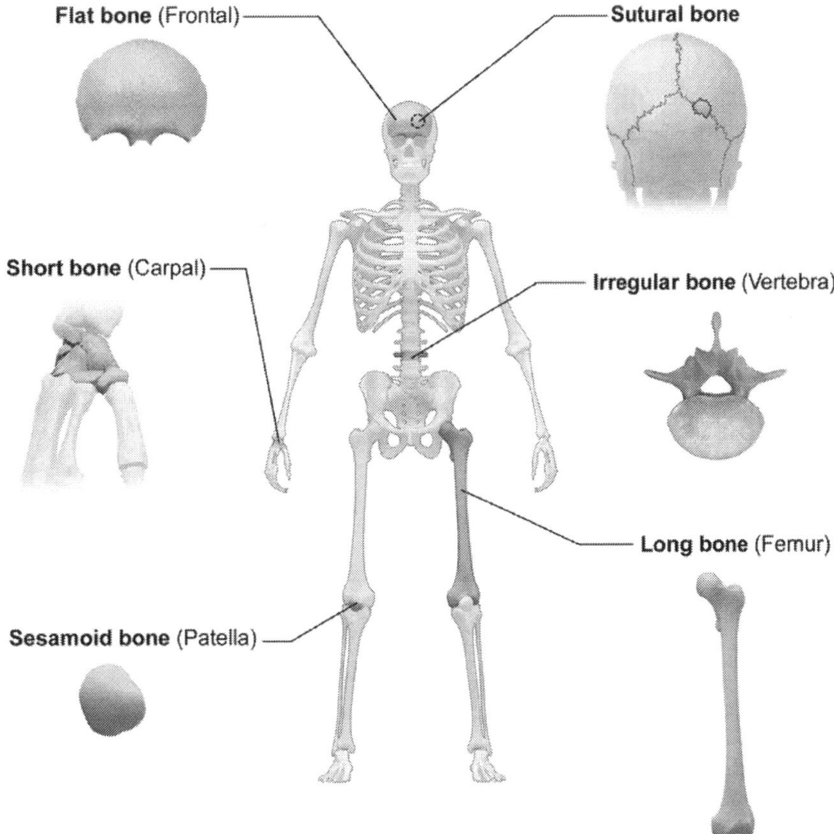

Classification of Bones by Shape

Joint Structures

Joints are the locations where two or more elements of the skeleton connect. They can be classified according to range of motion, as well as the material that holds the joint together.

Functional classification		
Type of Joint	**Description / Range of Motion**	**Examples**
Synarthrosis	Immovable—either fibrous or cartilaginous	Skull sutures, teeth/mandible
Amphiarthrosis	Slight range of motion—either fibrous or cartilaginous	Intervertebral discs, distal tibiofibular joint
Diarthrosis	Moves freely—always synovial	Wrist, knee, shoulder

Structural classification		
Type of Joint	**Description / Material**	**Types / Examples**
Fibrous	Held together by fibrous connective tissue	Suture: immovable, ex: skull Gomphosis: immovable, ex: teeth/mandible Syndesmosis: slightly movable, ex: distal tibiofibular joint
Cartilaginous	Held together by cartilage	Synchondrosis: hyaline cartilage, nearly immovable, ex: first rib/sternum Symphysis: fibrocartilage, slightly movable, ex: intervertebral discs, pubic symphysis
Synovial	The most common type of joint; characterized by a joint cavity filled with synovial fluid	Pivot: allows rotation, ex: atlantoaxial joint Hinge: allows movement in one plane, ex: knee Saddle: allows pivoting in two planes and axial rotation, ex: first metacarpal/trapezium Gliding: allows sliding, ex: carpals Condyloid: allows pivoting in two planes but no axial rotation, ex: radiocarpal joint Ball and socket: have the highest range of motion, ex: hip

Endoskeleton Vs. Exoskeleton

An **endoskeleton** is an internal framework that supports an organism. It is derived mainly from the mesoderm, and produces bone and cartilage. Bones are made mostly of calcium and phosphorus, but they are still living tissues with various types of cells and a blood supply. An endoskeleton grows as the body grows, and is able to support a large body size.

An **exoskeleton** is a nonliving outer covering that encloses an organism. It is derived from the ectoderm, and can produce a chitinous cuticle (as seen in insects and arthropods) or calcified shells (as seen in oysters or snails), though shells are not considered "true" exoskeletons. A chitinous exoskeleton does not grow with the body, and must be shed so that a larger one can be made. These hardened coverings protect the softer living tissues that they enclose.

Bone Structure

Compact (or cortical) bone is the hard, dense tissue that forms the outer surfaces of bones, as well as the shafts of long bones. It consists of cylindrical structures called **osteons**, also called Haversian systems. Each osteon consists of a central **Haversian canal** that contains nerve fibers and blood vessels, and these canals connect to each other via **perforating canals** (or **Volkmann's canals**). The Haversian canal is surrounded by concentric layers of calcified **lamellae** with small spaces called **lacunae**, each of which contains an **osteocyte**. Tiny channels called **canaliculi** connect the lacunae to allow oxygen and nutrients to reach the osteocytes, and wastes to be removed.

Spongy (or cancellous) bone is the porous tissue found at the ends of long bones and inside the vertebrae and flat bones. It is not as strong or abundant as compact bone, and does not contain osteons. Instead, it consists of flattened, interconnected plates called **trabeculae**. Within the spaces of the trabeculae is the **red bone marrow** that produces blood cells. There are no central canals, but osteocytes do reside in lacunae that are connected by canaliculi.

Compact Bone & Spongy (Cancellous Bone)

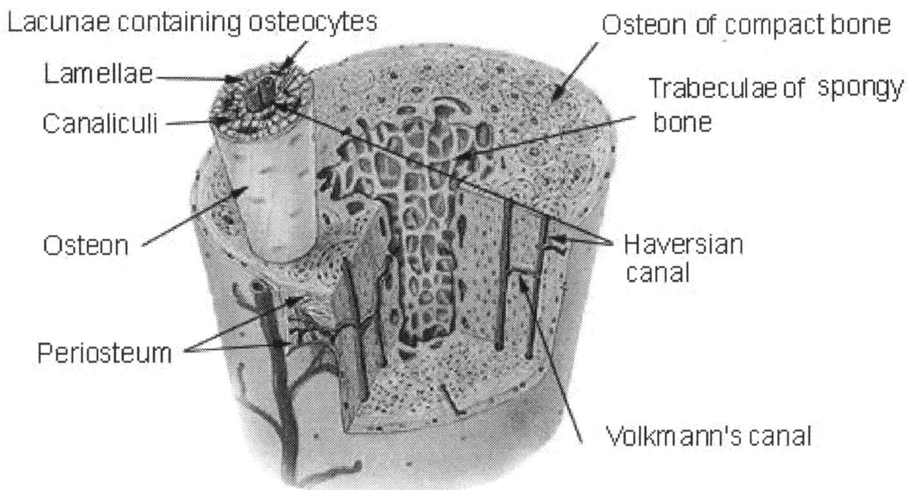

Cellular Composition of Bone

Bone consists of an extracellular matrix that surrounds bone cells and functions much like reinforced concrete. The matrix consists of about 2/3 inorganic matter; mostly calcium phosphate (hydroxyapatite) with calcium carbonate and other minerals. The organic portion makes up about 1/3 of the matrix. It consists mainly of collagen, which adds strength and flexibility to the matrix, as well as ground substance proteins such as glycosaminoglycans (GAGs).

There are three types of bone cells. **Osteoblasts** (derived from osteoprogenitor cells) take calcium from the blood, and produce the matrix (including collagen fibers) that forms bone. When it is completely encased in matrix, the osteoblast differentiates into a mature bone cell called an **osteocyte**. Osteocytes are the most abundant bone cells, and they maintain the matrix by recycling calcium salts. **Osteoclasts** are large multinucleate cells that are formed by the fusion of monocytes (large white blood cells). They reside on bone surfaces and secrete acid and digestive enzymes that break down bone and return calcium to the blood.

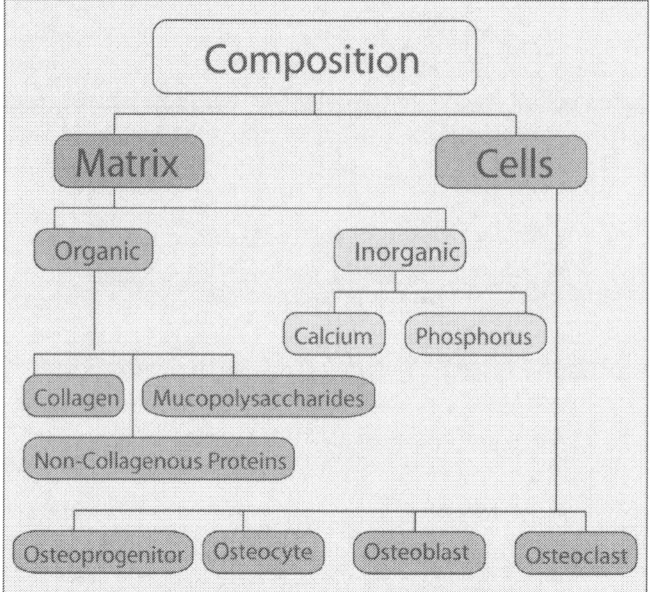

CARTILAGE: STRUCTURE AND FUNCTION

Cartilage is a connective tissue with a matrix that is flexible yet resistant to stretching. Cartilage is not innervated, nor does it have a blood supply, except for the **perichondrium** that forms the surfaces of nearly all cartilage. The immature cartilage cells that secrete the matrix are called **chondroblasts**. Chondroblasts give rise to mature cells called **chondrocytes** that reside in lacunae.

There are three types of cartilage: hyaline, elastic, and fibrocartilage. **Hyaline cartilage** is the most common cartilage in the body. It consists of evenly distributed collagen fibrils that explain its glassy appearance. It is found in locations that require strong support with some pliability, such as the ribs, nose, trachea, and articular surfaces. **Elastic cartilage** is similar to hyaline cartilage but is more flexible due to the presence of elastic fibers. It is found in the epiglottis and external ear.

Fibrocartilage has collagen arranged into thick fibers, which allows it to withstand tension and compression. It is found in the jaw, in the knee, and between the vertebrae.

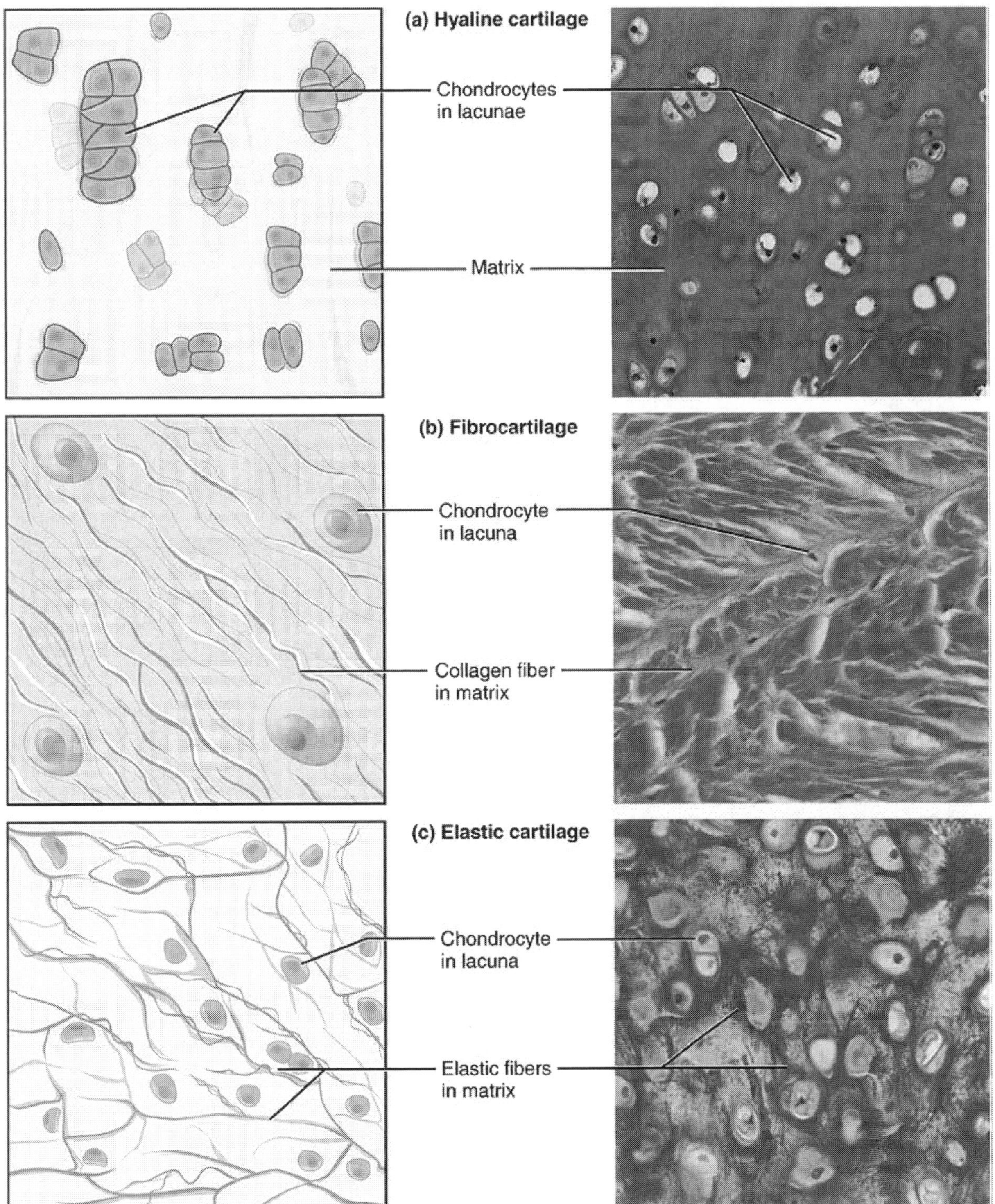

LIGAMENTS, TENDONS

Ligaments connect bones to bones, and help to stabilize joints. **Tendons** connect muscles to bones or other structures such as the eyeballs, and facilitate movement. They are both composed of **dense**

regular connective tissue, which consists of bundles of collagen fibers as well as elastic fibers. This gives them strength and resistance to stretching. The collagen fibers of tendons are more densely packed than those of ligaments. They are also arranged in parallel bundles, while the fibers of many ligaments are not. Tendons are tougher, but ligaments are more elastic. The yellowish color of certain ligaments results from the protein elastin.

Endocrine Control

The calcium-regulating hormones of the endocrine system are responsible for breaking down and reabsorbing bone tissue. The kidneys produce 1,25-hydroxyvitamin D, a biologically active form of vitamin D also known as **calcitriol**. This hormone regulates levels of calcium by promoting the absorption of dietary calcium in the intestines, which increases the level of calcium in the blood. Calcitriol also stimulates osteoclasts to break down bone, which moves calcium into the blood. When blood calcium is high, the peptide hormone **calcitonin** is secreted by the parafollicular cells of the thyroid gland. Calcitonin inhibits the activity of osteoclasts, and stimulates the activity of bone-forming osteoblasts. When blood calcium is low, parathyroid glands secrete a peptide hormone known as **parathyroid hormone (PTH)**. This increases the quantity and also the activity of osteoclasts.

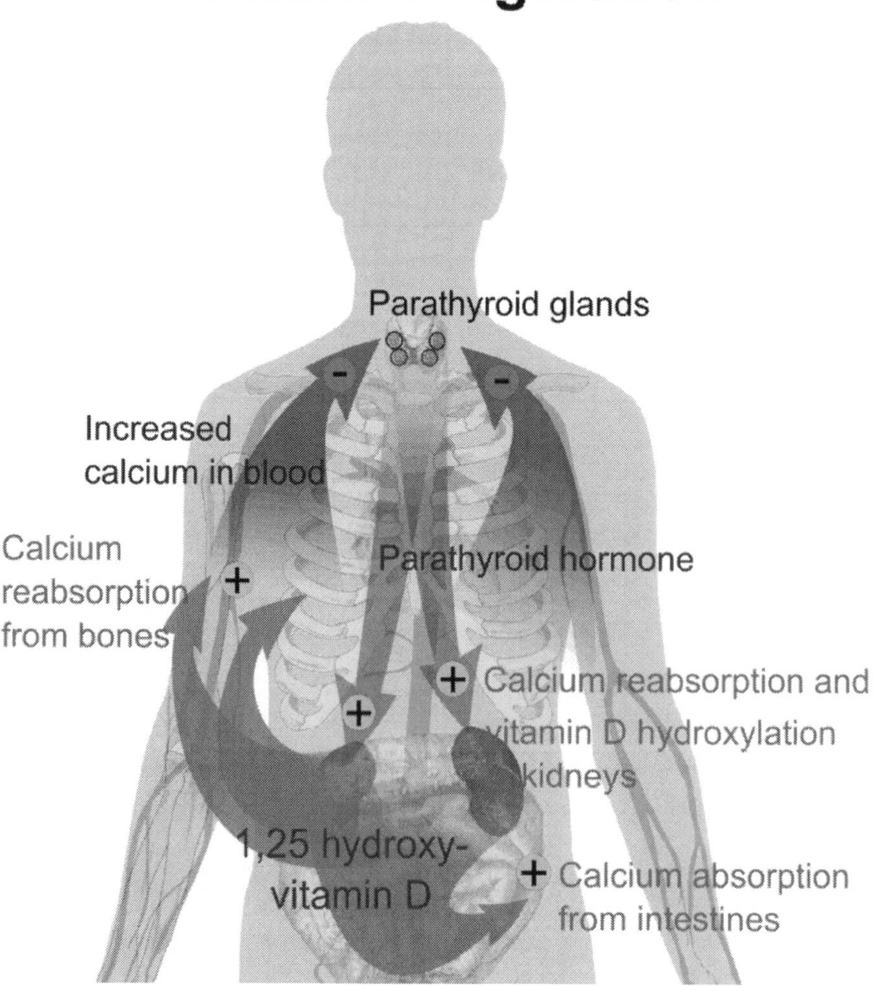

Skin System

Structure

Layer Differentiation, Cell Types and Relative Impermeability to Water*

The types of cells found in the epidermis and dermis:

Cell Type	Location	Description
Keratinocytes	Epidermis	The most common type of cell in the epidermis Arise from stem cells in the stratum basale They flatten and die as they move toward the surface of the skin Produce keratin—a fibrous protein that hardens the cell and helps make the skin water resistant
Melanocytes	Epidermis	Produces melanin—a pigment that gives skin its color and protects against UV radiation
Langerhans cells	Epidermis	Antigen-presenting cells of the immune system (phagocytes) More common in the stratum spinosum than in any other layer of the epidermis
Merkel cells	Epidermis	Cutaneous receptors, detect light touch Located in the stratum basale
Fibroblasts	Dermis	Secrete collagen, elastin, glycosaminoglycans, and other components of the extracellular matrix
Adipocytes	Dermis	Fat cells
Macrophages	Dermis	Phagocytic cells that engulf potential pathogens
Mast cells	Dermis	Antigen-presenting cells that play a role in the inflammatory response (release histamine)

The **epidermis** is the outermost layer of skin. The keratinocytes of the stratum basale are the stem cells of the epidermis. The give rise to cells that differentiate as they move toward the surface.

The **stratum basale** is the deepest layer of the epidermis. It usually contains just a single layer of cuboidal or columnar cells that adhere to the basement membrane. These are the most nourished cells because they are closest to the capillaries of the dermis. The **stratum spinosum** consists of eight to ten layers of spiny cells that are connected by structures called **desmosomes**. There is limited mitotic activity in the deeper portion of this layer. The **stratum granulosum** consists of two to five layers of slightly flattened cells containing granules of keratohyalin. The cells in the superficial portion of this layer lose their nuclei. The **stratum lucidum** consists of two to five layers of dead, flattened keratinocytes, and is only present in the palms and the soles of feet. These cells contain **eleiden**—a translucent, water-resistant protein derived from keratohyalin. The **stratum**

corneum is the most superficial layer, and it consists of 15 to 30 layers of dead, keratin-containing squamous cells. This layer helps to prevent water loss from the body.

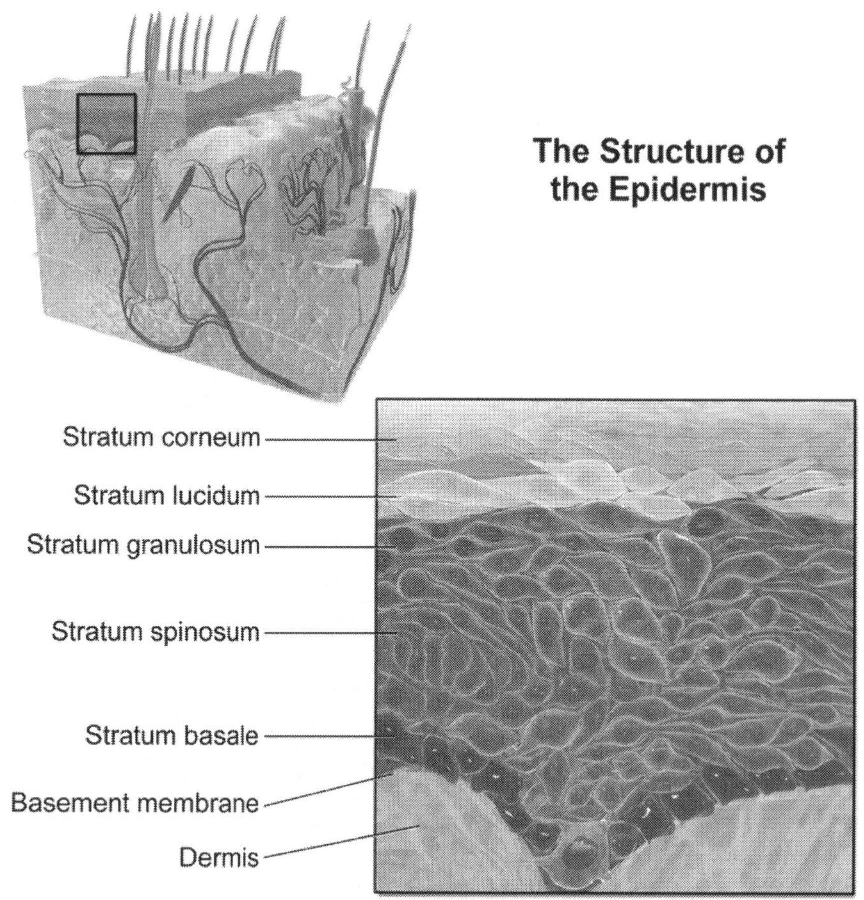

Functions in Homeostasis and Osmoregulation

The skin functions in homeostasis in a variety of ways. Different types of *sensory receptors* in the skin can detect touch, pressure, temperature, and pain. This system allows the body to sense changes in the environment and to respond appropriately. As a *physical barrier*, the skin can prevent infectious microbes or harmful substances from entering the body. (Pathogens that do manage to enter are subject to a second line of defense: macrophages and other cells of the immune system.) The skin also helps to shield the body from ultraviolet radiation. When the body is exposed to the sun, melanocytes respond by increasing the production of melanin. The integumentary system has many mechanisms for *thermoregulation*, including vasoconstriction and vasodilation of superficial capillaries, and sweating and evaporation. While the skin is not the primary organ involved in *osmoregulation*, it does play an important role. The skin helps prevent water loss from the underlying tissues, as well as the excessive uptake of water from outside the body. It also excretes salts and metabolic wastes such as urea and ammonia through sweat. The ducts of eccrine sweat glands reabsorb many of the sodium ions before they are lost during perspiration.

FUNCTIONS IN THERMOREGULATION

HAIR, ERECTILE MUSCULATURE AND FAT LAYER FOR INSULATION

When the body is cold, it responds by contracting a small smooth muscle in the dermis called the **arrector pili**. This muscle pulls on the hair follicle, causing the hair to stand erect. When many hairs stand up simultaneously, it helps to trap a warm layer of air which has an insulating effect. However, this effect may be minimal in humans.

A better insulator comes in the form of adipose tissue. Beneath the dermis is a layer of subcutaneous tissue known as the **hypodermis** (which is considered separate from the skin). It helps to anchor the skin to the underlying organs, and consists mainly of loose connective tissue, specifically adipose tissue. This layer of fat cells provides insulation from heat and cold.

SWEAT GLANDS, LOCATION IN DERMIS

There are two types of sweat glands (also called sudoriferous glands) in the body: eccrine glands and apocrine glands. The secretory portion of these glands lies in the dermis. Apocrine sweat glands tend to lie deeper in the dermis than eccrine sweat glands because eccrine sweat glands secrete sweat directly onto the skin, while the ducts of apocrine glands empty into hair follicles. Apocrine sweat glands are found only in certain regions of the body, and their function is not clear; they play no role in thermoregulation. They only activate at the onset of puberty in response to sex hormones. Eccrine glands, however, are found nearly everywhere, and the secretion and evaporation of sweat helps to cool the body. The release of sweat is regulated by the hypothalamus. When body temperature rises above normal, the hypothalamus sends signals telling the eccrine sweat glands to secrete until enough heat has been removed. Hormones play a role in the degree to which the body sweats, which may explain why men sweat more than women.

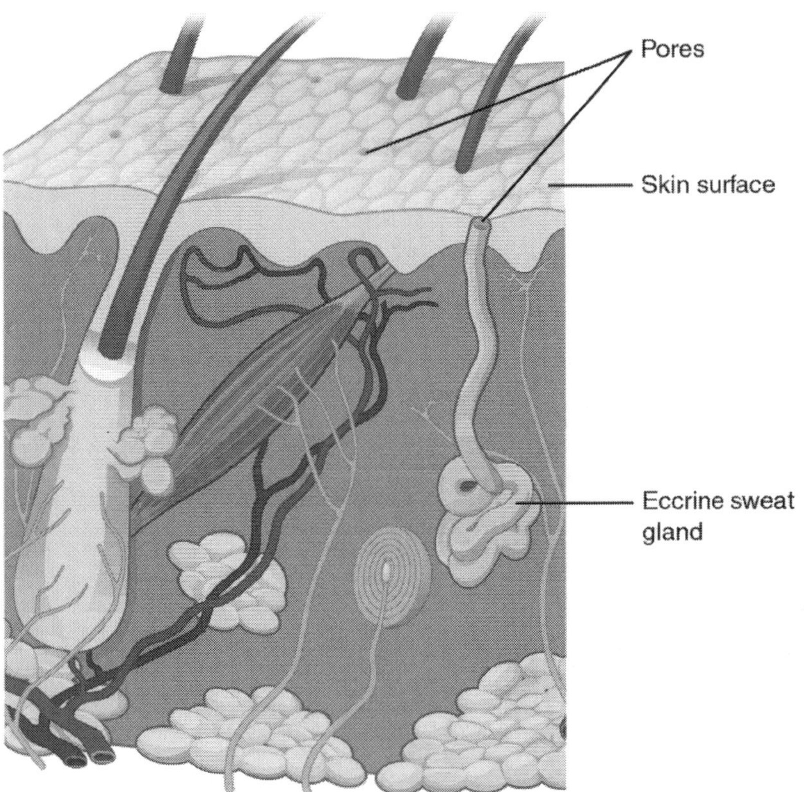

Vasoconstriction and Vasodilation in Surface Capillaries

When body temperature rises, arterioles in the dermis can promote heat loss by dilating in response to signals from the hypothalamus. This allows more blood to enter capillary beds near the surface of the skin, and heat is lost to the surroundings, primarily through radiation. Conduction and convection can also cool the body, assuming the surrounding temperature is cooler than the body. If the body temperature is too low, the adrenal medulla secretes the hormones epinephrine and norepinephrine, which act on the arterioles, causing them to constrict. This reduces the volume of warm blood that flows near the body's surface, minimizing heat loss at the skin surface.

Physical Protection

Nails, Calluses, Hair

Nails are dense plates of hardened keratinocytes that protect the distal ends of fingers and toes. Each nail is composed of modified epidermal tissue that grows from the nail matrix. The nail itself does not have sensory receptors, but pressure can still be detected. Nails also aid in the grasping and manipulation of objects, while protecting delicate tissues beneath.

When a region of the skin experiences repeated mechanical abrasion, the stratum basale responds by increasing the rate of mitosis, which soon leads to an overdevelopment of the stratum corneum (hyperkeratosis). The buildup of dead cells forms a protective pad called a callus.

Hair provides a variety of protective functions as well. It shields the scalp from ultraviolet light, and offers some cushioning in case of injury. It also helps to insulate the skull. Hairs of the nostrils, ears, eyebrows, and eyelashes help to trap foreign particles. Hairs can also act as sensory receptors, allowing a quick response to possible injury.

Protection Against Abrasion, Disease Organisms

The skin is continually subject to minor abrasions, but it is protected by the keratin-filled cells of the epidermis. The outer cells of the stratum corneum lose their connection to neighboring cells and slough off when exposed to mechanical stress. Keratinocytes, along with glycolipids produced by the stratum granulosum, form a seal that keeps harmful chemicals and pathogenic organisms from entering the body. The secretions of sweat and sebaceous glands mix together on the surface of the skin to form the **acid mantle**. The low pH of these secretions, along with antimicrobial agents and enzymes, helps to prevent infection. There are also beneficial microorganisms that populate the surface of the skin that outcompete harmful microbes. Within the layers of skin are dendritic cells and other white blood cells that are ready to engulf disease-causing organisms.

Chemical and Physical Foundations of Biological Systems

Translational Motion, Forces, Work, Energy, and Equilibrium in Living Systems

Translational Motion

Units and Dimensions

The standard unit of length is the meter, abbreviated m. The meter is currently defined as the distance that light travels in a vacuum in $\frac{1}{299{,}792{,}458}$ seconds.

The standard unit of mass is the kilogram, abbreviated kg. The kilogram is currently defined as being equal to the mass of a particular reference weight kept in the International Bureau of Weights and Measures in Sèvres, France. (It is the only standard metric unit defined in terms of a specific object rather than fundamental physical constants.)

The standard unit of time is the second, abbreviated s. The second is currently defined as being equal to 9,192,631,770 times the time associated with the transition between two specific states of the cesium 133 atom.

Derived units based on these units include the units of velocity, m/s; the units of acceleration, m/s^2; the units of force, N or kg m/s^2; the units of energy, J or kg m^2/s^2; the units of pressure, Pa or kg/m^2, and the units of frequency, Hz or s^{-1}.

Vectors, Components

If a vector has a magnitude of v and its angle from the x-axis is θ, then the x component of the vector is $v \cos \theta$, and the y component of the vector is $v \sin \theta$.

These aren't formulas that need to be memorized—although it doesn't hurt to memorize them to speed up your work. They can be derived straightforwardly through trigonometry. The vector v, its x component v_x, and its y component v_y can be arranged to form a right triangle, with θ as one of its angles:

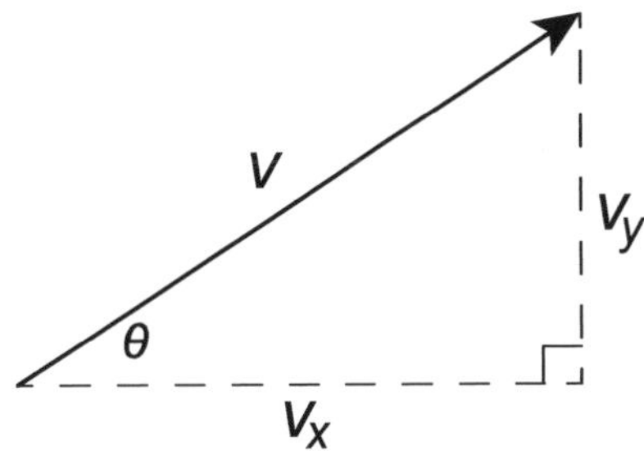

Because the cosine of an angle in a right triangle is equal to the length of the adjacent side over the length of the hypotenuse, that means $\cos \theta = \frac{v_x}{v}$; solving for v_x gives $v_x = v \cos \theta$. A similar argument for the sine yields $v_y = v \sin \theta$.

If a vector has an x component of v_x and a y component of v_y, then the magnitude of the vector is $\sqrt{v_x^2 + v_y^2}$, and the angle from the x axis satisfies the formula $\tan\theta = \frac{v_y}{v_x}$.

Note that it is not necessarily the case that $\theta = \tan^{-1}\frac{v_y}{v_x}$: the arctangent is always by definition in the first or fourth quadrant, so this equation holds if the angle is in one of those quadrants, but if the angle is in the second or third quadrant, then it is 180° off. This can be accounted for by considering the sign of the x component: if $v_x > 0$ then $\theta = \tan^{-1}\frac{v_y}{v_x}$, whereas if $v_x < 0$, then $\theta = \tan^{-1}\frac{v_y}{v_x} + 180°$. And if $v_x = 0$, then $\theta = 90°$ if $v_y > 0$ or $270°$ if $v_y < 0$.

Vector Addition

It is possible to add two vectors graphically by drawing them to scale and joining them from head to tail. A vector drawn from the tail of the first vector to the head of the second vector will then represent the sum of the two vectors.

However, adding two vectors graphically can lead to considerable imprecision. A more precise way of adding vectors is to add the components. Suppose the first vector has a magnitude of v_1 and an angle from the x-axis of θ_1, and the second vector has a magnitude of v_2 and an angle from the x-axis of θ_2. The x and y components of the first vector are $v_1\cos\theta_1$ and $v_1\sin\theta_1$, respectively, and the components of the second vector are $v_2\cos\theta_2$ and $v_2\sin\theta_2$. To find the components of the sum, just add together the individual components: $v_x = v_{1x} + v_{2x} = v_1\cos\theta_1 + v_2\cos\theta_2$ and $v_y = v_{1y} + v_{2y} = v_1\sin\theta_1 + v_2\sin\theta_2$. Finally, if you need the magnitude and angle of the total angle, you can find those from the components: $\sqrt{v_x^2 + v_y^2}$ and $\tan\theta = \frac{v_y}{v_x}$.

Speed, Velocity (Average and Instantaneous)

Velocity is the rate of change of position over time. The average velocity is, as the name implies, the average velocity over an interval of time; it can be found by finding the change in position over that interval and dividing by the change in time. In other words, if the position at time t_1 is x_1 and the position at time t_2 is x_2, then the average velocity over the interval (t_1, t_2) is equal to $\frac{x_2 - x_1}{t_2 - t_1}$.

The instantaneous velocity is equal to the rate of change of the position at a particular point in time. It can be found from the slope of a graph of position versus time. This follows from the definition of velocity: the slope of a graph is the rate of change of the dependent variable relative to the independent variable, and velocity is the rate of change of position over time. If the portion of the graph at that time is linear, then the instantaneous velocity is simply the slope of that linear segment of the graph. If the graph is not linear, then the instantaneous velocity is equal to the slope of the tangent line at that point.

Acceleration is the rate of change of velocity over time. The average acceleration is, as the name implies, the average acceleration over an interval of time; it can be found by finding the change in velocity over that interval and dividing by the change in time. In other words, if the velocity at time t_1 is v_1 and the velocity at time t_2 is v_2, then the average acceleration in the interval (t_1, t_2) is equal to $\frac{v_2 - v_1}{t_2 - t_1}$.

The instantaneous acceleration is equal to the rate of change of the velocity at a particular point in time. It can be found from the slope of a graph of velocity versus time. This follows from the definition of acceleration: the slope of a graph is the rate of change of the dependent variable relative to the independent variable, and acceleration is the rate of change of velocity over time. If the portion of the graph at that time is linear, then the instantaneous acceleration is simply the slope of that linear segment of the graph. If the graph is not linear, then the instantaneous acceleration is equal to the slope of the tangent line at that point.

The change in velocity is the area under the graph of acceleration versus time. More specifically, it is the area between the graph and the *x*-axis, where areas under the *x*-axis are counted as negative. The following diagram shows an example:

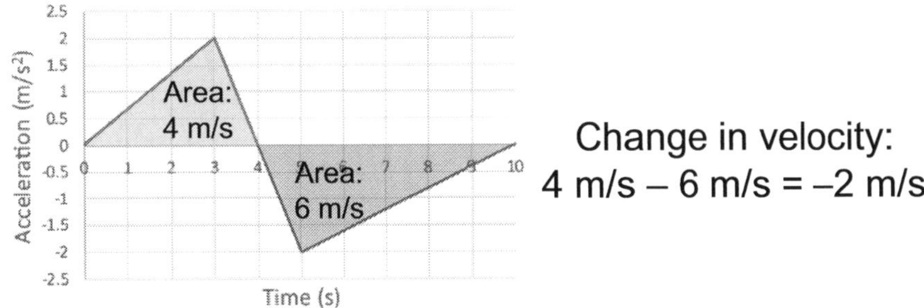

It is important to note that this area gives the change in velocity over a particular interval, which is not the same thing as the absolute velocity. To find the velocity at the end of this interval, you would have to add this change in velocity to the initial velocity at the beginning of the interval.

The change in position is the area under the graph of velocity versus time. More specifically, it is the area between the graph and the *x*-axis, where areas under the *x*-axis are counted as negative. The following diagram shows an example:

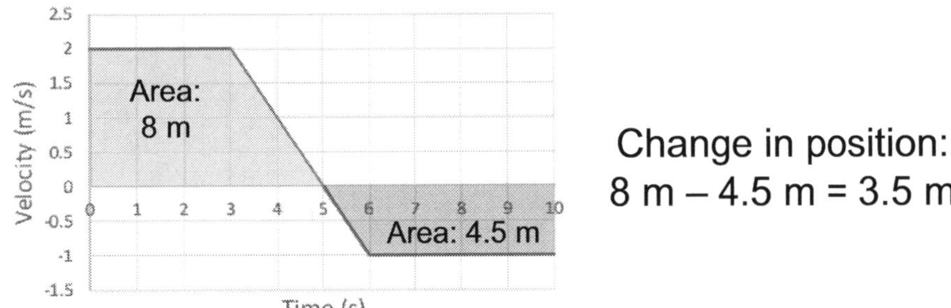

It is important to note that this area gives the change in position over a particular interval, which is not the same thing as the absolute position. To find the position at the end of this interval, you would have to add this change in position to the initial position at the beginning of the interval.

FORCE

NEWTON'S FIRST LAW

Newton's First Law, also called the Law of Inertia, is often stated as follows: An object at rest tends to remain at rest, and an object in motion tends to remain in motion, unless acted on by an outside force. Although Newton's First Law is purely qualitative, it has important consequences; the idea that only external forces can change the motion of an object contradicts previous ideas such as Aristotle's theory that a force was necessary to keep an object in motion and that objects without force acting on them would gradually slow and stop.

Technically, Newton's First Law (like Newton's other laws) only applies in an inertial reference frame—a reference frame that is itself either stationary or moving at a constant velocity (relative to other inertial reference frames). For example, a ball on the floor of a car may seem to move on its own when the car turns, but that's because while it is turning, the car is not an inertial reference frame—relative to the street below the car, the ball is still moving at constant speed (ignoring friction and until the ball hits the side of the car).

Newton's Second Law

Newton's Second Law states that the net force on an object is equal to the product of the object's mass and its acceleration. It is often written in the simple equation form $\vec{F} = m\vec{a}$. Newton's First Law follows directly from Newton's Second Law; in fact, Newton's Second Law can be thought of as a quantification of the first.

Newton's Second Law is very useful in physics because it can be used to predict the acceleration of an object if the net force on the object is known or vice versa. If the force and acceleration are known, it can be used to predict the mass—this is, in fact, how a typical spring scale works; what it is actually measuring is the gravitational force on an object, and the mass it displays is this force divided by the known acceleration of gravity. A special case that frequently occurs is when the object is not moving or when the object is moving at a constant velocity. In this case, the acceleration of the object is zero, so Newton's Second Law shows that the net force on the object must also be zero.

Newton's Third Law

Newton's Third Law is often stated as follows: For every action, there is an equal and opposite reaction. This wording, however, is somewhat misleading because it implies that one force applies first and the other is a later reaction in response to it. In fact, the two forces apply simultaneously, and which one is the "action" and which is the "reaction" is entirely semantic. A more accurate phrasing of the law, then, is that forces always occur in equal and opposite action/reaction pairs. Action/reaction pairs of forces reverse the object acting and the object being acted on: If object A exerts a force on object B, then the reaction force is exerted by object B on object A.

For example, the gravitational force the Earth exerts on you is paired with the gravitational force you exert on the Earth. When a man pushes a car, the car pushes back on the man with an equal force. When a block slides along a table, the block and the table exert equal frictional forces on each other but in opposite directions.

Friction, Static and Kinetic

Whenever two objects are in contact and there exists a normal force between them, then there is a frictional force between those objects. If the two objects are in motion relative to each other—such as a block sliding across a table or a child going down a slide—then this is *kinetic* friction. If the two objects are *not* in relative motion—such as a book resting on a shelf, or a car parked on a slope—then it is *static* friction.

One significant difference between static and kinetic friction is that the coefficient of static friction between two objects is always greater than the coefficient of kinetic friction. It takes more force to overcome friction and start moving an object than it does to keep it moving despite friction once it is already in motion.

The coefficient of friction is a value that characterizes the frictional force between two objects depending on their materials and textures. It is not equal to the force of friction between the objects because the force of friction depends not only on the materials of the objects but also on the normal force between them. However, there is a simple relationship between the coefficient of friction μ and the force of friction f: $f = \mu n$, where n is the normal force. More specifically, this relationship always holds for kinetic friction, $f_k = \mu_k n$; for *static* friction this formula gives the maximum force before friction is overcome and the objects start moving: $f_s \leq \mu_s n$. As long as the net force excluding friction is less than this threshold, the static friction is just enough to balance this force and make the total net force equal to zero. However, as soon as the net force excluding friction on an object exceeds $\mu_s n$, friction is no longer sufficient to prevent it from moving.

Review Video: Friction
Visit mometrix.com/academy and enter code: 716782

Center of Mass

One way to find the object's center of mass experimentally is to suspend it from a point (e.g., by tying a string to the object at that point). The center of mass will always be directly below the point from which it is suspended. This locates a line along which the center of mass lies; to find the exact location of the center, repeat the process by suspending the object from a different point, determining another such line. The center of mass is located at the intersection of these two lines.

Finding the center of mass mathematically involves dividing the object into pieces that are considered separately. Define a system of axes, multiply the mass of each part by its position along the x-axis, add those products together, and divide by the total mass. Formulaically, $x_{CM} = \frac{\sum m_i x_i}{\sum m_i}$. Repeat for the other axes. If the object consists of a collection of point masses, this formula is exact; otherwise, finding the center of mass exactly requires calculus.

Units of Force

The units of force are newtons, abbreviated N. The unit takes its name after the English mathematician and physicist Sir Isaac Newton, who is credited with discovering the laws of motion that relate force to mass and acceleration.

One newton is equal to 1-kilogram times meter per second squared (kg m/s^2). This relationship can be derived by considering Newton's second law: because force equals mass times acceleration, the units of force must be equal to the units of mass (kg) times the units of acceleration (m/s^2).

Equilibrium

Free Body

A free body diagram is a diagram showing all the forces acting on an object with their magnitudes and directions. The forces are drawn as arrows radiating from a point that represents the object. The lengths of the arrows are in proportion to the magnitudes of the forces they represent, and their directions match the directions of these forces. The following is an example representing perhaps the forces on an object being pulled by a rope up an incline, and therefore subject to the force of gravity, the normal force from the incline, the tension in the rope, and kinetic friction:

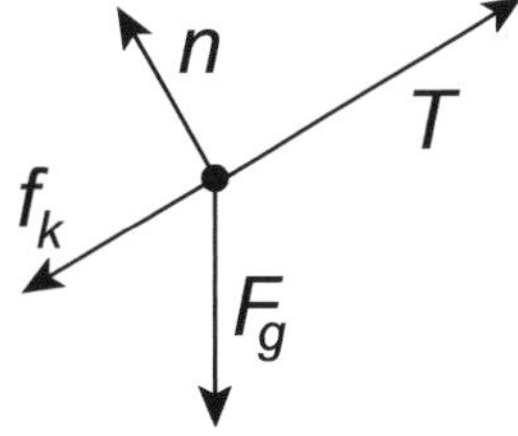

Free body diagrams are useful because they make it easy to visualize the forces acting on the object and to write a formula for the net force based on the individual components. For instance, for the free body diagram drawn here, the net force parallel to the incline would be equal to $T - f_k - F_g \sin\theta$ (where θ is the angle of the incline), and the net force perpendicular to the incline would be $n - F_g \cos\theta$—which, because the object is not accelerating along this direction, should be equal to zero.

Static Equilibrium vs. Dynamic Equilibrium

An object is in equilibrium if the net force (or torque) on the object is zero. This means that the acceleration (or angular acceleration) of the object must also be zero, and therefore the object is not moving (or rotating). This is certainly true if the object is stationary, but it is also true if the object is moving at constant velocity (or angular velocity). In the former case—if the object is not moving (or rotating) and if its velocity (or angular velocity) is zero—the object is said to be in *static equilibrium*. If the object is moving (or rotating), but its velocity (or angular velocity) is constant, then the object is said to be in *dynamic equilibrium*.

Translational Equilibrium vs. Rotational Equilibrium

Equilibrium refers to the balance of opposing influences. In physics, these influences can be forces or torques.

If the forces on an object are balanced—that is, the net force on the object is zero—then the object is said to be in translational equilibrium. An object in translational equilibrium is either not moving or moving at constant velocity.

If the torques on an object are balanced—that is, the net torque on the object is zero—then the object is said to be in rotational equilibrium. An object in rotational equilibrium is either not rotating, or rotating at constant angular velocity.

It is possible—and indeed quite common—for an object to be in both translational and rotational equilibrium. In fact, when an object is said to be in equilibrium, this is often assumed to be the case.

Vector Analysis of Forces Acting on a Point Object

The net force on an object is simply the total force on the object, that is, the sum of all the individual forces. However, because force is a vector, the forces on the object must be added as vectors; it is not sufficient to simply add their magnitudes. For example, if there are two forces acting on an object, one of 3 N and one of 4 N, then the net force on the object may be anywhere from 1 N to 7 N, depending on the directions. If the two forces are acting in the same direction, then the net force is 7 N; if they're acting in opposite directions, the net force is 1 N in the direction of the larger force; if they're acting at right angles to each other, the net force is 5 N at an angle of about 37° from the larger force.

No, if the net force on an object is zero, it does not necessarily follow that the object is motionless. According to Newton's Second Law, $\vec{F} = m\vec{a}$, which means if the net force on an object is zero, then the acceleration of the object is zero. However, acceleration is equal to change in velocity over time, so all this means is that the velocity is not changing. If the net force on the object is zero, its velocity must be constant, but not necessarily zero, which means the object may still be moving—it just can't be accelerating.

Torques, Lever Arms

Torque is something of a rotational analogue of force. Just as a greater force will, all else being equal, produce a greater acceleration, a greater torque will, all else being equal, produce a greater angular acceleration. However, torque is not simply equal to force; there are other factors affecting it. For instance, if you try pushing on a door's outer edge, you will close the door faster than if you exert the same force near the hinges. So, the distance between the axis of rotation and the point at which the force is exerted also matters. A vector pointing from the axis to where the force is exerted is called the lever arm, and the length of the lever arm is the distance in question. There's one more factor that also matters: the angle at which the force is exerted. You'll get the most angular acceleration by exerting a force perpendicular to the lever arm, whereas a force parallel to the lever arm will produce no angular acceleration. The full formula is $\tau = r\,F\sin\phi$, where τ is the torque, r is the lever arm, F is the force, and ϕ is the angle between the force and the lever arm.

Qualitatively, the greater the torque, the greater the angular acceleration—just as for linear motion, the greater the force, the greater the acceleration. In fact, the quantitative formula is similar as well: just like for linear motion we have Newton's Second Law, $\vec{F} = m\vec{a}$, for rotational motion, we have the analogous relationship $\tau = I\alpha$, where τ is the torque and α is the angular acceleration. The remaining factor is not the mass, however, because the torque required for a given angular acceleration depends not just on the mass of an object but on the mass distribution as well and also on the axis of rotation: it is much easier, for instance, to rotate a sledgehammer about a lengthwise axis than it is to rotate it about a crosswise axis through the end of the handle. Therefore, the mass is replaced in this equation by another value, the moment of inertia, abbreviated I, that takes these other factors into account. The units of the moment of inertia are $kg{\cdot}m^2$.

Units of Torque

The units of torque are N·m, newtons times meters. Because a newton is equal to a kg m/s^2, an N·m is equal to kg m/s^2 times m, which comes out to kg m^2/s^2. This is the same combination of units as the unit of energy, joules, but joules are never used as units of torque. Even though they have the same units, in terms of their relationship to fundamental units, torque and energy are two very different things, and the joule is reserved for energy. The units of torque are simply written N·m, and unlike many other derived units (including joules and newtons themselves), they are not given a shorthand name.

Work

Work Done by a Constant Force

The work done by a constant force depends on the magnitude of the force and on the distance over which the object that the force is acting on moves. Specifically, if the object is moving in the same direction as the force, the work done by the force is just $W = F\,d$. If the motion is not in the same direction as the force, then the angle between the force and the distance also becomes a factor: then the work done by the force is $W = F\,d\cos\theta$. For example, suppose a boy exerts a 50-N force to pull a wagon 3 meters along the ground by a rope that makes an angle of 30° with the horizontal. The total work the boy does pulling the wagon is then $F\,d\cos\theta = (50\text{ N})(3\text{ m})(\cos 30°) = 75\text{ J}$.

Mechanical Advantage

Mechanical advantage is the factor by which a machine decreases the necessary force to perform a task; it is the ratio of the force produced to the force applied. Pulleys, inclined planes, and other simple machines are useful because they grant a mechanical advantage; they allow a task to be done with a smaller force than would be necessary without the machine. The smaller force must be exerted over a larger distance, however, so the total work done remains the same.

For a lever, the mechanical advantage is simply the ratio of the distance from the fulcrum to the point where the force is applied to the distance from the fulcrum to the point where the force is exerted. For example, if an object is placed 10 cm from the fulcrum of a lever, and a force is exerted 30 cm from the fulcrum, the mechanical advantage is 3; the object can be lifted with a force one-third the object's weight.

For a pulley system, the mechanical advantage is equal to the number of rope systems that hold up the object being lifted. (The rope that the force is being applied to doesn't count.)

Work Kinetic Energy Theorem

The work kinetic energy theorem states that the work done on an object by the net force on that object is equal to the change in the object's kinetic energy. This can be used either to find the work given the change in kinetic energy, or to find the kinetic energy given the work, and then possibly to use these results to find other unknown values. For example, suppose a 2.0 N constant horizontal force pushes a 5-kg object 8 meters across a table against friction, accelerating it from rest to a final speed of 2 m/s. This means the object's change in kinetic energy is $\frac{1}{2}(5\text{ kg})(2\text{ m})^2 = 10\text{ J}$. The work kinetic energy theorem tells us that this is also equal to the work done by the net force. For a constant force in the direction of motion $W = F\,d$, we can derive that $F_{net} = \frac{10\text{ J}}{8\text{ m}} = 1.25\text{ N}$. Because this net force must be the applied force minus the force of friction, we can conclude that the force of friction on the object must be 2.0 N – 1.25 N = 0.75 N.

Conservative Forces

The work done on an object by some forces depends on the path it takes, whereas for other forces the work only depends on the start and end points. A force of the latter type is called a conservative force. For example, gravity is a conservative force; gravity does the same amount of work on an object that falls directly as it does on an object that slides down a ramp of the same height. Friction, on the other hand, is not a conservative force; friction does much less work on an object sliding straight across a table than it does on one that reaches the same point along a longer, zigzag path.

Aside from gravity, other conservative forces include electric force and the elastic force of a spring.

Aside from friction, other non-conservative forces include tension and air drag.

Units of Energy

The units of energy are joules, abbreviated J. They are named after the English physicist James Prescott Joule, best known for his discovery of the equivalence between heat and mechanical work.

One joule is equal to 1-kilogram times meter squared per second squared: kg m^2/s^2. This can be derived by considering any of the various equations for work or energy. For example, the work done by a constant force is $W = F\,d\cos\theta$, so the units of work must be equal to the units of force times the units of distance. (The cosine is unit-less.) That means the units of force are newtons times meters, or kg m/s^2 times m, which comes out to kg m^2/s^2.

Energy of Point Object Systems

Kinetic Energy

The kinetic energy of an object depends on its mass and its velocity. Specifically, the equation for the kinetic energy is $K = \frac{1}{2}mv^2$: the kinetic energy is equal to half the mass of the object times the square of its velocity. Although velocity is a vector, its square is a scalar, so the kinetic energy is a scalar quantity.

One way to derive this formula is by starting with the formula for the gravitational potential energy and considering an object that falls through a distance y. The potential energy lost is mgy because gravity is a conservative force that must be equal to the kinetic energy gained. Because the gravitational acceleration is a constant g (as long as the distances are sufficiently small), we can calculate the final velocity of the object: $v_f^2 = v_0^2 + 2ay = 0 + 2gy = 2gy$, so $gy = \frac{1}{2}v_f^2$, so $mgy = \frac{1}{2}mv_f^2$.

For example, a 2000-kg car moving at 30 m/s has a kinetic energy of $K = \frac{1}{2}mv^2 = \frac{1}{2}(2000\text{ kg})(30\text{ m/s})^2 = 900{,}000\text{ J}$.

Potential Energy

Gravitational, Local

The gravitational potential energy of an object can be calculated as $U = mgy$, where m is the mass of the object, g is the acceleration of gravity (which is equal to about 9.8 m/s^2 on Earth), and y is the altitude of the object. Where the altitude is calculated from (the ground, the surface of the table, etc.) is not important as long as you're consistent within a given problem; it is really the change in potential energy that's important.

This formula can be derived simply from the equation for work due to a constant force. Because the force of gravity on an object is mg, when an object falls a distance Δy, then the work gravity does on it is equal to $Fd = mg\Delta y$. Because gravity is a conservative force, this must be equal to the change in potential energy.

For example, a 10-kg weight at the top of a 2.0-m ladder has a potential energy of $mgh = (10\text{ kg})(9.8\text{ m/s}^2)(2.0\text{ m}) = 196\text{ J}$, assuming that you consider the height to be zero at the bottom of the ladder.

Spring

The spring constant is a value related to the elasticity of a spring: the harder it is to stretch the spring, the higher the spring constant. As such, despite the name, it is not a universal constant; it is only constant for a given spring.

An equation defining the spring constant is Hooke's law: $F = -k\Delta x$: the greater the force applied, the greater the displacement of the end of the spring from the equilibrium position (where it would be with no force applied), with the spring constant as the constant of proportionality. The negative sign in this equation arises because F and Δx are in opposite directions; the spring constant itself is always positive. (Hooke's law only holds as long as the spring is not stretched too far; there is a threshold called the elastic limit beyond which Hooke's law breaks down, and the spring may become permanently deformed.)

Solving for k in Hooke's law gives $k = -\frac{F}{\Delta x}$. From this we can determine the units of the spring constant: it must have units of force (newtons) over units of displacement (meters), so its units are N/m, or kg/s^2.

The potential energy of a spring is equal to $\frac{1}{2}k(\Delta x)^2$, where Δx is the displacement of the end of the spring from its equilibrium position (where it would be with no force applied), and k is the spring constant. As one would expect, a spring in its equilibrium state has no potential energy, whereas the more the spring is stretched or compressed, the higher its potential energy.

For example, consider a spring with a spring constant of 10.0 N/m. If this spring is stretched by 5.0 centimeters, its potential energy is $\frac{1}{2}(10.0\text{ N/m})(0.050\text{ m})^2 = 0.013\text{ J}$. If it is compressed by 20.0 centimeters, its potential energy is $\frac{1}{2}(10.0\text{ N/m})(0.200\text{ m})^2 = 0.200\text{ J}$.

Review Video: Potential and Kinetic Energy
Visit mometrix.com/academy and enter code: 491502

Conservation of Energy

Saying that energy is conserved means that whereas energy may be changed from one form to another (such as kinetic energy to potential energy), the total amount of energy in a system does not change. For a closed system, energy is always conserved, if you include thermal energy and other dissipative forms of energy (at least, on the macroscopic scale—technically in certain reactions involving subatomic particles it is possible for energy to be converted to mass, or vice versa, but that's beyond the scope of what's covered here.)

However, thermal energy is not generally easy to convert to another form, or easy to measure, and often it is more useful to exclude it and refer only to the conservation of mechanical energy—where mechanical energy refers only to kinetic and potential energy. Mechanical energy is conserved only when the only forces acting on the system are conservative forces—that is, in the absence of friction and air resistance and other dissipative forces.

Generally, conservation of energy can be used to solve for physical quantities by writing expressions for the total energy of a system at two different times, setting these two expressions equal to each other (because the total energy isn't changing), and then solving for unknown quantities. For example, consider a block starting from rest and sliding down a frictionless ramp 2.0 meters tall. At the top of the ramp, the block has a potential energy of $mgh = m\ (9.8\text{ m/s}^2)(2.0\text{ m}) = (19.6\text{ m}^2/\text{s}^2)\ m$ and a kinetic energy of zero, so its total energy is $(19.6\text{ m}^2/\text{s}^2)\ m$, where m is the (unknown) mass of the block. At the bottom of the ramp, the block has a potential energy of zero and a kinetic energy of $\frac{1}{2}mv^2$, so its total energy is $\frac{1}{2}mv^2$. Because mechanical energy is conserved in this situation, we can set these total energies equal: $(19.6\text{ m}^2/\text{s}^2)\ m = \frac{1}{2}mv^2$; the mass cancels, and we can solve for the velocity to get $v = \sqrt{2(19.6\text{ m}^2/\text{s}^2)} = 6.3\text{ m/s}$. Note that this result is independent of the mass of the block or the angle of the ramp.

Units of Power

The units of power are watts, named after the Scottish engineer James Watt, best known for his popularization of the steam engine. Although Watt did not invent the steam engine, it was his refinements to its design that allowed its use to become widespread.

In terms of the fundamental metric units, 1 watt is equal to 1-kilogram times meter squared per second cubed: $1\text{ W} = 1\text{ kg m}^2/\text{s}^3$. This can be derived from the definition of power: power is change in energy over time, so the units of power must be the units of energy divided by the units of time: joules divided by seconds, or $(\text{kg m}^2/\text{s}^2) / \text{s} = \text{kg m}^2/\text{s}^3$.

One simple equation to calculate power derives from the definition of power: power is change in energy over time, so $P = \frac{\Delta E}{\Delta t}$ or $P = \frac{W}{\Delta t}$ (where W is work). For instance, a machine that uses 30 kJ of energy per hour is using a power of $\frac{30{,}000\text{ J}}{3600\text{ s}} = 830\text{ W}$.

Another equation can be used to determine the power exerted by a constant force: $P = F\ v$. This can be derived from the previous equation: because $W = F\ d = F\ \Delta x$, that means $P = \frac{W}{\Delta t} = \frac{F\ \Delta x}{\Delta t} = F\frac{\Delta x}{\Delta t} = F\ v$. For instance, if a man pushes an appliance across the floor, exerting a force of 150 N to keep it moving at 0.2 m/s, then the power he exerts is (150 N)(0.2 m/s) = 30 W.

Periodic Motion

Amplitude, Frequency, Phase

The frequency, *f*, is the number of waves that pass a point per unit of time. The wavelength, λ, is the length of one wave. The speed, *v*, is, of course, how fast the wave is moving. (This does not refer to how fast the particles of the medium are moving, which may be very different; *v* is the speed of the wave itself.) To see how these quantities are related, consider this: the reciprocal of the frequency is the period, *T*, the amount of time it takes one wave to pass a given point. By definition, then, because exactly one wave passes in one period, the distance that the wave travels in one period is its wavelength. Because speed is distance over time, the speed of the wave must therefore be equal to $v = \frac{\lambda}{T}$. And because $T = 1/f$, this reduces to $v = \frac{\lambda}{1/f} = f\lambda$: the speed of the wave is equal to its frequency times its wavelength.

The phase of a wave is its shift along its own direction of propagation, or where in the cycle the wave starts. Two waves with the same frequency and wavelength have different phases if they start at different parts of the wave's cycle, as in these examples:

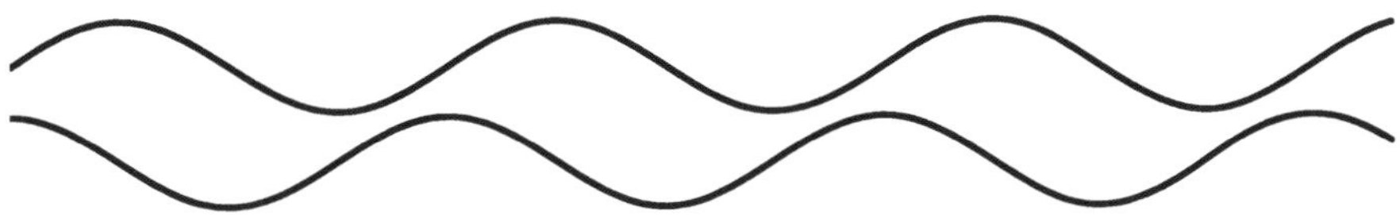

The phase is usually given as an angle, where one full wave corresponds to an angle of 360° or 2π radians. The difference in phase between two waves is called the phase shift. Two waves with a phase shift of zero are said to be in phase. Two waves with a phase shift of 180° or π radians are maximally out of phase. In the previous diagram, the lower wave is shifted left by about a quarter cycle relative to the upper wave, so it has a phase shift of $-\frac{360°}{4} = -90°$ or $-\frac{\pi}{2}$ radians.

Roughly speaking, the amplitude of a wave is a measurement of how "big" the wave is—not in the sense of the wavelength but in the sense of how much the medium moves to create the wave. More specifically, for a transverse wave, the amplitude is the difference between the maximum displacement and the equilibrium position—between the crest of a wave and its center line. The amplitude in this case is measured in units of distance. For a longitudinal wave, the amplitude is often measured not in units of distance but in units of pressure and represents the difference in pressure between the regions of maximum compression or rarefaction and the equilibrium pressure.

The amplitude of a wave can be easily determined from a graph of displacement versus time (or pressure vs. time, in the case of a longitudinal wave): it is the vertical distance between the crest of the wave and its center, or half the distance between the crest and the trough. For example, the wave graphed here would have an amplitude of 10 centimeters:

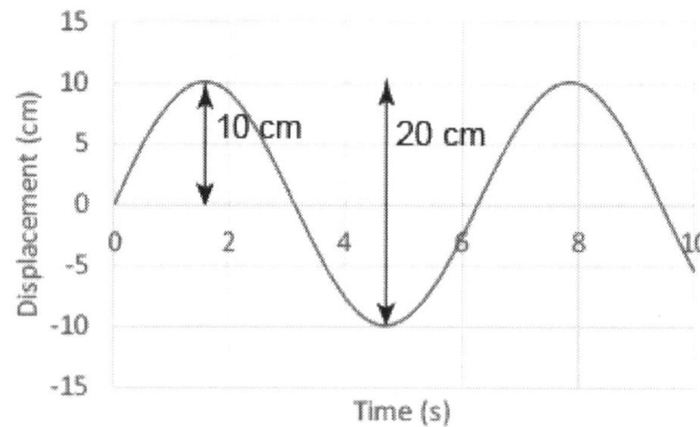

The frequency of a wave, abbreviated *f*, is the number of waves that pass a point per unit time. The standard metric unit of frequency is the Hertz, abbreviated Hz, named after the nineteenth-century German physicist Heinrich Rudolph Hertz, best known for proving the existence of electromagnetic waves. One Hertz is simply equal to one inverse second: that is, 1 Hz = 1 s^{-1}.

The period of a wave, abbreviated *T*, is the time it takes for a wave to pass a particular point, or equivalently, the time for a wave to complete one full cycle. Because the period is just a time, it is measured in seconds. There is a simple reciprocal relationship between the period and the frequency: $T = \frac{1}{f}$.

Transverse and Longitudinal Waves

A transverse wave is a wave in which the displacement of the medium (the object or substance the wave is traveling through) is perpendicular to the velocity of the wave itself. For example, if the wave is traveling left to right, the displacement of the medium occurs either up and down or forward and backward (or at some angle between the two). A wave on a string is a transverse wave; the wave travels along the string, but the points on the string itself oscillate perpendicular to the string. Electromagnetic waves are also transverse waves, though the vibration is of the intangible electric and magnetic fields and can't be perceived directly.

A longitudinal wave is a wave in which the displacement of the medium is along the same axis as the wave itself. They are also called compression waves because they involve an alternating compression and rarefaction of the medium. Sound waves are perhaps the most common example of compression waves.

It is not hard to produce both kinds of wave in a slinky: transverse waves by moving an end of the slinky side to side, longitudinal by moving it forward and backward. Earthquakes also combine transverse and longitudinal waves.

Importance of Fluids for the Circulation of Blood, Gas Movement, and Gas Exchange

Fluids

Density, Specific Gravity

The specific gravity of a fluid is the ratio of its density to the density of some reference substance—most commonly water for liquids or air for gases. (More specifically, it is water at the temperature at which it is densest (about 4°C) or air at room temperature (25°C).) Because specific gravity is a ratio between two quantities with the same units, the specific gravity itself is unit-less.

For instance, the density of mercury is about 13,500 kg/m^3, whereas the density of water is 1,000 kg/m^3. This means mercury is 13.5 times as dense as water, so the specific gravity of mercury is 13.5.

Buoyancy

Any time that an object is immersed in a fluid, there is a buoyant force exerted on it that acts upward, against gravity. If the buoyant force is greater than the object's weight, the object floats; if less, the object sinks. If the buoyant force is equal to the object's weight, the object will neither float nor sink but remain at the same height within the fluid; in this case, the object is said to have neutral buoyancy.

The buoyant force results from the difference in pressure on the top and bottom of the object. Because the hydrostatic pressure increases with depth, the pressure on the bottom of the object is slightly more than the pressure on the top of the object. This in turn means that the force on the bottom of the object will be slightly greater than the force on the top of the object, which results in an upward net force.

An object can float in a less dense liquid provided that the object displaces a weight of water greater than its own weight—which requires it to displace a greater volume of water than its own volume. This is possible if the object has a cavity or depression in it that increases its fluid displacement; metal boats can float because they are hollow, whereas a solid block of metal would sink.

For instance, consider a hemispherical shell of lead, 1.000 meter in diameter and 1 millimeter thick. Lead is much denser than water: 22,600 kg/m^3 as opposed to 1,000 kg/m^3 for water. The volume of the lead shell would be $\frac{1}{2}4\pi[(0.500\text{ m})^3 - (0.499\text{ m})^3\,)] = 0.0047\text{ m}^3$; its weight would be (0.0047 m^3)(22,600 kg/m^3)(9.80 m/s^2) = 1,040 N. However, if it is placed in the water up to its rim, open side up, the volume of water it displaces is $\frac{1}{2}(4\pi(0.500\text{ m})^3) = 0.196\text{ m}^3$; the weight of water (and thus the buoyant force) is (0.0196 m^3)(1,000 kg/m^3)(9.80 m/s^2) = 1,920 N. The buoyant force is greater than the weight of the lead shell, so the shell would float!

(Be careful not to confuse P and ρ—the symbols look similar but have very different meanings!)

Archimedes' Principle

Archimedes' Principle states that the buoyant force on a body immersed in a fluid is equal to the weight of the fluid the body displaces. Equivalently, $B = \rho V g$, where B is the buoyant force, ρ is the density of the fluid, V is the volume of fluid displaced, and g is the acceleration of gravity.

This principle can be derived by considering a cube of side length s immersed at a depth h under the fluid. The hydrostatic pressure on the top of the cube is $\rho g h$, so the downward force is the pressure times area, ρghs^2. On the bottom of the cube, the pressure is $\rho g(h+s)$, and the upward force is $\rho g(h+s)s^2$. The net force is the difference between the two, which is $pgs^3 = \rho gV$. Although this was derived for the special case of a cube, it holds for objects of any shape.

For example, consider a sphere with a radius of 1.00 meter submerged in water. Its volume is $4\pi r^3 = 12.6\text{ m}^3$, so the buoyant force on it is $\rho Vg = (9.81\text{ m/s}^2)(1{,}000\text{ kg/m}^3)(12.6\text{ m}^3) =$ 123 N. Note that the mass of the sphere is irrelevant—that affects the weight of the sphere but not the buoyant force on it.

Hydrostatic Pressure

The hydrostatic pressure within a fluid is the pressure exerted by a fluid at equilibrium. The hydrostatic pressure arises because of gravity; as gravity exerts a downward force on each part of the fluid, the fluid will therefore also exert a downward force on the fluid below it. This implies that the hydrostatic pressure increases with the depth in the fluid as there's more fluid above to press down.

To derive a formula for the hydrostatic pressure, consider a small cube of fluid a distance h below the surface, with an area of A on each face. Directly above the cube is a column of fluid with a height h and an area A, which means its volume is Ah. The mass of the column of fluid pressing down on the cube is the density times the volume, ρAh, and its weight—the force of gravity acting on the column—is its mass times gravity, ρAhg. The pressure on the small cube of fluid is the force exerted on its top surface divided by the area of that surface, $\frac{\rho Ahg}{A} = \rho gh$. So, the hydrostatic pressure at a depth h within a fluid is equal to ρgh.

Pascal's Law

Pascal's Law states that a change in pressure exerted anywhere in an incompressible fluid in a closed container is propagated throughout the fluid. In other words, if the pressure of a fluid is increased at one point in the fluid, it increases everywhere in the fluid.

One of the best-known applications of Pascal's Law is hydraulics. Hydraulic brakes in a car, for instance, work because pushing down on the brake pedal exerts a pressure on the brake fluid below, and then that pressure is transmitted through the fluid to the brakes themselves, causing the brake pads to press against the rotor. A hydraulic lift works by a piston exerting a downward pressure on a fluid, and the pressure is then transmitted through the fluid to exert upward pressure elsewhere.

Viscosity

The viscosity of a fluid is a measurement of how readily it flows; the more viscous the liquid, the "thicker" it is and the more it tends to stick together. More precisely, the viscosity can be defined in terms of the force necessary to make two layers of fluid move at different speeds. For example, honey and oil have high viscosities; they flow slowly and take time to spread out. On the other hand, alcohol and water have low viscosities; they flow readily and quickly fill the bottoms of their containers. The units of viscosity are the Pascal times second, or kg m/s, sometimes called the poiseuille (PI). (Technically, this is true of the dynamic viscosity, and there are other slightly different ways of defining viscosity, but they're beyond the scope of this discussion.)

Aside from the material, the principal factor that affects viscosity is temperature; the higher the temperature, the less viscous the fluid. The viscosity of a compressible fluid also depends slightly on pressure, and some non-Newtonian fluids vary in viscosity depending on the applied forces.

Poiseuille Flow

The Poiseuille flow equation, named after the French physicist Jean Léonard Marie Poiseuille, relates the flow rate of liquid through a tube to other known or measurable parameters. It can be written as $\Delta P = \frac{8\mu LQ}{\pi R^4}$, where Q is the volumetric flow rate of the fluid, ΔP is the pressure difference between the ends of the tube, μ is the (dynamic) viscosity of the fluid, L is the length of the tube, and R is the tube's radius. The fact that the radius is raised to the fourth power is notable; this shows that the flow rate is highly sensitive to the radius of the tube. All else being equal, doubling the radius of the tube would multiply the flow rate by 16!

The Poiseuille flow equation is most commonly used to predict the flow rate Q of the fluid, when other factors are known or to determine what length, radius, and so on would be necessary to achieve a particular flow rate. It is important to note, however, that the Poiseuille flow equation holds only for laminar flow. If the radius is too large, the viscosity is too small, or other factors lead to turbulent flow, then the Poiseuille flow equation no longer applies.

Continuity Equation

In fluid dynamics, the continuity equation states that the total volumetric flow rate Q of an incompressible fluid through a channel must be constant. This volumetric flow rate is defined as the volume of fluid that passes a point in the system per unit time. Because the volume of fluid in a section of a channel is equal to the cross-sectional area of the section times the length of the section, we can find an equation for Q: $Q = \frac{\Delta V}{\Delta t} = \frac{A\Delta x}{\Delta t} = A\frac{\Delta x}{\Delta t} = Av$, leading to the most common way of writing the continuity equation: $A_1 v_1 = A_2 v_2$.

The continuity equation is useful because it allows us to solve for the area or velocity at a given point in the channel, providing that the other quantity is known at that point and that both quantities are known at another point. For instance, if a fluid has a velocity of 6 m/s at a point where the channel has an area of 0.1 m^2, then where the channel has an area of 0.3 m, the velocity must be $\frac{(6\text{ m/s})(0.1\text{ m}^2)}{0.3\text{ m}^2} = 2\text{ m/s}$.

Concept of Turbulence at High Velocities

Fluid flow is said to be laminar if the fluid flows in continuous, parallel layers; each particular part of the fluid moves parallel to each other part (although not necessarily at the same speed). Otherwise, if the fluid flow is chaotic and multidirectional, the flow is said to be turbulent. A broad, smooth river is an example of laminar flow; whitewater rapids are turbulent.

In general, fluid flow tends to be laminar if the effects of viscosity and friction are dominant over those of inertia and turbulent if the reverse is true. High fluid density, low fluid viscosity, and high velocity all are factors that tend to lead to turbulent flow. The ratio of inertial forces to viscous forces is called the Reynolds number and can be used to estimate whether or not flow will be turbulent; in general, if the Reynolds number is less than 2,000, the flow is likely to be laminar; if it is much more than 2,000, it is turbulent.

Surface Tension

Surface tension is the tendency of the surface of a liquid to "stick together," as if the liquid were enclosed in a thin film or membrane. It is a consequence of the attractive forces between molecules of the liquid: because the molecules of the liquid are more strongly attracted to each other than they are to the molecules of the air or other surrounding gas, the molecules at the surface of the liquid are subject to a net inward force. Because of the relatively strong hydrogen bonds between water molecules, water has a higher surface tension than most liquids.

It is because of surface tension that small quantities of water and other liquids tend to form into rounded droplets rather than spreading evenly over a surface. Surface tension also can be sufficient to support small objects that are too dense to float because of the buoyant force—it is possible, with care, to place a paper clip such that it floats on a glass of water. Some small animals, such as water striders, are able to walk on the surface of water due to surface tension.

Bernoulli's Equation

Bernoulli's equation relates the speed, pressure, and height of a fluid flowing through a channel at different points. It can be written as $P_1 + \rho g h_1 + \frac{1}{2}\rho v_1^2 = P_2 + \rho g h_2 + \frac{1}{2}\rho v_2^2$, where P_1 and P_2 are the pressures of the fluid at the two points, h_1 and h_2 the heights (above some consistent baseline), and v_1 and v_2 the velocities; ρ is the density of the fluid. Bernoulli's equation can be derived from principles of conservation of energy, although the derivation is too lengthy to include here.

Bernoulli's equation can be used to solve for an unknown quantity, given the other quantities. For example, suppose water flows through a tube with an open end (so the pressure there is equal to the atmospheric pressure, 101,300 N). At the open end, the water's speed is 1.0 m/s; at an interior point 10.0 meters above the open end, it is 2.0 m/s. We can find the pressure at this interior point: 101,300 Pa + (1000 kg/m^3)(9.8 m/s^2)(0.0 m) + ½(1000 kg/m^3)(1.0 m/s)^2 = P_2 + (1000 kg/m^3)(9.8 m/s^2)(10.0 m) + ½(1000 kg/m^3)(2.0 m/s)^2; solving for P_2 yields 1,800 Pa.

Venturi Effect

The Venturi effect refers to the fact that the pressure in a fluid decreases as it moves through a narrower section in a vessel. This is a consequence of the continuity equation and the Bernoulli equation: from the continuity equation, $A_1 v_1 = A_2 v_2$, where the vessel is narrower (has a smaller area), the fluid's velocity is greater; Bernoulli's equation shows that where the velocity is greater, the pressure must be lower (if there is no change in height).

The Venturi effect can be used to measure the flow rate of a fluid by measuring the pressure at two points with different known areas; from the difference in pressure, the velocity of the fluid at either point can be calculated using Bernoulli's equation and the continuity equation. The Venturi effect also plays a role in the operation of spray bottles, gas stoves, and carburetors.

Pitot Tube

A pitot tube is a simple instrument used to measure the velocity of an incompressible fluid. It is named after the French hydraulic engineer who invented it, Henri Pitot. A pitot tube often looks like a simple bent tube with a hole in the end; the hole is faced into the flow of the fluid, and the instrument gives a velocity reading.

A pitot tube works by measuring the pressure of the moving fluid that enters the tube and comparing it to the pressure of unmoving fluid—either taking this as a known quantity, or measuring the pressure of fluid that enters through channels perpendicular to the direction of flow. From Bernoulli's equation (taking the heights to be the same for both), we have $P_{moving} + \frac{1}{2}\rho v^2 = P_{static}$; assuming the fluid density is known, this can be solved for the velocity of the fluid to give $v = \sqrt{\frac{2(P_{static} - P_{moving})}{\rho}}$; it is this value that the pitot tube reading shows.

Units of Pressure

The units of pressure are pascals, abbreviated Pa, named after Blaise Pascal, a French mathematician and physicist also known for his contributions to the fields of probability theory and fluid flow. Because pressure is defined as force over area, the units of pressure must be equal to the units of force divided by the units of area: newtons divided by meters squared. So, 1 Pa = 1 N/m^2. Because a newton is equal to a kg m/s^2, this can be expressed in terms of fundamental units as 1 Pa = 1 kg $/(m \cdot s^2)$, although it is rarely written this way.

GAS PHASE

ABSOLUTE TEMPERATURE, (K) KELVIN SCALE

The size of 1 Kelvin is the same as the size of 1° Celsius; the only difference between the two scales is where the zero is: 0°C corresponds to 273.15 K, so to convert from degrees Celsius to Kelvins, it is only necessary to add 273.15. Conversely, Kelvins can be converted to degrees Celsius by subtracting 273.15. For example, the typical room temperature of 25°C corresponds to 298.15 K.

What makes the Kelvin scale particularly useful in science is the fact that 0 K corresponds to the absolute zero of temperature. Multiplying or dividing temperatures is only meaningful in such a scale; it doesn't make sense, for instance, to double a temperature expressed in degrees Celsius because doubling a negative temperature would result in a lower temperature (among other reasons). The Kelvin scale has no negative temperatures, and such an operation is entirely reasonable. In any calculation that involves multiplying or dividing by temperatures (such as some applications of the Ideal Gas Law), the temperature must be expressed in Kelvins, not degrees Celsius. If only differences of temperature are involved, however, then the two scales are interchangeable.

PRESSURE, SIMPLE MERCURY BAROMETER

A mercury barometer in its simplest form consists of a tube closed at one end and filled with mercury inverted in an open container of mercury. The pressure of the surrounding air will press on the mercury in the open container; due to Pascal's Law, this pressure is propagated throughout the mercury. At equilibrium, the hydrostatic pressure due to the mercury column will precisely equal the atmospheric pressure of the surroundings, so the atmospheric pressure can be calculated from the height h of the column of mercury: $P_{atm} = \rho_{Hg} g h$.

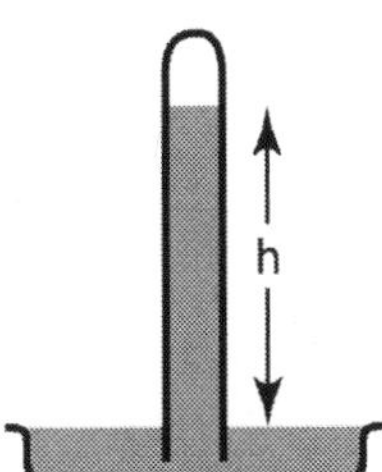

In principle, this would work the same with any incompressible liquid, not just mercury. In practice, mercury is chosen because of its high density. The higher the density of the fluid, the lower the height of the column, so for fluids of low density, the height becomes impractical. At normal atmospheric pressure, the column of mercury in a mercury barometer is about 76 centimeters high. A similar instrument using water instead of mercury would require a column more than 10 meters high!

MOLAR VOLUME

Molar volume is the volume occupied by one mole of a substance: by definition, the number of molecules or atoms in one mole of a substance is Avogadro's number, about $6.022 \cdot 10^{23}$. Although the molar volume cannot be measured directly (you can't count $6.022 \cdot 10^{23}$ atoms), it can be calculated from the molar mass and the mass density: $V_m = \frac{M}{\rho}$, where V_m is the molar volume, M is the molar mass, and ρ is the mass density. Because the mass density varies with temperature and pressure, so does the molar volume; it is therefore not correct to say that a particular substance has a specific molar volume but rather that it has a specific molar volume at some particular temperature and pressure.

For instance, nitrogen gas has a molar mass of 28.0135 g/mol and a mass density at 25°C of 1.145 kg/m^3, or 0.001145 g/cm^3. This means that at 25°C, nitrogen gas has a molar volume of $\frac{28.0135 \text{ g/mol}}{0.001145 \text{ g/cm}^3} = 24470 \text{ cm}^3\text{/mol}$, equivalent to 0.02447 m^3/mol or 24.47 L/mol.

At a temperature of 0°C and a pressure of 1 atm, an ideal gas has a molar volume of 0.0224 m^3/mol, or 22.4 liters/mol.

Ideal Gas

An ideal gas is a gas made up of particles with the following characteristics:

- Their volume is negligible compared to the volume of the container.
- They do not interact except during collisions.
- All collisions are perfectly elastic (no kinetic energy is lost).
- Between collisions, the particles travel at constant speed in straight lines.

Although an ideal gas is an abstract concept, and no real gases have exactly these characteristics, the ideal gas concept is useful because it allows certain calculations and predictions to be made about the gas's properties and behavior—and these predictions turn out to hold to a high level of precision for many real gases, even if they aren't exactly ideal. Essentially, a real gas behaves as an ideal gas to a very good approximation as long as its pressure isn't too high and its temperature isn't too low.

Ideal Gas Law

The Ideal Gas Law is an equation that relates the pressure, volume, temperature, and number of moles or molecules of an ideal gas. It combines Boyle's Law, Charles's Law, and Avogadro's Law, although each of these laws was originally separately determined on empirical grounds. Like these other laws, and like its name implies, the Ideal Gas Law only holds exactly for a nonexistent ideal gas, but for most real gases it is a very good approximation.

The Ideal Gas Law can be stated as $PV = nRT$, where P is the pressure of the gas, V is the volume, n is the number of moles, T is the temperature (in Kelvins!), and R is the ideal gas constant, equal to about 8.314 J/(mol K) or 0.08205 L atm/(mol K).

The Ideal Gas Law can be used to solve for the pressure, volume, temperature, or number of moles of gas if the other quantities are known. For instance, consider a room with a volume of 60.0 m^3 filled with air at 25°C and a pressure of 1.000 atmosphere. We can use the Ideal Gas Law to determine the number of moles of air in the room: $n = \frac{PV}{RT} = \frac{(1.013 \cdot 10^5 \text{Pa})(60.0 \text{ m}^3)}{(8.314 \text{ J/(mol K)})(298 \text{ K})} = 2450 \text{ mol}$.

By definition, the particles of an ideal gas have negligible volume and do not interact except during collisions. The particles of a real gas, of course, do have some finite volume, and there are long-range forces between them, such as the van der Waals forces arising due to their charge distributions. The difference from ideal behavior is most notable at high pressures and low temperatures. At very high pressures, the effect of the volume of the particles may become important and $PV > nRT$, whereas at very low temperatures the intermolecular forces play a role and $PV < nRT$.

The Dutch physicist Johannes Diderik van der Waals derived a generalization of the Ideal Gas Law that takes these features of a real gas into account: what is now called the van der Waals equation, $\left(P + \frac{an^2}{V^2}\right)(V - nb) = nRT$. Although still not exact, this equation gives closer results for real gases for a broad range of circumstances. Unfortunately, however, it relies on two constants, a and b, that are not universal and must be determined separately for each gas.

Review Video: Ideal Gas Law
Visit mometrix.com/academy and enter code: 381353

BOYLE'S LAW

Boyle's Law states that for a gas at constant temperature, the pressure of the gas is inversely proportional to the volume: all else being equal, $P \propto \frac{1}{V}$, or $P_1V_1 = P_2V_2$. It is named after the Irish chemist and physicist Robert William Boyle, who was among the first to define the modern study of chemistry.

Boyle's Law can be used to solve for an unknown pressure or volume, when the other is known and when both quantities are known at a different time. For instance, consider an air bubble deep under the ocean at a pressure of 20 atm. As it rises to the surface, the bubble will expand due to the decreased pressure. If the bubble initially has a volume of 1.0 cm^3, we can find its volume at the surface using Boyle's Law: (20 atm)(1.0 cm^3) = (1.0 atm)V_2, so we can solve for V_2 yielding V_2 = 20 cm^3.

Review Video: Boyle's Law
Visit mometrix.com/academy and enter code: 115757

CHARLES'S LAW

Charles's Law states that for a gas at constant pressure, the volume of the gas is proportional to the temperature: all else being equal, $V \propto T$, or $\frac{V_1}{T_1} = \frac{V_2}{T_2}$. The law is named after French physicist and inventor Jacques Alexandre César Charles, also known for his development of hydrogen balloons.

Charles's Law can be used to solve for an unknown volume or temperature, when the other is known and when both quantities are known at a different time. For instance, consider a balloon that at room temperature (25°C) has a volume of 12.0 m^3. If the gas inside the balloon is heated, the balloon will expand. If the gas is heated to a temperature of 300°C, we can find the balloon's new volume using Charles's Law, $\frac{12.0 \text{ m}^3}{298 \text{ K}} = \frac{V_2}{573 \text{ K}}$, so V_2 = 23.1 m^3. Note that we had to convert the temperatures from degrees Celsius into Kelvins—this is necessary whenever we're multiplying or dividing by temperatures.

Review Video: Charles's Law
Visit mometrix.com/academy and enter code: 537776

AVOGADRO'S LAW

Avogadro's Law states that at constant temperature and pressure, the volume of gas is proportional to the number of molecules or moles. That is, all else being equal, $V \propto n$, or $\frac{V_1}{n_1} = \frac{V_2}{n_2}$. Alternatively, we can write $V \propto N$, or $\frac{V_1}{N_1} = \frac{V_2}{N_2}$. (In gas equations, it is common to use n for the number of moles and N for the number of molecules.)

Avogadro's Law can be used to solve for an unknown volume or number of molecules or moles when the other is known and when both quantities are known at a different time. For instance, consider two chambers filled with gas at equal pressure and temperature. One chamber has a volume of 500 m³, the other 200 m³. If we are given that the larger chamber contains 20,000 moles of gas, we can use Avogadro's Law to determine the number of moles of gas in the smaller chamber: $\frac{500\text{ m}^3}{20000\text{ mol}} = \frac{200\text{ m}^3}{n_2}$, so $n_2 = 8{,}000$ mol.

Kinetic Molecular Theory of Gases

Heat Capacity

Heat capacity is a measurement of the amount of heat that must be transferred to an object to raise its temperature by a specific amount (or, equivalently, the amount of heat that is released when its temperature lowers). It can be expressed as $C = \frac{Q}{\Delta T}$, where Q is the heat and ΔT the change in temperature. (Technically, the heat capacity itself varies slightly by temperature, so this equation isn't exactly valid, but it holds well for relatively small changes in temperature.) Because heat capacity depends on the amount of material, however, it is also useful to define the specific heat capacity, or specific heat, $c = \frac{C}{m} = \frac{Q}{m\Delta T}$. (Heat capacity is represented by an uppercase *C*, specific heat by a lower-case *c*.) The specific heat capacity depends only on the material and not on the quantity present.

Because heat has units of joules and temperature has units of Kelvins or degrees Celsius, the units of heat capacity are J/K or J/°C. For differences in temperature, Kelvins and degrees Celsius are interchangeable, so these two units are equivalent. Because $c = \frac{C}{m}$, the specific heat has units of J/(kg K) or J/(kg °C)

For a gas, the heat capacity is not a constant; it depends on what other quantities are changing. The Ideal Gas Equation, $PV = nRT$, shows that temperature cannot change without affecting other properties of the gas; assuming that the amount of gas (the number of molecules) doesn't change, then either the pressure or the volume must change or both. The heat capacity depends on which of these is changing, and so a gas is said to have a heat capacity at constant pressure, C_P, and a heat capacity at constant volume, C_V.

These two heat capacities are not the same—the heat capacity at constant pressure is always higher than the heat capacity at constant volume because some energy is required to do work on the gas as it expands. However, for an ideal gas there is a simple relationship between the two. The derivation is a bit complicated, but it can be shown that for an ideal gas $C_P - C_V = nR$, where n is the number of moles of gas and R is the ideal gas constant.

Boltzmann's Constant

Boltzmann's constant, abbreviated k or k_B, is a constant that arises in multiple places in thermodynamics. It is named after Austrian physicist Ludwig Eduard Boltzmann, best known for his development of statistical mechanics. Boltzmann's constant is equal to about $1.38 \cdot 10^{-23}$ J/K.

One place Boltzmann's constant arises is as the ratio of the ideal gas constant to Avogadro's number: $k_B = \frac{R}{N_A}$. In fact, by using the number of molecules instead of the number of moles, it is possible to rewrite the Ideal Gas Law in terms of Boltzmann's constant instead of the ideal gas constant: $PV = Nk_BT$. This may be useful if you actually know (or want to determine) the number of molecules rather than the number of moles. Boltzmann's constant also turns up in the relationship of kinetic energy to temperature: the average kinetic energy of a molecule in a gas at temperature T turns out to be equal to $\frac{3}{2}k_BT$.

Deviation of Real Gas Behavior from Ideal Gas Law

The main property of an ideal gas that is affected by the number of atoms per molecule is the gas's heat capacity. It can be shown that the heat capacity of a gas at constant pressure is equal to $\frac{1}{2}nR$ for each degree of freedom of the gas particles—roughly, each direction in which the gas particles can meaningfully move or rotate. A single atom is spherically symmetrical, so rotations don't matter, but it can move along any of three axes, so it has three degrees of freedom: its heat capacity at constant pressure is therefore $\frac{3}{2}nR$. A diatomic molecule, on the other hand, has in addition two axes of rotation, so it has five total degrees of freedom and a heat capacity at constant pressure of $\frac{5}{2}nR$. (There's a sixth degree of freedom in the ability of the bond to change its length, but near room temperature it can be ignored due to energy limitations.) Because for an ideal gas $C_P = C_V + nR$, we can also find the heat capacities at constant pressure: $\frac{5}{2}nR$ for a monatomic gas or $\frac{7}{2}nR$ for a diatomic. Once the molecules have more than two atoms, the degrees of freedom become more difficult to determine.

Most instruments that measure the pressure inside a container, including manometers, the gauges used to check tire pressures, and the sphygmomanometers doctors use to measure blood pressure, don't actually measure the total pressure. What they're really measuring is the difference in pressure between the inside of the container and the outside. Because this is the pressure read by gauges, this is called the gauge pressure.

Although the gauge pressure is often useful, at other times it is important to know not just the difference in pressure but the total pressure of the gas inside a container—for example, if one has to use that pressure to calculate some other property using the Ideal Gas Law. This pressure is called the absolute pressure. There is a simple relationship between the two pressures: the absolute pressure is equal to the gauge pressure plus the atmospheric pressure.

For instance, if a gauge used to measure the pressure in a car's tire gives a reading of 32.5 psi, then the gauge pressure is 32.5 psi, but the absolute pressure is $P_{gauge} + P_{atm} = 32.5\text{ psi} + 14.7\text{ psi} = 47.2\text{ psi}$.

Partial Pressure and Mole Fraction

The partial pressure of a gas in a container is the pressure that a particular gas within a mixture of gases would have in the absence of the other gases in the mixture. For example, if two ideal gases are mixed together in equal quantities, the partial pressure of each gas is just half the total pressure of the two gases.

The mole fraction of a particular element or compound in a mixture is the ratio of the number of moles of the substance in question to the total number of moles of all the substances in the compound. In a mixture of 10 moles of oxygen and 30 moles of nitrogen, for instance, the mole fraction of oxygen would be $\frac{10}{10+30} = 0.25$, and the mole fraction of nitrogen would be $\frac{30}{10+30} = 0.75$.

For an ideal gas, or rather a mixture of ideal gases, the partial pressure of any constituent is proportional to the mole fraction of that constituent. This follows from the ideal gas law: $PV = nRT$, and the volumes and temperatures of all the constituent gases are the same, so $P_i \propto n_i$.

Dalton's Law

Dalton's Law states that the sum of the partial pressures of all the constituents of a particular mixture of (ideal) gases is equal to the total pressure of the gas. It is named after the English chemist and physicist John Dalton, perhaps best known for his seminal role in the development of modern atomic theory.

Dalton's Law has applications to medicine and meteorology, among other fields. In medicine, it is often important to know the partial pressures of individual gases because it is that partial pressure that determines its effect on the body; this also applies, for instance, to scuba divers, who can't let the partial pressure of nitrogen in the mixture they're breathing get too large without risking adverse effects. In meteorology, the partial pressures of different gases in the atmosphere are responsible for many weather phenomena.

Review Video: Dalton's Law of Partial Pressure
Visit mometrix.com/academy and enter code: 355830

Units of Pressure

The standard SI unit of pressure is the Pascal, Pa, where 1 Pa = 1 N/m^2. However, there are several other units of pressure in common use under certain circumstances. Some other common units of pressure include the following:

- *Atmospheres* (atm): one atmosphere is the (approximate) mean atmospheric pressure at sea level on Earth. It is defined as exactly 101,325 Pa.
- *Pounds per square inch* (psi): this is the standard unit of pressure in traditional avoirdupois (English) units, and although rarely used in science, is still often seen elsewhere: pressure in car tires, for instance, is usually measured in psi. One psi is about 6890 N; 1 atm = 14.70 psi.
- *Millimeters of mercury* (mmHg): this is a pressure scale based on the height of a column of mercury in a standard mercury barometer. One mmHg is about 133.3 Pa; 1 atm is about 760 mmHg. Historically, the mmHg was also called a torr; now these units have been redefined to be slightly different but still very close to the same: 1 torr is about 0.99999985 mmHg.

Electrochemistry and Electrical Circuits and Their Elements

Electrostatics

Charge, Conductors, Charge Conservation, Insulators

To say that charge is conserved means that the total charge in a closed system does not change. Charge may be transferred from one object to another, but the total must remain the same. If a system is initially electrically neutral, for instance, one part of the system cannot become positively charged without another part becoming negatively charged.

Charge conservation is important because it allows prediction of unknown charges. If an object initially has a charge of 2 C, and after touching another (initially neutral) object it has a charge of 3 C, the other object must have acquired a charge of −1 C for the total charge to remain the same. Charge conservation also places restrictions on possible events; it is because of charge conservation, for instance, that we know that the total current flowing into a point in a circuit must be equal to the total current out because otherwise a charge would be building up at that point.

An electrical conductor is a substance that conducts electricity—that is, a substance through which electrical charge is able to freely flow. Electrical conductors tend to have loosely bound electrons, or free ions. For instance, metals are good conductors because they share their electrons in such a way that it is easy for electrons to move between atoms; solutions of ionic compounds such as saltwater are also good conductors because the positive and negative dissolved ions are themselves free to move through the solution.

An electrical insulator is a substance that does not conduct electricity; an electrical charge does not easily flow through it. Rubber is known as a good insulator; other insulating materials include glass, asbestos, and PVC.

Whether a material is a conductor or an insulator is not an all-or-nothing affair; there are no perfect insulators, and the only perfect conductors are special superconductor materials that only hold that property under certain circumstances (most notably, all known superconductors require very low temperatures). Therefore, when we call a material a conductor or an insulator, these are relative terms, and there are some materials—semiconductors—that lie right in between and can't easily be classified as one or the other.

Coulomb's Law

Coulomb's Law is an equation giving the electric force between two charged particles: $F = \frac{kq_1q_2}{r^2}$, where q_1 and q_2 are the magnitudes of the charges, r is the distance between them, and k is Coulomb's constant, equal to about $8.99 \cdot 10^9$ N m^2 / C^2. The direction of the force on either particle is directly toward the other particle if their charges have opposite signs or directly away from the other particle if the charges have the same sign. Like the coulomb, the SI unit of charge, Coulomb's Law is named after the French physicist Charles-Augustin de Coulomb.

For example, the charge on an electron is about $-1.602 \cdot 10^{-19}$ C. Suppose we have two electrons separated by the diameter of a hydrogen atom, about $5 \cdot 10^{-11}$ m. The electric force these atoms exert on each other would then be $\frac{(8.99 \cdot 10^9 \text{ N m}^2/\text{C}^2)(1.602 \cdot 10^{-19}\text{C})^2}{(5 \cdot 10^{-11}\text{m})^2}$ = about $9 \cdot 10^{-8}$ N. Because the electrons are both negatively charged, the force on each electron would be directed away from the other.

Electric Field

Field Lines

The electric field lines are lines that trace the direction of the electric field in space. Although the exact places the lines are drawn are arbitrary, the direction of the electric field lines represents the direction of the electric field, and the density of the electric field lines represents its magnitude.

The equipotential lines are lines that connect points in space with the same electrical potential in much the same way that the lines in a topological map connect points of equal altitude.

The most salient relationship between the electric field lines and the equipotential lines are that they are always perpendicular. This stands to reason from the definition of electrical potential: the electrical potential is the amount of work done in moving a unit charge from one point to another. The electrical force is in the same direction as the electric field and does work on the charge in that direction. Therefore, if there were any component of the electric field parallel to the equipotential line, there would be work done on the charge in that direction, which means there would be a difference in potential, which contradicts the definition of the equipotential line.

The electric field at a given point in space is defined as the force that would be exerted on a positive unit charge at that point. Turning that around and solving for the force, the force on a unit charge at a particular point is equal to the field at that point times 1 C. Because the electric force is proportional to the charge, for a charge of a different magnitude we have to multiply by that charge instead of by 1 C, so in general the force on an arbitrary charged particle at a given point is equal to the field times that charge: $\vec{F} = q\vec{E}$. For instance, a 3.0 C charge in an electric field with a magnitude of 0.4 N/C would experience a force of (3.0 C)(0.4 N/C) = 1.2 N. (Note that the force and the field are both vectors, whereas the charge is a scalar, so the force will simply be in the same direction as the field.)

FIELD DUE TO CHARGE DISTRIBUTION

The electric field lines point in the same direction as the electric force on a positive particle. Positively charged particles repel each other, so the electric force—and therefore the electric field—points directly away from a positively charged particle. A negatively charged particle attracts a positively charged particle, so the electric field points toward a negatively charged particle. So, the electric field lies near a positively charged particle point radially away from the particle, whereas the electric field lines near a negatively charged particle point radially toward the particle.

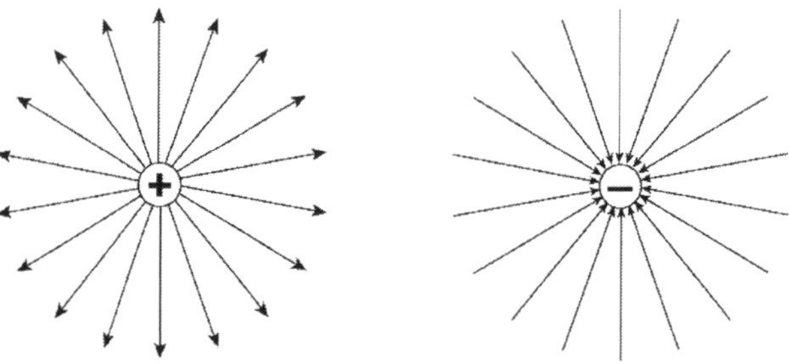

ELECTROSTATIC ENERGY, ELECTRIC POTENTIAL AT A POINT IN SPACE

To find the electric field near a point charge Q, we can consider a hypothetical charge q at that point and use Coulomb's Law to determine the force on that charge: $F = \frac{kQq}{r^2}$. Because the field at a point is equal to the force on a charge at that point divided by the magnitude of the charge, we can find the field by dividing the force by q, giving $E = \frac{kQ}{r^2}$. This field points directly away from the point charge if it is positive or toward the point charge if it is negative.

In the case of a distribution of multiple point charges, we have to find the contribution to the electric field of each charge and then add those fields together. Because the electric field is a vector, we have to add the component fields as vectors, not just add their magnitudes. For example, the net electric field at a point directly between two equal charges is zero because the contributions from each charge are equal in magnitude but opposite in direction, so they cancel each other out.

UNITS OF ELECTRIC POTENTIAL AND ELECTRIC FIELD

We can determine the units of the electric potential by considering the relationship between electric potential and electric potential energy: $U_E = qV$, so $V = \frac{U_E}{q}$. Because the electric potential energy has units of joules and the charge has units of coulombs, the electric potential must have units of J/C. This unit—joules per coulomb—is also known as a volt, abbreviated V and named after the Italian physicist and chemist Alessandro Giuseppe Antonio Anastasio Volta.

As for the electric field, we can determine its units from the equation relating electric field to electric force: $\vec{F} = q\vec{E}$, so $\vec{E} = \frac{\vec{F}}{q}$. Because the force has units of newtons and the charge has units of coulombs, the units of electric field must therefore be N/C, or equivalently, V/m. (That these are equivalent is not immediately obvious but can be shown by expressing both in terms of the fundamental metric units.)

Circuit Elements

Current

Current is the rate of flow of charge past a given point. In other words, it is equal to the amount of charge that passes through a given point per unit of time.

The unit of current is the ampere, abbreviated A. The ampere is named after the French mathematician and physicist André-Marie Ampère, considered one of the pioneers of the study of electromagnetism. We can see what the ampere must be in terms of the fundamental units by considering its definition. Because current is the rate of flow of charge, the units of current must be units of charge divided by the units of time: coulombs per second. So, 1 A = 1 C/s. (The coulomb is itself a fundamental unit and cannot be broken down further.)

Sign Conventions

The current is defined to be positive in the direction that positive charge is flowing. This may seem a little backward because in solid conductors what's actually moving is the electrons, which are negatively charged—so the direction of the current is in the opposite direction that the electrons are moving! However, the sign convention for the current was defined before it was understood exactly what particles were moving to cause the current.

The voltage is defined to have the same sign as the potential energy that a positively charged particle would have at that point. As with gravitational potential energy, however, it is really the difference in potential energies that matters, and where to set the zero is arbitrary; by convention, the potential energy of a particle is usually defined to be zero when it is infinitely far away from other charged particles.

Electromotive Force, Voltage

Electromotive force is a bit of a misleading term because what it describes is not a force in the usual sense and not measured in newtons. Rather, it is a measurement of voltage but specifically the voltage produced by a source of electrical energy in a circuit. Electromotive force is often abbreviated to EMF, or simply to $\mathcal{E}$. (Note that this is always a script $\mathcal{E}$, not a block E; in electromagnetism, the symbol E conventionally refers to electric field.)

One common source of electromotive force is a battery, which uses its stored chemical energy to produce a potential difference across its terminals. Other possible sources of electromotive force include solar cells and electric generators.

The voltage, also known as electrical potential, is defined as the potential energy difference that a unit charge would experience between two points. Its units are equal to the units of energy divided by the units of charge, joules per coulomb, which—unsurprisingly—is equivalent to volts.

For example, if a 2 C charge had a potential energy of 30 J at one point and a potential energy of 20 J at another point, then the voltage between the two points is $\frac{30\text{ J}-20\text{ J}}{2\text{ C}} = 5$ J/C, or 5 V.

Note that formally voltage is defined only in terms of the voltage difference between two points. In practice, however, it is common to designate one particular point as having a voltage of zero (e.g., the ground of a circuit) and to state the voltage difference between another point and this point as the voltage at the other point.

The voltage difference is defined as the difference in potential energy experienced by a unit charge as it travels between two points. A uniform electric field exerts a force on the charge of $F = qE$. From the equation for work done by a constant force, the work done by this force is equal to $F\ d \cos\theta = q\ E\ d \cos\theta$. The electrical force is a conservative force, so this work must be equal to the change in potential energy. The voltage difference is therefore equal to the potential energy divided by the charge, or $\Delta V = E\ d \cos\theta$, where d is the distance between the two points and θ is the angle between the electric field and a line drawn between the two points.

For example, consider two points 5.0 cm apart in an electric field with a magnitude of 0.20 N/C. If a line drawn between the points is parallel to the electric field, then the voltage difference between the points is $\Delta V = (0.20\ \text{N/C})(0.05\ \text{m})(\cos 0) = 0.01\ \text{V}$. If, on the other hand, a line drawn between the points is perpendicular to the electric field, then the voltage difference is $\Delta V = (0.20\ \text{N/C})(0.05\ \text{m})(\cos 90°) = 0$—the two points are at the same voltage.

Electrical Circuit Ground

The ground in an electrical circuit is a part of the circuit that is connected to a large electrically neutral reservoir that can absorb or provide charge as needed without its own charge changing appreciably. This prevents the circuit from building up too much charge itself. If an excess negative charge builds up in the circuit, electrons flow to the ground; if an excess positive charge builds up, electrons flow from the ground into the circuit. In either case, the circuit itself remains neutral. A circuit or object connected to the ground is said to be grounded. Many electrical appliances are grounded when in use; in a standard three-prong plug, the third plug connects to the ground.

The ground gets its name from the fact that generally it is literally the ground; the ground wire connects ultimately to the Earth itself, which is certainly a very large neutral reservoir. Likewise, a person working on a sensitive electrical project who doesn't want to risk any buildup of static electricity can ground himself or herself by touching some conductive object that is in contact with the Earth, such as a metal faucet.

Resistance

Ohm's Law

Ohm's Law is an equation relating some of the most important properties of an electrical circuit. It is usually written in the form $V = IR$ or sometimes $\mathcal{E} = IR$ if the voltage is provided by a battery or other source of electromotive force. V (or $\mathcal{E}$) is the voltage, I is the current, and R is the resistance.

Ohm's Law can therefore be used to solve for any of these three quantities if given the other two. For instance, if 45 mA of current flow through a lightbulb attached to a 9 V battery, then the resistance of the lightbulb must be $R = \frac{V}{I} = \frac{9\ \text{V}}{0.045\ \text{A}} = 200\ \Omega$.

Resistance

Electrical resistance is the tendency of a material to oppose the passage of current. The higher the resistance, the less current will be produced by application of a given voltage. Conductors have a low resistance; insulators have a high resistance.

The units of resistance are ohms, abbreviated by the upper-case Greek letter omega, Ω. The ohm is named after Georg Simon Ohm, the German mathematician and physicist credited with discovering the relationship between the voltage and current in a circuit. It is this relationship that shows how the ohm is related to other units: because $V = IR$, the units of resistance must be units of voltage over units of current, that is, volts over amperes. So $1\ \Omega = 1\ \text{V/A}$ or, put in terms of the fundamental metric units, $1\ \text{kg m}^2 / (\text{C}^2\ \text{s})$.

Resistors in Parallel

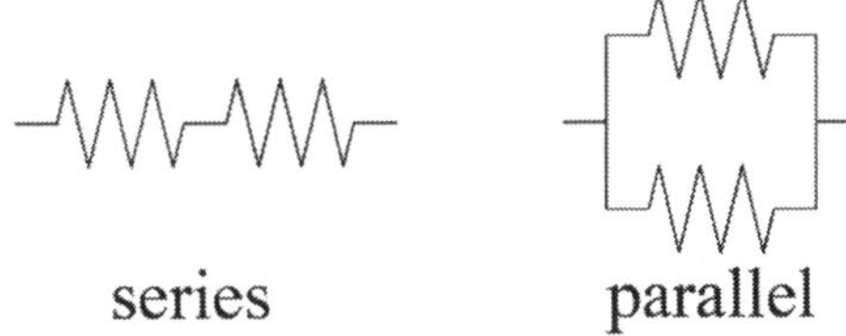

For resistors in series (joined linearly end to end so current must pass sequentially through each of them), the resistances simply add together: $R_{net} = R_1 + R_2 + \cdots$. For example, if you connect a 200 Ω and a 300 Ω resistor in series, their net resistance is 200 Ω + 300 Ω = 500 Ω.

For resistors in parallel (with each end of each resistor connected to the corresponding end of the others so that current may pass through any of the resistors), the reciprocals of the resistances add together: $R_{net} = \frac{1}{\frac{1}{R_1}+\frac{1}{R_2}+\cdots}$. For example, if you connect a 200 Ω and a 300 Ω resistor in parallel, the net resistance is $\frac{1}{\frac{1}{200\ \Omega}+\frac{1}{300\ \Omega}} = 120\ \Omega$.

Note that when the resistors are joined in series, the net resistance is greater than any of the individual resistances, whereas when they're connected in parallel, the net resistance is smaller than any of the individual resistances. This makes sense because for resistors in series, the current must flow through all of the resistors, meaning it is affected by each one, whereas for resistors in parallel, the current has more paths it can take and isn't wholly affected by any one resistor.

Resistivity

Resistivity is the tendency of a particular material to prevent the flow of current through it. The higher the resistivity of a material, the more voltage it takes to produce a given current, all else being equal. The difference between resistivity and resistance is that the resistivity depends only on the material; an object's resistance also depends on its shape and dimensions. (Technically, resistivity may also be affected by temperature, but it is independent of the material's shape and size.) Specifically, for a wire or other cylindrical (or prism-shaped) object, $R = \frac{\rho L}{A}$, where R is the object's resistance, ρ is its resistivity, L is its length, and A its cross-sectional area. We can also use this equation to figure out the units of resistivity: for the units on both sides of this equation to match, resistivity must have units of $\Omega \cdot \text{m}$, or ohms times meters.

Capacitance

Capacitance is the ability of an object to store electrical charge. Although almost any object can store some charge and technically has a nonzero capacitance, the term is typically used mostly in relation to circuit elements called capacitors, which are specially designed for this purpose. In the case of parallel-plate capacitors, it is used not for the total charge of both plates (which remains zero) but for the charge stored by each plate of a capacitor, in which case it is technically called mutual capacitance. The units of capacitance are farads, abbreviated F, and named after Michael Faraday, an English physicist and chemist who was responsible for many fundamental discoveries regarding electromagnetism.

As capacitance can be thought of as the ratio of the charge of an object to the voltage across it, the units of capacitance are equal to the units of charge over the units of voltage: 1 F = 1 C/V. In terms of the fundamental metric units, $1\ \text{F} = 1\ \text{s}^2\,\text{C}^2 / (\text{m}^2\ \text{kg})$. Compared to the capacitances of the capacitors traditionally used in circuits, the farad is a very large unit, and in practice capacitances have been usually stated in millifarads, microfarads, nanofarads, or even picofarads.

Parallel Plate Capacitor

One way to conceive of capacitance is as the amount of charge that can be induced in an object by a unit voltage. This definition leads directly to the equation relating charge to voltage in a capacitor: $Q = CV$, where Q is the charge, C is the capacitance (the ability of the particular capacitor or object to store charge), and V is the voltage. This means that for a given capacitor, the charge is directly proportional to the voltage across the capacitor. Of course, this only holds as long as the voltage is not too large; if the voltage exceeds a quantity known as the breakdown voltage of the material, the proportional relationship no longer applies.

For instance, if a 2.0 μF parallel-plate capacitor has a charge of 5 mC on each plate, then the voltage across the capacitor is $V = \frac{Q}{C} = \frac{5 \cdot 10^{-3} \text{C}}{2.0 \cdot 10^{-6}\ \mu\text{F}} = 2{,}500$ V.

Energy of Charged Capacitor

The energy stored in a charged capacitor is equal to $U = \frac{1}{2}\frac{Q^2}{C}$, where Q is the charge of the capacitor and C is the capacitance. The most straightforward way to derive this formula is through calculus, but it is possible to justify it without use of calculus, using the equation for the work done in moving a charge across a potential difference: $W = qV$. Because the voltage changes as the charge accumulates, we can't simply assume that the work is equal to the total charge Q times the voltage, but as the voltage changes linearly with the charge, we can use the average voltage. The initial voltage is zero, and the final voltage is $V = \frac{Q}{C}$, so the average voltage is $\frac{1}{2}\frac{Q}{C}$. The potential difference is then $Q\left(\frac{1}{2}\frac{Q}{C}\right) = \frac{1}{2}\frac{Q^2}{C}$.

The relationship among charge, voltage, and capacitance, $Q = CV$, can be used to rewrite the equation for the energy in several different ways: $U = \frac{1}{2}\frac{Q^2}{C} = \frac{1}{2}CV^2 = \frac{1}{2}QV$.

Capacitors in Parallel

In a parallel-plate capacitor, two conductive plates are separated by a thin layer of vacuum or polarizable insulating material (dielectric). The electric field within the capacitor depends on the charge on each capacitor and the area of the plates: for a capacitor where the plates are separated by a vacuum, it is equal to $E = \frac{Q}{\varepsilon_0 A}$, where Q is the charge on each plate, A is the area of the plates, and ε_0 is a constant called the permittivity of free space, equal to $8.854 \cdot 10^{-12}$ F/m.

Knowing the electric field within the capacitor, we can use this to determine the capacitance. We know from the relationship between voltage and electric field that the voltage across the capacitor must be $V = Ed$, where d is the distance between the plates, and we know that for a capacitor $Q = CV$. So $C = \frac{Q}{V} = \frac{Q}{Ed} = \frac{Q}{\left(\frac{Q}{\varepsilon_0 A}\right)d} = \frac{\varepsilon_0 A}{d}$.

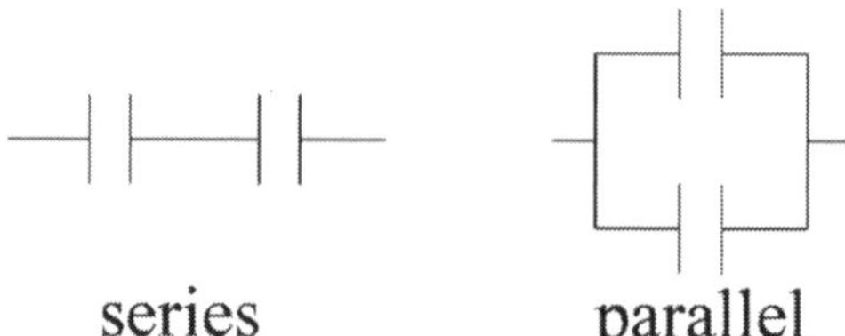

For capacitors in series (joined linearly end to end), the reciprocals of the capacitances add together: $C_{net} = \frac{1}{\frac{1}{C_1}+\frac{1}{C_2}+\cdots}$. For example, if you connect a 200 μF and a 300 μF capacitor in series, the net capacitance is $\frac{1}{\frac{1}{200\ \mu F}+\frac{1}{300\ \mu F}} = 120\ \mu F$.

For capacitors in parallel (with each end of each the capacitor connected to the corresponding end of the others), capacitances simply add together: $C_{net} = C_1 + C_2 + \cdots$. For example, if you connect a 200 μF and a 300 μF capacitor in series, their net capacitance is 200 μF + 300 μF = 500 μF.

Note that this is reversed from how resistors join together: mathematically, capacitors in series work like resistors in parallel, and capacitors in parallel work like resistors in series.

Dielectrics

A dielectric is a polarizable insulating material that can be placed between the plates of a capacitor to increase its capacitance. In fact, although capacitors are often introduced by first discussing those with vacuums between the plates, in practice most real-world capacitors do include a dielectric, largely because keeping the plates of a capacitor separated with nothing between them but a vacuum is impractical.

Dielectrics are characterized by a quantity called the dielectric constant—sometimes also called the relative permittivity—that measures the strength of the dielectric: how much it affects the properties of the capacitor. The dielectric constant, commonly abbreviated k, is a unit-less value. The dielectric constant of vacuum is 1, that of air is very close to 1 (about 1.00059 at room temperature), but other materials may have dielectric constants in the thousands.

Because of the polarization of the dielectric, the effective electric field inside a capacitor with a dielectric is divided by the dielectric constant. It follows that the dielectric also affects the capacitance: $C = kC_0$, where C_0 would be the capacitance without the dielectric. For a parallel plate capacitor, $C = \frac{k\varepsilon_0 A}{d}$. The energy stored in the capacitor is likewise multiplied by the dielectric constant.

Conductivity

Metallic vs. Electrolytic Conductivity

Metallic conductivity is conductivity due to the flow of electrons. It is so called because it is this process that leads to the conductivity of solid metals; the nuclei of the metal atoms stay in place, while electrons flow between them.

Electrolytic conductivity is conductivity due to the flow of ions. It is this that leads to the conductivity, for example, of saltwater; not just electrons but entire Na^+ and Cl^- ions (and H^+ and OH^- ions) flow through the solution.

Among the differences in the effects of these two kinds of conductivity, electrolytic conductivity leads to chemical change as different ions accumulate at the positive and negative terminals; there is no chemical change involved in metallic conductivity as the nuclei of the atoms remain in place. Furthermore, the conductivity of a metallic conductor tends to decrease with temperature, whereas the conductivity of an electrolytic conductor tends to increase with temperature.

METERS

There are a number of kinds of meters that can measure properties of electric circuits, but perhaps the most common are these:

- Voltmeters are used to measure the voltage across a circuit element or a part of the circuit. Voltmeters are always connected in parallel to the circuit element(s), the voltage of which they are measuring.
- Ammeters are used to measure the current through a particular part of the circuit. The ammeter must be connected in series; the circuit is broken and the ammeter inserted. An ammeter that works by generating a magnetic field in a coil is called a galvanometer.
- Ohmmeters measure the resistance of a circuit element; they are connected across individual elements or collections of elements when the circuit is disconnected and no current is flowing.

Now, instruments are common that depending on their settings, can work as voltmeters, ammeters, or ohmmeters; these versatile instruments are called multimeters.

Other less common types of meters include capacitance meters, which as their name implies measure the capacitance of a circuit element, and wattmeters, which measure electric power.

MAGNETISM

DEFINITION OF MAGNETIC FIELD

The magnetic field, abbreviated $\vec{B}$, is a measurement of the magnetic effect on a moving charged particle. (The B doesn't stand for anything; this letter is used only because the Scottish physicist James Clerk Maxwell, who determined some of the basic laws of electromagnetism, arbitrarily used the letters A through H to stand for various quantities, and his use of B for the magnetic field happened to catch on and stick.)

The units of the magnetic field strength are the Tesla, abbreviated T and named after the Serbian-American engineer and inventor Nikola Tesla. One Tesla is equal to 1 kilogram per coulomb second: 1 T = 1 kg / (C s). This can be rewritten in a number of different, equivalent ways: 1 T = 1 kg / (C s) = 1 V s / m^2 = 1 N / (A m) = ...

MOTION OF CHARGED PARTICLES IN MAGNETIC FIELDS

The magnitude of the force on a moving charged particle due to a magnetic field can be calculated from the equation $F = qvBsin\ \theta$, where q is the charge of the particle, v is its speed, B is the magnitude of the magnetic field, and θ is the angle between the particle's velocity and the field.

This equation, however, gives the magnitude but not the direction. This can be found by a vector form of the equation using vector cross-products: $\vec{F} = q\ \vec{v} \times \vec{B}$. It can also be found through the right-hand rule. This rule takes many forms, but one is this: if you point the thumb of your right hand in the direction of the particle's velocity, and your index finger in the direction of the field, then the palm of your hand will face the direction of the force.

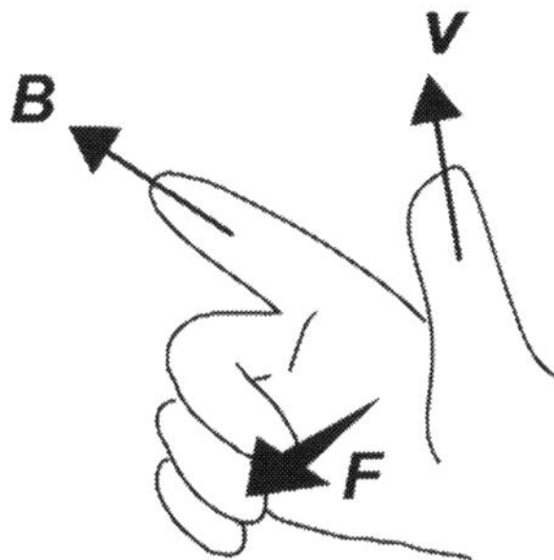

Note that the direction of the force is always perpendicular to both the velocity of the particle and the field.

Lorentz Force

The Lorentz force is the total force on a charged particle due to electromagnetic fields. It is named after Dutch physicist Hendrik Antoon Lorentz, who is also known for developing the coordinate transformation equations that later played an important part in Einstein's theory of relativity.

The Lorentz force can be calculated by simply adding together the formulas for the electric force and magnetic force: $\vec{F} = q\vec{E} + q\vec{v} \times \vec{B}$. Note that if the electric field and magnetic field are perpendicular, then it is possible for the electric and magnetic forces on a charged particle moving perpendicular to both to cancel and leave a Lorentz force of zero – but only on particles of a particular velocity equal in magnitude to $\frac{E}{B}$. This can be used to filter particles of specific velocities.

The force on a moving charged particle in a magnetic field is equal in magnitude to $F = qVB \sin \theta$ and is always perpendicular to the particle's velocity and to the field. When the velocity is perpendicular to the field, a force will be produced that changes the particle's velocity, but because the force is perpendicular to the field, the velocity will also remain perpendicular to the field, and the particle will keep turning in the same direction until its trajectory traces a circle. (It is easier to visualize this in small discrete steps, but of course in reality the particle's path will be smooth and continuous.)

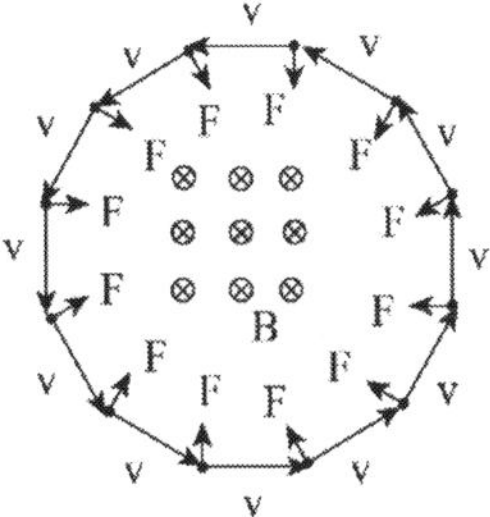

If the velocity is parallel to the field, $\sin \theta = 0$ and no force is produced; the particle continues moving at constant velocity.

For a velocity at some angle in between, the component of the velocity parallel to the field is unaffected, but the component perpendicular to the field is altered into a circle, as before. Putting these two together, the total trajectory of the particle is in a helical path, like the threads on a screw.

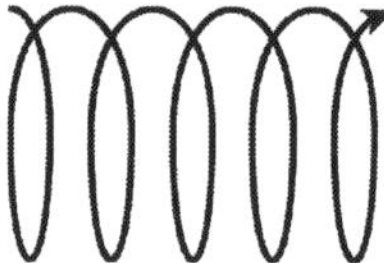

ELECTROCHEMISTRY

ELECTROLYTIC CELL

ELECTROLYSIS

Electrolysis is the use of current to induce a chemical reaction that would not otherwise occur. For instance, passing a sufficiently strong current through pure water can split it into hydrogen and oxygen, $2H_2O \rightarrow 2H_2 + O_2$.

Electrolysis is used to purify metals, to deposit thin films of metal on other materials (electroplating), and to produce useful chemicals, including sodium hydroxide and potassium chlorate. The electrolysis of water also has applications; it is used to create hydrogen fuel and to produce breathable oxygen for the International Space Station.

ELECTROLYTE

An electrolyte is a substance that separates into positive and negative ions when dissolved in water. The resulting solution remains electrically neutral because the total charge of the positive ions equals the total charge of the negative ions, but the presence of the ions makes the solution electrically conductive.

One of the most familiar everyday electrolytes is table salt, sodium chloride, NaCl, which when dissolved in water separates into sodium ions (Na^+) and chlorine ions (Cl^-). Other common electrolytes include hydrochloric acid (HCl); sodium hydroxide, or lye (NaOH); and baking soda, or sodium bicarbonate ($NaHCO_3$). Electrolytes play an important role in the body; the charge they carry is important for the working of nerves and muscles and to regulate fluid balance.

ELECTRON FLOW; OXIDATION, AND REDUCTION AT THE ELECTRODES

In electrolysis, current is passed through an electrolytic substance to cause a chemical reaction to occur. The electrodes are the conductors that connect the substance to the rest of the circuit. The current flows from the voltage source to one electrode, called the anode, through the solution to another electrode, called the cathode, and back to the voltage source.

Because current is defined as the flow of positive charge, the direction that electrons travel through the circuit is opposite the current. The electrons, therefore, move from the anode into the voltage source and from the voltage source into the cathode. This means that the anode tends to accumulate a positive charge as electrons move from it and the cathode a negative charge as electrons move into it. Each electrode attracts from the solution ions of the opposite charge. Positive ions flow toward the cathode and negative toward the anode. Because of the excess of electrons at the cathode, the ions there tend to undergo reduction reactions, reacting with electrons and reducing their oxidation numbers. On the other hand, the ions at the anode tend to undergo oxidation reactions.

Galvanic or Voltaic Cell

Half-Reactions

A galvanic or voltaic cell is a device that uses oxidation and reduction reactions in electrolytic solutions to produce electrical current. (There is no difference between a galvanic cell and a voltaic cell; these are two words for the same thing.) Electrical batteries consist of one or more galvanic cells.

A voltaic cell consists of two electrodes of different metals in different solutions. The electrodes are connected by a wire, and the solutions are either separated by a permeable membrane or connected by a "salt bridge" that allows some ions to flow between them and maintain the electrical neutrality of the solutions. The metals and solutions are chosen so that an oxidation reaction will occur at the electrode in one solution (the anode) and a reduction reaction will occur at the electrode in the other (the cathode). We refer therefore to the "half reaction" at each electrode. Essentially, as the metal atoms at the anode are oxidized, they release electrons that flow through the wire to the cathode, where they react to reduce metal ions at the cathode there. (Technically, single electrons don't make the entire circuit, but the effect is as if they did.)

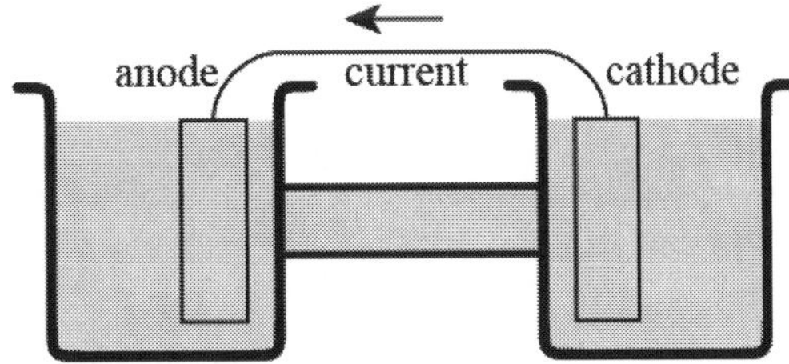

Reduction Potentials and Cell Potentials

The reduction potential is a measurement of how strongly a particular chemical substance tends to acquire electrons and undergo a reduction reaction. It is measured in volts, the units of electrical potential. A substance with a much stronger reduction potential will tend to take electrons from a substance with a much weaker reduction potential, causing the latter to be oxidized.

The cell potential is the electrical potential produced by a galvanic cell. It is equal to the difference between the reduction potentials of the materials making up the two electrodes. In fact, because the reduction potential of a material can't readily be measured directly; it is generally cell potentials that are used to determine reduction potentials, with the reduction potential of a "standard hydrogen electrode" defined as zero as a baseline.

Concentration Cell

A concentration cell is a type of galvanic cell in which both half-cells contain the same chemicals but differ in their concentrations. Concentration cells work because although the chemical compositions of the two half-cells are the same, the different concentrations still generate a potential difference. To equalize the concentrations and bring the system to equilibrium, ions undergo a reduction reaction at the electrode in the higher-concentration solution (which therefore acts as the cathode), and metal atoms undergo an oxidation reaction at the electrode in the lower-concentration solution (the anode).

The potential of a concentration cell can be determined by the Nernst equation, named after the German chemist Walther Hermann Nernst, known for his work in thermodynamics and electrochemistry. The Nernst equation states that at room temperature, the potential of an electrical cell is $E_{cell} = E^0_{cell} - \frac{0.0257}{z}\ln Q$, where E^0_{cell} is the standard cell potential if the concentrations were equal, z is the number of electrons transferred in each reaction, and Q is the reaction quotient, which is essentially equal to the ratios of the concentrations of the reactants and products. For a concentration cell, $E_{cell}^0 = 0$, and this reduces to $E_{cell} = -\frac{0.0257}{z}\ln Q = -\frac{0.0592}{z}\log_{10} Q$.

Batteries

Lead-Storage Batteries

A lead-storage battery is a galvanic cell in which the anode consists of lead, the cathode consists of lead dioxide (PbO_2), and the electrodes are surrounded by dilute sulfuric acid (H_2SO_4). Because both electrodes are immersed in the same electrolyte, it isn't necessary to have separate half-cells divided by a membrane or connected by a salt bridge. As the lead-storage battery discharges, the lead at the anode is oxidized and reacts with HSO_4^- ions in the solution to generate lead (II) sulfate ($PbSO_4$), while the lead dioxide at the cathode is reduced and reacts to also produce lead (II) sulfate. The full half-reactions are as follows:

- Anode: $Pb(s) + HSO_4^-(aq) \rightarrow PbSO_4(s) + H^+(aq) + 2e^-$
- Cathode: $PbO_2(s) + HSO_4^-(aq) + 3H^+(aq) + 2e^- \rightarrow PbSO_4(s) + 2H_2O(l)$

Lead-storage batteries are commonly used in cars. They have the advantage of being relatively lightweight and inexpensive and, importantly, of being rechargeable: because the lead sulfate generated in the redox reactions is not soluble, it remains available for reaction, and driving a current through the battery can reverse the discharge reactions and recharge its potential.

Nickel-Cadmium Batteries

A nickel-cadmium battery is a type of rechargeable battery commonly used in cordless power tools, although these batteries are becoming less common than they used to be as their place is being taken by nickel metal hydride batteries and lithium ion batteries. They have the advantage over alkaline batteries and lead-storage batteries of delivering a more or less constant voltage over time rather than having their voltage decrease significantly as the battery is depleted.

A nickel-cadmium battery consists of galvanic cells with cadmium anodes and nickel oxide hydroxide NiO(OH) cathodes. They are immersed in an alkaline electrolyte, commonly potassium hydroxide (KOH). The following are the half-reactions occurring at each electrode:

- Anode: $Cd(s) + 2OH^-(aq) \rightarrow Cd(OH)_2(s) + 2e^-$
- Cathode: $2NiO(OH)(s) + 2H_2O(l) + 2e^- \rightarrow 2Ni(OH)_2(s) + 2OH^-(aq)$

Because the electrolyte is not consumed in the net reaction, and because both the products cadmium hydroxide and nickel (II) hydroxide are insoluble in alkaline solutions, the battery is rechargeable; when a current is run through the battery, these reactions will occur in reverse.

How Light and Sound Interact with Matter

Sound

Production of Sound

Sound is, in essence, a vibration in a medium that propagates through the medium as a compression wave. All that is necessary to produce a sound, therefore, is to produce a vibration in some medium. Sound can pass from one medium to another; so, for example, a sound wave in air could have originated from the vibration of a metal plate in contact with the air. In fact, often when we produce a sound, it isn't by generating a vibration in the air directly but by producing a vibration in some solid object, which vibration is then transmitted to the air.

For example, when the skin of a drum is hit, it vibrates, producing a characteristic sound. Plucking a string, or drawing a bow across it, causes the string to vibrate, which is the basis of the working of pianos and string instruments. We produce sound with our voices by blowing air across taut mucous membranes in our larynges called vocal cords. In a wind or brass instrument such as a flute or trumpet, the air is more or less set in motion directly, but the shape of the instrument affects how the waves interfere and build up.

Relative Speed of Sound in Solids, Liquids, and Gases

Sound is a compression wave that travels through a medium. It is transmitted through the medium as particles collide and interact. Therefore, the greater the forces between the particles, the more readily the disturbance will propagate through the medium, and the faster the wave will travel. In a solid, the atoms or molecules are subject to significant intermolecular forces, which is why a solid tends to hold its shape. In a liquid, the intermolecular forces are smaller than those in a solid, but they are still sufficient to cause the liquid to maintain its volume. In a gas, the intermolecular forces are very small, and the particles may be very far apart. Therefore, sound will tend to travel faster through solids than through liquids and faster through liquids than gases.

The speed of sound also depends on the density—all else being equal, the denser the material, the slower sound travels through it because it takes more energy to set the material in motion. In practice, however, this effect tends to be less significant than the effect of the intermolecular forces.

Intensity of Sound

The absolute intensity of a sound, abbreviated I, is the amount of power contained in the sound per unit area: $I = \frac{P}{A}$. This intensity is measured in watts per square meter. However, we don't really hear a sound with twice the intensity as twice as loud; the apparent volume of a sound, or intensity level, has a logarithmic relationship to the intensity. This intensity level is measured in a unit called decibels. The decibel, abbreviated dB, originated as one-tenth of a now rarely used unit called the bel, named after Scottish-American engineer and inventor Alexander Graham Bell, most famous for inventing, or at least being first to patent, the telephone.

The relationship between the intensity I and the intensity level L_I is $L_I = 10\text{ dB}\log_{10}\frac{I}{I_0}$, where I is a reference intensity, conventionally 10^{-12} W/m^2 (approximately the lowest intensity of sound that the average human can hear). For instance, a sound with an absolute intensity of 0.5 W/m^2 would have an intensity level of $10\text{ dB}\log\frac{0.5\text{ W/m}^2}{10^{-12}\text{W/m}^2} = 10\text{dB}\log(5 \cdot 10^{11}\text{W/m}^2) = 117\text{ dB}$.

Attenuation (Damping)

A sound is attenuated, or damped, when there are dissipative forces that turn some of the energy of the wave into thermal energy. In a substance such as an ideal gas with no intermolecular forces, or with perfectly elastic intermolecular forces, no attenuation will occur, and the sound will propagate indefinitely at the same intensity. In reality, of course, no such perfect substances exist, and the internal forces between molecules will tend to dissipate some of the energy and cause the sound to be attenuated over time. (Even in a superfluid, an exotic liquid with zero viscosity, sound attenuation occurs due to interactions between pairs of particles.) Of course, it is possible to intentionally damp a sound by applying an external force—such as pressing down on a vibrating guitar string with a finger to stop its vibration.

The effect of attenuation is to decrease the sound's amplitude. Due to attenuation, a damped sound will gradually "die out" over time, its amplitude decreasing until it can no longer be detected. In most cases, the amplitude of the sound follows an exponential decay model.

Doppler Effect

Moving Sound Source or Observer

If a source is emitting a sound as it moves toward an observer, the successive crests of the sound wave will reach the observer at a higher frequency than if the source were stationary because when the source emits each wave, it is slightly closer to the observer than it was when it emitted the last one, so each new wave has a shorter distance to travel. A careful consideration of the quantities involved shows that the apparent frequency of the sound to the observer is $f = \left(\frac{v}{v-v_S}\right) f_0$, where v is the velocity of sound in the medium, v_s the velocity of the source, and f_0 the frequency of the sound as it is emitted. By similar arguments if the source is moving away from the observer or the observer is moving toward or away from the source, ultimately, we get the general equation $f = \left(\frac{v+v_o}{v-v_S}\right) f_0$, where v_o is the velocity of the observer, and v_o and v_s are each considered positive if the source or observer is moving toward the other and negative if it is moving away.

In general, then, a sound seems higher pitched if the source is moving toward the observer, or vice versa, and lower-pitched if it is moving away.

Reflection of Sound from a Moving Object

If a sound is reflected off a moving object, its frequency appears to change—the frequency seems higher if the object is moving toward the source and lower if it is moving away. To see why this is the case, and to quantify it, we can consider two adjacent crests hitting a moving object. We'll call the speed of the object v_s and the speed of sound in the medium v. Suppose a crest of the sound wave emitted at time $t = 0$ hits the object when it is at a distance D_1 from the observer; this will occur at time $t_1 = \frac{D_1}{v}$. A second crest is emitted at time T_0, where T_0 is the period of the wave, and will hit the object at a distance D_2 from the observer at time $t_1 + \Delta t = T_0 + \frac{D_2}{v}$. Using the fact that $D_2 - D_1 = v_S \Delta t$, some algebraic manipulation yields $\Delta t = \frac{T_0}{1-\frac{v_S}{v}}$. But the time for each reflected crest to return to the source is twice the time it takes to reach the object, so the apparent period $T = 2\Delta t = \frac{2T_0}{1-\frac{v_S}{v}}$. The apparent frequency is then $f = \frac{1}{T} = \frac{1}{T_0}\left(1 - \frac{v_S}{v}\right) = f_0\left(1 - \frac{v_S}{v}\right)$, where v_s is positive if the source is moving away from the object and negative if it is moving toward it.

Pitch

The pitch of a sound is how high or low it seems to the ear. A siren has a very high pitch and a foghorn a very low pitch. The keys to the right on a piano produce higher-pitched sounds than the keys to the left.

The pitch of a sound depends on the frequency of the sound wave—the number of vibrations per second. The higher the frequency, the higher the pitch. The frequency of a wave can in turn be affected by other factors. For a wave in a string, for instance, all else being equal, the higher the tension in the string, the higher the frequency, and the heavier the string, the lower the frequency. (Technically, these factors directly affect the velocity of the wave in the string, but this has an indirect effect on the frequency.) This is why the lower-pitched strings of a string instrument are thicker than the higher-pitched strings and why the instrument can be tuned by altering the strings' tensions.

Resonance in Pipes and Strings

The resonant frequencies on a string are frequencies at which the waves will constructively interfere and reinforce each other, leading to "standing waves" that have consistent points of zero amplitude (nodes). An important constraint on the resonant frequencies is that the ends of the string must be nodes because they are stationary. Because each full wave contains one node at each end and one in the middle, the only way for standing waves in the string to be possible is if the string contains an integral or half-integral number of wavelengths: $L = \frac{n\lambda}{2}$, where L is the length of the string, λ the wavelength of the waves, and n an arbitrary positive integer.

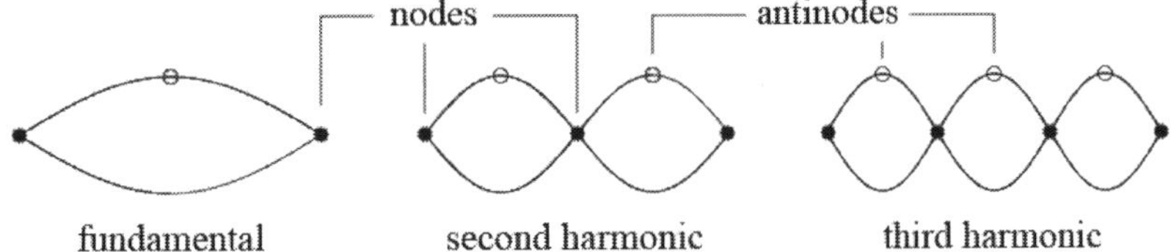

The frequency is related to the wavelength by the equation $v = f\lambda$. So $f = \frac{v}{\lambda} = \frac{v}{\frac{2L}{n}} = \frac{nv}{2L}$. This can be rewritten as $f = nf_0$, where f_0 is the lowest possible frequency, $f_0 = \frac{v}{2L}$. This lowest frequency is called the fundamental frequency, whereas higher resonant frequencies are called the harmonics. We can even go a little further: the velocity of a wave in a string is $v = \sqrt{\frac{T}{\mu}}$, where T is the tension in the string and μ its mass per unit length, so $f_0 = \frac{1}{2L}\sqrt{\frac{T}{\mu}}$.

A resonant frequency is a frequency at which reflected waves constructively interfere, producing standing waves and waves with fixed positions of zero amplitude (nodes) and of maximum amplitude (antinodes). A standing wave in a pipe must have a node where the pipe's end is closed and an antinode where it is open. Therefore, a pipe with open ends must have an antinode on each end; a pipe with closed ends must have a node on each end; and a pipe with one open and one closed end must have a node on one end and an antinode on the other.

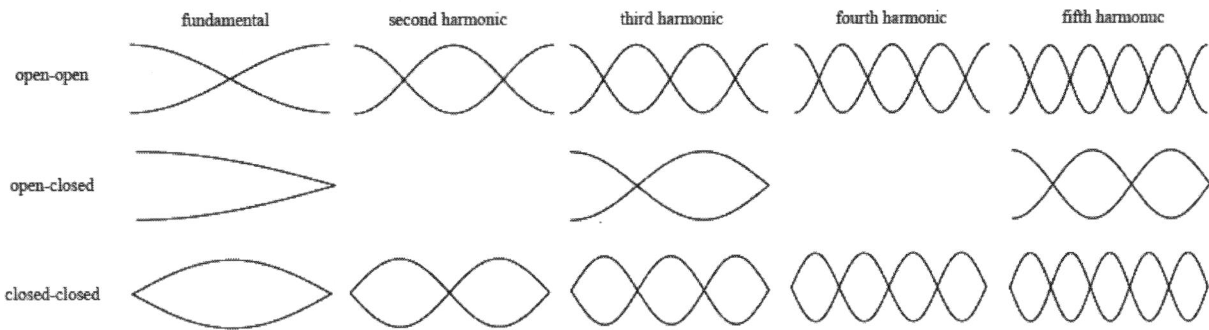

A pipe with open ends and a pipe with closed ends both must have a length that is an integral number of half-wavelengths: $L = \frac{n\lambda}{2}$, so $\lambda = \frac{2L}{n}$. For an open/closed pipe, there's a quarter wavelength between a node and an antinode, but because antinodes and nodes alternate, we have to have an odd number of quarter wavelengths. Thus, for this case $L = \frac{n\lambda}{4}$, or $\lambda = \frac{4L}{n}$, with the additional constraint that n must be odd.

Now, using $v = f\lambda$, we can find the frequency: $f = \frac{nv}{2L}$ for an open-open or open-closed pipe and for an open-closed pipe $f = \frac{nv}{4L}$, where n must be odd.

Ultrasound

Ultrasound is sound with a frequency too high for humans to hear. The typical range of human hearing is from about 20 Hz to 20,000 Hz, although the upper end of this range tends to decline with age. Ultrasound includes frequencies above 20,000 Hz.

Although it is inaudible, ultrasound has many applications. High-frequency sound waves can travel efficiently through solid and liquid matter, so ultrasound can be used to generate an image of the interior of an object—most famously, ultrasonic imagery can be used to "look at" fetuses still in the womb. Ultrasound is also useful for range finding; sonar works by sending out ultrasonic pulses, detecting their return, and using the time elapsed to determine how far they had traveled before encountering and reflecting off an object.

Shock Waves

A shock wave is an abrupt pressure difference that propagates through a medium; it is similar to a single, very intense sound wave, although the sharp, almost discontinuous nature of the pressure change makes it qualitatively different from ordinary sound waves. A shock wave in air is heard as a loud cracking or booming sound.

A shock wave occurs whenever a disturbance in a fluid travels faster than the speed of sound in that fluid. Essentially, the particles of the medium can't "keep up" with the change, so instead of the gradual, continuous change in pressure that would normally occur, the pressure and other properties change nearly instantaneously. An object moving through the fluid faster than the speed of sound will disturb the fluid enough to produce a shock wave. This is why supersonic air craft produce "sonic booms"—the "boom" is the effect of a shock wave produced by the plane's supersonic disturbance of the medium. On a smaller scale, the crack of a whip is produced by the tip of the whip traveling at supersonic speeds and producing a similar sudden disturbance in the air.

Light, Electromagnetic Radiation

Concept of Interference

Young Double-Slit Experiment

Named after English physicist and physiologist Thomas Young (although others had done versions of the experiment earlier), the Young Double-Slit Experiment is an experiment in which, in its usual modern form, a coherent light source such as a laser beam is shined through two thin slits onto a screen some distance behind them. Rather than an image of the slits, what is produced on the screen is an interference pattern of dark and light bands, their spacing dependent on the wavelength of the light and on the distance between the slits. Specifically, for a distant screen, the bright bands appear at the positions $y_m = \frac{m\lambda L}{d}$, where λ is the wavelength, L the distance to the screen, d the distance between the slits, and m an arbitrary integer.

Young's purpose in performing a version of this experiment was to demonstrate the wave nature of light. Although the experiment is still considered a classic demonstration of this principle, later variations involving particles instead of waves suggested wave-particle duality and laid some of the foundation for the theory of quantum mechanics.

Wave Interference

Wave interference occurs when two waves overlap and combine. Essentially, the displacements of two overlapping waves add together at each point. It can be classified into constructive interference, in which the combined wave is larger than either individual wave, and destructive interference, in which it is smaller. If two identical waves are perfectly in phase, they will constructively interfere into a wave twice as large; if they are perfectly out of phase, they will destructively interfere and completely cancel.

Wave interference is fundamental to the understanding of resonance and standing waves. The interference of light waves is responsible for the colors of bubbles and thin films of oil. Interference also has applications such as noise-cancelling headphones and interferometry, the use of interference between two beams of light following different paths to measure very small distances.

Thin Films, Diffraction Grating, Single-Slit Diffraction

Light shined through a thin single slit onto a screen some distance behind it will form an interference pattern of bright and dark lines. The positions of the dark lines are given by the equation $y_m = \frac{m\lambda L}{a}$, where λ is the wavelength, *L* the distance to the screen, *d* the distance between the slits, and *m* a nonzero integer. This occurs because the slit, although thin, still has a finite width, and the light passing through some positions in the slit interferes with the light passing through others.

The single-slit diffraction equation is very similar to the equation for double-slit diffraction but differs in that whereas the single-slit equation shows the position of the dark lines, the double-slit diffraction equation gives the positions of the bright lines—as well as, of course, the constraint in the single-slit case that *m* cannot be zero. In practice, light shined through a double slit shows not a perfect single-slit pattern but the superimposed patterns from the single- and double-slit interference because single-slit interference occurs at each slit.

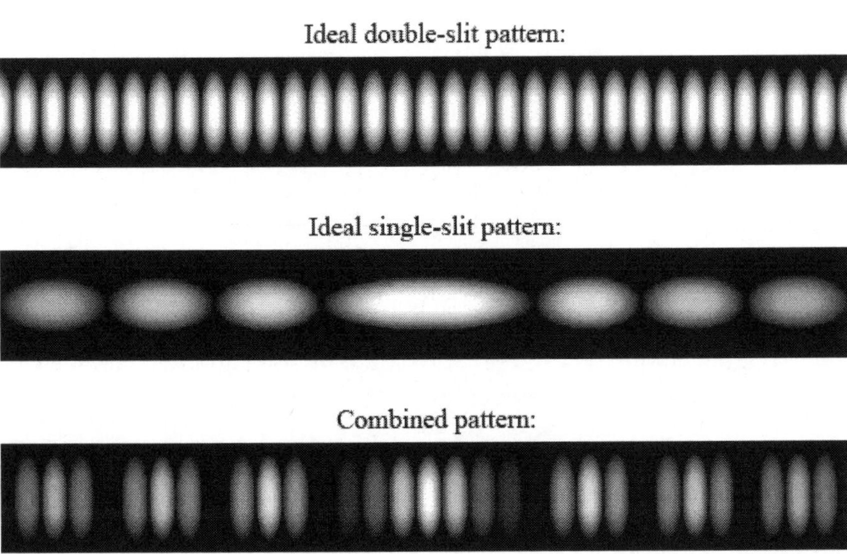

Thin-film interference refers to the interference between light that reflects off the surface of a thin film of a transparent material and light that passes through the film and reflects off a surface behind it. Because the light that passed through the film has traveled a slightly larger distance, it will be slightly out of phase with the light that reflected from the surface of the film, which is what causes the interference. In terms of the thickness of the film *t*, the film's index of refraction *n*, the angle of incidence *θ*, and the wavelength of the light *λ*, the condition for constructive interference is either

$2nt \cos\theta = m\lambda$ if the index of refraction of the film is greater than the index of refraction behind it (like an anti-reflective coating or a soap film on water) or $2nt \cos\theta = \left(m - \frac{1}{2}\right)\lambda$ if the index of refraction of the film is less than the index of refraction behind it (like a soap bubble in air or an oil film on water). In these equations, m is an arbitrary positive integer. The difference in the equations arises because the light reflecting off a material with a greater index of refraction undergoes a 180° phase change.

Other Diffraction Phenomena

A diffraction grating is an instrument consisting of an opaque plate with a number of very thin open or transparent slits or grooves, evenly and closely spaced. Typical diffraction gratings used in labs may have hundreds or thousands of slits per millimeter.

Diffraction gratings produce diffraction patterns like double slits, but the large number of slits allows the patterns to be brighter and more easily measurable. The spacing of the bright lines on the diffraction pattern follows the same relationship as for the double slit: $m\lambda = d\sin\theta$, where d is the spacing of the grating, λ is the wavelength of the light, θ is the angle at which the light is deflected from the slit to the position on the screen, and m is an arbitrary integer. When the distance L of the grating to the screen or detector is very large compared to d, this can be rewritten as $y_m = \frac{m\lambda L}{d}$, where y_m is the distance from the center of the diffraction pattern to the mth bright line on that side.

Because diffraction gratings diffract different wavelengths to different positions, they are useful for separating wavelengths of light and for finding what wavelengths of light are present in a source.

Polarization of Light

Light waves are transverse waves, and as such the oscillation of the electromagnetic fields in a light wave occurs in some particular direction perpendicular to the direction of propagation. In an ordinary beam of light, the directions of oscillation of different waves that make up the beam are randomly distributed; there are likely to be just as many waves oscillating in one direction as another. Light is said to be polarized if the directions of oscillation of the waves match up with each other if all the waves are oscillating in the same direction.

Although our eyes can't easily detect a difference between polarized and non-polarized light (although this isn't true of the eyes of bees and some other animals), it is possible to make filters that only let through light oscillating in a particular direction. Light reflecting in certain ways off flat surfaces is naturally polarized, such as the glare off of water or concrete. Polarized sunglasses eliminate the glare by filtering out the light polarized parallel to the ground. Polarization also is commonly used in 3-D movies; the light intended for the left and right eye is polarized in perpendicular directions and filtered accordingly by the 3-D glasses.

Linear vs. Circular Polarization

Most of the time, when one speaks of polarization of light, it refers to linear polarization. Light, as a transverse wave, oscillates in a direction perpendicular to the direction of propagation; if all the light waves from a source oscillate in the same direction, the light is linearly polarized.

However, what is oscillating in light is the electromagnetic fields, and waves in these behave a little differently than, say, waves in a string. Instead of just oscillating in a constant direction, it is possible for the oscillations in a light wave to rotate over time. (This can be conceived of as two superimposed linear oscillations equal in magnitude but in perpendicular directions and 90° out of phase.) If all the light waves from a particular source are rotating in the same direction, then the light is said to be circularly polarized. There is also an intermediate case (similarly corresponding to two superimposed linear oscillations but with a phase shift less than 90°) called elliptical polarization.

PROPERTIES OF ELECTROMAGNETIC RADIATION

ELECTROMAGNETIC RADIATION

The speed of propagation of electromagnetic radiation, otherwise known as the speed of light, abbreviated *c*, is about $3.00 \cdot 10^8$ m/s. More specifically, it is 299,792,458 m/s; this value is exact because the meter is currently defined as the distance traveled by light in 1/299,729,458 seconds.

Technically, this value is the speed of light in a vacuum. Under these circumstances, it is invariant; perhaps counterintuitively, the speed of light in a vacuum is always the same regardless of the relative motion of the source and observer. However, when passing through a medium, the speed of light is slower due to interaction between the light and the medium. The ratio of the speed of light in a vacuum to the speed of light in a transparent material is called that material's index of refraction, n. The index of refraction of air is very close to one; light travels at almost the same speed in air as in a vacuum. The index of refraction of water is about 1.33; light travels about three-quarters as fast in water as it does in a vacuum.

In electromagnetic radiation, the electric and magnetic fields and the direction of propagation are all mutually perpendicular. As the light wave moves, the electric and magnetic fields both oscillate perpendicular to the direction of propagation (as is usual for a transverse wave) as well as perpendicular to each other. This is true even for circularly polarized waves in which the field direction rotates; the electric and magnetic fields both rotate in the same direction at the same speed and maintain their perpendicularity.

We can be more specific about the relationship between these quantities. The magnitudes of the electric and magnetic fields in electromagnetic radiation are related by the equation $E = cB$, where c is the speed of light in a vacuum. The direction of propagation is the same direction as the vector $\vec{E} \times \vec{B}$, where "×" represents the vector cross product.

CLASSIFICATION OF ELECTROMAGNETIC SPECTRUM

Electromagnetic radiation comes in a broad range of wavelengths. Although the spectrum is continuous, different ranges have different effects on living things and the environment, so certain ranges of wavelengths and frequencies are given names. From longest to shortest wavelength (smallest to highest frequency), the conventional divisions include the following:

- Radio (roughly 100 cm to 100 km)—these waves can travel large distances and are useful for communication
- Microwave (10 mm to 100 cm)—aside from their use in microwave ovens, these can also be used for communication
- Infrared (700 nm to 1 mm)—objects at human body temperature radiate infrared light, which is why night vision goggles work
- Visible (400 to 700 nm)—this very small range of wavelengths comprises what we see as visible light; not coincidentally, the radiation from the sun peaks in this range
- Ultraviolet (10 nm to 400 nm)—ultraviolet light plays a part in the phenomenon of fluorescence as well as causing sunburn

- X-ray (10 pm to 10 nm)—these rays can penetrate many solid objects, which is why they are used in X-ray machines
- Gamma ray (less than 10 pm)—often produced in nuclear reactions, gamma rays can be very hazardous to living tissue

PHOTON ENERGY

The energy of a photon depends on its frequency. The exact equation that can be used to calculate the energy of a photon is $E = hf$, where h is a constant called Planck's constant, equal to $6.626 \cdot 10^{-34}$ J·s. (Planck's constant, which also plays a large part in quantum mechanics, is named after the German physicist Max Karl Ernst Ludwig Planck, best known for the pioneering role he played in the development of quantum theory.) Sometimes the symbol ν, the lowercase Greek letter nu, is used instead of f to stand for the frequency of light, and this equation is written $E = h\nu$.

Note that this equation implies that the higher the frequency of light, the greater the energy of the photons. This relationship is responsible for many of the different effects of different frequency ranges of light. X-rays can penetrate animal tissue because they have a very short wavelength and therefore a high frequency and consequently a high energy. Gamma rays have an even shorter wavelength and an even higher energy, which is what makes them dangerous; their energy is high enough to damage important molecules within cells, including DNA.

VISUAL SPECTRUM

The color of light depends on the wavelength of the electromagnetic radiation. Equivalently, it could be said to depend on the frequency because the two are related: in a vacuum, $f = c/\lambda$. (This follows from the general wave equation $v = f\lambda$, putting c in for v and solving for f.) Light near the low-wavelength end of the visible spectrum, 400 nm, appears violet. The colors then progress through blue, green, yellow, and orange, till reaching the high-wavelength end of the visible spectrum, about 700 nm, which appears red. Other colors not in this progression (such as reddish-purple, brown, or gray) do not correspond to individual wavelengths but to mixtures of colors.

Ultraviolet, the range of electromagnetic radiation with a wavelength slightly shorter than the visible range, gets its name from the fact that it has a frequency above ("ultra-") violet. Similarly, infrared, the range of electromagnetic radiation with a wavelength slightly longer than visible, has a frequency slightly below ("infra-") red.

GEOMETRICAL OPTICS

REFLECTION FROM PLANE SURFACE

Total internal reflection occurs when light hitting a boundary between transparent materials at a sufficiently large angle of incidence completely reflects off the boundary rather than being partially reflected and partially transmitted. Total internal reflection is the principle behind fiberoptics; the light hits the side of the optical fiber at a large enough angle to be reflected down the fiber rather than leaking out of the fiber and being lost. Some reflectors in streets also work by this principle.

Total internal reflection occurs when Snell's Law cannot otherwise be satisfied. By Snell's Law, $\sin\theta_r = \frac{n_i \sin\theta_i}{n_r}$. Because the sine of an angle cannot be greater than one, this suggests that refraction cannot occur when $\frac{n_i \sin\theta_i}{n_r} > 1$, that is, when $\sin\theta_i > \frac{n_r}{n_i}$. It is worth noting that this shows that total internal reflection can occur only when passing from a material of higher index of refraction into lower, never the reverse.

ANGLE OF INCIDENCE AND ANGLE OF REFLECTION

The relationship between the angle of incidence and the angle of reflection from a smooth surface is very simple: the angle of incidence equals the angle of refraction. Although this relationship may seem trivial, it can be useful; knowing that the angle of reflection equals the angle of refraction allows the use of ray tracing to locate the images formed by a mirror and even allows the treatment of more complicated scenarios such as reflections in curved mirrors, concave or convex.

For example, one can apply this principle to show that a mirror must be at least half a person's height for the person to see his or her whole body in it. Light rays from the top of the person's head reflect off the mirror to enter the person's eye, and because of the equal angles, the vertical distances from the top of the head to the point the light hits the mirror and from that point to eye level must be equal, and the top of the mirror must be halfway between the person's eye level and the top of the person's head. The same argument applies to the light from the bottom of the person's feet.

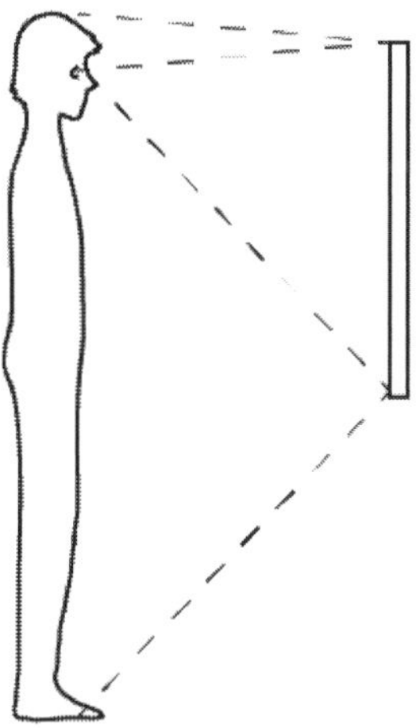

REFRACTION

REFRACTIVE INDEX

Although the index of refraction of a material is often given as a single number, it actually has some dependence on wavelength as well. For example, the index of refraction of pure water at room temperature is generally given as 1.33, but it actually varies from about 1.342 for 400 nm to 1.330 at 700 nm.

As this example shows, the dependence of index of refraction on wavelength is not necessarily large, but it still can have notable effects. It is because of this, for instance, that a prism splits white light into a spectrum because each wavelength is refracted a slightly different amount. The same phenomenon leads to rainbows, with tiny drops of water each acting like miniature prisms.

SNELL'S LAW

Snell's Law relates the amount that light is refracted (bent) on passing through the interface between two different materials to the respective indices of refraction of the materials. If the index of refraction of the material in which the light begins is n_i, that of the material in which the light ends up is n_r, and the angles of incidence and refraction are θ_i and θ_r respectively, then Snell's Law states that $n_i \sin\theta_i = n_r \sin\theta_r$.

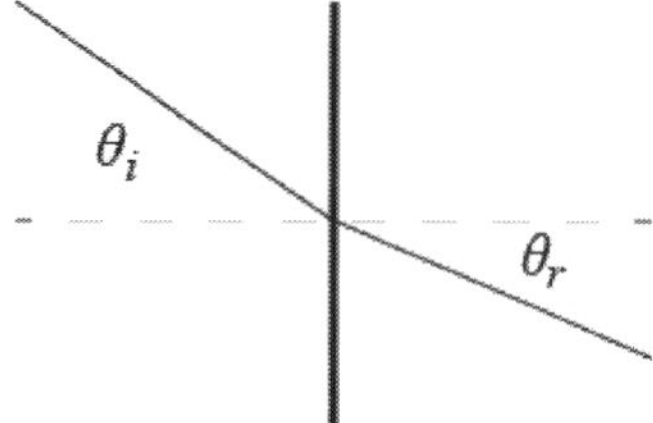

Snell's Law follows from the definition of the index of refraction as the ratio of the speed of light in a vacuum to its speed in the material. Because the frequency of the light does not change as it passes into a different material, $v = f\lambda$ implies that the wavelength must change proportionately to the speed, and it is possible (although nontrivial) to show geometrically that for the wavefronts to be continuous at the boundary, Snell's Law must hold.

Snell's Law can be used to determine an unknown index of refraction; by measuring the angles of incidence and refraction when light passes between two materials, one of which has a known index of refraction, the unknown n of the other material can be calculated.

Spherical Mirrors

Focal Length

The focal length of a spherical mirror is approximately half the radius of the mirror (i.e., the radius of the spherical surface of which the mirror is a section). This is true for both convex and concave mirrors, but the focal point will be in a different place. For a convex mirror, the focal point will be one focal length in front of the mirror (and for the purposes of the thin lens equation, the focal length can be regarded as positive). For a concave mirror, the focal point will be one focal length behind the mirror (and for the purposes of the thin lens equation, the focal length can be regarded as negative).

Real and Virtual Images

Real and virtual describe two kinds of images that can be formed by lenses or curved mirrors. A real image is an image that is formed where the reflected or refracted light rays actually converge. A virtual image is formed when the reflected or refracted rays diverge, but tracing their paths back reaches a point on the other side of the lens or mirror that they seem to be diverging from; this point is the location of the virtual image.

For an image formed by a single lens, a real image is always inverted (upside-down) and on the opposite side of the lens from the object, whereas a virtual image is always upright and on the same side of the lens as the object. For an image formed by a curved mirror, a real image is always inverted and on the same side of the mirror as the object, whereas a virtual image is upright and on the opposite side of the mirror (seeming to be behind the mirror).

Thin Lenses

Converging and Diverging Lenses

Applied to a lens, the words "converging" and "diverging" refer to the effect of the lens on parallel, incident light rays. In the case of a converging lens, these rays will converge on the opposite side of the lens. In the case of a diverging lens, the rays will diverge. Generally, converging lenses are thicker in the middle than they are at the edges, whereas diverging lenses are thicker at the edges and thinner in the middle.

Converging and diverging lenses differ in the way they form images. A diverging lens always forms a virtual image, regardless of the location of the object. A converging lens, however, can form either a real or a virtual image, depending on whether the object is closer or farther away from the lens than one focal length.

When an optical system includes more than one lens, the effective focal length and magnification of the system can be determined by considering the lenses in the order that the light passes through them and taking the image from each lens as the object of the next.

For instance, suppose you have a converging lens with a focal length of 25 cm and a diverging lens of 40 cm. The lenses are 50 cm apart, and the object is 30 cm in front of the converging lens. We first apply the thin lens equation for the converging lens: $\frac{1}{30\text{ cm}} = \frac{1}{25\text{ cm}} + \frac{1}{d_i}$; solving for d_i yields an image position of 150 cm. Because the two lenses are 50 cm apart, an image 150 cm behind the converging lens is 100 cm behind the diverging lens, so now we apply the thin lens equation again for the second lens, with an object position of –100 cm. (A multiple-lens problem like this is the only time the object distance can be negative.) So $\frac{1}{-40\text{ cm}} = \frac{1}{-100\text{ cm}} + \frac{1}{d_i}$; $d_i = -31.0$ cm. The image is 31.0 cm behind the diverging lens.

For thin lenses in contact, the effective combined focal length satisfies the equation $\frac{1}{f_{eq}} = \frac{1}{f_1} + \frac{1}{f_2}$.

Thin Lens Equation

The thin lens equation relates the focal length f of a lens to the position of an object d_o and the position of the image of the object formed by the lens, d_i, where both d_o and d_i are measured from the center of the lens: $\frac{1}{f} = \frac{1}{d_o} + \frac{1}{d_i}$. (Other choices of symbol are common; instead of d_o and d_i, one often sees s_o and s_i or p and q.) Despite the name of this equation, it also works for curved, spherical mirrors.

By convention, f is positive for a converging lens (or mirror) and negative for a diverging lens (or mirror); d_i is positive for a real image (one formed where the light rays actually converge), and negative for a virtual image (one formed where the light rays only seem to converge as traced back through the lens or mirror). Note that for a lens, a real image is on the opposite side from the image, and a virtual image is on the same side. For a mirror these are reversed; d_o is always positive except in the special case of a "virtual object" that is the image from a previous lens in a multiple-lens system and that is on the far side of the lens in question.

Lens Strength, Diopters

A diopter, abbreviated *D*, is a unit used to measure the optical power of a lens (or a curved mirror)—a measurement of how much it bends the light passing through it and how markedly it causes the light to converge or diverge. As such, the optical power has an inverse relationship to the focal length: the longer the focal length, the lower the optical power, and the shorter the focal length, the higher the optical length. As a matter of fact, the optical power is just the reciprocal of the focal length, and one diopter is simply equal to one inverse meter: $1\text{ D} = 1\text{ m}^{-1}$. For example, a lens with a focal length of 20 cm has an optical power of $\frac{1}{0.20\text{ m}} = 5.0\text{ m}^{-1} = 5.0\text{ D}$.

The diopter is not an official metric unit and is not commonly used by scientists but remains in use by optometrists and photographers.

Lens Aberration

Lens aberration is the tendency of lenses to not form perfect images. Although mathematically lenses are often treated as if they cause parallel rays to all converge to or diverge from a single point, in reality not all the parallel rays will meet at the same point. For the same reason, an image of an object in a single lens will not necessarily be perfectly clear and focused.

There are two main causes of lens aberration: spherical aberration and chromatic aberration. Spherical aberration occurs simply because a spherical lens does not form a perfect focus. It can be avoided by using lenses of other shapes; a parabolic lens, for instance, actually will focus parallel rays at a single point. Chromatic aberration occurs because the index of refraction is different for different wavelengths, so if the lens is perfectly focused for one wavelength, it can't be perfectly focused for others. Chromatic aberration can't be eliminated by using a lens of a different shape, but it is possible to arrange a system of a converging and diverging lenses so that their chromatic aberrations more or less cancel out.

Finding an Image of an Object by Ray Tracing

The image of an object can be found by choosing a point on the object and tracing three principle rays from it. Where these rays intersect—or, in the case of a virtual image, where the rays would intersect if traced back—is the location of the image. Technically, only two of the rays are sufficient to locate the object, but the third acts as a useful check.

The general principles of ray tracing work the same for any lens or mirror, but there are slight differences depending on whether it is a lens or mirror and whether it is converging or diverging. For a convex lens, these rays are the following:

- One ray that passes through the center of the lens and continues straight
- One ray that begins parallel to the optical axis (the line perpendicular through the center of the lens) and then refracts directly toward the focus on the other side
- One ray that begins by passing through the focus on the near side and then reflects or refracts parallel to the optical axis.

Depending on the position of the object, this can result in either a real or a virtual image:

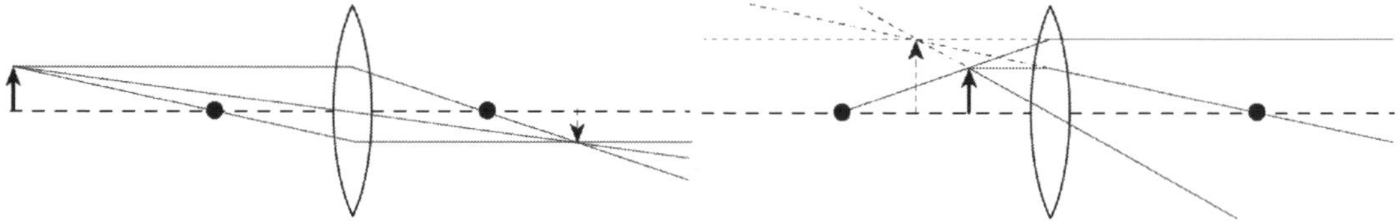

The image of an object can be found by choosing a point on the object and tracing three principle rays from it. Where these rays intersect—or, in the case of a virtual image, where the rays would intersect if traced back—is the location of the image. Technically, only two of the rays are sufficient to locate the object, but the third acts as a useful check.

The general principles of ray tracing work the same for any lens or mirror, but there are slight differences depending on whether it is a lens or mirror and whether it is converging or diverging. For a concave lens, these rays are:

- One ray that passes through the center of the lens and continues straight
- One ray that begins parallel to the optical axis (the line perpendicular through the center of the lens) and then refracts directly away from the focus on the near side
- One ray that begins by going toward the focus on the far side and then refracts parallel to the optical axis.

For a concave lens, this always results in a virtual image.

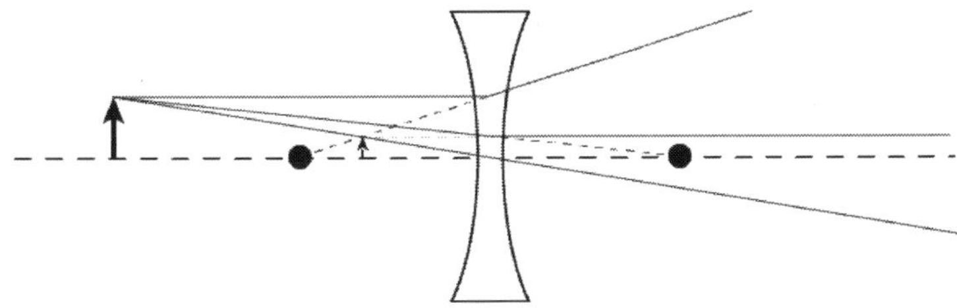

The image of an object can be found by choosing a point on the object and tracing three principle rays from it. Where these rays intersect—or, in the case of a virtual image, where the rays would intersect if traced back—is the location of the image. Technically, only two of the rays are sufficient to locate the object, but the third acts as a useful check.

The general principles of ray tracing work the same for any lens or mirror, but there are slight differences depending on whether it is a lens or mirror and whether it is converging or diverging. For a spherical mirror, these rays include the following:

- One ray that passes through the center of the mirror and reflects at the same angle
- One ray that begins parallel to the optical axis (the line perpendicular through the center of the mirror) and then reflects directly toward (convex) or away from (concave) the focus
- One ray that begins by going toward (convex) or through (concave) the focus and then reflects parallel to the optical axis.

For a convex mirror, this always results in a virtual image.

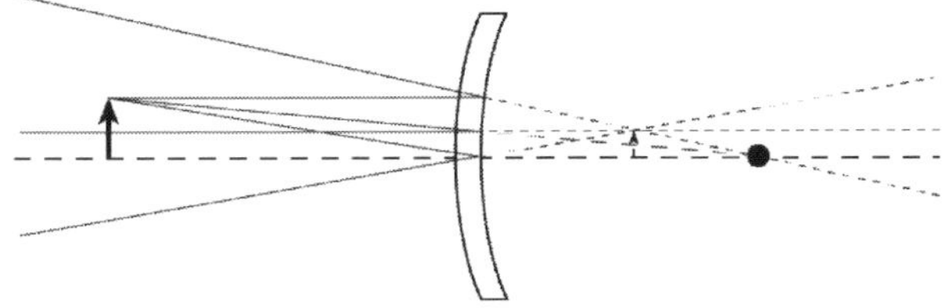

For a concave mirror, it can result in either a real or a virtual image.

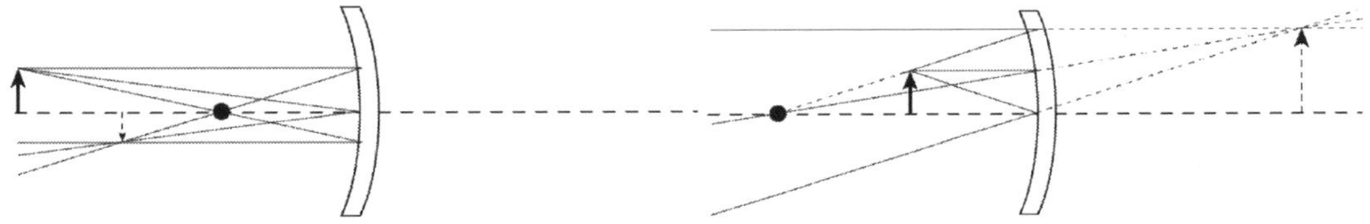

The magnification of an image is the ratio of the size of the image to the size of the object. The sign of the magnification is positive for an upright image and negative for an inverted image.

The magnification can be found by the same ray tracing techniques that are used to find the image position; the sizes of the object and the ray-traced image can be measured and their ratio calculated. The magnification can also be found more accurately from the equation $\frac{s_i}{s_o} = -\frac{d_i}{d_o}$, where s_i and s_o are the sizes of the image and object, respectively, and d_i and d_o their distance from the lens or mirror. The ratio on the left, $\frac{s_i}{s_o}$, is equal to the magnification. This means that the magnification is the same as the ratio of the image distance to the object distance but with the sign flipped. For example, if when an object is placed 20 cm in front of a given lens a real image is produced 50 cm behind it, then $\frac{s_i}{s_o} = -\frac{50\text{ cm}}{20\text{ cm}} = -2.5$: the image will be inverted and 2.5 times the size of the object. If the object is 4.0 cm tall, the image height will be $(-2.5)(4.0\text{ cm}) = 10.0\text{ cm}$.

Optical Instruments

As an optical instrument, the human eye focuses images on the retina, where they can be sensed by the rods and cones and the information transmitted to the brain. The specific part primarily responsible for the focusing is the lens, which sits in the front of the eye and acts as exactly that. Because the distance of the lens to the object depends on the distance of the lens to the image, the lens must adjust its focal length to the distance of the object; this is why your eye refocuses depending on the distance of the object you're looking at and why you won't see a distant object and a close-up object in focus at the same time. (The cornea in front of the lens also helps focus light on the retina, but unlike the lens its focal length is not adjustable.)

Some eyes are incapable of focusing the full necessary range, which leads to certain optical disorders. If the eye cannot focus properly on distant objects, then the eye is said to be nearsighted; if the eye cannot focus properly on close-up objects, the eye is said to be farsighted. Both conditions are treatable with corrective lenses.

A compound microscope, which includes most of the optical microscopes used in labs and classrooms, contains two convex lenses, an eyepiece and an objective lens. (This is something of a simplification because the eyepiece and the objective lens each often consist of multiple lenses, and there may be additional components such as mirrors to direct the light, but the basic working of the microscope can be explained in terms of these two lenses.) The object to be viewed is placed very close to the focal point of the objective lens, which then produces a virtual image at the focal point of the eyepiece; this virtual image then acts as the object of the eyepiece, which forms an image that the eye sees as infinitely far away.

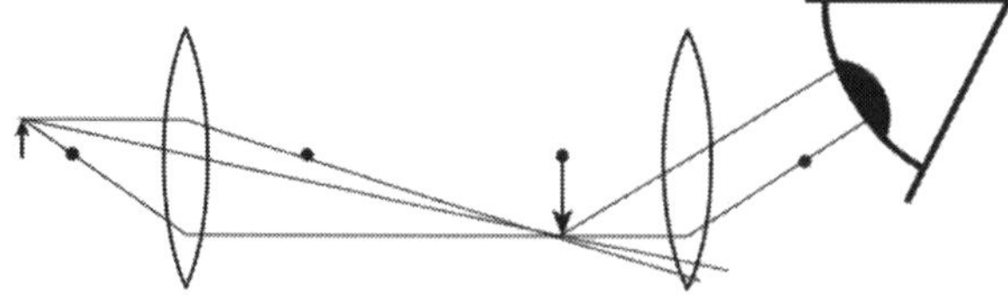

A microscope with an eyepiece of focal length f_e, an objective lens of focal length f_o, and a distance L between the two lenses is capable of magnifying an image by a factor of $M = -\frac{(25\text{ cm})L}{f_o f_e}$. (The 25 cm comes about from the near point of the average human eye.)

A telescope is used to increase the apparent size of very distant objects. Simple refracting telescopes do this with a pair of convex lenses, an eyepiece and an objective lens. The two lenses are placed a distance apart equal to the sum of their focal lengths. The light rays from the distant object are nearly parallel, which means that as they pass through the objective lens, they are focused at its focal point. The eyepiece, which has a shorter focal length, then forms a magnified image at infinity. If the telescope's objective lens has a focal length of f_o and the eyepiece of f_e, then the magnification of the telescope as a whole is just $M = -\frac{f_o}{f_e}$.

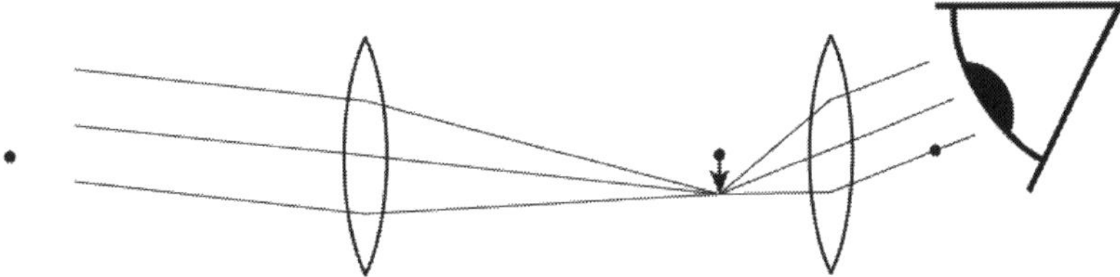

In practice, the largest telescopes in use today are not refracting telescopes but reflecting telescopes, which rely not just on lenses but on converging mirrors. The primary reason for this is because larger objective lenses are better for gathering light, but there is a limit on how large a high-quality lens can be made; large mirrors are much more practical.

Atoms, Nuclear Decay, Electronic Structure, and Atomic Chemical Behavior

Atomic Nucleus

Atomic Number, Atomic Weight

The three primary components of an atom are protons, neutrons, and electrons. Protons and neutrons are collectively called nucleons and form the nucleus of the atom; electrons orbit the nucleus at a distance—although they aren't really orbiting in the classical sense, like planets orbit a sun; rather, they are spread out in a probabilistic electron cloud. A neutral atom has the same number of electrons as protons; negative ions have more electrons; positive ions have fewer.

The atomic number of an atom is its number of protons. It is this that determines what element it is; carbon has an atomic number of six, so all carbon atoms have six protons. The mass number is the number of protons plus the number of neutrons. The number of electrons has no effect on the atomic number or the mass number. (The mass of an electron is only about 1/1800 the mass of a proton or neutron.) The number of electrons does determine the charge of the atom or ion, but an atom can gain or lose electrons and change its charge without altering its atomic number or mass number.

The atomic weight of an atom is the mass of the atom in atomic mass units (u), defined as 1/12 the mass of a carbon-12 atom (which contains six protons and six neutrons). Because the proton and the neutron have almost the same mass, the atomic weight is very close to the mass number—but because the protons and neutrons don't have exactly the same mass, and because the electrons also have some mass, they are not precisely equal. (There is also a little mass tied up in the binding energy of the atom.)

For the atomic weights of elements as given on a periodic table, however, there's a further factor to consider. The atomic weight of chlorine, for instance, is given as 35.45—much farther from an integral value than the slight differences in mass between protons and neutrons can account for. This is because the atomic weight given for each element in the periodic table is the average weight of the different isotopes of that element, weighted by their abundance in nature. Most chlorine atoms are chlorine-35, with some chlorine-37 and much smaller amounts of other isotopes; the weighted average of their weights comes out to 35.45.

The binding energy of a system in general is the energy required to separate a system into its component parts. In the case of an atom, the atomic binding energy is the energy required to separate the electrons from the atomic nucleus. Because the nth ionization energy of an atom is defined as the energy required to remove one electron after $n - 1$ have already been removed, the atomic binding energy can be thought of as the sum of the ionization energies of an atom for all possible values of n (up to the atom's atomic number).

The nuclear binding energy is the energy that would be required to completely separate the nucleus of the atom into isolated protons and neutrons. The nuclear binding energies are much larger than the atomic binding energies; the forces holding the atomic nucleus together are very large. For example, the atomic binding energy of a carbon-12 atom is about $7.85 \cdot 10^{-17}$ J (490 eV), whereas its nuclear binding energy is about $1.5 \cdot 10^{-11}$ J (92 MeV)—almost a million times as great. This is why a nuclear fission reaction releases so much energy; a part of the nuclear binding energy is released.

Neutrons, Protons, Isotopes

An isotope of an element is an atom of that element with a particular number of neutrons. Two atoms of the same element are said to be different isotopes if their number of neutrons differs. A specific isotope is named in terms of the atomic number and mass number, either by stating the mass number after the element name or writing the atomic number to the lower left and the mass number to the upper right of the chemical symbol. An atom with six protons and eight neutrons, for instance, would be called carbon-14 or ${}^{14}_{6}C$.

Two isotopes of the same element differ in their mass, of course but often also in their stability. For example, carbon-12 and carbon-13 are stable; carbon-14 is radioactive with a half-life of 5,700 years (making it useful in carbon dating); carbon-15 is extremely radioactive with a half-life of only 2.45 seconds.

Radioactive Decay

The three kinds of radioactive decay are alpha, beta, and gamma decay, named after the first three letters of the Greek alphabet. In alpha decay (α), an atomic nucleus emits an alpha particle, consisting of two protons and two neutrons; the atom's atomic number then decreases by two and its mass number by four, altering the atom into a different element. Beta decay actually comes in two varieties: in beta minus decay (β^-), a neutron turns into a proton, emitting an electron (and a very light particle called an antineutrino), whereas in beta plus decay (β^+) a proton turns into a neutron, emitting a positron, the antimatter version of an electron (along with a neutrino—the very light particle of which the antineutrino is the antimatter version). The atom's atomic number goes up (β^-) or down (β^+) by one, whereas its mass number is unchanged. In gamma decay (γ), the atom emits a very high-energy photon; this itself has no effect on the atom's atomic number or mass number, but gamma decay often accompanies one of the other kinds of radioactive decay.

Half-Life

The half-life of a radioactive material is the time it takes for half of the atoms in a sample to undergo radioactive decay. This does not mean that after two half-lives there is none of the sample left. Rather, after one half-life half of the original atoms have decayed, and after another half-life, half of the remaining atoms have decayed, which means that one-quarter of the original atoms remain. In general, the amount of a radioactive substance over time decays exponentially. The number of atoms of a radioactive sample remaining after a time t is equal to $N(t) = N_0 \left(\frac{1}{2}\right)^{t/t_{1/2}}$, where N_0 is the number of atoms originally present and $t_{1/2}$ is the half-life. This can be expressed in a base e exponential as $N(t) = N_0 e^{\ln 2(t/t_{1/2})}$.

For example, the radioactive isotope nitrogen-13 has a half-life of 9.965 minutes. This means that if you start with 100.0 moles of nitrogen-13, after one hour you would be left with $(100.0 \text{ mol})\left(\frac{1}{2}\right)^{(60 \text{ min})/(9.965 \text{ min})} = 1.540$ moles of the isotope that have not yet decayed.

Mass Spectrometer

A mass spectrometer is a device used to separate molecules by mass. Although the spectrometer relies on the particles being charged, uncharged molecules can be separated by a mass spectrometer if they are first ionized. (Technically, the spectrometer separates particles by the mass-to-charge ratio, but it can often be assumed that the charges of most of the particles are the same.)

In a mass spectrometer, charged particles are first accelerated by a voltage that gives all the particles the same kinetic energy. The moving particles are then subjected to a magnetic field. Because the magnetic field deflects some particles more than others, particles of a specific mass (or mass-to-charge ratio) can be selected out. Specifically, the voltage accelerates the particles to an energy of $U = qV$; setting that equal to the kinetic energy gives $qV = \frac{1}{2}mv^2$, and hence $v = \sqrt{\frac{2qV}{m}}$. The magnetic field produces a force of qvB, deflecting the particle in a circular path; setting this equal to the centripetal force yields $qvB = \frac{mv^2}{r}$; putting in our previous formula for v and solving for the radius of the path gives $r = \frac{1}{B}\sqrt{2V\left(\frac{m}{q}\right)}$—the deflection depends on the mass-to-charge ratio.

Electron Volt

The electron volt, abbreviated eV, is a unit of energy equal to the change in potential energy of an electron when it moves across a potential difference of one volt. Because this change in potential energy is equal to $U_E = qV$, one electron volt is equal to the magnitude of the charge of an electron multiplied by one volt: $(1.602 \cdot 10^{-19} \text{ C})(1 \text{ V}) = 1.602 \cdot 10^{-19} \text{ J}$.

Although it is not an official metric unit, the electron volt is frequently used in atomic and nuclear physics. The energies involved in single atoms are inconveniently small numbers when expressed in Joules but have more manageable values when expressed in electron volts. For instance, the energy of a ground state electron in a hydrogen atom is $-2.18 \cdot 10^{-18}$ J, which is equal to just −13.6 eV. For energies significantly larger than an electron volt but smaller than a joule, such as nuclear binding energies, units such as megaelectron-volts (MeV) and gigaelectron-volts (GeV) are commonly used.

Electronic Structure

Orbital Structure of Hydrogen Atom, Principal Quantum Number N, Number of Electrons Per Orbital

According to quantum mechanics, each electron in an atom can be completely described by four quantum numbers. The values of these quantum numbers are important for the shapes of the electron orbitals, for the electron energies, and for other properties. Each quantum number is constrained to only a discrete set of possible values. The four quantum numbers and their possible values are the following:

- The principle quantum number, n, can be any positive integer. This is the only quantum number that can (in principle) have infinitely many possible values, although in practice it will seldom exceed 9 or 10.
- The angular quantum number, l, can be any integer between 0 and $n - 1$. Thus, if an electron has a principal quantum number of 1, l must be 0; if $n = 2$, then l may be 0 or 1, and so on.
- The magnetic quantum number, m, can be any integer between $-l$ and l. If $l = 0$, then m must be 0; if $l = 1$, then m may be −1, 0, or 1, and so on.
- The spin quantum number is always ½ or −½; it does not depend on the other quantum numbers.

The principal quantum number of a hydrogen atom, abbreviated n, is a number characterizing the potential energy of the single electron in the atom. The principal quantum number is always an integer greater than or equal to 1; the higher n, the higher the energy of the hydrogen atom. One of the basic principles of quantum mechanics—in fact, the one that gives the theory its name—is that the energy of atoms, among other quantities, is quantized; rather than being able to take on any value in a continuous range, it is restricted to a discontinuous set of possible values, or quanta. More specifically, if the potential energy of an atom in the lowest state, E_1, is appropriately defined at a certain negative value ($-2.18 \cdot 10^{-18}$ J for a hydrogen atom, or −13.6 eV), then the potential energy of the state with principal quantum number n is $E_n = \frac{E_1}{n^2}$. As usual with potential energy, it is only the difference in energy between states that really matters, so the assignment of a negative value to the energy is not physically problematic and is done for mathematical convenience.

An atomic orbital is a possible state that a pair of electrons can be in in an atom. Therefore, strictly speaking, there are at most only two electrons per orbital. However, the word "orbital" is sometimes used interchangeably with "shell" or "subshell," the former referring to the collection of electrons with the same principal quantum number n, the latter to electrons that also share the angular quantum number l. The subshells are successively symbolized by the letters s, p, d, f, g, and so on; the s subshell contains only one orbital, the p three, the d five, and so on. The first shell contains only an s subshell and so only one orbital. The second contains an s and a p subshell for a total of 1 + 3 = 4 orbitals. The third contains an s, p, and d, for 1 + 3 + 5 = 9 orbitals, and so on through 16 and 25, and in general the nth subshell contains n^2 orbitals, and thus $2n^2$ electrons. Because the principal quantum number n corresponds to the energy level of the atom, it would also be correct to say that there are $2n^2$ electrons in each energy level of the hydrogen atom.

Ground State and Excited States

The ground state of an atom is the state with the lowest energy. In a ground-state atom, all the electrons are in the lowest-energy states possible, subject to the Pauli Exclusion Principle and the maximum number of electrons in an orbital. That is, no orbitals in a ground-state atom contain electrons unless all orbitals of lower energy are already full.

An atom that is not in the ground state is said to be in an excited state. An atom is in an excited state if there is at least one orbital that is not full despite at least one higher-energy orbital containing electrons.

An atom can change from its ground state to an excited state by one electron moving into an unoccupied, higher-energy state. This can occur if the atom is given energy by, for example, a high-energy photon colliding with it. The excited state is not stable, and an atom in an excited state will after some time spontaneously return to the ground state by the higher-energy electrons dropping back into unoccupied, lower-energy states. This is usually accompanied by emission of a photon.

Absorption and Emission Line Spectra

Emission line spectra are produced by photons emitted as electrons in excited atoms drop back down to lower energy states. The atoms may be put into excited states by high temperatures or electrical currents. Each element or compound has a characteristic emission line spectrum that depends on its possible energy levels. Essentially, there is an emission line corresponding to each possible transition between energy levels—although some transitions are more likely than others, which means the corresponding emission lines will be accordingly more prominent. The frequency of the emission line can be determined by taking the difference in energies between the two energy levels and dividing by Planck's constant, *h*, $6.626 \cdot 10-34\, J \times s$.

For example, the emission spectrum of mercury vapor has a prominent blue line; this arises from an electron dropping from an excited energy level of 7.70 eV to a still excited but lower energy level of 4.87 eV; then $\Delta E = 7.70\text{ eV} - 4.87\text{ eV} = 2.83\text{ eV} = 4.55 \cdot 10^{-19}\text{J}$; $f = \frac{\Delta E}{h} = 6.87 \cdot 10^{14}\text{Hz}$; $\lambda = \frac{c}{f} = 4.36 \cdot 10^{-7}\text{m}$ or 436 nm, in the blue range of visible light.

Absorption line spectra are produced by the absorption by a gas or other transparent medium of photons of particular frequencies from a continuous spectrum. When an atom or molecule absorbs a photon, the absorbed energy puts the particle into an excited state. It is not possible for the atom or molecule to partially absorb the photon; the photon must be absorbed completely or not at all. This places a constraint on the frequencies of photons that can be absorbed: only the photons that have the exact amount of energy to raise the particle to an excited state can be absorbed. Therefore, the energies of photons in the absorption line spectrum correspond to differences in energy between the ground state and the possible excited states; from this energy, the frequency and wavelength of the photons can be determined from the relationships $E = hf$ and $c = \lambda f$.

Unlike the emission line spectrum, the absorption line spectrum does not include lines corresponding to transitions between different excited states. The time that a particle spends in an excited state before returning to its ground state is generally small enough that the chances of its being further excited by another photon while in that state are negligible.

Fluorescence is a phenomenon in which certain materials absorb light at one wavelength and emit light at a wavelength of a lower frequency (and therefore a lower energy). This occurs because each photon of the absorbed light excites an electron in an atom of the material, but rather than fall immediately to the ground state and emit a photon of the same energy as it absorbs, the electron first passes through an intermediate, lower-energy excited state, emitting a photon for each transition and therefore ultimately emitting two or more photons with a total energy equal to the energy of the single-incident photon.

The best-known examples of fluorescence involve materials that absorb ultraviolet light and emit light in the visible range. Because the initial ultraviolet light is not visible to the human eye, the materials when they emit visible light seem to glow. Fluorescent dyes and paints that seem to glow under "black light" (i.e., ultraviolet light) are used for decorative purposes and on amusement park rides as well as in security features on some bills and credit cards. Fluorescence also occurs in nature and even in some living things; many fish and other organisms exhibit biofluorescence.

Pauli Exclusion Principle

The Pauli Exclusion Principle is a principle in quantum mechanics named after the Austrian theoretical physicist Wolfgang Ernst Pauli, who discovered it. It states that for a certain class of particles *called fermions*, two such particles in the same system cannot be the same state at the same time. Photons, for example, are not fermions, and the Pauli Exclusion Principle does not apply to them. Protons, neutrons, and electrons, however, are all fermions, and it is in electrons that the consequences of the principle are most obvious—and in terms of which Pauli first formulated the principle.

It is the Pauli Exclusion Principle that limits the number of electrons per orbital and the number of orbitals per shell. Specifically, the Pauli Exclusion Principle states that no two electrons in an atom can have exactly the same quantum numbers. It is this fact that causes shells to be filled by particular numbers of electrons and that ultimately leads to the details of electron structure.

Paramagnetism and Diamagnetism

Ferromagnetism, paramagnetism, and diamagnetism all refer to a material's ability to be influenced by a magnetic field. Ferromagnetism is the type of magnetism present in familiar permanent magnets. Only a few materials are capable of ferromagnetism, including cobalt, nickel, and as the prefix "ferro-" implies, iron. In ferromagnetic materials, adjacent atoms tend to align so that their electrons' spins are in the same direction, causing their individual magnetic moments to build into a significant magnetic field. When the material is not magnetized, the atoms are aligned in parts of the material, called domains, but the magnetic fields of the domains point in different directions and cancel. It is when the domains line up and combine into one large domain that the object as a whole is said to be magnetized.

Paramagnetism and diamagnetism both apply to a broader range of materials but are much weaker effects. In paramagnetic materials, unpaired electrons are attracted by a magnetic field, and the rest of the atoms come with them. In diamagnetic materials, all electrons are paired, and an induced magnetic field causes the material to be repelled by a magnetic field. Aluminum and myoglobin are examples of paramagnetic materials; carbon and antimony are diamagnetic.

Conventional Notation for Electron Structure

The conventional notation for electron structure of atoms lists the number of electrons in each subshell from lowest to highest energy. The electron structure arises from the four quantum numbers that characterize the electron's state: the principal quantum number n, the orbital quantum number l, the magnetic quantum number m, and the spin quantum number, s.

The orbital quantum number determines the subshell, and each value for l is given its own letter: the $l = 0$ subshell is given the letter s; $l = 1$ is p; then d, f, g, h, and so on. Because m can go from $-l$ to l, there are $(2l + 1)$ possible values of m for each subshell, and given the two possible values for s, there are a total of $2(2l + 1)$ electrons on each subshell.

To list the electron structure, then, each subshell is listed by a number for n and the appropriate letter for l and then with the number of electrons in that shell as a superscript. For instance, carbon has two electrons in the $n = 1, l = 0$ subshell, and four in the $n = 1, l = 2$; its electron notation is $1s^2 1p^4$.

Bohr Atom

The Bohr atom was an atomic model developed by and named for Danish physicist Niels Henrik David Bohr. According to the Bohr model of the atom, electrons orbited the nucleus in circular paths, but only in specific, discrete stationary orbits, and were only able to absorb or emit quantities of energy that would transfer them from one stationary orbit to another.

This constraint was intended to explain the observed phenomenon that atoms only emit specific frequencies of light. It improved on the previous atomic model, the Rutherford model of electrons orbiting the nucleus with no constraint on their radii, both by providing this explanation and by avoiding the Rutherford model's problematic prediction that electrons would gradually lose energy and spiral into the nucleus. However, Bohr had no theoretical justification for why the electrons would be constrained to these orbits, and the Bohr model was eventually superseded by the modern Schrödinger model in which the electrons do not occupy specific positions but probabilistic electron clouds, or orbitals. Still, the Bohr model is important in prefiguring the quantization that plays an important part in quantum mechanics.

Heisenberg Uncertainty Principle

The Heisenberg Uncertainty Principle states that the position and momentum of an object cannot simultaneously be known with arbitrarily high precision. Quantitatively, it states that $\Delta x \Delta p \geq \frac{h}{4\pi}$, where Δx is the uncertainty in the position, Δp is the uncertainty in the momentum, and h is Planck's constant, $6.626 \cdot 10^{-34}$ J/s. This is often written $\Delta x \Delta p \geq \frac{\hbar}{2}$, where ⍰, the reduced Planck's constant, is defined as $h/2\pi$. Instead of position and momentum, the uncertainty principle can also be stated in terms of energy and time $\left(\Delta E \Delta t \geq \frac{\hbar}{2}\right)$ or certain other pairs of variables.

Although sometimes it is assumed that the Uncertainty Principle arises because in observing an object's position, one necessarily must disturb it, it is actually more fundamental than that—it is not just that the object's position and momentum can't be simultaneously measured; it is that—counterintuitively—a particle can't simultaneously have an exact position and momentum. Because Planck's constant is so small, the effects of the principle on macroscopic phenomena are negligible, but for objects on the atomic scale, it is significant. For instance, the Heisenberg Uncertainty Principle explains quantum tunneling, the ability of a particle to pass through a barrier that classically would be impermeable.

Effective Nuclear Charge

The effective nuclear charge on an electron, Z_{eff}, is the effective net nuclear charge experienced by the electrons given the presence of other electrons in the atom. Because each electron is both attracted to the nucleus and repelled by the other electrons present, the electrical force from the other electrons effectively cancels much of the force from a like number of protons. The effective nuclear charge of an atom is therefore always less than the atomic number: $Z_{eff} < Z$ (except in the case of an atom or ion with only one electron). Calculating the exact effective nuclear charge is nontrivial, however, because it depends not only on the number of electrons but also on the shapes of the orbitals.

The effective nuclear charge has a number of ramifications. It affects the atomic binding energy, or ionization energy, as well as the atomic and ionic radius. It is also the reason that in an atom with multiple electrons, different orbitals with the same principal quantum number do not have the exact same energy and that at relatively high n, some of the orbitals fill in a different order than might be expected: for example, the 4s orbital has lower energy than the 3d.

Photoelectric Effect

The photoelectric effect is the phenomenon in which light shined on certain materials causes them to emit electrons. Although this can partly be explained by assuming that the energy of the light knocks electrons from the atom, there are several observed aspects of the phenomenon that this classically failed to explain. The photoelectric effect does not occur when the light's frequency is below a certain threshold, regardless of the intensity of the light. Likewise, the phenomenon can be prevented by applying a stopping voltage, but the necessary voltage depends only on the material and the frequency of the light, not on its intensity.

It was Albert Einstein who recognized that the photoelectric effect could be explained if light came in distinct quanta, now called photons, with an energy dependent on the light's frequency. The number of photons determined the intensity, but only if individual photons had sufficient energy would they be able to remove electrons from atoms. The recognition that light came in discrete quanta helped pave the way for the development of quantum mechanics. Although Einstein is most famous for his theory of relativity, it was for his work on the photoelectric effect that he won his Nobel Prize.

The Periodic Table—Classification of Elements into Groups by Electronic Structure

Alkali Metals

The alkali metals occupy the leftmost column of the periodic table, Group I. They include lithium, sodium, potassium, and so on; hydrogen, however, despite being usually positioned atop the leftmost column, is not conventionally included among the alkali metals.

The alkali metals all have a metallic luster and are soft enough to be easily cut with a knife. One of their most famous properties is their extremely high reactivity. The alkali metals even react with ordinary water, often bursting into flame on contact. Samples of alkali metals must be stored in oil to prevent their oxidation and their reaction with water vapor in the air. All alkali metals have a single valence electron and therefore tend to form singly charged positive ions.

Alkaline Earth Metals

The alkaline earth metals occupy the second column from the left on the periodic table. They include barium, magnesium, calcium, and so on.

The alkaline earth metals have a metallic luster and are relatively soft. They tend to react easily, although to a lesser degree than the alkali metals. Still, they are reactive enough that they are never found in nature as pure elements but only in chemical compounds. Their melting points and boiling points are higher than those of the alkali metals but lower than those of most other metals. All the alkaline earth metals have two valence electrons and therefore tend to form doubly charged positive ions.

Halogens

The halogens occupy the second column from the right on the periodic table. They include fluorine, chlorine, bromine, and so on. By convention, all the halogens are given names ending in "-ine," and no other elements are, so you can tell from the name whether or not a particular element is a halogen.

The halogens are highly reactive elements, all of which can react with hydrogen to form acids. In their pure elemental state, halogens form diatomic molecules, although because of their reactivity, halogens are never found in their pure elemental state in nature. All of the halogens have seven valence electrons and therefore form singly charged negative ions.

Noble Gases

The noble gases occupy the rightmost column in the periodic table. Newly discovered noble gases are given names ending in "-on," but this convention is relatively recent, so there are exceptions among some of the elements discovered earlier: helium is a noble gas but does not have a name ending in "-on," whereas boron, carbon, and silicon have names ending in "-on" but are not noble gases.

The noble gases were formerly also called inert gases; both names come from the nonreactivity of these elements. Although it isn't true that they're completely inert—the noble gases can react with other elements and form compounds—their reactivity is extremely low, and they are almost always found in nature in their pure elemental form. As the name also implies, all known noble gases are in the gaseous state at room temperature, although their melting points increase with their atomic numbers.

Transition Metals

By convention, the transition metals are usually considered to be the elements in groups III through XII of the periodic table, starting with the column topped by scandium (Sc) on the left and usually ending with the column topped by zinc (Zn) on the right. Sometimes the lanthanides and actinides, usually shown in separate rows below the rest of the table, are also included and called inner transition metals. The elements that are not transition metals are called main-group elements or representative elements.

As the name implies, the transition metals are all metals and have the properties shared by most metals: ductility, high electrical and thermal conductivity, and metallic luster. However, they differ from main-group metals in their high electronegativity, which allows them to form covalent compounds and to exist in several different oxidation states. For instance, beryllium, a main-group metal, always forms Be^{2+} ions. On the other hand, iron, a transition metal, can exist in a compound as Fe^{2+} or as Fe^{3+}–or, rarely, as Fe^{4-} or in any state from Fe^{2-} to Fe^{7+}.

Metals and Nonmetals

Most of the elements in the periodic table are considered metals; the nonmetals occupy the upper right corner of the periodic table (plus hydrogen). Metals are characterized in their solid state by malleability and ductility—the former property referring to the fact that they can be reshaped by pressure or hammering, the latter by the fact that they can be stretched into thin wires. Nonmetals, on the other hand, tend to be brittle, cracking under stress or strain rather than reshaping. Metals are also good conductors of both heat and electricity, resulting from the fact that their outer electrons are relatively free to move between atoms. Nonmetals, in general, do not conduct heat or electricity well. Another characteristic of metals is their metallic luster—metals look shiny, whereas nonmetals tend to have a matte and dull appearance. Generally, metals have a higher density and higher melting and boiling points than nonmetals, although this is less reliable; there are metals with relatively low densities (such as lithium) and melting points (such as mercury) and nonmetals with high densities and melting points (such as carbon).

Oxygen Group

The oxygen group is the third column from the right in the periodic table. The elements in the oxygen group are also sometimes called chalcogens. The uppermost element in the group is oxygen, hence the name; the group also includes sulfur, selenium, tellurium, and polonium.

All the elements in the oxygen group have six valence electrons, and the lighter elements in this group usually form doubly negative ions, such as O^{2-} and S^{2-}. Other oxidation states are possible, however, especially for the heavier elements in the group that have smaller electronegativities—polonium more often attains Po^{2+} or Po^{4+} states.

Metalloids

The metalloids are elements that lie between the metals and the nonmetals in the periodic table and have properties intermediate between the two. From lowest to highest atomic number, the metalloids include boron (B), silicon (Si), germanium (Ge), arsenic (As), antimony (Sb), tellurium (Te), polonium (Po), and astatine (At), although the last two are not always included. All the elements above and to the right of the metalloids are nonmetals; all the elements below and to the left of the metalloids are metals, with the exception of hydrogen.

Metalloids are solid at room temperature, and have a metallic luster, but are brittle and for the most part behave chemically like nonmetals. Perhaps their most useful property, however, is the ability of some metalloids to act as semiconductors—they can behave either as conductors or as insulators depending on certain conditions. This makes them very useful for various electronic applications and is the reason that computer chips, for example, contain silicon, a semiconductor metalloid.

Review Video: Periodic Table
Visit mometrix.com/academy and enter code: 154828

The Periodic Table—Variations of Chemical Properties with Group and Row

Valence Electrons

Valence electrons are the electrons in the outermost shell of an atom. For a main-group element, it is under normal circumstances solely the valence electrons that are involved in chemical reactions; therefore, it is the number of valence electrons in an atom that primarily determines its chemical properties. This is why elements in the same group have similar chemical properties: elements in the same group have the same number of valence electrons. All the alkali metals have one valence electron, all the halogens have seven, and so on. As a general rule of thumb, atoms will tend to gain or lose electrons in such a way as to be left with a full outer shell of eight valence electrons; this principle is known as the octet rule.

In transition metals, some of the electrons in inner shells can also participate in chemical reactions. The concept of valence electrons is therefore less well defined for transition metals than it is for main-group elements.

First and Second Ionization Energy

The ionization energy of an element is the amount of energy needed to ionize an atom of that element—that is, to remove an electron from the atom. More specifically, the energy required to remove one electron from a neutral atom is the first ionization energy, the energy required to remove another electron from an atom that has already lost an electron (a singly charged positive ion) is the second ionization energy, and so on; the nth ionization energy is the energy required to remove one electron from an atom that has already lost $n - 1$ electrons.

In general, the closer the outermost electron is to the nucleus, the harder it is to remove, and therefore the greater the ionization energy. This means that the ionization energy increases as the atomic radius decreases. Therefore, the ionization energy within a group tends to decrease as the atomic number increases because the heavier elements in a group have a larger atomic radius. However, across a period the atomic radius decreases from left to right, and therefore the ionization energy increases. So, the atomic energy of elements in the periodic table tends to increase from left to right and from down to up.

ELECTRON AFFINITY

Electron affinity is a measurement of the change in energy when an atom or molecule in the gaseous state gains an electron. Equivalently, the electron affinity can be defined as the amount of energy required to remove an electron from a singly charged negative ion. The larger the electron affinity, the more stable the negative ion.

Electron affinity tends to increase from left to right on the periodic table, although there is no clear trend within groups: electron affinity decreases from top to bottom within the alkali metals, for instance, but mostly increases from top to bottom within the alkaline earths. A few elements do not form negative ions at all or require energy to be added to give them an electron; the electron affinity of these elements is considered to be negative or zero. These elements include the noble gases as well as beryllium, nitrogen, magnesium, manganese, zinc, cadmium, and mercury.

ELECTRONEGATIVITY

Electronegativity is the tendency of an atom to attract electrons. Electronegativity is a unit-less quantity that is only meaningful in terms of the difference in electronegativity between two atoms. It is therefore necessary to decide on a reference point; by convention, the electronegativity of hydrogen is defined as 2.20, and the electronegativities of other atoms are derived based on this. Generally, when two atoms or molecules of different electronegativity interact, the atom that has a smaller electronegativity will tend to "donate" an electron to the atom with a larger electronegativity—or, in the case of a covalent bond, the shared electron will tend to be more closely associated with the latter atom.

Generally, among elements in the periodic table, electronegativity increases from left to right and decreases from top to bottom. (The noble gases are a special case, and because of their nonreactivity are often considered not to have electronegativity.) There are exceptions to these trends among the transition metals and in the boron and carbon groups; lead, for example, has a higher electronegativity than tin despite being positioned below it on the periodic table.

Review Video: Electronegativity
Visit mometrix.com/academy and enter code: 823348

ELECTRON SHELLS AND THE SIZES OF ATOMS

The sizes of atoms of elements in the periodic table tend to increase from top to bottom within a column, and to decrease from left to right within a row. The former trend is easy to understand; as one goes down a row in the periodic table, the atoms have added electron shells that must lie outside the inner shells possessed by the higher atoms and must therefore increase the atomic radius.

The latter trend, however, may be more counterintuitive; as one goes from left to right along a row in the periodic table, the atoms gain more protons and electrons, and one might therefore expect them to become larger, not smaller. The key to understanding the trend is that it is not the size of the nucleus that determines the size of the atom but the size of the electron clouds; as the number of protons increases without adding a new electron shell, the effective nuclear charge on the electrons in the outermost shell increases, pulling these outermost electrons closer to the nucleus.

ELECTRON SHELLS AND THE SIZES OF IONS

In general, negative ions are larger than the neutral atom, whereas positive ions are smaller. Furthermore, the greater the charge of the ion, the greater the difference in size from the neutral atom; for instance, a Ti^{4+} ion is smaller than a Ti^{3+} ion, which is smaller than a Ti^{2+} ion.

The reason for this difference has to do with the effective nuclear charge on the outermost electrons. As an atom gains electrons to become a negative ion, the effective nuclear charge on the outermost electrons decreases because the extra electron partially cancels it; this results in less force holding the electrons to the nucleus, so the electrons' distance from the nucleus is greater. As an atom loses electrons to become a positive ion, the opposite occurs; the effective nuclear charge increases, and the outermost electrons are bound more tightly to the nucleus.

An electron shell is a collection of electrons with the same energy level—the same value of the principal quantum number, *n*. Very roughly, an electron shell can be thought of as a layer of electrons surrounding an atom. A shell in turn consists of subshells of electrons with the same angular quantum number *l*. Each shell can hold only a certain maximum number of electrons; the greater the energy of the shell, the more subshells it has, and the more electrons it can hold. The first shell holds up to 2 electrons, the second 2 + 6 = 8, the third 2 + 6 + 10 = 18, and so on. It is largely the electron shells that determine the arrangement of the atoms in the periodic table—each row of the periodic table has one more shell than the one above it.

Because each electron shell lies farther from the nucleus than the previous, the more electron shells an atom or ion possesses, the higher its radius. This is the reason that the atomic and ionic radii increase within a group as the atomic number increases.

Stoichiometry

Molecular Weight

The molecular weight of a compound, also called molecular mass, is the mass of a single molecule of the compound, generally given in atomic mass units. It can be determined using the periodic table by looking up the atomic weight of each atom in the compound and adding them together. For example, sodium sulfate has the chemical formula Na_2SO_4: it contains two sodium atoms, one sulfur atom, and four oxygen atoms. The atomic weights of sodium, sulfur, and oxygen are 22.990, 32.065, and 15.999, respectively; the molecular weight of sodium sulfate is therefore $2(22.990) + 32.065 + 4(15.999) = 142.04$.

Empirical Versus Molecular Formula

The molecular formula of a compound consists of the symbols for the elements in the compound, with a subscript indicating the number of atoms of that element if that number is greater than one. Water contains two hydrogen atoms and one oxygen atom, so its molecular formula is H_2O. Hydrogen peroxide contains two hydrogen atoms and two oxygen atoms, so its molecular formula is H_2O_2. Glucose contains six carbon atoms; 12 hydrogen atoms; and six oxygen, so it is $C_6H_{12}O_6$.

The empirical formula, on the other hand, only gives the ratios of elements in the compound. If the numbers of atoms of each element have no common divisor, then the empirical and molecular formula are the same: thus, the empirical formula for water is still H_2O. Otherwise, the subscripts are reduced by their common divisor: the empirical formula for hydrogen peroxide is HO, and for glucose is CH_2O. Two compounds may have the same empirical formula but different molecular formulas: the molecular formula for ethylene is C_2H_4, propylene is C_3H_6, and butylene is C_4H_8, but all would have the same empirical formula of CH_2.

Description of Composition by Percent Mass

The percent mass of an element in a compound is the ratio of the mass of the element in question to the total mass of the compound, expressed as a percentage. For example, in water, H_2O, the mass of the hydrogen in each molecule is 2(1.008 u) = 2.016 u; the mass of the oxygen is 15.999 u; the total mass of the molecule is 2.016 u + 15.999 u = 18.015 u. The percent mass of hydrogen in the molecule is then 2.016 u / 18.015 u = 0.1112 = 11.12%, and the percent mass of the oxygen is 15.999 u / 18.015 u = 0.8881 = 88.81%. The chemical composition of water can therefore be said to be 11.12% hydrogen and 88.81% oxygen by mass.

The percent mass of the elements in a compound and the empirical formula are related—if the percent mass of each element is known, the empirical formula can be determined by dividing the percent mass of each element by the atomic mass of that element and finding the ratios of the results. The full molecular formula, however, cannot be found from the percent masses without more information.

AVOGADRO'S NUMBER

Avogadro's Number, abbreviated N_A, is the number of atoms or molecules in one mole of a substance. It is a constant equal to about $6.022 \cdot 10^{23}$ mol^{-1}. Avogadro's Number is named after Italian physicist Lorenzo Romano Amedeo Carlo Avogadro, remembered for his contributions to molecular theory.

Avogadro's Number forms the basis of the definition of the mole, and it was not chosen arbitrarily. The number was originally defined as equal to the number of atoms in 1 gram of hydrogen and was later redefined as the number of atoms in 12 grams of carbon-12. As such, in addition to the number of atoms or molecules in a mole, Avogadro's Number is also the number of atomic mass units in 1 gram. Avogadro's Number is therefore useful in converting between microscopic and macroscopic units, including converting between moles and molecules or grams and atomic mass units.

DEFINITION OF DENSITY

Density is the amount of mass in a substance or object per unit volume. It is usually abbreviated in science by the lowercase Greek letter rho, ρ. It is important to note that although this letter looks somewhat like a lowercase P, it is a different symbol, with a different meaning, and the two should not be confused, especially because there are some significant formulae (such as Bernoulli's equation) in which both symbols appear.

The units for density are the units of mass divided by the units of volume, so in SI units they are kg/m^3.

Unlike mass and volume themselves, density is an intrinsic property, independent of the quantity of matter present. If you break a rock in two, the pieces have a smaller mass and volume than the original rock but the same density. Of course, for a gas, the density does depend on other properties, such as temperature and pressure; this is also true for liquids and solids but to a much smaller degree.

OXIDATION NUMBER

The oxidation number of an atom in a compound is a measurement of its effective charge within the molecule. Essentially, the oxidation number is the number of electrons that have been removed from or (for a negative oxidation number) added to the atom in question. The more electronegative atom in a compound generally has a lower oxidation state.

The oxidation state of a monatomic ion is the charge of the ion; the oxidation state of a neutral pure element is zero (even if the element forms polyatomic molecules, such as H_2 or S_8). Some elements have consistent oxidation states: the oxidation state of alkali metals in compounds is always +1 and of alkaline earths always +2. Hydrogen usually has an oxidation state of +1, halogens of −1, and oxygen of −2, although there are exceptions.

The oxidation states of the atoms in a neutral molecule must add to zero and in a polyatomic ion must add to the charge of the ion. This often makes it possible to solve for the oxidation states of elements where the oxidation states are not consistent by plugging in the oxidation states of atoms that are known and solving for the unknowns.

Hydrogen atoms in a compound usually have an oxidation number of –1. However, this is not the case when the hydrogen is bonded to a metal (which has a lower electronegativity), such as in sodium hydride, NaH, or lithium aluminum hydride, $LiAlH_4$.

Oxygen atoms in a compound usually have an oxidation number of –2. However, there are two important exceptions. In the peroxide ion, O_2^{2-}, the ion as a whole has an oxidation number of –2, so each atom in the ion has an oxidation number of –1. This still holds when the ion is part of a compound, as in hydrogen peroxide, H_2O_2. The other exception is when the oxygen is bonded to fluorine. Fluorine is even more electronegative than oxygen, so in this case the fluorine will get a negative oxidation number, and the oxygen's oxidation number will be positive. In a molecule of oxygen difluoride, OF_2, the oxidation number of the oxygen atom is +2.

Common Oxidizing and Reducing Agents

An oxidizing agent is an element or compound that takes electrons from another substance, causing it to be oxidized. A reducing agent is an element or compound that donates electrons to another compound, causing it to be reduced. Note that in an oxidation-reduction reaction, the oxidizing agent is itself reduced, whereas the reducing agent is oxidized.

Common oxidizing agents include oxygen, chlorine and other halogens, hydrogen peroxide, and sulfuric acid. Common reducing agents include hydrogen gas, sodium and other alkali metals, iron, and carbon monoxide.

Disproportionation of Reaction by Chemical Equations

A disproportionation reaction is a redox reaction in which the same chemical species is both oxidized and reduced: that is, some of the molecules of the compound are reduced, whereas others are oxidized. One well-known example of a disproportionation reaction is the decomposition of hydrogen peroxide: $2H_2O_2 \rightarrow 2H_2O + O_2$. Note that in the reactant, H_2O_2, the oxygen atoms have an oxidation number of –1. In the product H_2O, the oxygen atoms have an oxidation number of –2—these atoms have been reduced. But in the other product, O_2, the oxygen atoms have an oxidation number of 0—these atoms have been oxidized.

Other examples of disproportionation reactions are the disproportionation of copper(I) ions in solution, $2Cu^{+}$ (aq) $\rightarrow$ Cu (s) + Cu^{2+} (aq) (the oxidation number of the copper goes from +1 on the left to 0 and +2 on the right); the disproportionation of carbon monoxide, $2CO \rightarrow C + CO_2$ (the oxidation number of the carbon goes from +2 to 0 and +4); and the disproportionation of mercury chloride, $Hg_2Cl_2 \rightarrow Hg + HgCl_2$ (the oxidation number of the mercury goes from +1 to 0 and +2).

Conventions for Writing a Chemical Equations

When writing a chemical equation, the reactants—the elements and compounds initially present before the reaction—go on the left, separated by plus signs, and the products—the elements and compounds produced in the reaction—go on the right, likewise separated. An arrow points from the reactants to the products. The relative number of particles of each reactant and product is shown by a number preceding them, such that the reaction is balanced—each element is represented in equal numbers on the left and right. Optionally, a parenthetical after each species can be written for its state: (s) for solid, (l) for liquid, (g) for gas, and (aq) for aqueous (in solution with water).

For example, take the reaction of sulfuric acid (H_2SO_4) with sodium hydroxide (NaOH) in solution to form water (H_2O) and sodium hydroxide (Na_2SO_4). The first two are the reactants, and the last two the products, so we would write $H_2SO_4 + NaOH \rightarrow H_2O + Na_2SO_4$. This, however, is not balanced; there are, for instance, three hydrogen atoms on the left but only two on the right. The full balanced equation, with states, would be $H_2SO_4\ (aq) + 2NaOH\ (aq) \rightarrow H_2O\ (l) + 2Na_2SO_4\ (aq)$.

Balancing Equations

Balancing a chemical equation means putting the correct coefficient on each species in the reaction so that the total number of atoms of each element is the same on both sides of the equation. For complex equations, this may involve some trial and error, but there are some steps that make it easier. It is generally simplest to balance one element at a time and to start by balancing the elements that appear in the fewest species. One may end up with fractional coefficients; if this is the case, one can simply multiply all the coefficients by the lowest common denominator.

For instance, take the reaction $NH_3 + O_2 = NO + H_2O$. H only appears in one compound on each side, so we can start there: $2NH_3 + O_2 = NO + 3H_2O$. N likewise only appears in one compound on each side and can be balanced by writing 2 in front of NO. That leaves the oxygen. There are now five oxygen atoms on the right, so we need $\frac{5}{2}$ in front of the O_2 on the left. We can multiply all the coefficients by 2 to remove the fraction, giving finally $4NH_3 + 5O_2 = 4NO + 6H_2O$.

Redox Equations

Redox equation is short for reduction-oxidation equation, a chemical equation for a reaction involving the reduction of one element or compound and the oxidation of another. When balancing a redox equation, not just the number of atoms of each element on each side must match, but the total oxidation number of all the atoms must match on the left or right as well. Generally, this is done by separating the reaction into half-reactions for oxidation and reduction—adding electrons to the reactions as necessary—and then combining the two reactions such that the electrons cancel.

For instance, take the simple redox reaction $Fe^{3+} + Sn^{2+} \rightarrow Fe^{2+} + Sn^{4+}$. The number of atoms of each element on each side matches, but the oxidation numbers do not: we have a total of +5 on the left and +6 on the right. We first write the separate half-reactions $Fe^{3+} + e^- \rightarrow Fe^{2+}$ and $Sn^{2+} \rightarrow 2e^- + Sn^{4+}$. For the electrons to cancel when we combine the half-reactions, the first half-reaction must be multiplied by two. Our final balanced equation is then $2Fe^{3+} + Sn^{2+} \rightarrow 2Fe^{2+} + Sn^{4+}$, with a matching total oxidation number of +8 on each side.

Limiting Reactants

The limiting reactant is the reactant that determines how much of the product will be produced—essentially, it is the reactant that runs out first when the reaction takes place. The other reactants that remain after the limiting reactant has been expended are called excess reactants. One way to determine which reactant is the limiting reactant, given the quantities of each reactant, is to calculate how much of one of the products could be formed from each reactant (assuming that sufficient quantities of the other reactants are available). Whichever reactant yields the smallest amount of product is the limiting reactant.

For instance, consider the reaction $Si + 2NaOH + H_2O \rightarrow Na_2SiO_3 + 2H_2$, and suppose we are given that we have 20 grams of Si, 30 grams of NaOH, and 10 grams of H_2O. Dividing by the respective molecular masses, this means that we have 0.712 moles of Si, 0.750 moles of NaOH, and 0.555 moles of water. These would each be sufficient to produce, respectively, 0.712 moles, 0.375 moles, and 0.555 moles of Na_2SiO_3; 0.375 moles, the amount produced by the NaOH, is smallest, so NaOH is the limiting reactant.

THEORETICAL YIELDS

The theoretical yield of a chemical product is the amount that would be produced if the maximum amount of the reactants reacted—that is, if all of the limiting reactant participated. The theoretical yield can be determined by identifying the limiting reactant and determining how much of the product it would produce based on the ratios of the coefficients in the chemical equation. For example, consider the reaction $Fe_2O_3 + 3C \rightarrow CO + 2Fe$, and suppose that we know that the limiting reactant is carbon, of which we have 500 grams; we want to determine the theoretical yield of iron. Five hundred grams of carbon is 41.6 moles; because there are two atoms of elemental iron produced for every three atoms of elemental carbon that reacts, this would produce $\frac{2}{3}(41.6 \text{ mol}) = 27.8$ mol of iron, or 1.55 kg.

The experimental yield is the amount of product that is actually produced in a reaction and empirically measured. It is possible that not all the limiting reactant participates in the reaction—because other reactions occur or because the system reaches an equilibrium state. Therefore, the experimental yield may be (and generally is) less than the theoretical yield but never greater.

Unique Nature of Water and Its Solutions

ACID/BASE EQUILIBRIA

BRØNSTED-LOWRY DEFINITION OF ACIDS AND BASES

According to the Brønsted-Lowry definition of acids and bases—named after Danish chemist Johannes Nicolaus Brønsted and English chemist Thomas Martin Lowry—an acid is a substance that donates protons in a chemical reaction, and a base is a substance that accepts protons. This broadened the earlier Arrhenius definition, by which an acid dissociates in water to form H^+ ions, and a base dissociates in water to form OH^- ions. Because an H^+ ion is basically a proton, and because OH^- ions combine with H^+ ions to form water, in general an Arrhenius acid or base is also an acid or base by the Brønsted-Lowry definition. However, the Brønsted-Lowry definition also includes substances that are not acids or bases by the Arrhenius definition. For example, NH_3 in aqueous solution can accept a hydrogen ion from HCl to form NH_4^+ and Cl^-, making NH_3 a Brønsted-Lowry base even though it does not contain an OH^- ion.

Some substances can both donate and accept electrons and can therefore act as both acids and bases by the Brønsted-Lowry definition. Such substances are called amphoteric; the most prominent example is water.

IONIZATION OF WATER

PH

pH is a measurement of the concentration of hydrogen ions in an aqueous solution and therefore of the solution's acidity. More specifically, it is equal to the negative logarithm base 10 of the ion concentration. Technically, free hydrogen ions in an aqueous solution tend to combine with water to form hydronium ions, H_3O^+, so it is really the concentration of hydronium ions, not free H^+ ions, that the pH measures. For example, if the molar concentration of H^+ (or H_3O^+) ions in a solution is 10^{-4}, then the solution's pH is $-\log_{10} 10^{-4} = 4$.

The pH of pure water is 7, which is considered neutral, neither acidic nor basic. Acidic substances have a lower pH; the pH of most orange juice is between 3.5 and 4, and the pH of white vinegar is about 2.4. Basic substances have a higher pH; the pH of baking soda is about 9, and the pH of strong drain cleaners can be about 14.

EXAMPLES

Explain how the concentration of hydronium and hydroxide ions in an aqueous solution can be found given its pH, and vice versa.

The pH is equal to the negative log base 10 of the concentration of hydroxide ions in an aqueous solution: $\text{pH} = -\log_{10}[\text{H}_3\text{O}^+]$. Turning this around to solve for the concentration of hydronium ions, we get $[\text{H}_3\text{O}^+] = 10^{-\text{pH}}$. For example, in a solution with a pH of 10, the molar concentration of hydronium ions is 10^{-10}.

The dissociation reaction of water is $2H_2O \rightarrow H_3O^+ + OH^-$. The equilibrium condition for this reaction is $K_{eq} = \frac{[\text{H}_3\text{O}^+][\text{OH}^-]}{[\text{H}_2\text{O}]^2}$. Because the number of the ions for typical solutions is very small in comparison to the number of neutral water molecules, we can treat $[H_2O]$ as being essentially constant and write $K_{eq}[\text{H}_2\text{O}]^2 = [\text{H}_3\text{O}^+][\text{OH}^-]$. The left-hand side of this equation can be written as a single constant K_w; at room temperature $K_w = 1.0 \cdot 10^{-14}$, so the concentrations of hydronium and hydroxide ions must multiply to this number: $[\text{H}_3\text{O}^+][\text{OH}^-] = 10^{-14}$. Therefore, given either the concentration of hydronium ions or the concentration of hydroxide ions, you can find the other by dividing the known concentration into 10^{-14}. In the example with a concentration of hydronium ions of 10^{-10}, the concentration of hydroxide ions is $\frac{10^{-14}}{10^{-10}} = 10^{-4}$.

Explain what ions are present in pure water and in what concentrations.

Even in pure water, water molecules can spontaneously dissociate. Although this reaction is sometimes written as $H_2O \rightarrow H^+ + OH^-$, in practice free H^+ ions quickly join with other water molecules, so a more accurate rendition of the dissociation reaction is $2H_2O \rightarrow H_3O^+ + OH^-$. Therefore, pure water contains hydronium ions (H_3O^+) and hydroxide ions (OH^-).

The equilibrium condition for this dissociation reaction is $K_w = [\text{H}_3\text{O}^+][\text{OH}^-]$, where K_w is the water ionization constant, equal at room temperature to $1.0 \cdot 10^{-14}$. For pure water, because no other ions are present and the water as a whole is neutral, the concentrations of hydroxide and hydronium ions must be equal. We can then replace $[\text{OH}^-]$ in the equation by $[\text{H}_3\text{O}^+]$, and we get $K_w = [\text{H}_3\text{O}^+]^2$, so $[\text{OH}^-] = [\text{H}_3\text{O}^+] = \sqrt{K_w} = \sqrt{1.0 \cdot 10^{-14}} = 1.0 \cdot 10^{-7}$. In pure water, both hydroxide and hydronium ions are present at a concentration of 10^{-7} M.

CONJUGATE ACIDS AND BASES

In an acid-base reaction, under Brønsted-Lowry definitions, the acid donates a proton to the base, converting both the acid and the base into new compounds. In general, this reaction is reversible, which means that the new compound formed from the base can donate the proton it received, and the new compound formed from the acid can accept a proton. This means the new compound formed from the base is an acid, and the new compound formed from the acid is a base. The base formed from an acid when it donates a proton is called its conjugate base; the acid formed from a base when it accepts a proton is called its conjugate acid. An acid or base together with its conjugate are known as a conjugate base pair. The stronger an acid, the weaker its conjugate base and vice versa.

For instance, hydrochloric acid, HCl, can donate a proton to become Cl^-, its conjugate base, but because HCl is a very strong acid, Cl^- is a very weak base. On the other end of the range, S^{2-} is a strong base by the Brønsted-Lowry definition; it can accept a proton to become HS^-, a very weak acid.

Strong and Weak Acids and Bases

The strength of an acid or base refers to how readily it donates or accepts a proton. A strong acid dissociates completely in water, with practically every molecule losing a proton. A weak acid only partially dissociates; the smaller the proportion of molecules that donate protons, the weaker the acid is said to be. Similarly, in a strong base, practically every molecule will accept a proton—in most cases because the base dissociates into a cation and a proton-accepting hydroxide ion. A weak base can accept a proton but does so less readily.

Common examples of strong acids are nitric acid (HNO_3), sulfuric acid (H_2SO_4), and hydrochloric acid (HCl). Weak acids include acetic acid (CH_3COOH), citric acid ($C_6H_8O_7$), and hydrofluoric acid (HF). Some strong bases include sodium hydroxide (NaOH), lithium hydroxide (LiOH), and potassium hydroxide (KOH). Weak bases include ammonia (NH_3), calcium carbonate ($CaCO_3$), and ammonium hydroxide (NH_4OH).

Calculation of pH of a Solutions

A salt is a compound (other than water) formed in a neutralization reaction between an acid and a base. When dissolved in water, a salt undergoes hydrolysis, reacting with the water to split into two products.

A salt of a weak base and a strong acid is called an acid salt. To find the pH, given the molarity of the salt and the base dissociation constant K_b of the base, you can find K_a for the conjugate acid and use it to solve for the concentration of H_3O^+ ions. For a basic salt of a strong base and weak acid, the procedure is similar but using K_b for the acid's conjugate base.

A salt of a strong acid and a strong base forms a neutral solution.

For example, suppose you have a 2.00 M solution of potassium cyanide, KCN. Because KOH is a strong base and HCN is a weak acid, this is a basic salt. K_a for HCN is $5.8 \cdot 10^{-10}$, so K_b for its conjugate base is $\frac{1.0 \cdot 10^{-14}}{5.8 \cdot 10^{-10}} = 1.7 \cdot 10^{-5}$. The equilibrium equation is $K_b = \frac{[\text{HCN}][\text{OH}^-]}{[\text{CN}^-]}$; we can set [HCN] and [OH-] (which must be equal) to x and solve it to get $x = \sqrt{K_b[\text{CN}^-]} = \sqrt{(1.7 \cdot 10^{-5})(2.00)} = 0.0058$ M; thus the pH is $-\log_{10} \frac{1.0 \cdot 10^{-14}}{0.006} = 11.8$.

Equilibrium Constants K_a, K_b, pK_a, and pK_b

K_a and K_b are the acid dissociation constant and the base dissociation constant, respectively. They are constants that relate to the equilibrium condition for the dissociation of a particular acid or base. The equilibrium condition for the dissociation of an acid HA with conjugate base A^- is $K_a = \frac{[\text{H}^+][\text{A}^-]}{[\text{HA}]}$; for a base B with conjugate acid HB^+, it is $K_b = \frac{[\text{HB}^+][\text{OH}^-]}{[\text{B}]}$. These constants can be used to determine the concentration of one of the chemical species involved if the concentrations of the others are known—in particular, they can be used to find the concentration of H^+ or OH^- and therefore the pH of the solution.

In practice, these concentrations are typically very small, so it is often more convenient to refer to logarithmic versions of these constants, pK_a and pK_b. These hold the same relation to K_a and K_b as pH does to the concentration of H^+ ions: $pK_a = -\log_{10} K_a$, and $pK_b = -\log_{10} K_b$.

For an acid and its conjugate base, $K_a \cdot K_b = 10^{-14}$ and $pK_a + pK_b = 14$.

Buffers

A buffer is a solution that resists changes in pH. A buffer's pH remains almost constant even after the addition of a strong acid or base (in relatively small amounts). Generally, a buffer solution contains either a weak acid and its conjugate base or a weak base and its conjugate acid. When a strong base is added to a solution containing a weak acid, the weak acid will tend to give up a proton to the base, changing it into its conjugate acid. Because there is no significant change in the concentration of hydronium ions in solution, there is little change in pH. Similarly, when a strong acid is added to a solution containing a weak base, the weak base will accept a proton from that acid, again tending to stabilize the concentration of hydronium ions and therefore the pH.

Buffer systems are present in the human body (and other organisms) because many enzymes and other chemicals only work well at certain pH ranges. Blood, for example, is a buffer solution (with carbonic acid, H_2CO_3, and its conjugate base) that remains at a pH of about 7.4. Buffers are also used in shampoos and detergents, in breweries, and in textile dyeing processes. Some examples of weak acids or bases used in buffer systems include acetic acid (CH_3COOH), ammonia (NH_3), citric acid ($C_6H_8O_7$), and monopotassium phosphate (KH_2PO_4).

Review Video: Buffer
Visit mometrix.com/academy and enter code: 389183

Unique Properties of Water

Although water is so much a part of our lives that we may take it for granted, it has some important chemical properties that lend particularly well to supporting life. For one thing, water has a very high specific heat. This means that water tends to resist changes in temperature and moderate climates and helps maintain homeostasis within living systems. Water is also unusual in that it is less dense as a solid than as a liquid. This is why ponds and lakes freeze over but retain liquid water underneath, maintaining a habitat for underwater organisms.

Other properties of water are less unusual but still important. Water is a powerful solvent, which makes it useful as a medium to carry other chemicals through our bodies. Water has both a boiling point and a freezing point close to the average temperature of our surroundings, which means that it is present in all three states of matter and can easily be cycled through the environment. The hydrogen bonds present in water give it a high surface tension and a high cohesion, which among other things allows trees to draw water up their trunks by capillary action.

Ions in Solutions

Anion, Cation Common Names

A monatomic anion is named by the element of the atom with the suffix "-ide." For example, a monatomic chlorine ion is called chloride, a monatomic iodine atom iodide, a monatomic sulfur ion sulfide, and so on.

With rare exceptions, the charge of a monatomic anion depends on its group. A halogen (group 17) has a charge of −1, an element in the oxygen group (group 16) has a charge of −2, and an element in group 15 has a charge of −3. Elements of other groups do not generally appear as monatomic anions. So, for instance, because iodine is a halogen, it has a charge of −1 and iodide is I^-; sulfur is in the oxygen group, so a sulfide ion is S^{2-}; because nitrogen is in group 15, a nitride ion is N^{3-}.

The prefixes "hypo-" and "per-" are used for oxyanions, which consist of one or more oxygen atoms and one atom of another element. For a given element, the most common such anion is named with the suffix "-ate" and the anion with one less oxygen atom with the suffix "-ite." For some elements, however, there are more than two such ions, and in these cases the prefixes "hypo-" and "per-" are used for the additional anions. The prefix "per-" always accompanies the suffix "-ate" and identifies the anion with one more oxygen atom than the anion named with -ate. The prefix "hypo-" always accompanies the suffix "-ite" and identifies an anion with one fewer oxygen atom than the anion named with -ite.

The best-known anions using these prefixes are oxyanions of chlorine. Chlorine has four oxyanions: chlorate is ClO_3^-, chlorite is ClO_2^-, perchlorate is ClO_4^-, and hypochlorite is ClO^-. There are likewise four oxyanions of bromine: bromate is BrO_3^-, bromite is BrO_2^-, perbromate is BrO_4^-, and hypobromite is BrO^-. Iodine has the oxyanions iodate, IO_3^-; iodite, IO_2^-; periodate, IO_4^-; and hypoiodite, IO^-.

One of the most common types of anion is the oxyanion, consisting of one or more oxygen atoms and one atom of a different element. There are also some anions that are similar to oxyanions but with the addition of a hydrogen atom (and with one less negative charge). These anions are named by the name of the corresponding oxyanion preceded by hydrogen. For instance, CO_3^{2-} is carbonate, and HCO_3^- is hydrogen carbonate; PO_4^{3-} is phosphate, and HPO_4^{2-} is hydrogen phosphate; SO_4^{2-} is sulfate, and HSO_4^- is hydrogen phosphate. Hydrogen carbonate and hydrogen sulfate are also called bicarbonate and bisulfate, respectively.

The oxyanion may also have two hydrogen atoms added to it, in which case its name is preceded by dihydrogen. The only common example is dihydrogen phosphate, $H_2PO_4^-$.

As the prefix "di-" implies, the dichromate ion includes two chromium atoms. The suffix "-ate" is the same suffix used for oxyanions, and like an oxyanion, dichromate includes a number of oxygen atoms. Unfortunately, there's nothing in the name of the ion to specify exactly how many oxygen atoms it contains, or its charge, so those may have to be memorized. The dichromate ion is $Cr_2O_7^{2-}$.

The prefix "thio-" is applied to anions that are similar to oxyanions but have one of the oxygen atoms replaced by a sulfur ion. Cyanate is OCN^-—the cyanide ion, CN^-, with the addition of an oxygen atom. In thiocyanate, that oxygen atom is replaced by sulfur to make SCN^-. Sulfate is SO_4^{2-}; although it already contains a sulfur atom, in thiosulfate, one of the oxygen atoms is replaced by an additional sulfur atom to make $S_2O_3^{2-}$.

The suffixes "-ate" and "-ite" are used for oxyanions, a common class of polyatomic ions that combine one or more oxygen atoms with one atom of a different element. These ions are generally named after the non-oxygen atom, with the suffix "-ate" or "-ite." Different anions exist with the same element but with different oxidation values and different numbers of oxygen atoms. They are distinguished by the suffixes: the most common such ion, or the one considered in some sense the more fundamental, gets the suffix "-ate," whereas an anion with the same element but one less oxygen atom gets the "-ite" suffix.

Polyatomic cations are in general less common and less numerous than polyatomic anions (at least in terms of relatively simple ions, one can construct arbitrarily many complex examples of both). One important polyatomic cation, however, is ammonium, NH_4^+. Chemicals including ammonium include ammonium chloride, commonly used as in fertilizers; ammonium nitrate, used in fertilizers and explosives; and ammonium carbonate, used as a leavening agent (although today largely replaced by sodium bicarbonate).

Another important polyatomic ion *is hydronium,* H_3O^+, which is notable as one of the products of the dissociation of water: $2H_2O \rightleftharpoons H_3O^+ + OH^-$. Despite its importance in the chemistry of water, hydronium is not a component of any common stable compounds.

One other relatively common polyatomic ion is the mercury (I) ion, Hg_2^{2+}. This ion is found in compounds including mercury (I) chloride, also known as calomel, and is used in electrochemistry, and mercury (I) iodide, formerly used as a medicine despite its (then unrecognized) toxicity.

There are other polyatomic cations, but they are much less common. They include phosphonium (PH_4^+), arsonium (AsH_4^+), methanium (CH_5^+), and tropylium ($C_7H_7^+$).

As monatomic ions, metals are most likely to be cations, whereas nonmetals are most likely to be anions. This is because metals in general have only a few electrons in their outer shells, so they can most easily obtain full valence shells by donating electrons, turning them into positive ions. Nonmetals, on the other hand, have mostly filled valence shells, so they can most easily fill their valence shells by gaining electrons. (Carbon and silicon are exceptions because their valence shells are half full, but these elements do not commonly occur as monatomic ions.)

Hydrogen can be either a cation or an anion because it can fill its valence shell either by gaining one electron or by losing one electron. Most often it is a cation (as in hydrochloric acid, HCl, or hydrofluoric acid, HF), but it can also bond with a metal with a lower electronegativity to become an anion (as in lithium hydride, LiH).

Review Video: Anion, Cation, and Octet Rule
Visit mometrix.com/academy and enter code: 303525

There is, unfortunately, no easy way to tell from the name how many oxygen atoms a particular ion has, so it is useful to memorize some common ions. Some of the most important such anions include the following:

Carbonate:	CO_3^{2-}
Nitrate:	NO_3^-
Nitrite:	NO_2
Phosphate:	PO_4^{3-}
Sulfate:	SO_4^{2-}
Sulfite:	SO_3^{2-}

Formulas and Charges for Familiar Ions

Hydroxide is OH^-. Hydroxide ions are found in many strong bases including sodium hydroxide and potassium hydroxide as well as in water.

Cyanide is CN^-. Cyanide salts such as sodium cyanide are noted for their high toxicity.

Acetate is $C_2H_3O_2^-$. This organic anion is found in acetic acid, the main component of vinegar as well as in fatty acids and many other organic compounds.

Peroxide is O_2^-. Many peroxide compounds are used as bleaching agents. The simplest common peroxide compound is hydrogen peroxide, H_2O_2, used as a household disinfectant.

HYDRATION

Hydration refers to the addition of water to a chemical species. Although other reactions with water are sometimes called by this name, one common phenomenon referred to as hydration involves water molecules surrounding an ion or a polar molecule to form a hydration shell. The water molecules are attracted to the ion or molecule because the water molecules are themselves slightly polar—the oxygen atom slightly positive and the hydrogen atoms slightly negative—so the oxygen atoms in water are attracted to positive ions or to the positive ends of polar molecules, and the hydrogen atoms are attracted to negative ions or the negative ends of polar molecules.

Hydration helps polar molecules dissolve in water; when sodium chloride dissociates in water, for instance, the water molecules surrounding the ions help disperse them through the solution. Hydration also plays an important role in the functioning of proteins; the water molecules surrounding parts of the proteins affect their shapes.

SOLUBILITY

UNITS OF CONCENTRATION

Molarity, molality, and normality are all measures of the concentration of a solution, but they are measured in different ways. Molarity (abbreviated M) is a measurement of the number of atoms or molecules of solute by volume of the solution; it has units of moles per liter. Molality (abbreviated m) is a measurement of the number of atoms or molecules of solute by mass of the solution; it has units of moles per kilogram.

Normality (abbreviated N) is a measurement of concentration that is used for acids. It measures the number of H^+ ions—of donatable protons—per liter of solution. For monoprotic acids, which only donate one proton per molecule, the normality is equal to the molarity. For polyprotic atoms, which donate multiple protons per molecule, the normality is equal to the molarity times the number of protons potentially donated by each atom. For example, sulfuric acid, H_2SO_4, is diprotic; it can donate up to two protons per molecule. The normality of a sulfuric acid solution is therefore double its molarity.

SOLUBILITY PRODUCT CONSTANT

The solubility product constant, K_{sp}, is a constant that relates to the equilibrium conditions for the concentrations of ions in a slightly soluble ionic compound. It is a special case of the general equilibrium constant K_{eq}. In the case of an arbitrary ionic compound A_mC_n with anion A^{n-} and cation C^{m+}, the equilibrium condition is $K_{sp} = [A^{n+}]^m[C^{m-}]^n$. (The original compound A_mC_n does not contribute to the equilibrium condition because of its solid state; the concentrations of solids and liquids do not change in a reaction, so they do not appear in the equilibrium equation.)

If an ion is present from sources other than the dissolved chemical, the solubility product constant can be used to find out how much of the other ion is present. For example, consider calcium fluoride; CaF_2. K_{sp} for calcium fluoride is $3.45 \cdot 10^{-11}$. If all the calcium and fluoride ions in a solution come from dissolved CaF_2, then there must be twice as many fluoride ions as calcium. Setting the number of fluoride ions to x gives $K_{sp} = (x)(2x)^2 = 4x^3$, so $[Ca^{2+}] = x = \sqrt[3]{K_{sp}/4} = \sqrt[3]{3.45 \cdot 10^{-11}/4} = 2.05 \cdot 10^{-4}$. This must also be the moles per liter of the calcium fluoride that it dissolved; multiplying by the molar mass of CaF_2 gives a solubility of 0.016 g/mol.

The mass percent of a solution is a ratio of the mass of the solute in a solution to the total mass of the solution. Molarity is a measurement of the moles of solute to the volume of the solution in moles per liter. You can convert mass percent to molarity by first dividing by the molar mass to convert the mass of solution to moles and then multiplying by the density of the solution to convert the mass of solute to liters. To convert molarity to mass percent, just do the reverse.

For example, suppose you have a 4.00 M solution of NaCl, with a density of 1150 kg/m^3. The molar mass of sodium chloride is 58.443 g/mol, so the mass percent of this solution is $\frac{(4.00\ \text{mol/l})(0.058443\ \text{kg/mol})}{1.15\ \text{kg/l}} = 0.203$, or 20.3%.

Parts per million, sometimes abbreviated ppm, is a unit that is sometimes used for very dilute solutions when the concentration expressed in traditional units like molarity or mass percent would be an inconveniently small number. It literally refers to the number of grams of solute per million grams of solution. One ppm is therefore equal to 0.0001% as a mass percent. For an aqueous solution, which if sufficiently dilute will have essentially the same density as water, 1.00 g/mL; 1 ppm equals 1 mg/L.

For even more dilute solutions, other, similar units are sometimes used such as parts per billion (ppb), parts per trillion (ppt), and so on.

Common-Ion Effect

The common-ion effect refers to the fact that a slightly soluble ionic compound will become less soluble in a solution that contains one of the same ions as the compound. For example, calcium carbonate ($CaCO_3$) already has a low solubility in water, but in a solution of potassium carbonate (K_2CO_3), its solubility is even lower because the calcium carbonate and the potassium carbonate share the carbonate ion in common. The common ion effect follows from the solubility equilibrium condition that the product of the concentrations of the ions is constant. Therefore, an increase in the concentration of one ion must result in a decrease of the other; this is only possible if some ions combine to precipitate the solid compound. The effect can be considered a special case of Le Châtelier's Principle.

The common-ion effect is useful in preparing laboratory separations because it can be used to precipitate out a desired compound from a solution by adding another compound that shares an ion with it. For instance, sodium chloride (NaCl) can be precipitated out of saltwater by the addition of hydrochloric acid (HCl).

Complex Ion Formation

A complex ion is an ion consisting of a metal ion surrounded by other molecules or ions referred to as ligands. Each ligand acts as a Lewis base, donating one or more pairs of electrons to the metal ion at the center. Common ligands include water, ammonia (NH_3), hydroxide (OH^-), cyanide (CN^-) and various halide ions (Cl^-, F^-, etc.) For instance, two ammonia molecules bonded to a central silver (I) ion would form the complex ion $[Ag(NH_3)_2]^+$. The nomenclature of complex atoms is itself somewhat complex, including prefixes for the number of each ligand, followed by prefixes for the ligands, ending with the name of the metal. $[Ag(NH_3)_2]^+$, for example, would be called diamminesilver (I).

Complex ions are formed one ligand at a time. The central metal ion uses its empty orbitals to accept a pair of electrons from a ligand, and then the resultant single-ligand complex ion accepts a pair of electrons from another ligand, and so on. The maximum number of ligands depends on how many of the molecules or ions in question will fit around the metal ion. Six water molecules can fit around most metal ions, for instance, but only four chloride ions.

The formation constant K_f relates to the equilibrium condition for complex ions. It is arrived at the same way as any other chemical equilibrium constant: with the concentration of the product in the numerator—in this case, the complex ion—and the product of the concentrations of the reactants in the denominator—in this case, the separate metal ion and ligands (aside from water). For instance, for the complex ion $[Cu(NH_3)_4(H_2O)_2]^{2+}$—called tetraamminediaquacopper—the equilibrium condition would be $K_f = \frac{[Cu(NH_3)_4(H_2O)_2]^{2+}}{[Cu^{2+}][NH_3]^4}$.

The formation constant can be used as a measure of the stability of the complex ion: the higher K_f, the more stable the complex ion. Like other equilibrium constants, the formation constant can be used to determine an unknown concentration if other concentrations are known.

Complex Ions and Solubility

The formation of complex ions in a solution will tend to increase the solubility of a solute that shares an ion with the complex ion—whether it is the central metal ion or an ionic ligand. This is a consequence of Le Châtelier's Principle—the formation of the complex ion decreases the concentration of the ion in question; this shifts the equilibrium toward the formation of the ion, causing more of the solute to dissolve.

One application of this principle is in photography; some photographic film contains the photosensitive chemical silver bromide (AgBr), which can dissociate in the presence of light to form elemental silver and bromine. After the photograph is taken, the extra silver bromide must be removed. Silver bromide has a very low solubility, but that solubility can be increased dramatically by the use of a sodium thiosulfate ($Na_2S_2O_3$) solution—the thiosulfate ions react with silver ions to form the stable complex ion $[Ag(S_2O_3)_2]^{3-}$ (dithiosulfatoargentate [I]), removing free Ag^+ ions from the solution and therefore causing more AgBr to dissolve.

Solubility and pH

The pH of a solution will not affect the solubility of all chemicals. In particular, the solubility of neutral salts will generally not be affected by the pH of a solution. However, the solubility of acidic or basic salts will be pH dependent.

A basic salt—the salt of a weak acid—will have a greater solubility the lower the pH of the solution. This is because the H_3O^+ ions in the acidic solution will react easily with the relatively strong basic anions of the salt. By Le Châtelier's Principle, the removal of these ions from the solution will shift the equilibrium toward the production of more such ions, leading to more of the salt dissolving. For similar reasons, an acidic salt—the salt of a weak base—will have a greater solubility the higher the pH of the solution.

Titration

Indicators

An indicator is a substance that when added to a solution, changes color (or some other easily observable property) depending on the pH of the solution (or some other property not easily observed directly). One of the best-known indicators is litmus, a mixture of chemicals extracted from lichens that is red in acidic solutions and blue in basic. It is typically sold in the form of litmus paper, strips of paper impregnated with the chemical. Another class of indicators, anthocyanins, are found in red cabbage and certain other plants. Other widely used indicators include phenolphthalein, methyl orange, and bromothymol blue.

Indicators are useful in titration because they help the observer identify the moment at which the pH changes. Because different indicators differ in the range of pHs over which they change color, an appropriate indicator will be chosen for a given titration based on the pH of the expected change. Methyl orange, for instance, changes color at a low pH and phenolphthalein at a high pH; litmus and bromothymol blue both change color around neutral pH, although the range of pH for the color change of litmus is wider.

NEUTRALIZATION

Neutralization in chemistry refers to the reaction of an acid and a base to form a salt. In the case of Arrhenius bases—bases that include a hydroxide (OH^-) ion—the reaction also produces water. Despite the name, neutralization does not necessarily result in a neutral solution. The acid and base are said to be neutralized when no excess acid or base remains, but the resulting solution may be acidic, if it results from a strong acid and a weak base, or basic, if it results from a weak acid and a strong base.

For example, the strong acid hydrochloric acid and the strong base sodium hydroxide neutralize each other to form water and sodium chloride: $HCl + NaOH \rightarrow NaCl + H_2O$. (In this case, because HCl is a strong base and NaOH is a strong acid, the resulting solution is neutral.) Other neutralization reactions include $H_2SO_4 + 2KOH \rightarrow K_2SO_4 + 2H_2O$ and, for an example of a neutralization reaction involving Brønsted-Lowry acids and bases, $H^+ + NH_3 \rightarrow NH_4^+$.

INTERPRETATION OF THE TITRATION CURVES

Titration is the process of slowly adding small amounts of a solution of known concentration—the titrant—to a known volume of solution of unknown concentration—the analyte—until some reaction occurs. The volume of titrant added can then be used to find the concentration of the analyte. One common type of titration is acid-base titration, in which the titrant is acidic and the analyte basic, or vice versa, and the looked-for reaction is neutralization.

The titration curve is a curve used in acid-base titration to chart how the pH of the solution changes as more titrant is added. The independent variable is the total volume of titrant added, and the dependent variable is the pH.

The equivalence point of a titration curve is the point of maximum slope. Generally, a titration curve will start out with a relatively shallow slope, then at some point the slope will sharply increase, only to level off again. The equivalence point is where the curve is at its steepest.

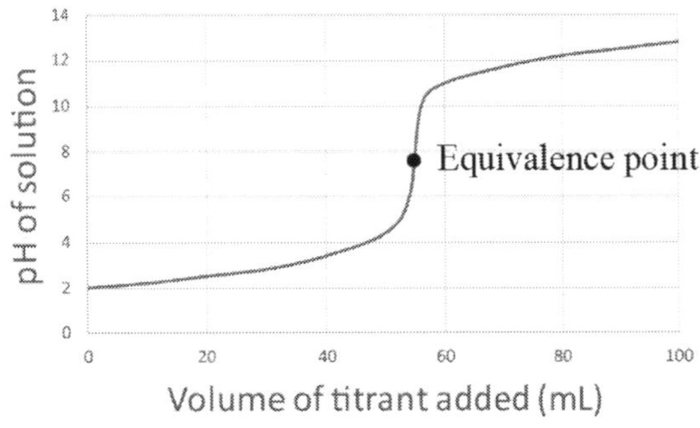

The equivalence point is important because it marks the moment where neutralization occurred. The slope of the titration curve of an acid-base titration indicates the rate of change of the pH of the solution as more titrant is added. It starts out shallow because when the solution is far from neutrality, adding small amounts of acid or base will have little effect. As the concentrations of acid and base become nearly equal, however, a small change in the amount of acid or base can have a large effect on pH, and the slope increases sharply. As the neutralization point is passed, and now the titrant is in excess, again a small increase in the amount of titrant has little effect on the pH, and the slope decreases again.

A monoprotic acid is an acid that can donate only a single proton or that has only a single H^+ ion. Monoprotic acids include hydrochloric acid, HCl; nitric acid, HNO_3; and acetic acid, $HC_2H_3O_2$. (Although acetic acid has four hydrogen atoms, three of them are part of the acetate anion and are not available for donation.) A polyprotic acid is one that has two or more protons or H^+ ions available for donation. Polyprotic acids include sulfuric acid, H_2SO_4; carbonic acid, H_2CO_3; and phosphoric acid, H_2PO_4.

Unlike a monoprotic acid, the titration curve of a polyprotic acid will have more than one equivalence point—the slope of the curve will become steeper and shallower several times. Specifically, it will have one equivalence point for each proton it can donate. This is because a polyprotic acid becomes a different acid when it donates a proton, and that acid has its own inflection point as well. For instance, when H_2SO_4 donates a proton, it becomes HSO_4^-, hydrogen sulfate, which is itself (weakly) acidic. The titration curve for H_2SO_4 shows both an equivalence point at which the H_2SO_4 itself is neutralized and then a second equivalence point where the HSO_4^- is neutralized.

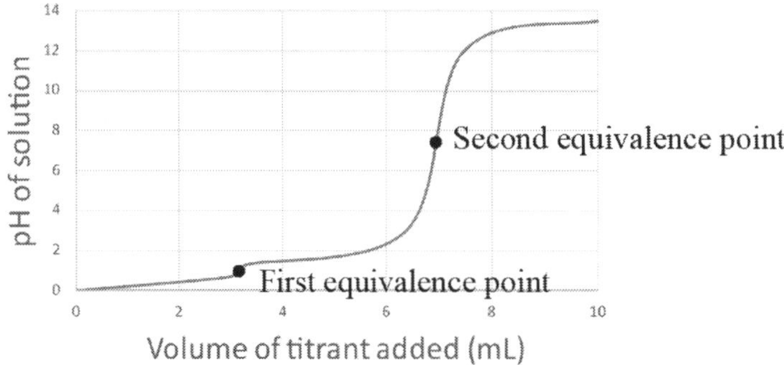

A titration curve with a strong acid or base will have a simple, well-defined sigmoid shape; the titration curve will rise or fall relatively slowly at the start, then become much steeper near the inflection point, and then return to a low rate of change. In the case of a weak acid or base, however, including a buffer solution, the shape will be slightly more complex. For a weak acid, at a pH below the equivalence point when the acid is of a higher concentration than the base, the solution will form a buffer, and the slope will become almost flat. Once the concentrations are nearly equalized, the slope will increase again, and the curve will reach an equivalence point as before. At the center of the flat region of the curve is the half-equivalence point, where half the acid has been converted to its conjugate base. At this point, the pH of the solution is equal to the pK_a for the weak acid.

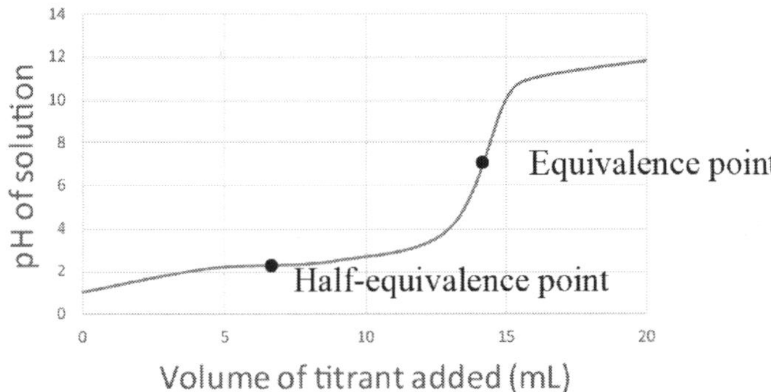

For a weak base, the situation is similar, except that the flat region of the curve and the half-equivalence point will be at a high pH, and at the equivalence point, the pH of the solution is equal to $(14 - pK_b)$.

Redox Titration

A redox titration is a titration based not on a neutralization reaction as with acid-base titration but on a redox reaction. As with other titrations, small amounts of a substance of known concentration (the titrant) are added to a fixed volume of a substance of unknown concentration (the analyte). In a redox titration, the titrant is a reducing agent, and the analyte is an oxidizing agent, or vice versa.

In a redox titration curve, the independent variable is the amount of titrant added, and the dependent variable is the cell potential of the system. A redox titration curve starts out with a shallow slope, as the titrant is almost completely oxidized or reduced by the more abundant analyte, then becomes steeper as the concentrations of titrant and analyte near equality, and then becomes shallower again as the titrant becomes more abundant than the analyte. The point of steepest slope is the equivalence point, where the amount of reducing agent and balancing agent are just enough for each to react completely with the other.

Review Video: Titration
Visit mometrix.com/academy and enter code: 550131

Nature of Molecules and Intermolecular Interactions

Covalent Bond

Lewis Electron Dot Formulas

A Lewis Electron Dot formula is a method of visually portraying the bonds between atoms in a molecule or ion and the positions of unbonded electron pairs. In a Lewis formula, each atom is represented by its chemical symbol; a line drawn between atoms represents a bond—with two lines for a double bond and three for a triple—and a dot represents an unbonded electron.

One method to derive Lewis structures starts with totaling the number of valence electrons in all the atoms. Then sum the electrons needed to surround each atom—usually eight for most atoms (the octet rule) and two for hydrogen. Total these electrons, subtract the valence electrons (and the charge, for an ion), and divide by two to find the number of bonds required. Find a way to place this many bonds between the atoms (which may involve some trial and error), and then place the remaining electrons to satisfy the octet rule.

For instance, formic acid is CH_2O_2. There are 4 + 2(1) + 2(6) = 18 valence electrons; 8 + 2(2) + 2(8) = 28; (28 – 18) / 2 = 5. Five bonds are needed, which can be arranged as follows, with the additional electrons:

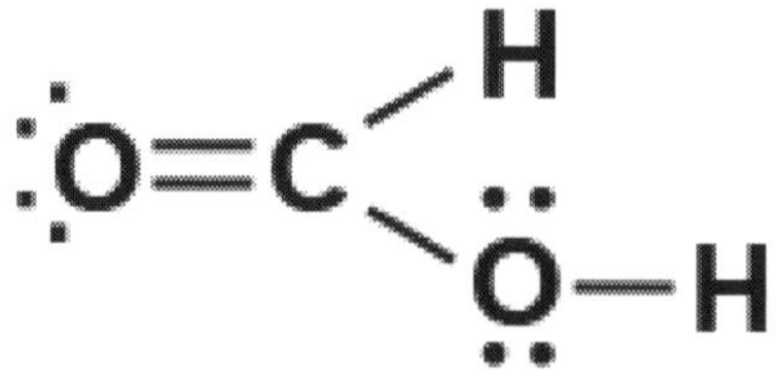

RESONANCE STRUCTURES

Sometimes when deriving a Lewis dot formula, it turns out that there is more than one possible way to arrange the bonds and electrons so that the necessary conditions are satisfied, without changing the overall structure of the molecule (which atoms are bonded to which other atoms). In this case, the molecule or ion is said to have resonance, and the different possible arrangements are called resonance structures. For example, consider the thiocyanate ion, CNS^-. There are 4 (from C) + 5 (from N) + 6 (from S) + 1 (from the charge) = 16 total valence electrons; 3(8) = 24 are needed, so we need (24 – 16) / 2 = 4 bonds. There are three ways to achieve this:

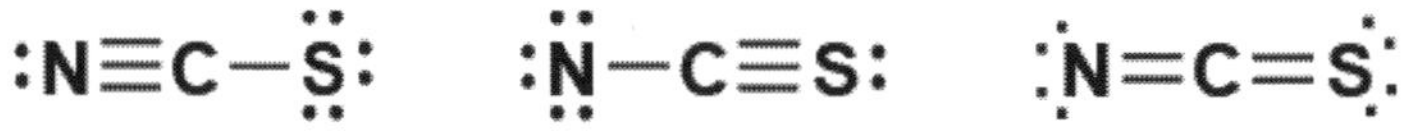

In this case, the third structure is the most accurate; the formal charges are minimized, and the most electronegative atom has the lowest formal charge. But often there is no preferred structure. For the carbonate ion CO_3^{2-}, we need ([4(8) + 2] – [4 + 3(6)] / 2 = 4 bonds, leading to the following structure:

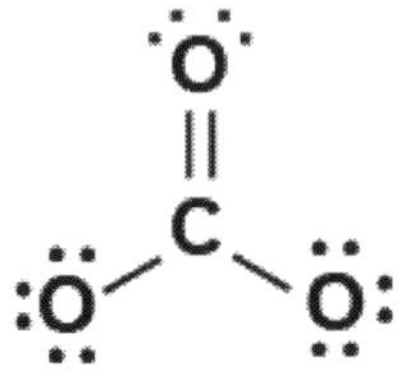

But there's no reason to choose any particular oxygen atom for the double bond; there are three resonant structures:

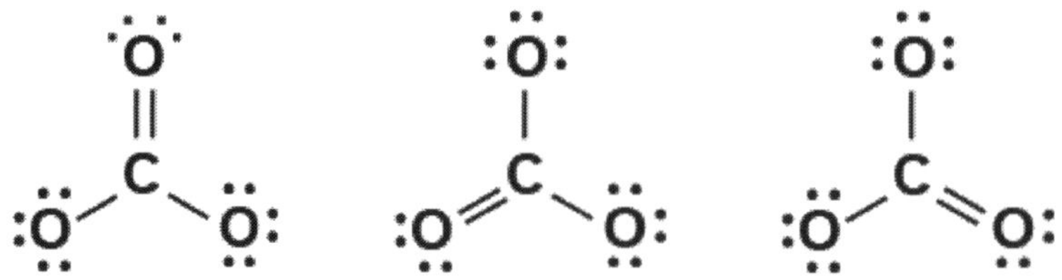

In practice, the ion's structure is a hybrid of all of these.

FORMAL CHARGE

To find the formal charge of an atom in a Lewis Electron Dot formula, take the number of valence electrons in a free atom of the element, subtract the number of unbonded electrons, and then subtract half the number of bonded electrons—which is equivalent to subtracting the number of bonds. The total of the formal charges of all the atoms is equal to zero for a neutral molecule or, for an ion, the charge of the ion. If there are multiple possible Lewis structures (resonances), the preferred structure is the one where the atoms have the smallest magnitudes of formal charges, and the most electronegative atom has the most negative formal charge.

For example, consider carbon dioxide, which has three resonances:

:O≡C—O: :O—C≡O: :O=C=O:

In all three, the carbon atom has a formal charge of 4 (valence electrons) – 0 (bonded electrons) – 4 (bonds) = 0. In the first, the oxygen on the left has a formal charge of 6 – 2 – 3 = +1 and the oxygen on the right of 6 – 6 – 1 = –1. In the second, these are reversed. In the third, both oxygen atoms have a formal charge of 6 – 4 – 2 = 0, so the third is preferred.

Lewis Acids and Bases

The Lewis theory of acids and basis is named after American physical chemist Gilbert Newton Lewis, noted for his work in thermodynamics and chemical bonding. (This is the same Lewis who developed the Lewis Electron Dot formula.) A Lewis acid is a substance that can accept a pair of electrons. A Lewis base is a substance that can donate a pair of electrons. The Lewis definition of acids and bases further expands the concept beyond the Brønsted-Lowry definition, allowing consideration of chemicals as acids and bases that don't qualify under that theory. Any molecule or ion with an unshared pair of electrons can be a Lewis base, and any with an atom that requires one or more pairs of electrons to fill its valence shell can be a Lewis acid. This means that the H^+ ion qualifies as a Lewis acid because it needs a pair of electrons to fill its valence shell, but so do other molecules and ions, such as boron trifluoride, BF_3, in which the boron molecule has only six electrons in its valence shell.

Formation of Covalent Bonds

Unlike an ionic bond, in which one atom "donates" one or more electrons to another and then the two atoms are attracted to each other by their opposite charge, in a covalent bond two atoms share a pair of electrons. Covalent bonds usually occur between nonmetals; the elements in group 14 (carbon, silicon, etc.) are especially prone to form covalent bonds because their valence shells are half full: this makes it impractical to form an ionic bond as they would have to donate or accept four electrons.

It is possible for two atoms to share more than one pair of electrons. If they share two pairs of electrons, then there is said to be a double bond between them. If the atoms share three pairs of electrons, this is said to be a triple bond. Double bonds are shorter than single bonds—that is, the atoms are closer together—as well as stronger—and harder to break. Triple bonds are shorter and stronger still.

Lewis Electron Dot Formula Exceptions

One of the fundamental rules of creating Lewis Electron Dot formulas is the octet rule that each atom must be surrounded by eight electrons. Nevertheless, this rule has exceptions. The most common exception is that concerning hydrogen—unlike the heavier elements, hydrogen needs only two electrons to fill its valence shell, not eight. But exceptions sometimes occur, not including hydrogen as well. Most commonly, a compound will have too many electrons to make it possible to satisfy the octet rule, leaving one or more atoms with more than eight electrons surrounding them. Usually these excess electrons will surround the central atom. For instance, in thionyl chloride ($SOCl_2$), the sulfur atom has 10 electrons; in iodine pentafluoride (IF_5) the iodine atom has 12. Other compounds may have too few electrons; this is most common for compounds involving boron and beryllium. (These compounds generally act as Lewis acids.) In boron trichloride (BCl_3), the boron atom has only six electrons; in beryllium iodide (BeI_2) the beryllium has only four. Finally, some molecules contain an odd number of electrons, which makes it impossible to satisfy the octet rule; examples include nitrous oxide (NO) and chlorine dioxide (ClO_2).

Partial Ionic Character

Role of Electronegativity in Determining Charge Distribution

Although electrons are shared between atoms in a covalent bond, they are not necessarily shared equally. Generally, the electron is more closely associated with the atom with higher electronegativity. If the two atoms have the same electronegativity, then the electron will be shared equally; thus, in a molecule of H_2 or O_2, the electrons in the covalent bonds are shared equally between both atoms. On the other hand, in hydrochloric acid (HCl), the chlorine has a much higher electronegativity than the hydrogen (3.16 vs. 2.20). The electron will thus be more closely associated with the chlorine atom, and although the atom as a whole will be neutrally charged, the chlorine atom will have a slight negative charge, whereas the hydrogen atom is slightly positive. Similarly, because oxygen has a higher electronegativity than hydrogen (3.44 vs. 2.20), the oxygen atom in a molecule of water (H_2O) will have a slight negative charge, and the hydrogen atoms will have a slight positive charge. A covalent bond in which the electrons are shared unequally is called a polar covalent bond.

Dipole Moment

The dipole moment of a molecule is a measurement of the polarity of a molecule—the difference in charge between the ends. More specifically, the magnitude of the dipole moment of an atomic bond in a molecule is equal to the charge difference between the bonded atoms times the length of the bond. It is a vector quantity, pointing from the positive toward the negative charge. For a molecule with more than two atoms, the overall dipole moment can be found by adding together as vectors the dipole moments of each bond.

Polar molecules—molecules with nonzero dipole moments—tend to align themselves to electric fields and to other polar molecules and ions. This makes it possible to determine the dipole moment experimentally by measuring this alignment. For instance, a polar substance placed between the two charged plates of a parallel-plate capacitor will tend to align to the electric field of the capacitor and in doing so will alter the capacitance of the system; by measuring the capacitance, one can in principle derive the dipole moments of the particles.

A polar molecule is a molecule in which two sides of the molecule have opposite charges. A nonpolar molecule is a molecule in which in any orientation of the two sides of the molecule are equally charged. Equivalently, a polar molecule is a molecule with a nonzero dipole moment; a nonpolar molecule has a dipole moment of zero. Thus, for instance, H_2 is a polar molecule; the electrons are shared equally, and the dipole moment is zero. HF is polar; the hydrogen atom has a positive charge, and the fluorine negative.

Note that a molecule can be nonpolar even if the individual bonds are polar. For example, oxygen has a higher electronegativity than carbon, so in a carbon dioxide molecule, the oxygen atoms are slightly negative and the carbon atom positive. However, because the oxygen atoms are positioned symmetrically on either side of the carbon atom, the dipole moments of the bonds cancel, and the carbon dioxide molecule as a whole is nonpolar. The same is true of methane, CH_4, in which each bond is polar but the molecule has tetrahedral symmetry. It is not true, however, of molecules such as water and ammonia, which lack such symmetry and are polar.

Σ AND Π BONDS

A sigma bond is a bond formed by two atomic orbitals of similar orientation overlapping end to end. Overlapping s-orbitals always form sigma bonds because they are spherically symmetrical and their orientation is irrelevant, but p-orbitals and higher orbitals can also form sigma bonds if they overlap along their axes of symmetry. A pi bond forms when two atomic orbitals overlap along their sides, such as two p-orbitals that are displaced along a line perpendicular to their axes of symmetry.

Single bonds between atoms are almost always sigma bonds (although the bond in B_2 is an exception). Double bonds comprise one sigma bond and one pi bond, whereas triple bonds contain one sigma bond and two pi bonds. Although sigma bonds are stronger than pi bonds, the fact that double bonds consist of a sigma bond and a pi bond make them stronger than single bonds that consist of just a sigma bond, and for the same reason triple bonds are stronger still.

HYBRID ORBITALS SP, SP2, AND SP3 AND RESPECTIVE GEOMETRIES

Hybrid orbitals occur when atomic orbitals combine into new configurations to facilitate the pairing of electrons and the formation of bonds by orienting the electrons in such a way as to minimize the repulsive forces between them.

In a sp hybrid orbital, one s orbital mixes with one p orbital to form two sp orbitals. This often occurs in molecules that include a triple bond. Ethylene (C_2H_2) is an example of a simple molecule with sp orbitals: the 2s orbital of each carbon atom mixes with one of the 2p orbitals to form two sp orbitals, one of which bonds to the hydrogen atom and the other with the other carbon atom; and the remaining two 2p orbitals bond to the other carbon atom in pi bonds.

In a sp2 hybrid orbital, one s orbital mixes with two p orbitals to form three hybrid orbitals. This often accompanies a double bond and occurs, for example, with the carbon atoms in ethene, C_2H_4. Finally, a sp3 hybrid orbital mixes one s orbital and three p orbitals to form four symmetrically arranged hybrid orbitals; this occurs where bonds have tetrahedral symmetry, such as, for instance, in methane, CH_4.

VALENCE SHELL ELECTRON PAIR REPULSION AND THE PREDICTION OF SHAPES MOLECULES

Valence shell electron pair repulsion, or VSEPR, refers to the tendency of electrons around a given atom to arrange themselves in such a way as to put them maximally distant from each other, including both bonds and unpaired electrons. This can be used to predict the geometry of a molecule. The key to using this technique is to count the number of electron groups around the atom, which is sometimes called the VSEPR number. Any pair of unbonded electrons counts as one electron group; so does an unpaired electron; and so does a bond, regardless of its multiplicity (single, double, or triple). This VSEPR number determines how the electron groups are distributed: linear for 2, in an equilateral triangle for 3, tetrahedrally for 4, and so on. For example, the carbon in CO_2 has two (double) bonds and no unbonded electrons; its VSEPR number is 2. This means carbon dioxide is linear. On the other hand, the oxygen in water has two bonds plus two pairs of unbonded electrons for a VSEPR number of 4. Its electron groups are arranged tetrahedrally, with unbonded electron pairs on two corners of the tetrahedron and the bonded hydrogen atoms on the other two.

MULTIPLE BONDING

The geometries of bonds around atoms in molecules mostly fall into a few classes. A linear geometry describes an atom with another atom bonded on either side, the three forming a straight line. This generally occurs when the atom has two bonds and no unbonded electrons, such as in carbon dioxide (CO_2) or beryllium fluoride (BeF_2). This contrasts with a bent geometry that occurs when there are two bonds but also one or two unbonded electron pairs, as in water (H_2O) or sulfur dioxide (SO_2). A trigonal planar geometry occurs when an atom has three bonds and no unpaired electrons and involves the three bonds all being in a plane and forming (something close to) an equilateral triangle. Examples include the nitrate ion NO_3^- and formaldehyde, CH_2O. In a trigonal pyramidal geometry, the atom's three bonds are all in the same direction, making the central atom the apex of a pyramid; this occurs when the atom has three bonds and one pair of unbonded electrons, as in ammonia (NH_3) and the sulfite ion (SO_3^{2-}). Finally, tetrahedral geometry involves four bonds arranged tetrahedrally, as in methane (CH_4) or the sulfate ion (SO_4^{2-}).

Rigidity in Molecular Structure

In general, single bonds are able to freely rotate, which may lead to some decrease in molecular rigidity. In some simple molecules, the rotation of a bond may not make a difference; rotating the bonds in a water molecule or a molecule of HF will not change the structure of the molecule at all. On the other hand, rotating the bond between oxygen atoms in a molecule of hydrogen peroxide, H_2O_2, will change the geometry of the molecule significantly. Double and triple bonds do not have this rotational freedom, so a molecule with many double or triple bonds will tend to be more rigid than a molecule of similar size with only single bonds.

Number of Bonds for Atoms

Hydrogen only has a single electron and needs one more electron to fill its valence shell, so it generally makes only one bond in a molecule.

Oxygen is in group 16 and has six valence electrons. It needs two more to fill its valence shell, so it will typically make two bonds, counting multiplicity—that is, it will make two single bonds or one double bond.

Nitrogen is in group 15 and has five valence electrons. It needs three more to fill its valence shell, so it will typically make three bonds, counting multiplicity—that is, it can make three single bonds, or one single bond and two double bonds, or one triple bond. It can form up to four bonds in some circumstances.

Carbon is in group 14 and has four valence electrons. It needs four more to fill its valence shell, so it will typically make four bonds, counting multiplicity. It is the fact that carbon makes so many bonds, and can bond in so many ways (four single, two double, one single and one triple, etc.) that enables it to form into complex organic molecules and form the foundation of life on Earth.

Fluorine and chlorine are both halogens in group 17. They have seven electrons in their valence shells and need one more to fill their shells; they therefore generally form one bond.

Silicon is in group 14, along with carbon; like carbon, it has four valence electrons, and needs four more to fill its valence shell, and so typically makes four bonds, counting multiplicity (i.e., counting a double bond as two bonds and a triple bond as three—although silicon rarely forms double or triple bonds). The bonds formed by silicon are weaker than those formed by carbon, however, and it isn't quite as versatile in the molecules it can make up.

Phosphorus is in group 15; it has five valence electrons and needs another three electrons to fill its valence shell. It often forms three bonds but can form up to five bonds—the reason nitrogen, in the same group, can't form as many bonds is simply because phosphorus is larger and can fit more atoms around it.

Sulfur is in group 16 and needs two electrons to fill its valence shell, but although it often forms two bonds, it can form anywhere from two to six.

Drawing the Structural Formula of a Molecule

The structural formula of a molecule is a diagram that shows the atoms of the molecule and the bonds between them. Each atom is represented by its chemical symbol, and a line is drawn between bonded atoms—two lines for a double bond and three lines for a triple bond. Unlike a Lewis Electron Dot formula, the structural formula does not necessarily show unbonded electrons. Common groups of atoms may be depicted as a unit rather than with their bonds; OH and CH_3 may appear in structural formulas in this way.

For complex organic molecules, the structural formula is often simplified by not explicitly representing carbon and hydrogen atoms. The carbon atoms are implied where the lines representing the bonds end and intersect, if no atom is explicitly shown there. Hydrogen atoms bonded to carbon atoms are omitted and can be inferred to exist wherever there are fewer than four bonds shown. This simplified structural formula is also called a skeletal formula.

As examples, shown below are the structural formulas for ammonia, NH_3, and acetaldehyde, C_2H_4O. The latter is shown in three ways: with all bonds shown, with the CH_3 compacted, and as a simplified (skeletal) formula.

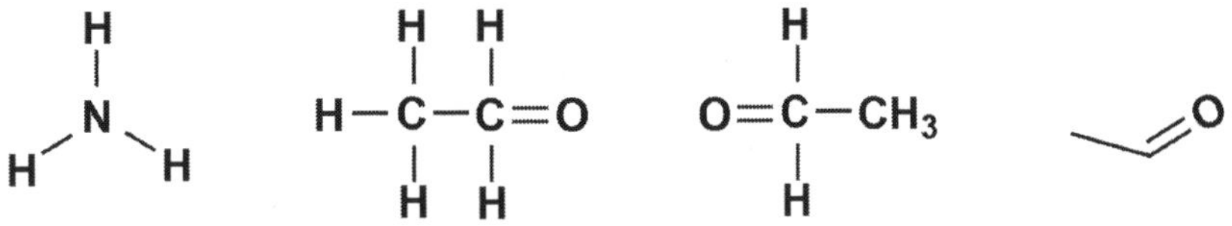

Delocalized Electrons

A delocalized electron is an electron that may pertain to a particular molecule or ion but is not associated with any one atom or bond. Because of their mobility, the presence of delocalized electrons tends to lead to greater electrical and thermal conductivity. Delocalized electrons are common in metals, which form metallic bonds in which the valence electrons move freely among the atoms in a sort of "electron sea" rather than remaining near one or two atoms. They also can occur under some circumstances, however, in other molecules. When a molecule or ion has two or more resonance structures, no one of which is highly favored over the others, this generally represents one or more electrons being delocalized to combine the resonance structures. One important example of such a structure is the benzene ring, which consists of a ring of six bonded carbon atoms. Although the benzene ring is sometimes depicted with alternating single and double bonds, a more accurate representation involves one electron from each carbon atom becoming delocalized and being free to move around the entire ring; each bond between atoms in the ring is not a "pure" single or double bond but something in between.

Review Video: Metallic Bonds
Visit mometrix.com/academy and enter code: 230855

Stereochemistry of Covalently Bonded Molecules

Isomers

Isomers: Structural Isomers

When two molecules have the same elements and the same number of atoms of each element, but have the atoms bonded together in different ways, they are said to be structural isomers. Structural isomers have the same molecular formula but different structural formulas. One of the simplest examples is C_2H_2O, which describes three different structural isomers: ethenone, ethynol, and oxirene. The structural formulas for these are depicted below:

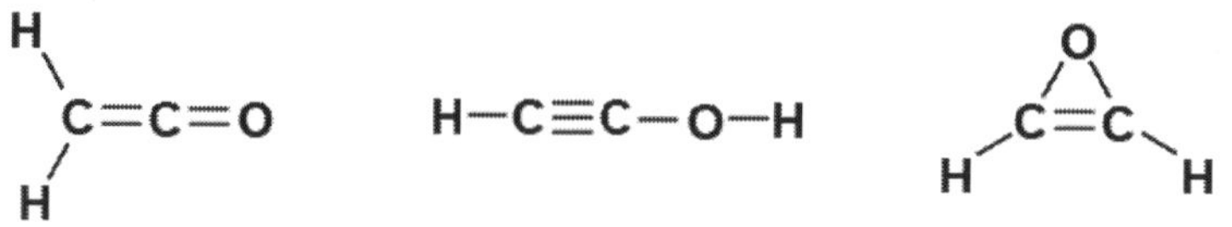

More complex organic molecules may have many more structural isomers. The molecular formula $C_6H_{12}O_6$, for instance, describes the sugars glucose and fructose but also hundreds more structural isomers with six carbon, twelve hydrogen, and six oxygen atoms (most of which have no simple names but are given complicated names like alpha-L-altropyranose and (2S,3R,4R,5S)-2,3,4,5,6-pentahydroxyhexanal).

Isomers: Stereoisomers

Two molecules are enantiomers if they are mirror images of each other—but are not identical—so a symmetrical molecule would not be said to be an enantiomer of itself; the term only applies to chiral molecules. For example, the compound chlorofluoroiodomethane, CHClFI, exists in two different forms that are enantiomers. Both versions of the molecule are tetrahedral, with the carbon atom in the center and the hydrogen, chlorine, fluorine, and iodine atoms at the points of the tetrahedron. But there are two different ways of choosing the placement of the outer atoms that result in two different mirror-image molecules that cannot be rotated into each other. Despite their structural similarity, enantiomers may be very different in their interactions with biological systems.

There are, of course, much more complicated examples of enantiomers than chlorofluoroiodomethane. Amino acids, for example, are chiral—asymmetrical—and so each amino acid also has a corresponding mirror-image form. However, life on Earth uses almost exclusively only one form of each amino acid; their enantiomers are rarely found in nature.

In general, two molecules are stereoisomers if they have the same molecular and structural formulae, but they nevertheless differ in the orientation of the bonds and in their three-dimensional shapes. Enantiomers—different molecules that are mirror images of each other—are one kind of stereoisomer. Two molecules are diastereoisomers (or just diastereomers) if they are stereoisomers but not enantiomers—they differ in their three-dimensional structure but are not just mirror images. Diagrams of diastereomers are sometimes distinguished by drawing them in a sort of quasi-perspective, with black triangles representing bonds coming "out of the page" and dashed triangles representing bonds going "into the page."

For instance, 2,3-butanediol consists of a line of four carbon atoms, with an oxygen atom bonded to each of the middle two atoms, and hydrogen atoms filling all the remaining bonding locations. This chemical has three different stereoisomers, depicted below. (These are skeletal diagrams, so the carbon atoms and the hydrogen atoms bonded to them are implicit.)

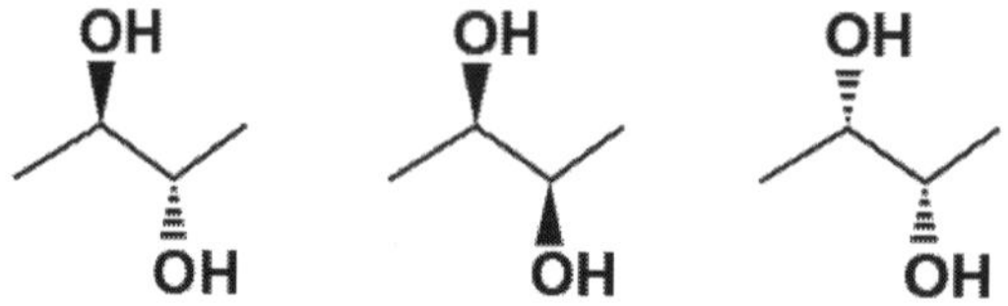

Note that the two molecules on the right are enantiomers of each other, but they are both diastereoisomers of the molecule on the left (meso-2, 3-butanediol), which is symmetrical and has no enantiomer.

Two molecules are cis/trans isomers if they are stereoisomers that contain a chain of carbon atoms and that differ as to whether two like atoms or groups of atoms are on the same side (cis) or opposite sides (trans) of the central carbon chain. By definition, all cis/trans isomers are diastereoisomers, but not all diastereoisomers are cis/trans isomers. Note that in all cis/trans isomers, the carbon chain contains at least one double bond or ring structure; this is because parts of molecules can freely rotate around a single bond so that the same molecule can easily change between forms with like parts on the same or opposite side of the central carbon chain if it has only single bonds.

One simple compound that exhibits cis/trans isomerism is 1, 2-dichloroethene, a molecule with two carbon atoms connected by a double bond, and with one chlorine and one hydrogen atom connected to each carbon molecule. The cis and trans forms are shown symbolically below:

cis trans

A slightly more complicated is 2-butene, a molecule consisting of four carbon atoms with a double bond between the center two and with hydrogen atoms filling the remaining bonding locales:

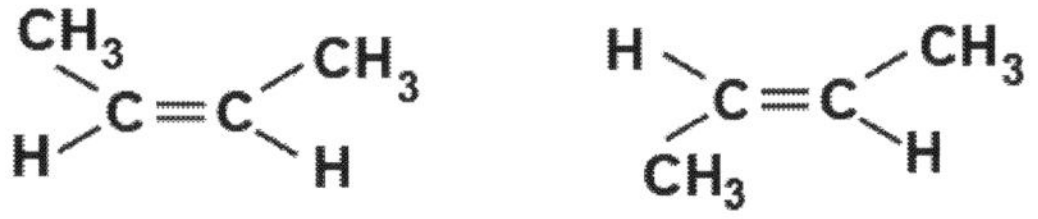

cis trans

Isomers: Conformational Isomer

Two different molecular structures are conformational isomers if they have the same molecules with the same bonds (they are stereoisomers), but they can be converted between each other without breaking any bonds. In other words, the molecules are identical except for rotation around single bonds (double and triple bonds are more rigid and do not allow free rotation). However, this does not necessarily mean that the same molecule can freely change between conformational isomers; it may happen that only certain rotation angles are stable and that an energy barrier inhibits the molecule from readily changing from one stable state to another.

One simple molecule that has different conformational isomers is ethane, C_2H_6. The ends can be rotated about the single bond in the middle to form a so-called eclipsed conformation, in which the hydrogens on each side are directly lined up with each other; a "staggered" conformation, in which the hydrogen atom on one side is in the middle of the gap between hydrogen atoms on the other or anywhere in between.

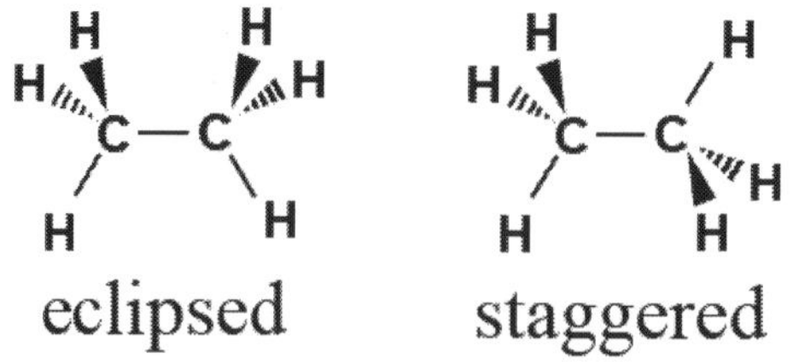

eclipsed staggered

In practice, the staggered conformation is much more stable than the eclipsed, so ethane molecules will most often be found in or near this conformation.

Polarization of Light, Specific Rotation

A molecule is said to be optically active if the polarization direction of linearly polarized light is rotated when it passes through a substance composed of this molecule. Such molecules can be further classified based on which direction they rotate the light: molecules that rotate light clockwise are said to be dextrorotary; those that rotate light counterclockwise are levorotary.

Molecules are optically active only if they are chiral—that is, they are asymmetrical; they have a mirror image form. If a molecule is levorotary, its enantiomer—the mirror-image version—is dextrorotary and vice versa. An equal mixture of both enantiomers of a compound is said to be racemic and is not optically active because the rotation due to the levorotary and dextrorotary molecules tends to cancel out.

Specific rotation is a measurement of how much an optically active substance rotates linearly polarized light that passes through it. More specifically, it is a measurement of the angle by which the light rotates when it travels 1 decimeter (0.1 m) through a solution of the substance in question with a mass concentration of 1 gram per milliliter. The units of specific rotation are therefore degrees times milliliters (grams times decimeters) but are sometimes given in just degrees, the other units being implied.

The specific rotation of a substance can be measured by a device called a polarimeter, which measures the change in angle of polarization of light after it passes through a solution. Dividing this angle by the light's path length in decimeters and the solution's concentration in grams per milliliter yields the specific rotation.

Absolute and Relative Configuration

Absolute and relative configuration are terms that refer to the arrangement of atoms in chiral molecules—asymmetrical molecules that exist in two mirror-image forms, or enantiomers. The relative configuration of the molecule is its configuration relative to another molecule from which it can be produced. Historically, relative configuration was often stated relative to glyceraldehyde, a particular simple sugar which could be converted into many different compounds (without affecting the configuration of key parts of the molecule). The enantiomers were labeled with the prefix D- if they had the same configuration as the dextrorotary enantiomer of glyceraldehyde (which did not necessarily imply that the molecule in question was itself dextrorotary) and L- if they had the same configuration as levorotary glyceraldehyde. Absolute configuration refers to the precise known geometrical arrangement of the atoms, not relative to any other compounds.

Absolute and Relative Configuration: Conventions for Writing the R and S Forms

The enantiomers of a simple chiral molecule (i.e., the two mirror-image forms of an asymmetrical molecule) can be distinguished by calling one form the R form and one the S form. For a more complex molecule, this terminology can be applied not to a molecule as a whole but to each stereocenter—location in the molecule where there is an atom (usually carbon) with asymmetrical bonds.

To distinguish between the two, determine the "priority" of each constituent bonded to the central atom. The higher the atomic number of the atom bonded directly to the carbon, the higher the priority. If the atom immediately bonded is the same, follow the chain of atoms until you reach a difference. If there's still a tie, double bonds have higher priority than single bonds. Now, picture the lowest-priority constituent pointing away from you, and trace a circle through the others from highest to lowest priority. If this circle runs clockwise, it is an R form; if counterclockwise, it is L.

For instance, consider lactic acid:

Although this has three carbon atoms, only the central one is asymmetrical, so this is our stereocenter. The priority goes $H < CH_4 < COOH < OH$, so we have:

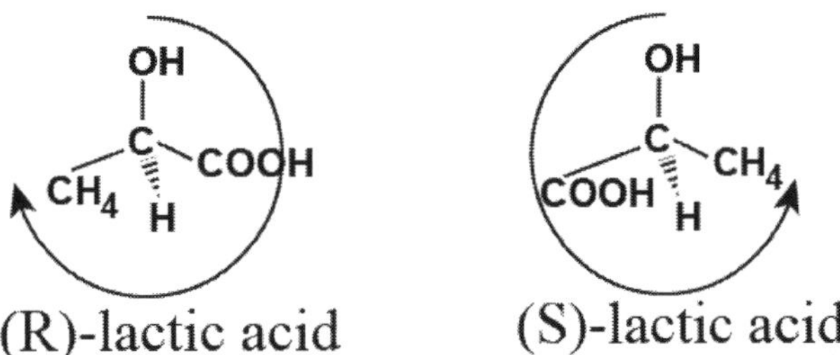

Absolute and Relative Configuration: Conventions for Writing the E and Z Forms

The E and Z terminology is used to distinguish stereoisomers with double bonds, based on the relative positions of the constituents on each side. When there are only two different constituents, they can be distinguished by calling the one with matching constituents on the same side of the central carbon chain cis and the other trans; with more than two constituents, however, these terms are ambiguous, and the E–Z terminology is used.

To distinguish between (E) and (Z) isomers, determine which constituent on each end has a higher "priority." The higher the atomic number of the atom directly connected to the double-bonded atom, the higher the priority; in case of a tie, consider the next atom out, and so on. If the higher priority constituents on each end are on the same side of the double bond, it is a (Z)-isomer; if not, it is an (E)-isomer.

For instance, consider the molecules tiglic acid and angelic acid: two chemicals that are (E) and (Z) isomers:

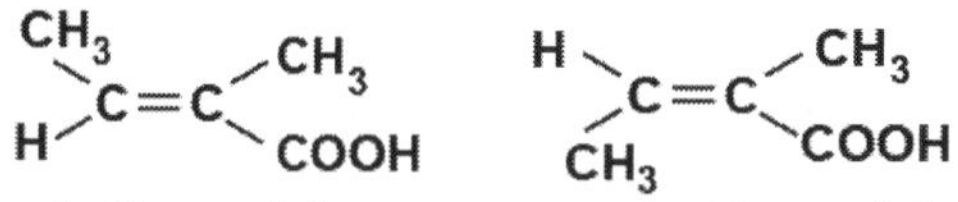

CH_3 has a higher priority than H, but COOH has a higher priority than CH_3. So tiglic acid is the (E)-isomer, and angelic acid is the (Z)-isomer.

Liquid Phase - Intermolecular Forces

Hydrogen Bonding

Hydrogen bonding refers to an intermolecular force between two polar molecules arising because a hydrogen atom with a partial positive charge in one molecule is attracted to an atom in another molecule with a partial negative charge. Although hydrogen bonds are not as strong as molecular covalent bonds, the fact that they do cause the molecules to "stick together" better is responsible for increasing the boiling points and viscosities of the compounds in which hydrogen bonds occur. For example, water molecules form hydrogen bonds—between a hydrogen atom in one molecule and the oxygen atom in another—and it is this that gives water its relatively high boiling point and viscosity as well as allowing it to form an open lattice in the solid form that gives solid water (ice) its low density.

When two molecules form a hydrogen bond, due to a positively charged hydrogen atom in one molecule being attracted to a negatively charged atom in the other, the negatively charged atom that the hydrogen atom is attracted to is called the hydrogen bond acceptor, whereas the atom bonded to the hydrogen atom in the first molecule (not the hydrogen atom itself) is called the hydrogen bond donor. The hydrogen bond acceptor must have an unbonded electron pair for the hydrogen atom to be attracted to. Both the donor and the acceptor tend to be highly electronegative atoms—the acceptor because it is this electronegativity that results in the atom remaining negatively charged while part of a molecule, the donor because the electronegativity of the atom the hydrogen is bonded to results in the hydrogen atom being positively charged. Oxygen, nitrogen, and fluorine, due to their high electronegativities, are common as both hydrogen bond donors and hydrogen bond acceptors.

Dipole Interactions

A dipole-dipole interaction is an intermolecular force arising because of the attraction between the negative end of one polar molecule and the positive end of another. Generally, the more polar the molecules, the stronger this force, although dipole-dipole interactions are never as strong as covalent or ionic bonds. Hydrogen bonding is one kind of dipole-dipole interaction, but dipole-dipole interactions can occur between any polar compounds—molecules in which one end has a partial positive charge and one end has a slight negative charge. Dipole-dipole interactions play important parts in biological systems; for example, the shape of a protein is largely determined by the dipole-dipole interactions between its parts.

Van der Waals' Forces

London dispersion forces are weak forces that arise between molecules because of temporary polarization—even if a molecule is nonpolar, it may have a temporary dipole moment at a given time because the electrons happen to be at that time distributed more toward one side of the nucleus, and two molecules with such temporary dipole moments may be attracted to each other similarly to a dipole-dipole interaction. London dispersion forces and dipole-dipole interactions, the other main kind of intermolecular force, are collectively called Van der Waals forces (although sometimes this term is used to refer only to dispersion forces).

Although London dispersion forces can occur between any molecules, polar or nonpolar, they tend to be stronger between larger molecules and atoms than smaller ones and stronger in long, thin molecules than in more compact ones. That is because the larger the molecule or atom, and the less compact it is, the easier it is for the electrons to become displaced and for the molecule to become temporarily polar—this property is referred to as the molecule's polarizability.

Principles of Chemical Thermodynamics and Kinetics

Energy Changes in Chemical Reactions – Thermochemistry, Thermodynamics

Thermodynamic System

A state function in thermodynamics is a quantity describing a thermodynamic system that depends only on the current state of the system and not on its history. If a state function changes, the magnitude of that change is entirely determined by the beginning and end states of the system, independent of the path it took between them. Pressure, volume, and temperature are all state functions; the current values of these properties of a system can be measured without requiring any knowledge of a system's past states. Other state functions include internal energy, entropy, enthalpy, and free energy. In contrast, non-state functions include work and heat. The work done by a system as it changes between two states very much depends on the path it takes; it cannot be calculated solely on the basis of the start and end states.

Zeroth Law

The Zeroth Law of Thermodynamics states that two bodies both in thermal equilibrium with a third body are also in thermal equilibrium with each other. Two objects are in thermal equilibrium if they are in contact—or at least they are connected by some method that would allow heat to flow between them—but there is no net heat flow between the objects.

The importance of the Zeroth Law of Thermodynamics is that it establishes that temperature is a meaningful quantity. Two objects in thermal equilibrium can be defined as having the same temperature; two objects in thermal contact but not in thermal equilibrium have different temperatures. The Zeroth Law guarantees that this definition leads to no contradictions. In fact, sometimes the Zeroth Law is written directly in terms of temperature: systems in thermal equilibrium are at the same temperature.

First Law

The First Law of Thermodynamics states that the total energy of an isolated thermodynamic system is constant. For a non-isolated system, energy may be added or taken away from the system in the form of work or heat, but this means the system's internal energy will change by the same amount. The First Law is also written mathematically as $\Delta U = Q + W$, where ΔU is the change in internal energy of the system, Q is the heat added to the system, and W is the work done on the system. (Sometimes it is instead written in the form $\Delta U = Q - W$, in which case W represents the work done by the system.)

The First Law of Thermodynamics is essentially a restatement of the law of conservation of energy or at least an application of that law to thermodynamics. Among other things, it is the first law that proves the impossibility of perpetual motion machines that provide "free energy." Energy cannot be created arbitrarily; it can only be transferred between systems in the forms of work and heat.

Review Video: First Law of Thermodynamics
Visit mometrix.com/academy and enter code: 340643

pV Diagram

A pV diagram is a diagram of a thermodynamic system in which the pressure is plotted on the *y* axis and the volume on the *x* axis. The thermodynamic state of a system is uniquely determined by these two variables, so any state variable pertaining to the system can be determined from its position on the diagram. Changes in thermodynamic state can be drawn as lines or curves on the pV diagram, representing all the states that the system passes through; changes in non-state functions can be determined from this curve. For instance, the work done by a system as it undergoes a change in state is equal to the area under the curve in a pV diagram.

As an example, the following pV diagram shows a thermodynamic cycle as a system undergoes first an isothermal (constant temperature) expansion, followed by an isobaric (constant pressure) compression, and finally an isochoric (constant volume) increase in pressure:

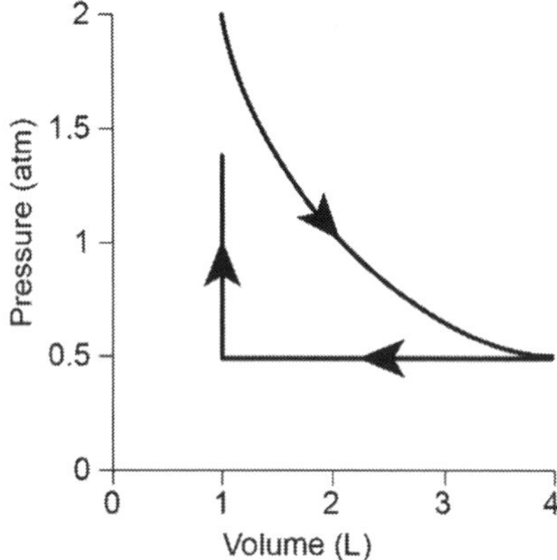

Second Law

The Second Law of Thermodynamics states that the total entropy of an isolated system can never decrease. Over time, the disorder in an isolated system must increase or stay the same. Note that this refers only to isolated systems; the entropy of part of a system can decrease as long as there is an equal or greater increase to make up for it. For instance, the entropy of the water in a pond decreases when it freezes over in winter, but this is countered by an increase in the entropy of the air the water's heat escapes to.

There are several other statements of the law that are (not obviously) equivalent and that do not explicitly refer to entropy. For instance, it is equivalent to the statement that it is not possible for heat to flow from a colder to a warmer body without work being done on the system.

The Second Law of Thermodynamics has many consequences. It determines the maximum efficiency of a heat engine and demonstrates why some chemical reactions and other processes occur preferentially in one direction (because that direction increases entropy).

Review Video: The Second Law of Thermodynamics
Visit mometrix.com/academy and enter code: 251848

ENTROPY AS A MEASURE OF "DISORDER"

Entropy is, roughly speaking, a measurement of the "disorder" in a system. It can be defined more rigorously in terms of the number of possible states that are in a certain sense equivalent. (As a quantitative value, the entropy is conventionally abbreviated *S*.) As an analogy, if you have a number of coins on the ground, there's only one state in which they are all showing heads, so this is a low-entropy state; there are many states in which roughly equal numbers of coins are heads and tails, so this is a relatively high-entropy state. Entropy tends to increase with temperature, and thanks to the Second Law of Thermodynamics the entropy of a closed system increases (or at best remains constant) over time.

In general, gases have higher entropy than liquids, and liquids have higher entropy than solids. This follows, again roughly speaking, from the fact that as a compound passes from solid to liquid to gas, its molecules or atoms become less constrained, and there are more possible states for them to be in. Crystals have particularly low entropy.

MEASUREMENT OF HEAT CHANGES (CALORIMETRY)

Calorimetry is the process of measuring the heat transferred to or from a system. Although the heat cannot be measured directly, it can often be calculated given the change in temperature and the specific heat capacity of the substance. A calorimetry problem is a problem involving heat flow to or from a system or different objects within a system. One common kind of calorimetry problem involves finding the final temperature of two objects in thermal contact. For instance, suppose you drop a 50-gram iron ball with an initial temperature of 500 °C into 100 grams of water with an initial temperature of 25°C in an insulated container. At thermal equilibrium, both will have the same temperature, T_f. Because no net heat is gained or lost by the system as a whole, we can write:

$$Q_{\mathrm{H_2O}} + Q_{\mathrm{Fe}} = 0$$

$$m_{\mathrm{H_2O}} C_{\mathrm{H_2O}} \Delta T_{\mathrm{H_2O}} + m_{\mathrm{Fe}} C_{\mathrm{Fe}} \Delta T_{\mathrm{Fe}} = 0$$

$$(100\text{ g})(4.184\text{ J/g°C})(T_f - 25\text{ °C}) + (50\text{ g})(0.450\text{ J/g°C})(T_f - 500\text{ °C}) = 0$$

$$\text{Solving for } T_f \text{ gives } T_f = 49\text{°C}.$$

More complex calorimetry problems may also involve changes of state of matter; this requires the inclusion of terms for the heat gained or lost due to this change of state (in terms of the heat of fusion or heat of vaporization).

HEAT TRANSFER – CONDUCTION, CONVECTION, RADIATION

Conduction is the transfer of heat between two objects in contact. If you put a pot of water on a hot electric stove, heat is conducted from the stove to the pot and from the pot to the water. Some materials conduct heat better than others; the reason that metal cooking pans often have wood or plastic handles is because these materials conduct heat much more poorly than metals, so you can touch the handle of the hot pan without burning your hand.

Convection is the transfer of heat within a fluid by the movement of the fluid. Warm and cold ocean and air currents are examples of convection. The churning of boiling water in a pan is a consequence of heat convection as the hotter parts of the water rise to the top.

Radiation is the transfer of heat by the emission of electromagnetic radiation. Any object loses heat by such radiation. Compared to conduction and convection, radiation is a very slow method of heat transfer. However, it does not require objects to be in contact and can therefore occur even between objects separated by the vacuum of space—heat from the Sun reaches the Earth through radiation.

Endothermic/Exothermic Reactions

Hess's Law

Hess's Law of Heat Summation states that if a chemical reaction can be broken down into smaller steps, then the total heat of the reaction is equal to the sum of the heats of reaction of each step. This can often be used to determine the heat of reaction of a particular chemical reaction if we have no feasible way to measure it directly but can find a way to break it down into sub-reactions with heats of reaction we know or can measure.

For instance, the heat of reaction of $2C + O_2 \rightarrow 2CO$ is not easy to measure directly, but we can measure those of the reactions $C + O_2 \rightarrow CO_2$ and $2CO + O_2 \rightarrow 2CO_2$. Doubling the first reaction and reversing the second, we can combine those into our original reaction:

$$\begin{array}{ccccccccccc} & & 2C & + & 2O_2 & \rightarrow & 2CO_2 & & & & \\ 2CO_2 & & & & & \rightarrow & & & 2CO & + & O_2 \\ \hline \cancel{2CO_2} & + & 2C & + & \cancel{2O_2} & \rightarrow & \cancel{2CO_2} & + & 2CO & + & \cancel{O_2} \\ & & 2C & + & O_2 & \rightarrow & & & 2CO & & \end{array}$$

The heat of reaction of $C + O_2 \rightarrow CO_2$ is –393 kJ/mol and the heat of reaction of $2CO + O_2 \rightarrow 2CO_2$ is –566 kJ/mol; therefore, the heat of reaction of $2C + O_2 \rightarrow 2CO$ is 2(–393 kJ/mol) – (–566 kJ/mol) = –220 kJ/mol.

Review Video: Hess's Law
Visit mometrix.com/academy and enter code: 329059

Bond Dissociation Energy as Related to Heats of Formation

The bond dissociation energy of a compound is the energy required to break a covalent chemical bond in such a way as to leave one of the two shared electrons with each resultant part. (This is called a homolytic cleavage, as contrasted with a heterolytic cleavage, in which both shared electrons go to the same part.) This can be thought of as a measurement of the strength of the bond—the higher the bond dissociation energy, the harder it is to break the bond, and so the stronger the bond.

Knowing the bond dissociation energy of all of the bonds in all the products and reactants of a chemical reaction allows the heat of reaction of any reaction to be determined: it is the sum of the bond dissociation energies of all the bonds in the reactants minus the bond dissociation energies of all the bonds in the products. In particular, the heat of formation of a compound—the heat of reaction of the compound from its elements—is the sum of the bond dissociation energies of all its bonds with the sign changed.

Spontaneous Reactions

The Gibbs free energy of a system, abbreviated *G*, was originally defined by the American chemist and physicist Josiah Willard Gibbs, best known for his work on thermodynamics. Gibbs defined it as the amount of available energy in a chemical system, the energy that could be used to do useful work. Specifically, the Gibbs free energy is equal to the enthalpy of the system minus the product of the temperature and the entropy: $G = H - TS$.

A chemical reaction is said to be spontaneous if it occurs in nature when the reactants are present without any necessary input of energy. A reaction is spontaneous if and only if the total free energy of the reactants is greater than the total free energy of the products—that is, if ΔG of the reactants is negative. This was, in fact, what led Gibbs to formulate this concept in the first place; he was looking for a relatively simple criterion to determine whether or not a reaction would spontaneously occur.

Coefficient of Expansion

The coefficient of (thermal) expansion is a measurement of how much an object or substance expands as heat increases. For a solid, this increase can be measured either linearly or volumetrically. The linear coefficient of expansion, α, is defined as $\alpha = \frac{\Delta L}{L_0 \Delta T}$, where L_0 is the initial length of the object in question, ΔL is the change in length, and ΔT is the change in temperature. (This assumes that the coefficient is independent of temperature, but this is generally a good approximation.) For a liquid, with no fixed shape, only the volume coefficient of expansion is meaningful; this is defined similarly but in terms of volume instead of length as $\beta = \frac{\Delta V}{V_0 \Delta T}$. For a solid, $\beta \approx 3\alpha$.

For example, the linear coefficient of expansion of steel is about $1.3 \cdot 10^{-5}$ K^{-1}. This means that if a steel wheel with a diameter of 0.5 meters increases in temperature from 0 °C to 80 °C, its diameter changes by an amount equal to $\Delta L = \alpha L_0 \Delta T = (1.3 \cdot 10^{-15} \text{K}^{-1})(0.5 \text{ m})(80 \text{ K}) = 0.00052 \text{ m}$, or about half a millimeter. That may not sound like much, but for some high-precision instruments, such a small change may be significant.

Heat of Fusion and Heat of Vaporization

The heat of fusion of a compound, abbreviated L_f, is the amount of heat released when a particular quantity of the compound changes from liquid to solid state—or, equivalently, the amount of heat required to change that quantity of the compound from solid to liquid. The heat of vaporization, L_v, is the amount of heat released when a particular quantity of the compound changes from gas to liquid state—or, equivalently, the amount of heat required to change that quantity of the compound from liquid to gas. Typically, in metric units, the quantity is taken to be 1 gram, and L_f and L_v are both measured in Joules per gram (J/g).

For instance, suppose we want to know the amount of heat required to convert 1.0 kilogram of ice into water vapor. This requires first melting the ice into water, then heating the water from 0 °C to 100 °C then vaporizing the water. Water has a heat of fusion of 334 J/g, a heat of vaporization of 2230 J/g, and a specific heat of 4.184 J/g°C; the total heat involved is therefore $mL_f + mC\Delta T + mL_v = (1000 \text{ g})(334 \text{ J/g}) + (1000 \text{ g})(4.184 \text{ J/g°C})(100 \text{ °C}) + (1000 \text{ g})(2230 \text{ J/g}) = 2.98 \cdot 10^6 \text{ J}$, or 2980 kJ.

Enthalpy, abbreviated H, is a measurement of the total energy of a thermodynamic system. Specifically, it is equal to the internal energy of the system plus the product of its pressure and volume: $H = U + PV$. (It should not be confused with entropy, which has a similar name but is an entirely different concept.)

During a process at constant pressure, the change in enthalpy is equal to $\Delta H = \Delta U + P\Delta V = \Delta U - W$, where W is the work on the system (or $\Delta U + W$, where W is the work done by the system). The First Law of Thermodynamics says that $\Delta U = Q + W$; therefore, $\Delta U - W = Q$, and the change in enthalpy is equal to the heat added to the system. Because of this, the heat of reaction of a chemical process is also called its enthalpy of reaction; the two terms are equivalent because the heat added to the system is equal to its change in enthalpy.

Phase Diagram

A phase diagram is a diagram that shows the phase (solid, liquid, or gas) that a particular compound or element is in at different pressures and temperatures. It is conventionally drawn with pressure on the *y* axis and temperature on the *x* axis; lines on the diagram mark the boundaries of the regions in the diagram where the compound is in each phase. At points on these lines, the two phases are in equilibrium; the points on these lines at particular pressures mark the compound's freezing or boiling points at those pressures. The point where all three phases are in equilibrium is the triple point, the unique pressure and temperature where all three phases of the compound are in equilibrium.

For example, below is a phase diagram of water, with the triple point marked as well as the boiling and freezing points at atmospheric pressure:

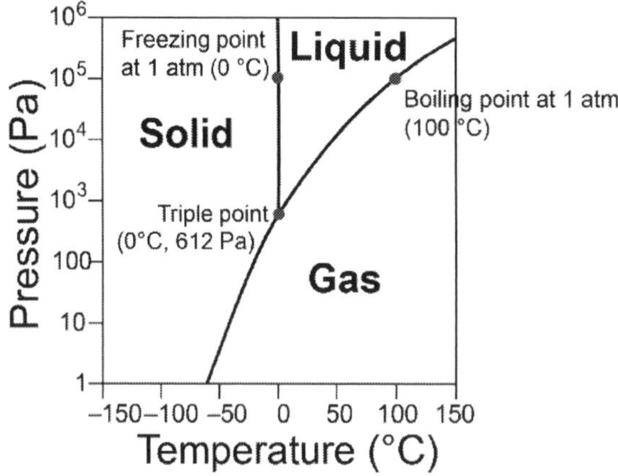

Note that in this diagram the pressure is given a logarithmic scale; this is common in phase diagrams to depict a wide range of pressures, but it is not required; phase diagrams can also be drawn with linear pressure scales.

Rate Processes in Chemical Reactions - Kinetics and Equilibrium

Reaction Rate

The reaction rate of a chemical reaction is a measurement of what quantity of the reactants reacts per unit time. It is typically measured in units of mol/(L s) so that a reaction rate *r* means that in each liter of the substance, *r* moles of the reactants react each second.

For chemicals to react, their molecules must come into contact. Therefore, increasing the concentration of the reactants will increase the reaction rate—the higher the concentration of the reactants, the more likely it is for molecules of the reactants to meet each other. Temperature affects reaction rate for similar reasons; the higher the temperature, the faster the molecules are moving, and the more frequently molecules of the reactants will collide. For solid reactants, the shape of the solid may also affect things; the larger the surface area, the more molecules of the reactant are exposed and available to contact the other reactants. (This is why finely ground flour is highly flammable, and even aluminum dust may be flammable if the particles are small enough.) In general, however, reactants in the liquid or gas phases have higher reaction rates than solids.

Furthermore, the reaction rate of a chemical reaction can be increased by the presence of a catalyst, another compound that facilitates the reaction without itself being consumed.

Dependence of Reaction Rate on Concentration of Reactants

Rate Law, Rate Constant

The rate law of a chemical reaction is an equation relating the reaction rate of a chemical reaction to the concentrations of its reactants. It generally (but not always) takes the form of a power law in which the reaction rate is equal to a reaction rate constant *k* times the product of the concentrations of the reactants, each raised to some exponent. These exponents are called the reaction orders of the associated reactants. That is, if a chemical reaction has reactants R_1, R_2, R_3, ..., then its rate law is $r = k\,[R_1]^{x_1}[R_2]^{x_2}[R_3]^{x_3}$ ..., where x_n is the reaction order of the reactant R_n.

For example, for the reaction $2NO + O_2 \rightarrow 2NO_2$, the rate law is equal to $r = k[\mathrm{NO}]^2[\mathrm{O_2}]$, where *k* is about 7100 $L^2/(mol^2{\cdot}s)$. (Note that whereas the reaction orders happen to be the same as the stoichiometric coefficients for this particular equation, this is not necessarily the case in general!) This means that if the concentration of NO is 0.02 mol/L and the concentration of O_2 is 0.1 mol/L, the reaction rate will be $r = \left(7100\ \mathrm{L^2/(mol^2 \cdot s)}\right)(0.02\ \mathrm{mol/L})^2(0.1\ \mathrm{mol/L}) = 0.284\ \mathrm{mol/(L{\cdot}s)}$.

Reaction Order

The reaction order of a reactant in a chemical reaction is the exponent to which the concentration of that reactant is raised in the rate equation for the chemical reaction. For instance, the reaction $BrO_3^- + 5Br^- + 6H^+ \rightarrow 3Br_2 + 3H_2O$ has the rate law $r = k\,[BrO_3^-][Br^-][H^+]^2$—the reaction order of BrO_3^- and Br^- is 1, and the reaction order of Br_2 is 2. The overall reaction order of the equation is the sum of the individual reaction orders; for this equation, it would be 1 + 1 + 2 = 4.

As shown in this example, unlike the exponents in a chemical equilibrium equation, the reaction orders of the reactants are not related to their coefficients in a balanced chemical equation. Rather, the reaction orders of the reactants must be determined experimentally. There is no straightforward way to figure out the reaction orders of the reactants just from the chemical equation.

There are some reactions with more complicated reaction laws and in which the reaction orders are not well defined. This may be because the presence of the product slows the reaction; for instance, the reaction $2O_3 \rightarrow 3O_2$ has rate law $r = k\frac{[\mathrm{O_3}]^2}{[\mathrm{O_2}]^3}$.

Rate Constant

The rate constant of a chemical reaction is the proportionality factor between the reaction rate and the product of the concentrations of the reactants raised to the powers of their reaction orders. That is, it is the constant *k* in the rate law equation $r = k\,[R_1]^{x_1}[R_2]^{x_2}[R_3]^{x_3}$ .... Like the reaction orders, the rate constant must be determined experimentally. In practice, the rate constant of a reaction is not really a universal constant but depends on the temperature; rate constants are frequently given at a reference temperature of 298 K.

The units of *k* are chosen so that the reaction rate *r* has the appropriate units, usually mol/(L·s). This means the units of *k* are $\mathrm{L}^{\sum x-1}/(\mathrm{mol}^{\sum x-1} \cdot \mathrm{s})$, where $\sum x$ is the reaction order of the reaction, which is equal to the sum of the reaction orders of all the reactants. For instance, the reaction $2ClO_2 + 2OH^- \rightarrow ClO_3^- + ClO_2 + H_2O$ has the rate law $r = k[ClO_2]^2[OH^-]$; the reaction order is 1 + 2 = 3, and the rate constant must have units of $L^2/(mol^2{\cdot}s)$.

Rate-Determining Step

When, as is often the case, a chemical reaction actually occurs not all at once but as a series of subsidiary reactions, or steps, the rate-determining step of a reaction is the step that has the slowest reaction rate. The reaction cannot proceed more quickly than its slowest step, so the rate of the overall reaction will be equal to the rate of this step—this slowest step determines the rate of the reaction.

If the steps of the reaction are known, and the reaction order of the equation is known, this is often sufficient to determine the rate-determining step—it is the step at which the total number of molecules of the reactants that have been involved so far is equal to the reaction order. For instance, the reaction $2NO + 2H_2 \rightarrow N_2 + 2H_2O$ proceeds through the following steps:

$$NO + NO \rightarrow N_2O_2$$
$$N_2O_2 + H_2 \rightarrow N_2O + H_2O$$
$$N_2O + H_2 \rightarrow N_2 + 2H_2O$$

The reaction order of this reaction is experimentally determined to be three. After the second step, three molecules are involved (two NO from the first step plus H_2), so the second step must be the rate determining step.

Dependence of Reaction Rate Upon Temperature

Activation Energy

The activation energy of a chemical reaction is the minimum energy required for the reaction to proceed. Even if the total energy of the reactants is less than the total energy of the products, it takes some energy to break bonds in the reactants so that they can form new bonds and make the products; there is some initial energy needed to start, even if the compounds end up getting that energy back when the products are formed. Of course, the higher the temperature of the compound, the more kinetic energy its molecules have that can be used to overcome the activation energy, which is part of the reason that the reaction rate increases with temperature.

The activation energy is usually given not as the energy needed for one molecule of each reactant to react (or a number of molecules each to the stoichiometric coefficient of the compound in the balanced equation), but for a mole of the molecule (or a number of moles equal to the stoichiometric coefficient). The units of the activation energy are therefore equal to joules per mole or, more often, kilojoules per mole.

Activation Energy: Activated Complex or Transition State

In a chemical reaction, the compounds do not change instantaneously from the reactants to the products but pass through a range of intermediate steps. These intermediate forms may have higher energies than either the initial reactants or the final products, which is why some activation energy is necessary to form them, and they may only exist for very brief periods of time before returning to a lower-energy state, either re-forming the reactants or becoming the products of the chemical reaction. These high-energy intermediate steps are known as activated complexes.

Of all the intermediate forms, there is one that has the highest energy. This form, which the molecules may pass through only briefly as they change from the reactants into the products, is known as the transition state. It is this form that determines the activation energy of the reaction—it is the difference in energy between the transition state and the initial state of the molecules.

Activation Energy: Interpretation of Energy Profiles

An energy profile is a representation of the energy that a chemical system goes through during a chemical reaction. The y axis of the energy profile is the energy of the system (in any appropriate units, but because it is the shape of the energy profile that's important, the units are often omitted); the x axis is the reaction coordinate, measuring progress of the reaction. (The x axis is not given in more concrete units such as time or concentration of reactants because the reactants may react at different rates, and the rate depends on concentration and other factors.) Usually an energy profile shows the energy increasing gradually from its initial value to a maximum and then falling back to a lower energy again; multistep reactions may also show some local minima.

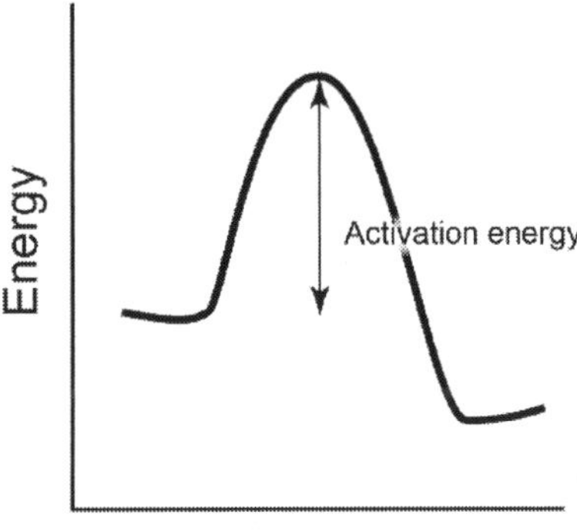

Several useful pieces of data can be drawn from the energy profile. Whether the final energy is higher or lower than the initial shows whether the reaction is endothermic or exothermic. The activation energy can be found as the difference between the maximum energy and the initial energy.

Arrhenius Equation

The Arrhenius equation is an equation showing the relationship between the reaction rate and the temperature. It is named after the Swedish scientist Svante August Arrhenius, who is credited as one of the founders of physical chemistry (and who also formulated the Arrhenius definition of acids and basis). The equation takes the form $k = Ae^{-\frac{E_a}{RT}}$, where A is a constant (which may be different for every reaction), E_a is the activation energy of the reaction, R is the ideal gas constant (8.314 J/[mol·K]), and T is the temperature in Kelvins.

Although it is not hard to see conceptually why the reaction rate increases with temperature, the Arrhenius equation quantifies the relationship and allows the calculation of the reaction rate at different temperatures as long as the relevant constants are known. The constant A, called the pre-exponential constant, is dependent on the frequency of collisions between molecules as well as their geometry but in practice is determined experimentally.

Kinetic Control Vs. Thermodynamic Control of a Reaction

In many cases, there is more than one set of products that could in principle be formed in a chemical reaction by a given set of reactants. Which products are formed depends on the rates of the related reactions as well as on the products' stability. A product produced by the reaction with the higher reaction rate (and generally the lower activation energy) is called a kinetic product. A product that is more stable (has the lower energy in its final form) is called a thermodynamic product.

Which products actually are formed in a given case, then, depends on which controlling factor becomes more important. At sufficiently low temperatures, there is not enough energy for the reaction forming the kinetic product to reverse despite its relative instability, so as this product has a faster reaction rate, it predominates, and the reaction is said to be under kinetic control. At higher temperatures, when the reaction forming the kinetic product can reverse, this limits the amount of those products that forms, and the thermodynamic product predominates; the reaction is said to be under thermodynamic control.

Catalysts

A catalyst is a compound that lowers the activation energy of a reaction and thus facilitates that reaction taking place without itself being expended in the reaction—it is said to catalyze the reaction. This may be because the catalyst does react in one step of a multistep reaction, but is then produced in another step, so that the total amount of the catalyst is unchanged. The highest activation energy of any step of the reaction involving the catalyst is smaller than the activation energy of the reaction without the catalyst, so the reaction can proceed at a greater rate.

For example, iron reacts with oxygen to form iron oxide (rust). However, the activation energy is high enough that this does not spontaneously occur at a noticeable rate when iron is exposed to oxygen. It does occur, however, in the presence of water because water acts as a catalyst to this reaction, lowering the activation energy. Important examples of catalysts in biological systems are enzymes, which ensure that metabolic processes occur at a high enough rate to sustain life.

Review Video: Catalysts
Visit mometrix.com/academy and enter code: 288189

Equilibrium in Reversible Chemical Reactions

Law of Mass Action

The Law of Mass Action states that the rate of a chemical reaction is directly proportional to the product of the concentrations of the reactants. If a reactant or product has a stoichiometric coefficient (a coefficient in the balanced chemical equation) other than 1, then its concentration appears that many times in the product—in other words, its concentration is raised to the power of its stoichiometric coefficient. In other words, the reaction rate is proportional to $[R_1]^{r_1}[R_2]^{r_2}$ ..., where R_1, R_2, ... are the reactants and r_n their respective stoichiometric coefficients. This has a number of applications—for instance, it says that we can increase a reaction rate by increasing the concentration of a reactant, although this also follows from Le Châtelier's Principle. It is especially useful for systems in equilibrium, in which case it can be used to derive the equilibrium expression $K_{eq} = \frac{[R_1]^{r_1}[R_2]^{r_2}...}{[P_1]^{p_1}[P_2]^{p_2}...}$, where P_1, P_2, ... are the products and p_n their respective stoichiometric coefficients.

Equilibrium Constant

The equilibrium expression is the constant K_{eq} that appears in the equilibrium expression $K_{eq} = \frac{[R_1]^{r_1}[R_2]^{r_2}...}{[P_1]^{p_1}[P_2]^{p_2}...}$, where R_1, R_2, ... are the reactants, P_1, P_2, ... the products, and r_n and p_n their respective stoichiometric coefficients. (Only gases and chemicals in solution are included in this equation; solid and liquid reactants and products are omitted.) A very large equilibrium constant implies that the products will predominate at equilibrium; a very small constant implies that the reactants will predominate.

The equilibrium constant can be used to determine an unknown concentration of a compound. For example, consider the reversible reaction $3H_2 + N_2 \rightleftharpoons 2NH_3$, which has an equilibrium constant at room temperature of $3.3 \cdot 10^8$, and suppose we know that at equilibrium the concentration of H_2 is 0.0050 M and of N_2 is 0.020 M. The equilibrium expression would be $K_{eq} = \frac{[NH_3]^2}{[H_2]^3[N_2]}$. This means we can find the concentration of NH_3 by solving for it in this equation: $[NH_3] = (K_{eq}[H_2]^3[N_2])^{1/2} = ([3.3 \cdot 10^8][0.0050]^3[0.020])^{1/2} = 2.9$ M. Note that the concentration of the product (NH_3) is much larger than the concentrations of the reactants (H_2 and N_2); this is expected because $K_{eq} \gg 1$.

Application of Le Châtelier's Principle

Le Châtelier's Principle states that a change in some property of a system in equilibrium will produce a shift in the equilibrium that counteracts the change. For example, if the concentration of one of the reactants is increased, the reaction will tend to proceed toward the right, using up some of the reactants and forming more of the product. A decrease in the concentration of a reactant (or an increase in the concentration of a product) will have the opposite effect. Increasing the pressure on a system of gases in equilibrium will shift the equilibrium toward the side of the reaction with fewer molecules. Increasing the temperature will shift the equilibrium toward the products, if the forward reaction is endothermic, or the reactants, if it is exothermic.

It is possible to take advantage of this principle to move a system's equilibrium in a desired direction. For instance, one step in the production of sulfuric acid involves the reversible reaction $2SO_2 + O_2 \rightleftharpoons 2SO_3$. This reaction can be made to proceed in the forward direction more efficiently by increasing the pressure or by adding oxygen. The reaction is also exothermic in the forward direction, so it works best at lower temperatures.

Relationship of the Equilibrium Constant and $\Delta G°$

The larger the equilibrium constant K_{eq} of a chemical reaction, the more the products will predominate, and the more the reaction will tend to proceed toward the right. The smaller K_{eq}, the more the reactants will predominate, and the more the reaction will tend to proceed toward the left. On the other hand, the reaction will tend to proceed in the direction that decreases the Gibbs free energy, so the larger the change in the free energy, ΔG, the more the equation will proceed toward the left, and the smaller ΔG, the more it will proceed toward the right. This suggests that the change in the Gibbs free energy and the equilibrium constant have an inverse relationship.

It is not, however, a simple matter of the two being inversely proportional (they can't be, because ΔG can be negative, and K_{eq} can't.) Rather, the relationship turns out to be logarithmic. The Gibbs free energy is equal to the negative product of the ideal gas constant $R = 8.314$, the temperature T in Kelvins, and the natural logarithm of the equilibrium constant: $\Delta G = -RT \ln K_{eq}$.

Psychological, Social, and Biological Foundations

Sensation, Cognition, and Response

Sensory Threshold

Sensory threshold is amount of strength needed for a stimulus to be perceived by an organism using one of the senses (sight, sound, taste, etc). For instance, if a person can hear everything above 20 hertz (Hz), but nothing below that frequency, their sensory threshold for sound would be 20 Hz. Different species, or even different organisms of the same species, may have different thresholds for the same stimulus.

Weber's Law

Weber's Law is based on the concept that an organism can sense a difference in a change in a stimulus. This change is known as the "just noticeable difference" and Weber's Law asserts that the proportion of this change must remain constant for the difference to be perceived, as opposed to the amount of change remaining constant. For instance, if you are waiting for your microwave popcorn to finish cooking, an extra 24 seconds added to the 2 minutes would be noticeable, a 20% increase in cooking time. However, if you were waiting 3 hours for a meal to finish cooking in the oven, the extra 24 seconds wouldn't be noticeable because the proportion of that difference in time is only .2%. Instead, you might notice a change in 36 minutes, because that would be a 20% increase in cooking time.

Signal Detection Theory

Signal detection theory explains methods for identifying a specific stimulus and being able to distinguish this signal from co-occurring signals that distort or disturb the desired stimulus. Using logic and probability through the signal detection theory, one should be able to identify the signal in question. Four possible outcomes determine whether or not a signal is present: hit, miss, false alarm, and correct rejection. If the signal is there and detected, hit. If the signal is there but undetected, miss. If the signal is not there but is detected, false alarm. If the signal is not there and is undetected, correct rejection. One example of the signal detection theory in action is when a doctor is diagnosing cancer. For instance, if the tumor is there but undetected, that would be a miss. But if the tumor is absent but detected, that would be a false alarm.

Sensory Adaptation

In short, sensory adaptation is the process of getting used to something. If exposed to a constant stimulus over a period of time, an organism gradually adapts to this stimulus and the signal becomes weaker. An example of this concept would be jumping into a swimming pool. At first, the water may feel cold and it might be a shock to be suddenly submerged in this cold water. But after a short amount of time, the water feels pleasant because the skin has become less responsive to this stimulus.

Psychophysics

Psychophysics refers to the field of study concerning both mental and physical aspects of sensation. More precisely, it is the branch of psychology that explains the relationships between external stimuli and the physical and mental sensations that occur in response to these stimuli.

Sensory Pathways

Sensory pathways allow the brain to receive sensory information from the rest of the body. This information travels either through the spinal cord or the thalamus and is delivered to the cerebral cortex or the cerebellum. Only the conscious cortex of the brain receives this information. Examples of these pathways may include pain and temperature information or touch and pressure information.

Sensory Receptors

Sensory receptors are nerve endings that detect certain stimuli and respond to these stimuli by sending impulses to the brain. There are multiple types of sensory receptors and they are often classified by where they are located. Exteroreceptors are closer to the surface of the skin and respond to touch or other stimuli that occur outside the body. Interoreceptors are inside the body and respond to internal stimuli such as stomach pain. Proprioceptors detect unconscious stimuli such as body position and movement. Other types of receptors are classified by stimulus. Thermoreceptors respond to temperature, nociceptors respond to pain, and baroreceptors respond to pressure. Vibrations and touch are detected by mechanoreceptors, and chemical stimuli are detected by chemoreceptors, while light and visual stimuli are detected by photoreceptors.

Structures of the Eye

The eye is composed of many parts that work together to send visual information to the brain through the optic nerve, translating the stimuli into images. The front of the eye is clear and called the cornea. This is where light travels through and into the pupil, which is the dark center of the iris. The iris is the color of the eye, such as brown, blue, or green, and filters the light that comes in. The clear, inside structure of the eye is called the lens, and it is responsible for focusing light on the retina. The retina is a layer of nerve cells, or photoreceptors, that respond to light stimuli. The ciliary muscles help focus this light by manipulating the shape of the lens. Lastly, the middle of the eye is filled with clear fluid known as vitreous.

Visual Pathway in the Brain

In order to process vision, eyes must send the information they receive to the brain. The photoreceptors in the retina capture the visual image and send nerve impulses through the optic nerve. Each eye sends its own messages that meet up at the optic chiasm and then split up on the way to the brain. Half of the left and right optic nerve travel to the left side of the brain, while the other half of each travel to the right side.

Parallel Processing and Feature Detection

Parallel processing is when the brain is presented with different stimuli and must process these stimuli at the same time. An example of this would be when the brain is sent an image and it must determine the color, size, texture, and movement simultaneously. Feature detection is a theory that explains the reasons why seeing certain images or words may elicit different parts of the brain. It asserts that the nervous system is able to distinguish between significant features of the environment and irrelevant information in the background.

Structure and Function of the Ear

The three main parts of the ear are classified as the external ear, the middle ear, and the inner ear. The ear canal, which is what sound travels through, and the outside of the ear drum, or tympanic membrane, are in the external ear. The bulk of the ear drum resides within the middle ear and is what sound bounces off on its way to the brain. Also in the middle ear are the malleus, incus, and stapes or stirrup bones. These bones respond to sound waves by vibrating together, amplifying the sound and creating a wave in the fluid of the ear. This fluid is housed in the cochlea, the structure shaped like a snail containing hair cells that is located in the inner ear. The hair cells of the cochlea then send the auditory signals to the brain where they are then processed.

Hair Cells

Hair cells are located in the cochlea of the ear and are auditory and vestibular sensory receptors. In response to movement, the hair cells bend and prompt a discharge of neurotransmitters that send signals to the brain. In humans, hair cells are unable to regenerate, so when they are damaged, hearing loss can occur.

Auditory Processing and Auditory Pathways in the Brain

Auditory processing is when sound enters through the ear and is delivered to the brain for interpretation. This sound passes through the ear canal and rebounds off the ear drum, creating vibrations in the cochlea, and is then transmitted via the auditory nerve. The message is sent to the brainstem where it can be translated into information regarding frequency, intensity, and position, and is then passed on through the temporal lobe, specifically the thalamus and auditory cortex. The auditory message is then interpreted to create a comprehensible meaning.

Somatosensation and Receptor Cells

When the body interacts with the environment, receptor cells transmit sensory information to the brain. This process is known as somatosensation. The following three types of receptor cells are involved in this process: mechanoreceptors, thermoreceptors, and nociceptors. Respectively, these receptors involve sensations of touch, temperature, and pain.

Sense of Taste

Taste receptors pick up signals from specific tastes, which are sent to the brain and translated into flavors. These different tastes include salty, sweet, bitter, sour, and "umami," also known as savory. Taste occurs through taste buds, which are spherical-shaped growths on the tongue and are linked to taste receptors. Certain chemicals in food are related to these different tastes, and if present in food, allow the brain to recognize the flavors via the taste hairs covering the taste buds. For a food to be sensed as sweet, it would contain sugar, while umami foods are meaty. Both can be detected by T1R2 and T1R3 receptors. Salt would be present and detected via sodium channels to be distinguished as salty. For bitter foods, basic chemicals such as quinine are present, and for sour foods, acidic chemicals would be present. Bitter taste is transmitted through the T2R receptors and sour taste through the transient receptor potential (TRP) channel.

Sense of Smell

Within the nasal cavity, olfactory cells detect smell, called olfaction. These cells are chemoreceptors and pick up on specific chemical stimuli in order to deliver messages to the brain about smell.

Olfactory Pathways in the Brain

When a person is exposed to something with a particular smell, this smell enters the nasal cavity. Inside the nasal cavity is the olfactory epithelium, close in proximity to the brain. Between the brain and the olfactory epithelium are the olfactory bulb and cribriform plate. The olfactory bulb has thousands of nerves and these nerves extend through the cribriform plate and into the olfactory epithelium. When a smell enters the olfactory epithelium, the cells at the end of these nerves detect the scent and send a message to the brain to interpret the particular smell.

Pheromones

Pheromones are a type of chemical that animals release, which work to communicate information to other animals of the same species. These pheromones help other animals avoid danger or find food by sending messages to their brain about the environment.

Kinesthetic Sense

Kinesthetic sense is detected by the type of sensory receptors known as proprioceptors. These sense movement and body position through muscles, ligaments, and tendons in the body.

Vestibular Sense

The ability to balance and perceive gravity is known as vestibular sense. This occurs through the hair cells within the inner ear. Because there is fluid within the cochlea, the body is able to sense when it moves and allows the brain to understand its position in space.

Bottom-up and Top-down Processing

Bottom-up processing is when the body is exposed to a stimulus and sensory receptors send information to the brain about this stimulus. Top-down processing is when a person is exposed to a stimulus but before the stimulus can send a signal to the brain, the brain remembers this specific stimulus and influences how the body reacts. The best way to explain these two different types of processing is through example. Imagine it is a hot day and you go to open your car door. When you touch the door handle, it burns your hand and sends a pain signal to your brain. This is bottom-up processing because the stimulus sent a signal that traveled from the hand to the brain. However, the next day is another hot day. You reach your car and remember yesterday when the handle burned your hand. You decide to use a jacket or other material to open the door in order to avoid burning your hand. In this scenario, you used top-down processing because the processing began in the brain when you remembered a previous experience with a hot door handle.

Perceptual Organization

Perceptual organization is the way by which our brain recognizes objects and the structure of objects in order to interpret this information. Some ways that this occurs are through depth, form, and motion. Depth is how we are able to see the position of objects in a three-dimensional space. Form is how we see the shape of the object, or its outline. Motion refers to the movement on an object. Using the knowledge that the word "gestalt" means "whole" in the German language; one can surmise that gestalt principles are related to perceiving something in its entirety. Understandably, the gestalt principles are a way of making sense of what our brains perceive in terms of its wholeness. For instance, when you are walking down a road, you perceive the street as a whole entity, as opposed to first seeing each pebble on the pavement, the texture of the road, and then the dark gray color of the street.

Selective and Divided Attention

Selective attention is when an individual must focus on a single event, task, or object when there are other things happening that are a distraction. For instance, if Joe needs to watch his daughter on the playground, he is using selective attention. He must focus on her playing and make sure she doesn't get hurt, without being distracted by the other children on the playground, other parents talking to him, or his phone. Divided attention is when an individual must focus on multiple things at once. In Joe's case, if he received an important phone call from work while he was watching his daughter, he would have to focus his attention on both of the tasks at hand.

Information-Processing Model

In the information-processing model, it is theorized that human memory works in a way similar to a computer. First the brain encodes sensory information that it receives and then it stores that information. When this information needs to be used, the brain has retrieval methods to bring that information to the mind once again.

Piaget's Stages of Cognitive Development

According to Piaget, there are stages of development that all children move through at around the same ages. The first stage, sensorimotor stage, spans from birth to 2 years of age. In this stage the infant moves through the world using sensory information and his or her emerging motor skills. The second stage, preoperational stage, occurs between the ages of 2 and 7. During this stage the child learns to view the world using symbolic representations and language. In the concrete operational stage, from ages 7 to 11, the child is less egocentric and is able to think logically. The principle of conservation is developed as well, which is the idea that just because a substance has a different outer appearance, the amount of the substance is constant. The last stage, formal operational stage, starts at the age of 12 and extends into adulthood. The child in this stage has reached cognitive maturity and is able to think deductively, as well as to think through arguments and abstract ideas.

Cognitive Changes in Late Adulthood

In adulthood, an individual will likely experience a decline in cognitive ability. Loss of memory, delayed reaction times, and difficulty speaking or following a schedule are common. This is due to the decline in information-processing abilities. The individual has difficulties encoding, storing, and/or retrieving information within the brain, and cognitive functioning is in turn negatively affected.

Roles of Culture, Heredity, and Environment in Cognitive Development

Cognitive development can be influenced by culture and the environment in multiple ways. How one interacts with others and the environment changes how they think about the world. This can occur through language, social ties, socioeconomic status, disabilities, life events, and many other cultural and environmental experiences. Heredity also plays a role in cognitive development through genetic phenomena and family upbringing.

Biological Factors That Influence Cognition

Biology plays a role in cognitive development in ways such as the formation of the frontal lobe, the hippocampus, and the amygdala. The frontal lobe is responsible for reason, organization, and future thinking. The hippocampus is pivotal in creating memories, while the amygdala gives humans the ability to sense danger while regulating emotions in response to certain stimuli.

Approaches and Barriers to Problem Solving

Problem solving, or finding a solution for an issue at hand, can be approached in many different ways. Using the trial and error method, experimenting until you find a method that works, is often used, but may be inefficient and time consuming. Another approach is using an algorithm. Algorithms give step-by-step instructions for solving a problem, usually relying on a computer to arrive at a solution by calculating the answer. Heuristics are also used to solve problems, and involve following a general guideline for achieving a desired result. These heuristics are numerous and have different rates of success, but also may be a barrier to effective problem solving by leading to an incorrect solution due to a using an inappropriate or faulty shortcut. Other barriers include biases and fixation. Having an inherent bias when it comes to problem solving may lead to a wrong answer or ignoring a correct answer. Fixation refers to relying on information and solutions that worked in the past, but might not be appropriate for the situation at hand. This is also known as a mental set. Function fixedness is also a form of fixation and refers to the idea that certain objects can only be used in a particular way, without realizing that they could be used differently to help solve a problem.

Availability Heuristic, Representativeness Heuristic, and Confirmation Bias

Availability heuristic refers to how easily one can call to mind an example of an event, and the assumptions that individual makes based on how the event is remembered. This might be based on how often the individual has heard of the event, how the media portray the event, or how significant the event might be to that individual. Representative heuristic is the idea that one may believe a certain sample shares the same qualities as the rest of the population, and assume certain characteristics about the population based on this sample. Confirmation bias refers to the idea that if you assume information about something and are very connected to this belief, you will recognize only the information that confirms that belief and not believe the opposing evidence. This is also known as belief perseverance.

Types of Intelligence

Linguistic intelligence refers to the ability to understand language, including speaking, reading, and writing. Logical or mathematical intelligence is related to numbers and using logic to find answers. Musical intelligence refers to understanding how to play and read music. Spatial intelligence is when one understands the world through its relationship to and position in space. Body or kinesthetic intelligence refers to one's athleticism or bodily movement. Interpersonal intelligence is how a person interacts and understands other people. Intrapersonal intelligence refers to understanding oneself, also known as self-perception. Lastly, nature or natural intelligence is the understanding of the biological world in terms of patterns and object recognition.

Triarchic Theory of Intelligence

Triarchic theory of intelligence includes three different aspects of one's intelligence: practical, analytic, and creative. Practical intelligence includes physical activity, learning from the world around you, and applying that knowledge to your life. This is also known as contextual intelligence. Analytic intelligence includes mathematical operations, logical reasoning, and abstract thinking. This is the type of knowledge commonly evaluated through IQ tests. The third aspect is creative intelligence, or experiential intelligence. One is considered to have this type of intelligence when they are inventive and creative, thinking outside the box. People who design things or are able to create new solutions are considered creatively intelligent.

Influence of Heredity and Environment on Intelligence

A common question in science is whether nature or nurture is responsible for a person's abilities or features. This concept also comes into play with intelligence. Although people have tried to pin down one or the other as the cause of intelligence, both have been found to influence this concept. Genetics play a large role in intelligence, as evidenced by twin studies, but this heritability of a trait is coupled with the effects of the person's environment. Experiences, culture, and learning have been shown to influence intelligence, especially negative events in one's life.

Variations of Intellectual Ability

Some individuals have variations in IQ, or intellectual ability, that are classified as either a form of intellectual disability or giftedness. Intellectual disability (previously called retardation) refers to someone with an IQ that is below average. Different forms of intellectual disability range from inability to perform academically past a sixth-grade level to being unable to function without a caretaker. This can be caused by both environmental factors and genetics. Another subset of the population is classified as intellectually gifted. These individuals have an IQ that is above average, or more than 2 standard deviations from the mean IQ score.

States of Consciousness and Alertness

States of consciousness occur when an individual is awake and aware of his or her surroundings. Being able to pay attention and respond to one's surroundings refers to the concept of alertness. Alertness can be affected by chemical substances or injuries to the head, as well as other medical conditions. Although one is in a state of consciousness, he or she may not necessarily be alert due to these various limitations. Examples of these circumstances are narcolepsy, sleep deprivation, or mental health conditions.

Stages of Sleep and the Sleep Cycle

The first stage of sleep is when the individual is able to wake easily because he or she is in between sleep and consciousness. It is also the first part of the non-REM sleep when the eye movements are slower than in REM sleep. This stage may last around 5 to 10 minutes and is when activity occurs in the muscles. Stage 2 of non-REM sleep is more difficult to wake from because the individual is in slightly deeper sleep. The next two stages are also non-REM sleep and where sleep is deepest. This is when delta waves are active and the body is able to repair itself. An hour and a half into this non-REM sleep is when the REM stage occurs, as well as when dreaming happens. This sleep cycle repeats itself about 4 or 5 times throughout the sleeping period, with the REM cycle getting longer each cycle, from 10 minutes to an hour long, and the deep sleep getting shorter.

Circadian Rhythms

In order to sleep, our bodies have a type of biological clock known as circadian rhythms. These rhythms control our sleep cycle by using light (both artificial and natural). This light sends information through the eye to the pineal gland in the hypothalamus. This gland releases hormones and enzymes, such as melatonin and adenosine, which cause sleepiness. Because of the important role light plays in the sleep cycle, one can reset these circadian rhythms by adjusting the light and dark cycles.

Sleep-Wake Disorders

Parasomnias are sleep disorders that involve the individual performing actions that are considered abnormal while a person is sleeping. Sleep walking, talking, and other actions are considered parasomnias. Dyssomnias also occur during sleep, but disturb a person's sleep cycle. Disruptions in breathing or falling asleep at abnormal times fit into this category with disorders known as sleep apnea and narcolepsy, respectively. Another disorder is called insomnia, which involves a person not being able to sleep when they need to.

Hypnosis and Mediation

Hypnosis is the process by which a person is put into a state of consciousness that makes them more suggestible. This state of consciousness is induced by a hypnotist and may lead people to say or do things they would otherwise not do. However, this does not mean the individual will do things against their will or that they would be morally opposed to, simply that they experience the world differently. Although many people use this technique to elicit forgotten memories, this also means that the patient is more open to suggestion and it has been found that some of these memories are inaccurate. Meditation also attempts to induce a different state of consciousness by using breathing or thinking techniques, usually in order to diminish stress.

Consciousness-Altering Drugs and Drug Addiction

Consciousness-altering drugs, or psychoactive drugs, affect the brain by changing the way an individual experiences or behaves in the world. Different drugs have different effects on the brain; depressants, barbiturates, and opiates help a person relax, stimulants induce energy, and hallucinogens make the user hallucinate and/or experience a vast array of emotions. These drugs work by changing how the neurons in the brain fire and in turn affecting the nervous system. Using these types of drugs excessively can lead to drug addiction. Many of these drugs create a pleasurable sensation by triggering the reward pathway in the brain. Dopamine is released when drugs are used and because this happens in the pleasure center of the brain, an individual may try to recreate that sensation by using drugs more often. When this happens, an individual may use drugs so frequently that their body depends on the drug (addiction) and reacts unpleasantly when the drugs are taken away (withdrawal).

Encoding

Memory encoding is a process in which our brains are able to transform sensory information into storable memories. The types of encoding are acoustic, visual, semantic, and tactile. Acoustic encoding uses sound to convert auditory signals into memory. Visual encoding converts images into memory, semantic encoding uses meaning to code information, and tactile encoding uses physical touch to create a memory.

There are many ways to help the brain remember certain information by encoding memories. Repeating words or information helps encode memories. In addition, visualizing information, placing information into separate categories (chunking), creating a narrative about the information, and using acronyms aid in encoding memories. Assigning meaning to a topic or making information relevant to your own life also helps memorize information.

Memory Storage

The different types of memory storage depend on how long information is stored in the brain. The first type of storage is sensory. This includes both iconic memory (also known as photographic memory) and echoic memory (sound memory). This type of memory is extremely short term and as soon as it is gone, it is replaced by a new sensory memory. The second type of storage is short-term, or working, memory. Using this sensory information, the brain often allows these memories to be stored for more processing. Performing math equations in your head, memorizing a list while you walk to the other room to write it down, or dialing a phone number that you were just given during another phone call all require this form of working memory. This type of memory only lasts for about 20 to 30 seconds. Long-term memories, on the other hand, can last anywhere from a few days to an entire lifetime. Long-term memory is also able to hold as much information as it needs, while the other forms of memory storage are more limited. Repeating information and focusing on the meaning of the information are some of the main ways to transfer short-term memories into long-term storage.

Semantic Networks and Spreading Activation

Semantic networks are based on the theory that long-term memory is organized by connecting related information into a type of web network. These relationships between ideas help us understand different concepts by relating them to things we have experienced or learned in our past. When a specific idea triggers different memories and concepts, this causes spreading activation. When you think of one idea, food, for example, it triggers thoughts about types of food (like cheese or bread) and the details about those foods. This helps to remember various details of a specific topic or event.

Recall, Recognition, and Relearning

Recall is defined as the ability to retrieve a memory. Three different types of tasks use recall. Free recall is when you can remember information without being cued, or asked, for it. Cued recall is when you remember something after being asked. The third type of recall task is serial recall, which is when you remember a list or sequence of events in a specific order. Recognition is defined as being able to remember information once presented with the correct option within a collection or range of information. An example would be when you answer a multiple-choice question, and can remember the information because you are presented with the correct answer among incorrect answers. Relearning is when you have already learned something, but have to familiarize yourself with the information once again.

Processes That Aid in Retrieving

One process that aids in retrieving memories is the use of retrieval cues. When trying to remember something, certain words, events, people, or images may trigger your brain to retrieve that memory. For instance, if you lose your train of thought and are trying to remember what you were thinking, it may help to retrace your steps by repeating topics or words that you were thinking of before this in order to retrieve your most recent train of thought. Another way to help retrieve memories is using emotion. It is easier to recall information when you have an emotion connected to it. For instance, if something makes you angry, feeling the emotion of anger again later may prompt you to remember this previous experience. By associating events and information with emotion it becomes easier to remember that material.

Effects of Aging on Memory

There are various and contradictory views on the effect aging has on memory. Many believe that the ability to recall information is hindered in late adulthood and that it is more difficult for older individuals to use free recall when retrieving a memory. Although this may be true and may be seen in the difference in brain structure as we age, it is also true that people who are older in age are still able to learn new information and recall old memories. Scientists and psychologists have also suggested ways to help people remember information as they age, including attributing meaning to new information and using other forms of memory aids.

Memory Dysfunctions

Memory dysfunctions occur when damage is sustained to parts of the brain and it negatively affects the brain's ability to store and recall memories. During late adulthood, a form of memory dysfunction, called dementia, may occur. This term refers to the rapid loss of memory function and can have many causes, ranging from biological abnormalities to environmental factors. The most common cause of dementia is known as Alzheimer disease. This disease is characterized by slow and subtle change in memory and personality, but it is irreversible and may lead to physical disability in an individual, which may result in death. Another memory dysfunction is amnesia, which is found in two forms: anterograde and retrograde. Anterograde is characterized by an individual not being able to create new memories, while retrograde is when the individual can't remember things that have occurred in the past. Another memory disorder, called Korsakoff syndrome, happens when a person doesn't get enough vitamin B1. Commonly caused by alcohol abuse, this disorder negatively affects memory, coordination, and speech.

Decay and Interference

Decay is defined as the fading of memory, especially short-term memory, due to the passage of time. The longer it is since you learned something or retrieved a memory, your ability to recall that memory is reduced. Long-term memory is less impacted by decay, likely because those memories are recalled more often, while short-term memories are new and less likely to be remembered after time has passed. Interference occurs when memories are unable to be retained because of a different memory. Proactive interference is when a new memory is impeded by an older memory and the new information is unable to be retained. The opposite is known as retroactive interference—when a new memory interferes with the ability to remember an older memory.

Constructing Memories and Monitoring Sources

The main way individuals are able to construct a memory is through something called a schema. This schema is a way that we are able to understand the environment based on biology and external influences. This framework can act on memories by skewing information to fit into the schema. Another way that we construct memories is through false memories, which happens when our imagination fills in gaps in our memories. Misinformation also influences our memories; when we are told false information, this changes our memories or creates new memories based on this misinformation. Lastly, remembering the source of the information helps make our memories more precise. Source monitoring errors occur when we are unable to remember how, when, or where we attained the information, despite still remembering the factual content.

Neural Plasticity

A person may experience many changes throughout his or her life that influence the brain's processes and abilities. The idea that the brain can adapt to these changes is known as neural plasticity. There are many different ways the brain is able to adapt to the changes. One way is through compensatory masquerade. This is when one area of cognitive functioning is negatively affected and the brain must find a way to compensate for this change. Another type of neural plasticity is cross-modal reassignment, which is when the brain is able to reorganize its processes or connections after one or more of the sensory systems is ineffective. For instance, if a person loses his or her sense of sight, the brain attempts to make up for this loss by strengthening other senses. Map expansion is another type of neural plasticity, and is the process of strengthening an area of the brain due to exposure or learning. An example of this is when a person takes a math class, the mathematical portion of the brain is strengthened. Lastly, homologous area adaption often occurs in early development when one area of the brain is damaged. In this type of neural plasticity, the function of the damaged area would be reassigned to another area of the brain, reorganizing and making room for these processes.

Memory, Learning, and Long-Term Potentiation

During the lifespan, an individual's brain is continually learning and growing. This growth does not take place in the literal sense of getting bigger, but it does strengthen the connections between different neurons with continued use. These connections are known as synapses and the processes of strengthening these synapses is known as long-term potentiation. The stronger the synapse, the quicker the brain is able to transmit information via this connection. This process is how we are able to learn new information and explains why we are able to do things at a faster pace when we have done something many times before.

Theories of Language Development

The main theories of language development explain how individuals acquire language. The nativist theory describes how individuals are born with genetic code that enables him or her to learn a language. This theory uses the idea of universal grammar to explain how different languages use similar rules of grammar and how children are able to understand language rules so easily. Another theory is the interactionist theory, which uses ideas from social and biological perspectives to explain how language is learned through a dependency on, and desire for, communication. In this theory, individuals learn through the environment and social interactions.

Language and Cognition

The Sapir-Whorf hypothesis explains how language influences cognition by stating that our thoughts are determined by language. The way we express our words and the grammar and patterns that we learn change the way we perceive the world. The utilization of objects or concept of time can often be seen differently in different languages around the world. The areas that control the processes of language and speech are known as Broca's area and Wernicke's area. Broca's area controls speech and is found in the left frontal lobe of the brain. Wernicke's area is in the left temporal lobe of the brain and is in charge of language comprehension.

Components of Emotion

Cognition, physiology, and behavior are the three components of emotion. The cognitive component includes how an individual thinks and evaluates different circumstances. Viewing a situation as dangerous, exciting, or another emotion is evaluated by using schemas and previous knowledge about the specific event. The physiological component of emotion is how your body experiences an emotion. Increased heart rate, sweating, or other bodily functions occur in certain situations in response to emotion. Lastly the behavioral component involves physical and vocal responses to an emotion. This component is observable and can include pacing, talking fast, or not talking at all.

Basic Universal Emotions and the Adaptive Role of Emotion

The universal emotions are sadness, happiness, disgust, surprise, anger, and fear. Some may also include joy and contempt. Joy is conceptualized to be long-lasting and derived from selflessness or spiritual connections, which is different than the temporary emotion of happiness. Facial expressions of these emotions involve changes in one's eyes, cheeks, jaws, and mouth corners. Emotion can also be adaptive, helping one to better interact with the environment. For instance, when surprised or fearful, individuals often open their eyes very wide, which may help them see everything around them. In addition, having a moderate amount of emotion, as opposed to excessive emotions or none at all, is shown to improve one's abilities and performance.

Theories of Emotion

The James-Lange theory of emotion endorses the concept that the cognitive component of emotion is directly influenced by behavior and physiology. For instance, if you have a fast heart rate and sweaty palms, this would lead you to think that you are fearful. On the other hand, Cannon-Bard theory states that behavioral aspects of emotion are the result of cognition and physiological emotion. Instead of interpreting your sweaty palms as evidence of fear, you would first interpret the situation as scary while also exhibiting physiological evidence of fear, and these would lead to screaming or running away from the scary situation. Lastly, Schachter-Singer theory focuses on the chronology of emotion being first physiological emotion, then cognitive emotion, and then experiencing an emotion. This means that an individual would have sweaty palms and a fast heart rate, and then think critically about the situation at hand. After having evaluated the situation, the emotion of fear would then be experienced.

Brain Regions Involved in Generating and Experiencing Emotions

The major brain regions involved in generating and experiencing emotions are the limbic system and the autonomic nervous system.

Role of the Limbic System in Emotion

The limbic system consists of the amygdala, the thalamus, the hypothalamus, and the cingulate gyrus. The amygdala is involved in the emotions an individual experiences when presented with certain stimuli. The amygdala is also responsible for the "fight or flight" response and helps the body be prepared when faced with a frightening or upsetting situation. The thalamus and hypothalamus control the neurotransmitters linked to emotions. The amygdala transmits information to the hypothalamus and this part of the brain is responsible for the physiological aspects of emotion. Lastly, the cingulate gyrus is responsible for experiencing emotions related to memories. Happy memories are related to that emotion, while upsetting memories trigger negative emotions.

Relationship Between Emotion and the Autonomic Nervous System

The autonomic nervous system consists of 2 different aspects: the sympathetic division and the parasympathetic division. The former of these is responsible for the release of adrenaline when faced with a stressful or surprising situation. This adrenaline leads to physiological changes such as increased heart rate, dilated pupils, increased blood sugar and blood pressure, and slowed digestion. This is also what is in charge of the flight or fight response. The parasympathetic nervous system controls the resting and relaxing aspects of the body with regard to emotion. In other words, when you are calm and relaxed, this part of the nervous system controls the constriction of pupils, increased digestion, and decreased heart rate and blood flow.

Physiological Markers of Emotion

Emotion can be detected by different types of physiological markers. For instance, a person will exhibit different bodily responses when he or she is calm versus when frightened. Heart rate, blood pressure, respiration, and muscle tension are increased when a person is scared, but decreased when relaxed and happy. Blood flow to certain areas of the body, such as the face, are also related to emotions of anger and embarrassment, while crying is indicative of sadness.

Concept of Appraisal in Relation to the Nature of Stress

Although some events throughout the course of an individual's life may generally be considered stressful, many people experience frustration in response to situations that others may not deem stressful. This phenomenon occurs by way of cognitive appraisals. A cognitive appraisal is how an individual perceives an event and therefore influences how he or she responds to such an event. This appraisal could be based on past events, personal beliefs, culture, or various other reasons, and is representative of the schemas at work for this individual. For example, let's say that Susan is given a new car. Many people would believe that this should be exciting and they might be grateful for this gift. However, after being given the car, Susan is unable to sleep and becomes angered by the gift. Susan had been in a car accident when she was younger, and her mother was killed by a drunk driver. This previous event altered Susan's perception of driving and cars, and therefore her cognitive appraisal of the gift was that it was dangerous, which caused her to feel stressed.

Stressors

Many different types of stressors impact individuals during their lives. Some are more difficult to overcome, some are easy, and some are even joyous. Cataclysmic events are recognized as being unpredictable and catastrophic. Events such as these are large and devastating, such as natural disasters and wars. Personal events are another category of stressors and involve life changes that may either be joyful or upsetting. These events range from getting married and having children, to losing a loved one or losing a job. Daily stressors are events and activities that a person experiences throughout the day. These types of stressors, also called hassles, include things such as traffic jams, paying bills, working, or running errands, which cause distress on a daily basis.

Effects of Stress on Psychological Functions

Stress can affect people in many different ways, from contributing to disease to causing psychological disorders. Stress can even help to increase productivity or motivation if experienced at a mild level. However, severe stress can lead to fatigue, depression, anxiety, post-traumatic stress disorder (PTSD), or lack of concentration.

Physiological Responses to Stressors

The body responds to stress in various ways. When experiencing a dangerous situation, the body may be triggered into the fight or flight response. This causes the heart rate to increase and releases glucose into the bloodstream. This in turn allows the individual to either "fight" against the stressor or run away ("flight"), as necessary. This is also the first stage when stress triggers the body to go through three stages of response: alarm, resistance, and exhaustion. Alarm is when adrenaline is pumped into the bloodstream and helps the individual respond to a situation. The resistance stage is when all of this adrenaline (or other hormones) is depleted and the body becomes fatigued. People are also likely to become ill at this stage because of the decreased resources. Lastly, the exhaustion stage is when these different side effects of stress (eg, depression, anxiety) are exhibited.

Emotional and Behavioral Responses to Stressors

When stress occurs, our emotions and behaviors are changed. Because of the strain on biological resources experienced during stress, the body is exhausted and this can impact the mind. It is likely that the individual experiencing stress may feel depressed or anxious and this may lead to a decreased resilience to difficult experiences, resulting in feeling increased stress to less stressful situations. Stress may also lead to poor judgment or bad decision making. It is also possible that a person changes his or her eating habits or consumes more alcohol. Disturbed sleep patterns and increased irritability are also likely side effects of stress.

Managing Stress

An individual can alter his or her behavior or mindset to manage stressful situations in many different ways. Eating healthier, sleeping more regularly, exercising, and avoiding alcohol and drugs help to keep stress away. It has also been shown that spending time doing pleasurable things with people that you enjoy leads to a reduction in stress. In terms of psychological changes a person can make to help manage stress, meditation is a common technique. Focusing on breathing and relaxing are common ways to reduce stress, as is working to increase patience and other positive emotions.

Influences on Behavior and Behavioral Change

Neurons and Neurotransmitters

Neurons are essential parts of the nervous system and work to transmit information using electrical impulses. Neurons are cells that have an axon and dendrites to help transmit and receive these impulses. The axon carries the information, while the dendrites receive it. This is done by way of neurotransmitters, which are chemicals that the neurons use in order to send and receive these messages. Neurons also play a role in reflexes. This is by way of a reflex arc, which consists of a sensory receptor and various neurons. The neurons involved in this process transmit sensory stimuli from the receptor to other neurons to the effector. This process does not send information to the brain for processing, but instead creates an instantaneous response by the body. For instance, when a person touches something hot, the sensory receptors send information through the neurons to the effector, producing an immediate response, causing the person to quickly move away from the source of heat.

Peripheral Nervous System

The peripheral nervous system is made of nerves and sensory organs that send sensory information through nerve impulses to the brain and spinal cord. These nerves and organs are found throughout the body, including everything outside the spinal cord and brain. The purpose of the peripheral nervous system (PNS) is to maintain communication with the central nervous system (CNS), but the PNS doesn't have the protection that the CNS has of bones that contain these vital organs. This means that the PNS is more susceptible to damage by environmental or biological factors.

Central Nervous System

The central nervous system (CNS) is made of the brain and spinal cord. The spinal cord is a column of nerve fibers that connects the brain to the rest of the body, while the brain is a complex organ responsible for our thoughts, memory, and other vital processes. The CNS receives sensory information from the peripheral nervous system, where the information is then processed. The CNS is also able to send this processed information back out in the form of motor output. This means the CNS is responsible for bodily movement and cognitive processing.

Forebrain, Midbrain, and Hindbrain

The forebrain is vital to the processes of problem solving, emotion, logic, and mood. It also controls temperature and sleep regulation. This part of the brain includes the cerebrum, the limbic system, the hypothalamus, and the thalamus. The midbrain includes the tegmentum, tectum, and cerebral peduncles. It is located in the middle part of the brainstem and is responsible for motor control, dopamine production, and motivation. It also is associated with visual and auditory processing. The hindbrain, located in the rear of the brain, includes the cerebellum, pons, and medulla oblongata. The processes that the hindbrain takes part in are arousal, digestion, balance, respiration, and other vital motor functions.

Lateralization of Cortical Functions

Lateralization of cortical functions refers to the separation of the left brain and right brain. The left-brain controls language, writing, positive emotion, and the right side of the body. The right brain controls the left side of the body, along with time and space processing, negative emotion, and nonverbal (facial and body movement) information.

Studying the Brain

One is able to understand the brain in more detail by use of imaging and measurement of chemical activity. Some of the imaging used for this is through computerized tomography (CT) and magnetic resonance imaging (MRI) scans that capture the structure of the brain. Positron emission tomography (PET) and functional MRI (fMRI) scans can also be used to capture the functions of the brain, while computer scans are also used to better understand these processes.

Neuronal Communication and Its Influence on Behavior

Neurons play a role in influencing behavior by communicating and releasing neurotransmitters. When these neurons send messages for the purpose of performing a certain behavior, neurons communicate with one another via chemical signals. One type of neuron that is involved in this process is called a dopaminergic neuron, which releases dopamine and influences mood and behavior. However, if there are issues with these neurons, the dysfunction may cause certain degenerative diseases such as Parkinson or Alzheimer disease. This leads to a decrease in motor skills and memory, and is often found in older individuals.

Influence of Neurotransmitters on Behavior

Neurotransmitters are the chemicals through which neurons communicate with one another. Many different chemicals are involved in this process and each one is related to different behavioral functions. One of these chemicals, endorphins, plays a role in experiencing pleasure or pain, reducing or numbing the pain when necessary. Norepinephrine is a neurotransmitter involved in learning and memory, and also energy and alertness. GABA (gamma-aminobutyric acid) is an inhibitor of neurons. Too little GABA in the brain can lead to anxiety and depression. Serotonin plays a role in sleep and mood, which also leads to anxiety and depression when deficient. Dopamine influences one's ability to concentrate and learn. If too little or too much, it can cause Parkinson disease or schizophrenia, respectively. Acetylcholine impacts memory, learning, and sleep, causing depression or dementia when out of balance. Lastly, epinephrine, also known as adrenaline, is helpful during stressful situations as it intensifies moods and emotions, allowing the individual to act quickly during fight or flight situations.

Endocrine System

The endocrine system plays an important part in the body and impacts a person's behavior through its use of hormones and neurotransmitters. These aspects of the endocrine system influence reproductive behaviors and sexual arousal, as well as sleep and mood. The main component of the endocrine system is the hypothalamus; it is important in the coordination and activity of this system and helps to control the pituitary gland. This gland, also known as hypophysis, releases hormones for growth and reproduction, as well as neurotransmitters. The adrenal gland releases adrenaline, while the thyroid controls energy and metabolism throughout the body. The parathyroid regulates the parathyroid hormone (PTH) and is responsible for bone development. The reproductive organs are also part of the endocrine system, and are responsible for either estrogen and progesterone or testosterone production, depending on the organs a person possesses. Lastly, the pineal gland connects the endocrine system to the nervous system, while controlling melatonin.

Review Video: Endocrine System
Visit mometrix.com/academy and enter code: 678939

Genes, Temperament, and Heredity in Relation to Personality

Personality is a result of a variety of factors including the environment and genetics. Genes are the biological coding that a person is born with and they interact with environmental factors to determine personality characteristics and other important behaviors and conditions. Temperament refers to the mood and overall character a person is born with. Whether they are inherently energetic, quiet, or intense is determined by temperament. This is also impacted by environmental influences, but still remains a part of the individual's personality. Heredity also plays a role in genetic personality as a person inherits personality traits and behaviors from their parents.

Adaptive Value of Traits and Behaviors

It is often necessary for individuals to alter their behavior due to the environment they are living in. Adaptation refers to the ability for the individual to adapt to the environment. Even though many traits and facets of personality are genetically determined, there is room for adaptation when needed. For instance, if Jane grew up not having to do the cooking or cleaning and her personality was somewhat lazy and entitled, then when she moved away to college she would have to adapt this personality to her new environment. She would need to learn to cook and clean for herself, and this would likely change her behavior, which in turn may have an impact on her personality.

Interaction Between Heredity and Environmental Influences

Environment and genetics both influence a person's behavior and personality, and these influences interact with one another as shown by twin studies. Twins who were raised separately shared more characteristics than two people unrelated. However, it was also shown that they had different personalities, giving evidence that environmental factors also have a significant influence on personality and behavior. For instance, a set of twins who were adopted by different parents may enjoy the same types of food, like the same clothes, or even have a similar haircut. However, despite having similar tastes, one may enjoy skiing, while the other would rather surf. These different preferences and behaviors contribute to personality and are impacted by multiple factors that interact with one another.

Influences of Experience and Genetics on Development of Behaviors

Experiences in an individual's life are often the cause of a change in behavior. For instance, if Billy was in a foreign country and his wallet was stolen by a robber, he may decide not to go back to that country, or begin to be more aware of his surroundings after. Also, because environmental and genetic factors both contribute to personality and behavior, there are instances where one can impact the other. Experiences can greatly influence a person's genetic code, while this genetic code may affect that person's behavior. In addition, genetics play a large role in how an individual behaves, and these genes may be expressed in different ways. Regulatory genes control how other genes are expressed, while epigenetics modify how a gene is expressed (a phenotype) without actually changing the genotype (genetic code). These epigenetics are influenced by experiences and environment, but also may be hereditary.

Genetically Based Behavioral Variation in Natural Populations

In natural populations, certain genes encode for certain behaviors. These genes are not found in all members of a particular species, group, or family, which means that there will inherently be differences in behavior for all of these individuals. These behaviors are likely to vary for a number of reasons, including social factors, the environment, and individual experiences.

Prenatal Development

Before a child is born, it goes through a process of development that begins with conception. After being fertilized by the sperm, the egg becomes a zygote, and then develops into a blastocyst. This then leads to an embryo, during which time the embryo develops organs and the cardiovascular system is grown. The next step is the fetus. During the fetal development, tissues and organs mature and the body of the fetus grows larger. Once the fetus is developed (or prior to this, depending on the circumstances of pregnancy), the baby is born.

Motor Development

Once a baby is born, he or she develops motor skills in order to better navigate and understand the world. First, the child learns how to roll over; this usually occurs after 4 months. After 6 months, it is common that the child is able to sit without needing assistance, and once he or she is a year old, walking skills are often developed. Being able to jump in place is the next milestone a child accomplishes, and this happens when the child is about 2 years old. Other motor skills continue to be developed after this time, including dexterity and being able to use utensils and scissors, using all of the fingers to hold an object, and being able to write and draw.

Developmental Changes During Adolescence

During adolescence, an individual will go through developmental changes, also known as puberty. This change is the signal of adulthood beginning and a time when both girls and boys are able to learn abstract problem-solving skills while discovering their identities and independence. For girls, the physical changes during puberty involve menstruation, growing hair on her underarms and pubis, acne, developing sweat glands, and breast formation. For boys, the voice begins to change and deepen, hair is grown around the pubis, underarms, and face, acne develops, and the testes and scrotum grow.

Personality Theories

Psychoanalytic Theory

Psychoanalytic theory was developed originally by Sigmund Freud in order to understand how our unconscious influences our behavior and personality. He developed a theory about the unconscious that included 3 major aspects: the Id, Ego, and Superego. The Id is believed to be the undeveloped part of the unconscious that is driven by basic instinct for survival and pleasure. The Ego regulates the Id and understands how to achieve goals realistically. This part of consciousness is rooted in the unconscious, but interacts with reality. The Superego is the conscience of a person and it is developed through learning morality from authority and parental figures. The Superego is based in the outside world and is considered a conscious entity. Psychoanalytic theory is also largely thought to revolve around psychosexual development. These development stages include the oral, anal, phallic, latency, and genital stages, which explain how an individual's personality is developed based on whether or not he or she successfully moved through these stages.

Humanistic Theory

Humanistic theory maintains that humans have control over their lives and are able to become self-actualized and aware of their behaviors if they put in the work to do so. This perspective is more optimistic in its view of the individual and was developed by the psychologists Abraham Maslow and Carl Rogers. Maslow believed that there was a hierarchy of needs that all people experienced, and that if basic needs such as food, shelter, and safety were unmet, the individual would not be able to move onto higher order needs, such as intimacy, work fulfillment, or self-actualization. Rogers developed a style of therapy known as person-centered, which allowed the therapist and client to develop a relationship in order to influence the client's personality and/or behavior. He stressed the importance of maintaining a self-concept that is congruent to reality in order to better understand one's identity.

Trait Theory

Gordon Allport and Raymond Cattell were the main contributors to the trait theory of personality, which endorsed the idea that traits and sequences of traits were better means to understand a person's personality, and that these traits were stable and observable. Allport theorized that the conscious was more useful than the unconscious in terms of assessing personality, and he explained the three different types of traits: cardinal, central, and secondary. The cardinal traits were the most important and overarching traits that a person exhibited, while central traits were more common among the rest of the population. Secondary traits were thought to be how a person responded to an event. Cattell proposed that the many different traits exhibited by people could be condensed into just 16 different factors of personality. He based this concept on his knowledge of statistics using factor analysis and created these factors, such as intelligence, discipline, assertiveness, and friendliness, to better understand personality.

Social Cognitive Theory

Social cognitive perspective theorizes that personality and behavior are determined by social and environmental influences. This theory proposes that observing the behavior of others, being told how to act, and understanding the motivations of our peers affects our own behavior, as do the situations we experience. Albert Bandura is the main contributor to this perspective, experimenting with children and their toys to better understand aggression. He showed that children learned how to be aggressive when exposed to someone modeling aggressive behavior, while the opposite was true of the children exposed to non-aggressive behavior. This theory also explains how cognition, behavior, and the environment are interconnected and affect one another to cultivate personality.

Biological Theory

The basis of the biological theory of personality is that our personality is somewhat determined by our genes and biology. Temperament and heritability are large parts of this theory, acknowledging that these are determined by how our genes and bodies are composed. This theory also includes the idea that behavior is influenced by the part of our brain responsible for reward and punishment, shaping our motivation based on what gives us pleasure or pain. Hans Eysenck is a main contributor to this theory and believed that genetics and the limbic system play a large part in personality. He suggested the three-factor model of personality that describes extraversion, neuroticism, and psychoticism as the aspects of a person's personality that are influenced by the various biological processes in the body.

Behaviorist Theory

The behaviorist approach to personality suggests that our behavior can be manipulated and influenced by observation and learning. The two main psychologists associated with this theory are B.F. Skinner and Ivan Pavlov. Skinner believed that our environment affects our behavior through operant conditioning. Being rewarded or punished for a specific behavior will lead to an increase or decrease in this behavior, respectively. Skinner's view on childhood and personality were notable for his time, as he didn't agree with other psychologists that the events of one's childhood shape personality. He also maintained that personality changes over the lifespan and that different events and experiences help to shape personality. Pavlov did not consider himself a behaviorist, but his contribution of classical conditioning was prominent in this perspective of psychology. He proposed that pairing a neutral stimulus with an unconditioned stimulus would create a conditioned response. For instance, imagine a person is afraid of loud noises, but feels indifferent towards dogs. If a dog approached that person at the same time a loud noise erupted, and this happened many times, the person would likely become afraid of dogs in addition to the loud noise.

Situational Approach to Explaining Behavior

The situational approach is related to the trait theory of personality. This concept explains that the way a person reacts to a situation is determined by both their personality as well as the situation. Some people will react to the same situation in very different ways, but there are also situations that tend to elicit a similar reaction from very different individuals. This approach also explains that a person will react differently from one situation to another depending on both the situation and the personality of that individual. Fritz Heider also contributed to this concept by proposing attribution theory. This theory is when people tend to interpret information about the world based on attributions. This tendency to interpret leads to people behaving differently because of the attributes of a situation or relationship.

Biomedical and Biopsychosocial Approaches to Psychological Disorders

In the biomedical approach to psychological disorders, the main concern is a focus on the body and bodily processes. This approach holds that illness can be traced back to biological causes, meaning there will be a biological treatment for such an illness. This approach does not believe social or psychological factors are important to diagnosing disease and the mind and body are considered unconnected. The biopsychosocial approach to psychological disorders is quite different. Instead of simply considering biological causes and treatments for illnesses, psychological and social factors are also thought to be significant. In addition, the mind and body are considered to be inseparable, influencing and changing one another.

Classifications and Rates of Psychological Disorders

Psychological disorders are classified in two main ways: using the International Classification of Diseases, Tenth Revision (ICD-10) from the World Health Organization or using the *Diagnostic and Statistical Manual of Mental Disorders, Fifth Edition* (*DSM-5*) from the American Psychiatric Association. The ICD-10 is based on 10 main groups of psychological disorders, including organic disorders, substance use, schizophrenia, mood disorders, neuroticism, behavioral syndromes, personality disorders, intellectual disability, psychological development disorders, and emotional disorders. The *DSM-5* now uses nonaxial documentation of diagnosis to identify psychological disorders that include clinical disorders, personality disorders and mental disability, general medical conditions, psychosocial and environmental problems, and the global assessment of functioning. It has also been found that about one-quarter of adults will experience some form of psychological disorder in their lifetimes. Age has an effect on psychological disorders, with prevalence increasing as people age and Alzheimer disease and dementia are the most common. Depression is also considered to be prevalent with between 6% and 8% of the population experiencing this disorder in their lifetimes. Anxiety rates are also high, with between 11% and 12% of people reporting anxiety in their lifetimes.

Anxiety, Obsessive-Compulsive, and Trauma- and Stressor-Related Disorders

Anxiety disorders are defined as a fear or worry about certain objects or situations. This fear or worry interferes with someone's ability to function in everyday situations and can cause different biological symptoms such as lack of sleep and indigestion. Anxiety disorders are categorized by type of disorder including panic disorder, phobias, and social anxiety disorder. Obsessive-compulsive disorder is also included under the umbrella of anxiety disorders and is defined as obsessive thoughts and compulsive behaviors revolving around a certain anxiety. Trauma- and stressor-related disorders are related to anxiety disorders as well, due to the anxiety symptoms (as well as depression symptoms) that are experienced after going through a traumatic or stressful event. A common disorder associated with this category of disorders is post-traumatic stress disorder (PTSD).

Somatic Symptom Disorders

Somatic symptom disorders are characterized by the physical problems and illnesses that are caused by psychological stressors. Having emotional difficulties or mental health issues, or experiencing a stressful event can trigger these physical symptoms, though there is no method of deriving the exact cause. If someone is experiencing a somatic symptom disorder, common symptoms the person will exhibit are difficulties speaking or using his or her senses, loss of strength, lack of balance, or difficulty moving certain parts of the body. Examples of these disorders are hypochondriasis, body dysmorphic disorder, conversion disorder, and pain disorder.

Depression, Bipolar Disorder, and Other Related Mood Disorders

Mood disorders are characterized by mood disturbances, changes, or difficulties. Depression is a mood disorder in which a person experiences feelings of extreme sadness, worthlessness, and a loss of hope for at least 2 weeks. This disorder may also lead to suicidal thoughts and actions. Bipolar disorder is another type of mood disorder in which individuals experience extreme mood swings and emotional instability. Those with bipolar disorder will have periods of depression or extreme sadness, followed by manic episodes with higher energy, positive thoughts, and increased activity levels, along with possible irritability.

Schizophrenia

Schizophrenia is a mental disorder that causes psychotic symptoms in an individual. These symptoms can include delusions, visual and auditory hallucinations, paranoia, unorganized speech and thinking, or difficulty with motor functions. This specific disorder causes the individual to lose touch with reality and is thought to be caused by a combination of genetics and environmental factors. Development of this disorder usually occurs in young adulthood, often when the individual is going through many social and physical changes.

Dissociative Disorders

Dissociative disorders are diagnosed when individuals have symptoms of memory loss, an altered view of their identity, are detached from the world and themselves, or exhibit depression and/or anxiety symptoms along with a dissociative state. This disorder is often marked by a traumatic life event, causing the individual's mind to protect him or her from psychological stress. Dissociative identity disorder (previously known as multiple personality disorder) is an example of such a disorder, characterized by different identities emerging from one individual, with each identity often having different memories or personalities to help cope with a stressful situation.

Personality Disorders

Personality disorders are a type of psychological disorder that are enduring, maladaptive, and rigid patterns of thoughts and behavior that make it difficult for an individual to function in a socially acceptable manner. Various types of personality disorders share these characteristics, often thought to be caused by life experiences and/or genetic abnormalities. Individuals with personality disorders have difficulties carrying out everyday behaviors or interacting with others and maintaining relationships. Examples of personality disorders include narcissistic personality disorder, in which a person has an inflated sense of self; paranoid personality disorder, in which a person is highly suspicious of those around him or her; schizoid personality disorder, in which a person avoids others and has little interest in establishing relationships; and obsessive-compulsive personality disorder, which differs from OCD in that a person is obsessively detail-oriented and strives for perfection, but does not exhibit obsessions and compulsions due to anxiety.

Biological Bases of Disorders

Schizophrenia

With schizophrenia, individuals are likely to have a genetic predisposition to the disorder. This means that if there is a predisposition, the individual is not guaranteed to be diagnosed with schizophrenia, but there are environmental factors that may contribute to developing the disorder because of the genetics involved. Schizophrenia is also thought to be related to elevated amounts of dopamine within the brain. Due to the effectiveness of antipsychotic drugs that block dopamine receptors, it is thought that dopamine dysregulation may be a biological basis for schizophrenia. The disorder is thought to be more likely associated with high numbers of dopamine receptors, as opposed to excessive levels of dopamine production. Brain abnormalities within the prefrontal cortex and the limbic system are also associated with schizophrenia and thought to be a cause for the disorder.

Depression

Depression has been shown to be associated with irregularities in neurotransmitters, such as serotonin, as well as abnormal levels of dopamine, norepinephrine, and cortisol. Serotonin is key in regulating mood, which leads scientists to believe that the abnormal levels of this neurotransmitter are related to the development of depression. In addition, antidepressants often increase serotonin levels, frequently leading to regulation in mood. It is also believed that some people are genetically predisposed to developing depression, meaning that those with this predisposition will not necessarily be diagnosed with depression, but environmental factors may influence the development of the disorder.

Alzheimer and Parkinson Diseases

Alzheimer disease is a nervous system disorder that is degenerative in nature and affects an individual's memory and functioning. Within the brain, plaques and tangles are formed that negatively impact the brain cells of a person. Plaques are likely to contribute to the death of brain cells and cause damage due to clusters of beta-amyloid protein. Tangles occur when strands of proteins are tangled within brain cells, preventing the essential nutrients needed for the brain from being transported. Parkinson disease is also degenerative in nature and negatively impacts motor function and mental processes. This occurs when the nerve cells within the brain (substantia nigra) are weakened. These nerve cells produce dopamine and the decline in functioning of these nerve cells leads to a drop in dopamine, affecting the ability for these nerve cells to communicate with the corpus striatum. The production of dopamine normally is how individuals are able to have coordination and muscle function, which is why Parkinson disease develops when the substantia nigra are weakened.

Stem Cell–Based Therapy to Regenerate Neurons

Many degenerative diseases are shown to be caused by the deterioration of neurons. Being about to regenerate these neurons would be essential to treating these diseases, such as Parkinson disease. Studies have shown that stem cells may be an effective tool in accomplishing this goal due to their ability to renew themselves, due to their efficacy in studies on animals. Brain cells are thought to be able to be restored by using neural stem cells, essentially repairing the damage caused by neurodegenerative diseases. These stem cells can be used to generate a significant amount of dopaminergic neurons, thus being a useful tool for this endeavor.

Influence of Instinct, Arousal, Drives, and Needs on Motivation

Instinct is behavior that is unlearned, but derived from biological influences. This behavior occurs throughout animals of the same species. The concept of arousal is seen as a level of awakening when an individual (or animal) is alert and stimulated, allowing him or her to be the most productive. Drives are known as mental and physical states that come from within the individual. These drives are helpful in creating a sense of urgency to carry out a specific behavior based on the drive involved. Hunger, thirst, exhaustion, and pain are all different types of drives that act in this manner. Lastly, needs are also internal states that influence behavior. Although needs may include different types of drives (needing to eat something, for instance, is an innate need), they can also incorporate higher level needs and learned goals in order to influence behavior. Wanting to earn money or power are examples of these learned needs, leading the individual to behave in ways that get him or her closer to this goal.

Drive Reduction Theory and Incentive Theory

Drive reduction theory uses the concept of drives to explain how motivation influences behavior. This theory suggests that humans will engage in behaviors that contribute to a reduction in drives. The discomfort involved in the drives motivate someone to find a way to reduce this discomfort, leading to the execution of certain behaviors. An example of this would be if someone is hungry. This hunger is a drive that creates a certain amount of discomfort, either psychologically or physically, and the individual experiencing this hunger will want to quell such a drive. In order to do this, the person decides to eat a sandwich, which in turn reduces his or her hunger. Incentive theory is thought to work in a similar way, but instead of being motivated by internal experiences, the individual is motivated by external sources. In this theory, it is proposed that the person is offered an incentive in some way to either increase or decrease a certain behavior. For instance, being rewarded with one's favorite food might be an incentive for that person to clean the house.

Cognitive and Need-Based Theories

Expectancy theory and goal-setting theory are examples of cognitive theories of motivation. Expectancy theory explains that individuals consciously behave in ways that they believe will decrease pain and increase pleasure. Goal-setting theory explains how individuals behave when they set goals for themselves. It proposes that when goals (even small goals) are accomplished and the individual receives positive feedback, this increases his or her performance later on. Need-based theories are also used to explain motivation and behavior. One example of this type of theory would be Maslow's hierarchy of needs. This theory explains how humans have 5 basic needs that include physiological needs, safety, social, esteem, and self-actualization. These are supposedly inherent needs, but in order to achieve the higher-level needs (esteem and self-actualization) one must first meet his or her physiological and safety needs, such as food, water, and shelter.

Biological and Sociocultural Motivators That Regulate Behavior

Certain behaviors, such as eating, having sex, and using substances, can be explained by both biological and sociocultural motivations. Eating, for instance, is necessary to survival, and the brain, digestive system, and hormones help to regulate this behavior. Hunger is signaled within the brain, leading a person to eat food. When full, the feeling of satiation comes from the ventromedial nucleus of the hypothalamus. Hormones, such as leptin and insulin, also aid in the digestion of the food. However, sociocultural motivators will also regulate eating; wanting to appear thinner or be healthier may lead a person to stop eating before they are full, or to wait to eat even when they are hungry. Sex is another behavior that is biologically influenced; hormones and sensory information may lead to an individual wanting to have sex. However, these desires may also be influenced by culture, social pressure, age, and emotion. Lastly, drug and alcohol behavior may be increased or decreased based on biological symptoms and experiences, such as dopamine levels or withdrawal symptoms. However, drug use may also be encouraged or discouraged based on the culture one is exposed to, curiosity, or events that they experience.

Components of Attitudes

Attitudes are composed of three different aspects: cognitive, affective, and behavioral. The cognitive aspect of attitude is how the individual thinks about something. Beliefs and knowledge about certain events or subjects fall into this category. For instance, if Jane knows that snakes are able to kill someone with just one bite, this may lead her to not like snakes, and possibly fear them. The affective aspect of attitude is how an individual feels about something. The feeling of love falls into this category; if Bob loves his wife, he is likely to have a positive attitude towards her. Lastly, the behavioral aspect of attitude is how someone acts in response to something. If a person has a negative attitude towards an issue, this will likely lead to that person behaving in a manner that exhibits this attitude. For instance, if Joe doesn't like Elaine and has a negative attitude towards her, this may influence his behavior in her presence. He may avoid her, or speak to her differently because of his dislike towards her.

Influence of Behavior on Attitudes

Behavior is a significant component of attitudes, and is likely to influence these attitudes. Foot-in-the-door phenomenon is one way in which behavior influences someone's attitude and works through the concept of compliance. When asked to do something simple, an individual may agree and fulfil this request. By engaging in this behavior, the individual is likely to agree to the next task, even if it is more difficult. After agreeing to these requests, the individual is likely to have a more positive attitude towards the person asking. Another way that behavior influences attitude is through role-playing effects. When asked to act in a way consistent with a type of person or character, the individual may internalize the behavior and have this influence his or her attitude. The most famous example of this is the Stanford prison study, when students were asked to act as either prisoners or prison guards. The student prisoners began to feel helpless or rebellious in face of their new role, while the prison guards began to feel more powerful and tough. The students had internalized these roles so extensively that the study was shut down after only 6 days.

Influence of Attitudes on Behavior

Often, a person acts in a certain way due to the attitudes he or she has about a situation. These attitudes can be influenced by personal experience, knowledge about a subject, or an expectation of a specific outcome. Icek Ajzen's theory of planned behavior is one way in which this process is explained. This theory holds that a person has a set of beliefs about a certain behavior, which influences his or her attitude towards that behavior. This in turn leads to the individual behaving in a way that coincides with this attitude. For example, if a student believes that she should be sitting quietly and alert in a class, it would make her happy to engage in this behavior, and she would sit quietly and alert in class. Another theory, the attitude-to-behavior process model, explains that a person's perception of an event will lead him or her to behave in a way that coincides with this perception. It also says that social norms are likely to affect a person's behavior. In this model, the event or situation prompts him or her to have an attitude about the situation, which in turn affects the social norms or individual perception of the event.

Cognitive Dissonance Theory

A common theme in our lives is thinking or feeling a certain way, but acting differently. Cognitive dissonance is the psychological explanation of this theme and can lead to anxiety if unresolved. This concept is best explained by an example. If George wants to lose weight, it would make sense that he would try to eat healthier. However, George loves ice cream, pizza, and other unhealthy foods. George may start to feel frustrated and angered at himself if he indulges in his favorite foods because of his goal of losing weight. These two opposing thoughts or feelings create a cognitive dissonance within George's psyche. Similarly, if George were to eat in an unhealthy manner while trying to lose weight, he may feel a certain tension within his mind. In order to resolve this cognitive dissonance, George would need to do one or more of three things: change his thoughts, change his behaviors, or introduce a new thought. George could either change his desire to lose weight, cease his indulgence in unhealthy foods, or decide to incorporate exercise into his routine. By making these alterations, George would resolve the tension created by his opposing thoughts and or behaviors, therefore alleviating his cognitive dissonance.

Social Facilitation

Social facilitation refers to how an individual performs better when there are other people around. Doing group activities, studying, exercising, and other simple tasks are often done better or more easily when done with two or more people. Having someone watch you or do an activity with you is likely to increase arousal/stimulation for that activity, making you work harder or more quickly on a simple task. However, because it increases arousal, this only works for easy behaviors; more complicated or difficult activities are done less easily when in the presence of others as it may make the individual more nervous and less able to focus on the task at hand.

Deindividuation

Deindividuation occurs when an individual is among a crowd and that individual loses his or her sense of self-awareness. A common term for this concept is also "mob mentality." When part of a "mob" or crowd, the individual may not feel responsible for his or her actions and participate in the actions of the group. This means that things that the individual would never do when he or she is alone may be easier to do when the rest of the group is doing it. For instance, Harold would never scream at a police officer when he is on his own, but when a crowd of people is yelling at the police in a protest, Harold also participates in the protest by yelling. Due to the anonymity and diffused responsibility, an individual is likely to feel more comfortable participating in the group activity than if he or she were alone. Not being able to be picked out of a crowd or held responsible for his or her actions may contribute to which behaviors the individual takes part in. The larger the group, the more anonymous the person is and the less responsibility her or she is likely to feel, and the more likely he or she will partake in the group behavior.

Bystander Effect

When something bad is happening in front of a large number of people, bystander effect may come into play. If someone is robbed in plain view of a group of people, and none of the people help or call the police, this is a bystander effect. This concept becomes more likely when there are more people around. For instance, if a single person is walking down the street and he or she witnesses a crime, he or she is likely to call for help or help the victim of the crime because there is no one else around. However, the more people are around to witness the crime, the less responsibility each individual person is likely to feel. Each person may assume that because there are so many people around someone else is likely to call the police. However, if everyone in the group assumes that someone else will take responsibility, then no one will actually help the victim, creating a bystander effect.

Social Loafing

When a group is given a project, each participant is likely to contribute less to the project than they would on their own. This concept is known as social loafing. Larger groups of people are more likely to lead to social loafing because each individual may feel as though they do not have as much responsibility when there are more people. In addition, if there is conflict within this group, group members are likely to contribute less to the project. Individuals also may fit into different categories when working on a group project. The in-group is comprised of individuals who are working hard and putting in more effort to finish the project. The out-group is comprised of individuals who aren't putting in as much effort and not taking responsibility for their part of the project. In order to reduce the phenomenon of social loafing, it is necessary to have smaller groups, as well as delegate responsibility to each individual member of the group.

Social Control

Social control is how society creates normative behaviors and formal rules for the way people should behave in order to prevent chaos. Informal social control is the category that unwritten social norms fall under. Not disrupting a funeral or not picking your nose in public are examples of informal social control that help keep society more organized. Formal social control refers to the laws placed on a society in order to keep society controlled. Behaviors that fall into this category are not committing crimes of murder or robbery because the individual will go to jail or be otherwise punished for disobeying these forms of formal control.

Peer Pressure

Peer pressure is when the people around you encourage you to participate in certain behaviors or decisions. This peer pressure can either be positive or negative depending on the behaviors performed. The people who are referred to as peers can be friends, family members, coworkers, team members, or other people who you relate to and want to spend time with. Peer pressure occurs when an individual doesn't necessarily want to participate in an activity or behavior, but feels pressured to do so by peers in order to "fit in" or follow norms of a certain group. Positive forms of peer pressure can include going to sporting events, volunteering, or other positive group activities. Negative forms of peer pressure include behaviors such as using drugs, committing crimes, or drinking alcohol illegally.

Conformity

Conformity is a way that individuals change their behaviors in order to be accepted into a group. Behaving in such a way is likely in response to feeling pressure to do so, but this pressure can be either real or imagined. The members of the group may explicitly tell the individual that participating in certain activities will make them fit into the group, but the individual may also infer from the group behavior how he or she is expected to act and subsequently feel pressured to act the same. Examples of conformity can include changing the way one dresses, engaging in risky behaviors such as drug and alcohol use, acquiring new hobbies, or going to events that the individual would normally not attend.

Obedience

Obedience can be defined as changing one's behavior in response to authority. This means that the individual may not normally engage in certain behaviors, but because they are being pressured by an authority figure to do so, the individual changes his or her behavior to obey. This occurs when an authority figure such as a boss, parent, teacher, or otherwise imposing person asks, commands, or instructs a person to perform a certain behavior, and the individual feels forced to comply with these instructions. Obedience can be viewed positively or negatively, depending on the context. For instance, obeying one's parents or a police officer may be considered socially acceptable or even required in order to maintain a sense of control or morality within a society. However, at times individuals may feel required to obey a person of power in order to keep their jobs or not be punished, which may lead to obeying orders that may be immoral or otherwise wrong.

Group Polarization

Group polarization is a concept that refers to groups of people making extreme decisions that don't necessarily align with the individual's original ideas. As an example, imagine that Joe originally felt that the pizza place should warn its customers that there are anchovies in certain menu items. However, when in the midst of a group of customers who also want a change in the menu items, they all decide that anything with anchovies should be taken completely off the menu. Joe originally did not want anchovies taken off the menu, but because of group polarization, the group made a more extreme decision. This concept also refers to the inclination of individuals to take greater risks when part of a group of like-minded individuals. Being part of this type of group may lead people to believe they share qualities and characteristics of a specific category of people, influencing the way they think and behave when part of a larger group.

Groupthink

Groupthink occurs when the members of a group agree to or accept the ideas and decisions of the larger group without bringing up their own individual ideas. This often leads to bad decisions made by the group because the decisions are not questioned or altered. For instance, imagine a group of people are trying to decide how to deal with a situation of unhealthy options at a fast food restaurant. Someone proposes the idea that they should take drastic action and vandalize the restaurant. Although this is a bad idea and one of the members, Sam, disagrees with this idea and thinks they should instead write a letter asking for healthy alternatives, everyone else in the group agrees with the idea of vandalism. This leads Sam to feel that he shouldn't disagree with the group and decides to support this proposal. The group then decides to vandalize the restaurant and the members of the group are arrested. This example of groupthink led to a bad decision even though there may have been better alternatives. Groupthink tends to occur when the group is more cohesive and lacks diverse opinions. In addition, strong group leaders also contribute to groupthink because people are less willing to disagree.

Sanctions

In society, people are expected to follow rules, whether explicit or implicit. These rules are called social norms and they can be laws that society has put in place or they can be unwritten rules that people have learned over the course of time. For these rules to work, there need to be punishments or consequences for individuals who fail to abide by these social norms. These punishments are known as sanctions. Sanctions can be punishments that individuals must endure for illegal behavior, such as jail time or being fined, but they can also be responses to violations of legal, but unwritten social norms, such as shame or ridicule from other members of a society. For instance, if someone were to wear a colorful and extravagant outfit to a funeral, instead of the traditional black clothing, that person may be judged by his or her peers or shamed into leaving early. These sanctions work to uphold the social norms and help people learn how to act in social settings.

Folkways, Mores, and Taboos

Multiple types of social norms are in place that individuals in a society must adhere to in order to maintain cohesion and control within the society. Three different types of social norms, folkways, mores, and taboos are used within a society to prevent chaos. Folkways are casual social norms that, if violated, cause less of an outrage than when more severe social norms are violated. For instance, wearing casual clothing to a formal event would be a violation of a folkway. Doing so may cause other people to stare or internally judge the individual, but consequences larger than that would be disproportional to the action. Mores are social norms that, if violated, lead to more severe social sanctions and stigmatization. The word "more" is derived from "morality," which helps understand what mores are: social norms based on a moral code. An example of a more would be living with a romantic partner before getting married. This type of more goes against certain religious moral codes that say couples must be married before cohabitating. Taboos are also a type of social norm that, when violated, elicit a strong response from society such as disgust or rejection. An example of a taboo is incest, which is not tolerated in certain societies and leads to extreme responses from society when it occurs.

Anomie

Social norms exist in order for a society to function in a controlled and predictable manner. However, when these social norms don't exist or when they are lacking, this concept is known as anomie. Anomie occurs when the social constructs of a community or group are broken down and the society no longer provides moral codes or laws for individuals to live by. Anomie can also refer to the phenomenon of individuals no longer accepting or abiding by the social norms, by way of individualism or isolation. Some believe that this is a form of anarchy and that the society can no longer exist with harmony among its citizens, while others may see it as freedom from oppression.

Deviance

Deviance can be defined as behavior that does not abide by social norms within a group. This deviance varies from culture to culture due to the various social norms that exist within each society. Something that is considered deviant in one culture does not necessarily mean that it is deviant in another. Some deviant behavior is against the law, while others may just be considered impolite or abnormal. Different theories also exist regarding deviance, including differential association, labeling theory, and strain theory. Differential association refers to the idea that when a person is associated with individuals who are considered deviant, that person will also be considered deviant. This form of deviation is thought to contribute to social change through more and more individuals becoming part of the deviant group, thereby changing how that behavior is viewed. Labeling theory refers to the idea that labels can influence how people view themselves, thereby potentially influencing their behavior. If someone is told he is an overachiever, for instance, he may either reject the label and become less motivated, or accept the label and embrace the motivation. Lastly, strain theory refers to how society is structured, and how it may put excessive pressure on individuals that lead to deviant behavior. For instance, if society is structured in a way that makes it difficult to afford rent or food, people may feel that robbery or committing other crimes is the only option for survival.

Collective Behavior

When large amounts of individuals engage in the same behavior, this is known as collective behavior. Collective behavior can include things such as fads, mass hysteria, and riots. Fads are defined as temporary trends that many people in a society follow. Collecting a specific item (Beanie Babies or Silly Bandz), saying certain phrases or words (selfie or psyche), or watching certain television shows (Care Bears or Jersey Shore) all fall under the category of a fad. Mass hysteria refers to a large amount of people worried about the same thing, whether real or imagined, due to media coverage or through rumors. An example of mass hysteria would be the Salem witch trials in the 1600s. Riots are also a form of collective behavior and can be in response to either positive or negative societal events. Riots may happen in a city where a professional sports team wins a national championship, or if there are accusations of racism in societal structures.

Socialization

Socialization can occur through many different societal structures with the goal of an individual learning the social norms of the community. The primary agent of socialization is family. This is the first place where an individual learns how to behave, and the different features of the family influence the individual's personality and belief system. How large the family is, how religious they are, and what culture they are part of are each part of the familial socialization. Another agent of socialization is the mass media. This is often where people get information about the world and how to perceive this information. Mass media includes television, Internet, radio, and other forms of communication and entertainment. These sources of media give individuals information about politics, religion, culture, and much more. Peers are also a way for an individual to learn social norms. How the peers are raised by their own family, their experiences and beliefs, and their interests influence how the individual perceives the world and their own interests. Peers are usually of the same age and share various interests that bring them together. Peers can be positive or negative depending on the behaviors they encourage, and are most influential during adolescence when the individual is attempting to create his or her own identity. Lastly, the workplace is also a main agent of socialization, and it is where individuals learn behaviors and knowledge that help them become a part of the workforce. Ethics, professionalism, and how to work in stressful situations are just some of the things an individual learns in the workplace in order to follow social norms.

Neutral, Conditioned, and Unconditioned Stimuli

The concept of classical conditioning uses specific terms to explain how behavior is learned through a biological response. A neutral stimulus is one that does not naturally produce a response from an individual, such as a bell ringing or a light flashing. An unconditioned stimulus is one that triggers a natural response, such as how a frightening loud noise causes an individual to feel scared, or how the smell of delicious food causes one to salivate. A conditioned stimuli is one to which an individual has developed a learned response. An example of this would be Pavlov's dogs: the dogs had no reaction to a ringing bell originally (neutral stimulus) and they would salivate when they smelled their food (unconditioned stimulus). Pavlov would ring the bell and serve the food at the same time, causing the dogs to become conditioned to this neutral stimuli. The conditioned stimuli became the ringing bell, which would cause the dogs to salivate before they could smell their food.

Conditioned and Unconditioned Responses

In the theory of classical conditioning, individuals are believed to learn certain behaviors through acquisition of conditioned responses to different stimuli. An unconditioned response is a naturally occurring response to an unconditioned stimuli. For instance, a natural reaction to a sudden loud noise would be fear or surprise. A person's response to that may be screaming, jumping back, or even running away. These responses are unconditioned responses to this specific stimulus. A conditioned response is one that does not occur naturally and the individual has acquired this response to a once-neutral stimulus through conditioning. An example of this would be Pavlov's dogs: The dogs in his study would salivate whenever they smelled their food. This salivation would be considered an unconditioned response because it is naturally occurring. The dogs originally had no response to a bell ringing (a neutral stimulus), but Pavlov decided to ring a bell at the same time he gave the dogs their food. Over time, because of the consistent pairing of the food with the bell, the dogs salivated when they heard the bell ring, even when there was no food. This salivation in response to the bell ringing is an example of a conditioned response.

Processes of Classical Conditioning

Classical conditioning explains the process of acquiring certain behaviors in response to certain stimuli. The process of learning the associations between certain stimuli is known as acquisition. Acquisition refers to developing a conditioned response to a stimulus through the pairing of a neutral stimulus with an unconditioned stimulus. However, if this pairing stops occurring, after a while extinction will occur. Extinction refers to the loss of the association of these stimuli. For instance, if a dog learns that a bell ringing signals food coming, he salivates in response to the bell (even when no food is presented). This is the acquisition of a conditioned response. However, if the bell rings consistently with no food presented, the dog may no longer salivate when the bell rings. This is known as extinction. After a response is extinguished, if there is a rest period (a couple hours or a day) where the bell does not ring, the next time the bell rings may elicit the same conditioned response: salivation. This reappearance of the conditioned response after extinction is known as spontaneous recovery. In addition, if the dog learns that the bell ringing means food, and therefore salivates, the dog may also salivate when the doorbell rings, or when a similar sound occurs. This is called generalization. However, there is also the possibility that the dog is able to distinguish between the bell ringing and the doorbell, which would be called discrimination. This is when the dog does not salivate when he hears a similar noise because he does not associate it with being given food.

Shaping and Extinction in Operant Conditioning

Operant conditioning is a theory in which behavior can be learned through punishments and rewards. When a behavior is learned through reinforcement, this is known as shaping. However, if the individual learns this behavior, but it is no longer being reinforced, the individual may not exhibit this behavior anymore. When this behavior declines, this is referred to as extinction.

Types of Reinforcement

Positive, Negative, Primary, and Conditional

In operant conditioning, one way of learning behavior is through reinforcement. There are different types of reinforcement, positive and negative, and they are used in order to increase a specific behavior. Positive reinforcement is when an individual is given a reward in order to encourage an increase in that behavior. For instance, if a parent wants a child to clean his or her room, the parent may reward a clean room by giving the child candy. The child then cleans his or her room more often in order to get more candy. Negative reinforcement is a bit more complex. Contrary to what one may think, negative reinforcement does not refer to a punishment; instead it refers to taking something away in order to increase a certain behavior. Using the example above, the parent may encourage the child to clean his or her room by saying that they will not make him or her clean the bathroom. Because the child does not want to clean the bathroom, he or she cleans the bedroom in order to avoid this extra chore. Primary and secondary reinforcers are rewards to help increase behavior. Primary reinforcers are rewards that a person desires naturally: food, water, and other pleasure, while secondary reinforcers are rewards that a person learns to desire, such as money or toys. These secondary reinforcers are not natural rewards, but instead things that a person has associated with a primary reward and learned to desire.

Fixed-Ratio, Variable-Ratio, Fixed-Interval, and Variable-Interval

In order to reinforce a behavior through operant conditioning, there are different schedules that this reinforcement can occur in, and these schedules may have different efficacy. Fixed-ratio schedules are when behavior is rewarded in a specific pattern. This could mean that each time the behavior occurs, it is rewarded, or it could mean that every fifth time the behavior occurs it is rewarded. This schedule is fairly predictable, especially compared to variable-ratio schedules. In this type of schedule, the behavior is rewarded at a different rate each time. For instance, instead of being rewarded for a behavior every time it occurs, the behavior is rewarded the first time, and then it is rewarded after 5 times, and then it is rewarded again after the fourteenth time. Another schedule of reinforcement is called fixed-interval. Similar to fixed ratio, the behavior is rewarded predictably after a certain amount of time has passed. For instance, the behavior is rewarded, and then it won't be rewarded again for another minute each time. Variable-interval schedule is similar to the variable-ratio, in that it is unpredictable; the behavior may be rewarded immediately, but then rewarded 4 minutes later, and then again 3 minutes later.

Punishment in Operant Conditioning

In operant conditioning, punishment is one way to shape a person's behavior. However, unlike reinforcement, punishment seeks to decrease a behavior. For instance, if a child is screaming, a parent may want to decrease this behavior through punishment. One type of punishment, positive punishment, introduces a stimulus in order to decrease a behavior. This means that the parent might spank his or her child, or scold them. This causes the child to stop screaming in order to avoid this punishment. Negative punishment works by taking something away in order to decrease a behavior. In this example, the parent might decide to take away the child's dessert in order to decrease his or her screaming. Because the child wants dessert and doesn't want to lose it, the child learns to stop screaming in order to avoid the punishment.

Escape and Avoidance Learning

Individuals often learn how to approach the world based on learning experiences that shape one's view of the world. For instance, escape and avoidance learning are ways that individuals learn about things that might do them harm or cause them discomfort. If something hurts a person, that person will likely try to get away as fast as possible. This is represented by the concept of escape learning. The next time the individual interacts with this thing that previously hurt them, they will try to avoid it. This concept is known as avoidance. The two concepts work together in escape and avoidance learning, and the individual learns that this thing must be avoided in order to evade discomfort. An example of this is if a person sees a cactus and decides to touch it, she may prick a finger. She reacts to the pain by jumping away from it, or escaping it. The next time she sees the cactus, she remembers being pricked by it previously and avoids touching it.

Associative Learning

Cognitive Processes

Associative learning is when a person learns that two things are associated and produce a specific response. Operant and classical conditioning are two ways that associative learning can occur. There are also different cognitive processes that influence associative learning including latent learning, problem-solving, and instincts. Latent learning is a passive type of association in which an individual is not rewarded for a behavior but learns to behave in this way naturally. Problem-solving is a process in which a person encounters a problem and must step back, observe the situation, think about it, and then decide how to solve the problem. Instincts are genetic or biological behaviors that are naturally occurring and difficult to change. Animals, especially mothers, have instinctual protectiveness of their young, making it difficult to teach these animals otherwise.

Biological Processes

Associative learning is a process of acquiring certain behaviors through learning, but this process may also be influenced by biology. One way this occurs is through instinctive drift. If an animal, for instance, has instincts that lead it to hunt for food in order to survive, this is the natural way for that animal to behave. However, if the animal in question is a domestic cat, a human may try to train the cat to stay at home, eat canned cat food, and sleep all day. However, the cat still has instincts to hunt, and when let outside, the cat reverts to these basic instincts and hunts and eats a mouse. This reversion back to hunting after being domesticated is known as instinctive drift. An individual or animal may also have biological predispositions that influence how they behave. This predisposition may make the individual more likely to develop certain diseases or various characteristics. An example would be a person who has parents who are alcoholics. This individual may be more likely to develop alcoholism based solely on this biological predisposition, in addition to being exposed to an environment and family that encourage drinking. Other examples would be personality traits, intelligence, diseases, and other similar behaviors.

Observational Learning

Modeling

Modeling is a process by which an individual learns how to do certain behaviors by watching other people engage in this behavior. Parents, teachers, friends, and other individuals that the person either relates to or is exposed to often can serve as these models of behavior. When an individual sees another person successfully engaging in a certain behavior, it increases the confidence of the individual also performing that behavior successfully. Being able to mimic another person's behavior through modeling allows the observer to understand how and when to act a certain way and increases the likelihood of successfully following in his or her footsteps.

Brain, Mirror Neurons, and Vicarious Emotions

In observational learning, there are different biological processes that impact learning different behaviors. Mirror neurons are one example of such a process; they originate in the frontal and parietal lobes of the brain and are activated when an individual is performing a certain behavior or exhibiting a certain emotion and that individual observes another person engaging in the same behavior. This allows an individual to learn how to perform certain behaviors and understand another person's feelings. The brain allows the individual to also feel emotions, despite not sharing the same emotion. Empathy is one way in which this occurs, and involves two individuals sharing an emotion and feeling that emotion together. Emotions can also be felt vicariously. This refers to the idea that even though two individuals don't share a certain emotion or experience, both feel the same emotion. For instance, if Rachel's friend gets married and is happy, Rachel may feel the same emotion because she is vicariously experiencing the happiness of her friend.

Applications of Observational Learning to Explain Individual Behavior

Individual behavior is often impacted by learning through observation. These observations are usually through family interactions, but may also refer to friendships, school life, the workplace, media, and other social environments. Some applications of this may be when a person is a part of an abusive family and they themselves develop an abusive personality and behavior, or if the individual has friends who are very loving and welcoming, the individual may learn to also be loving and welcoming through observation.

Elaboration Likelihood Model

The elaboration likelihood model explains the ways that people tend to make decisions. Taking time to think about a decision or following other peoples' decisions are ways in which people make a decision and these ways are explained in the elaboration likelihood model. The model evaluates how likely a person is to use either one of these methods for making a decision. Central route processing is the tendency for an individual to think hard about a decision. This person would read articles, talk to other people, and carefully examine each aspect of the decision at hand. Peripheral route processing refers to a person who is only paying attention to information that is not central to the decision at hand. This person would be more likely to look at how attractive something is to them, what their friends are doing, or what people tell them to do. An example of the elaboration likelihood model is when someone is deciding which computer to buy. A person using central route processing is more likely to pay attention to user reviews, the amount of hard drive, and the speed of the computer. Someone using peripheral route processing may be more likely to make a decision based on commercials, which computer looks better, or what a friend of theirs has.

Various Factors That Affect Attitude Change

Attitudes can be changed by different aspects. For instance, if a person's behavior were to change, this would be observed by others and then this would influence that person's attitude. An example of this would be if a person buys a new sweater, but then people don't compliment the sweater or they make fun of it, this may cause the individual to no longer like the sweater. Messages from others and the media also influence attitudes. These messages influence how the person feels about something, thereby affecting his or her attitude. In this scenario, the characteristics of the message and who the message is targeting would change a person's attitude. If that person were to see a movie and like it, he might change his attitude if he hears that other people didn't like it or he reads negative reviews about the movie. Attitudes can also be changed by social factors and the environment. For instance, if a person were to have friends that like certain types of food and going to specific social events that she originally didn't like, she may learn to like it or change her attitude to fit in with the friend group.

Self-Identity and Social Influences

Self-Concept and Self-Identity

Role of Self-Esteem

Self-esteem refers to how much an individual accepts and values themselves. People may have high or low self-esteem, and this influences their self-identity or self-concept. A person with high self-esteem may feel more confident and view themselves in a positive manner. This person is less likely to worry about what others say about him and other people's opinions are less likely to influence his self-identity. However, a person with low self-esteem is the opposite. This person does not view himself in a positive light, and has less confidence in how he is as a person. Other people's opinions of him are highly influential on how he sees himself, and this has a negative impact on his identity.

Role of Self-Efficacy

Self-efficacy can be defined as a person's belief in his or her ability to be successful or achieve a specific goal. Different tasks and circumstances are viewed to have different levels of self-efficacy for a person, and this level of self-efficacy can be either positive or negative. A person with high self-efficacy is more likely to have a positive view of the task at hand and have more confidence completing this task. This type of individual is also less fearful in taking risks and is able to evaluate themself more accurately. However, a person with low self-efficacy is more prone to negative thoughts regarding a specific task and has more doubts and fears of his or her ability to accomplish a goal. This person is less likely to take risks and believes she will fail, even when this evaluation of her abilities is incorrect

Role of Locus of Control

A person's self-concept and self-identity can be influenced by his locus of control. This phrase refers to how a person views his control of a situation and impacts the attitudes and behavior that are related to this situation. There are two different categories of locus of control: external and internal. A person with an external locus of control views the situation as being controlled by outside forces, and he doesn't believe that he has control over what happens. People who have this external locus of control tend to blame others or external causes for what happens, or feel hopeless about the situation. They may also say that if a problem is solved successfully, it was lucky or a fluke. Individuals with an internal locus of control have the opposite view of situations. These people tend to blame themselves if something goes wrong because they believe that they are able to control what happens. This type of person may also take more control over situations and work tirelessly to accomplish a goal because they have more confidence in their ability to control the situation.

Identity Types

People are likely to identify themselves in terms of different groups that they fit into. These groups form a basis for an individual's identity and can range from cultural identities to age or gender. Someone's racial or ethnic identity signifies their heritage or cultural background based on skin color or country of origin. Gender is another identity: males, females, transgendered people, and other groups fall under the category of gender. Age can also be an identity, not just by how old a person is, but by how old they act or feel internally. A person's religion, sexual orientation, or social class also signifies identity and may impact how an individual views him or herself.

Theories of Identity Development

There are many theories about the development of identity and they differ based on psychological fields of study and the theory's main focus. One theory, by Lawrence Kohlberg, is based on morality. This theory focuses on how an individual develops a sense of morality through cognition and resolution of moral dilemmas. This theory explains these moral dilemmas through consequences of certain actions, social order, and rules of social relationships throughout the lifespan. Freud also developed a theory of identity based on the different psychosexual stages. This theory explains that children go through a series of these psychosexual stages (oral, anal, phallic, latency, and genital) as the child ages, and if the child does not successfully move through these stages, he or she may become fixated at a certain stage, resulting in the formation of an identity or personality that is shaped by this fixation. Erik Erikson's theory of psychosocial identity development describes different stages of the lifespan wherein the individual must successfully resolve the conflict at each stage. These conflicts range from trust and autonomy to identity and intimacy. These different stages are different parts of an individual's psychology and formed through social interactions. Conflicts not fully resolved in this theory create difficulties in a person's life throughout time.

INFLUENCES ON IDENTITY FORMATION

INDIVIDUALS

A person's identity is formed through individual aspects in different ways. For instance, imitation is one way that a person can be influenced by the individuals around her. Mimicking the behavior of parents, siblings, friends, or other people in a person's life is the definition of imitation. These behaviors often occur because the person represents traits that you identify with and help to build your own identity. The looking-glass self is also a way that individuals shape another person's identity. For instance, if a Jon has friends who view him as fun, but his parents see him as a lazy person, these ideas shape the way that Jon thinks of himself, and therefore form his identity. Another way that individuals affect a person's identity is when the person takes on the roles or identity of the other individual. If Jon, for instance, pretends to be like a police officer on television, he is experimenting with that person's identity. By pretending to be someone else, this helps an individual figure out how his own identity coincides with that of another person.

GROUPS

Groups can have a large impact on how a person's forms his or her identity. The main way this occurs is through the use of reference groups. This means that an individual is exposed to groups that have different characteristics, interests, and personalities, and draws conclusions about these groups based on these traits. The individual is then able to see how his own identity fits into these groups to determine more information about his identity. An example of this would be Penny. Penny sees a group of girls at school who are very quiet and read many books. This group isn't very popular but they are very friendly and helpful to other people. Another group of girls at school is very popular and the girls in that group play sports and go to a lot of social events. However, this group isn't as friendly as the first group and they don't always treat people nicely. Penny doesn't play sports, but she does read a lot of books. This leads her to identify more with the first group of girls and use them as a reference group. This may shape more of her identity if she sees more things about this group that she can identify with. If Penny identifies with this group and they are very good students, she may also strive to be a good student and evaluate her own test scores on what the test scores of that group are.

CULTURE AND SOCIALIZATION

A person's identity may be influenced by the culture he lives in as well as the ways in which he socializes. Culture is often defined as the way people live and act within a certain group. These groups share characteristics such as religion, race, sexual orientation, ability, and language. These characteristics of a culture help individuals define themselves in relation to this culture, but also within a variety of cultures that they identify with. For instance, a person may have Japanese heritage and share characteristics of Japanese cultural groups, but also be sexually attracted to someone of the same sex, which would lead them to identify with homosexual groups. Some of these cultures may range in how accepted they are within a larger society, which may also shape the way an individual identifies with that culture. Socialization is also a way in which a person forms his or her identity based on their social experiences throughout the lifespan. This person may have to learn different rules and skills for maneuvering this society and also use others as a reference for how to behave.

Attributional Processes

Attributional processes happen when a person assigns meaning to behavior and events, and these meanings, or attributions, influence and represent the cognitive processes and actions of that person. There are different types of attributions: internal and external. Internal attributions are when a person attributes meaning based on internal motives such as beliefs and emotions. External attributions are more situational and assign meaning based on the events and external characteristics. Fundamental attribution error is a process that occurs when an individual uses internal attribution for something that is a cause of the environment or situation. For instance, if Bill is angry and yells at Karen, Karen may believe this is because Bill is simply an angry person. However, Karen was unaware that Bill was angry because he had been fired from his job that day. This is an example of fundamental attribution error. Culture also plays a role in attributions; some cultures are more individualistic and may attribute more behaviors to internal processes such as personality, while other cultures are more collectivist and are more likely to attribute behaviors to external sources.

Influences on Our Perceptions of Others

Self-Perceptions

Self-perception can be defined as how an individual sees themselves. They use their own experiences and beliefs, as well as cultural characteristics to better understand how they behave and interact with others. These self-perceptions also come into play when perceiving others. This means that how a person views his or her own behavior, morals, or social roles influences how he or she understands the behavior, morals, or social roles of another person. For instance, Jim believes that he is smart because he reads a lot of books. If Jim were to find out that his friend doesn't read as many, this may lead him to believe that his friend is not very smart.

Perceptions of the Environment

Perceiving others can be influenced by a variety of factors. The environment we live in can affect how we see others, how they see us, and how we behave. Different environments (eg, work, school, parties, funerals) may have different sets of social rules that people are expected to follow in order to maintain cohesion and understanding. How individuals see this environment may depend on the different social rules they understand, as well as other factors such as time and place. For instance, Gary thinks that wearing bright colors to a dance club or party is normal and expected of most people. But Gary also has come to understand that these outfits are not appropriate for all settings. If Gary were to see Wendy wearing a bright pink dress at a club, he may not even notice, but if she wore the same outfit to a funeral, his perception of Wendy would change. In addition, how a person feels in a certain situation may also influence their perception of others. If a person is comfortable, they may perceive others more positively than if they were in an uncomfortable environment.

Contributing Factors to Prejudice

Power, Prestige, and Class

Having power often refers to being able to control situations and other people. This ability is also a factor that contributes to prejudice. Prejudice is when a person has different opinions about a person or group of people based on the social, cultural, or other marginalized group they belong to. Political power, economical power, and personal power are different examples of these and each may contribute to prejudice by putting the needs of oneself in front of others. Having one's own opinions and being in a position of power make this easier and it is more likely to let biases control one's thoughts and behaviors. Prestige is also a contributing factor to prejudice and refers to the amount of recognition or fame a person has. Different occupations (e.g., doctors, lawyers) have more recognition and better reputations than others, giving them more prestige and different perceptions of the world. These perceptions may contribute to prejudicial opinions. In addition, social or economic class may also contribute to prejudice because of how a person views others. For instance, people with more money may view those of lower economic classes less intelligent or lazy simply based on the amount of money they make.

Emotion

Prejudice can be influenced by a variety of factors, such as emotion. Having stronger emotions, or being emotionally aroused, when something happens contributes to how one feels about that event. If someone were to be physically assaulted by someone of a different race or a different social class, this would likely trigger strong emotions during the assault. Seeing people who share characteristics with the assailant may also trigger those same emotions in other situations. This strong emotion may lead to prejudicial opinions based on the event.

Cognition

Cognition is defined as the thought processes that an individual has, and can be an influential factor in prejudice. When you hold certain beliefs or learn different information, this may influence your perception of others. Race, class, culture, and other characteristics are ways that people define others, and if we have certain beliefs and understandings of these characteristics, it is likely that we will jump to conclusions about others based on these cognitive processes. For instance, if Harry reads that certain races are arrested for more crimes than other races, this may lead him to believe that particular race is more prone to criminal behavior. Because of this knowledge, Harry may also treat people of that race differently.

Stereotypes

Stereotypes are a way that people can understand others based on generalizations about that person's class, gender, race, culture, religion, or other category. Although these stereotypes allow people to process information about groups of individuals more quickly and predict behavior, they also may be based on incorrect information or lead to people ignoring individual differences. These stereotypes are often based on specific experiences and are shared by many people. There can be positive or negative stereotypes, but both types can be detrimental to the understanding of different cultures and groups of people. Positive stereotypes explain the good characteristics of groups, such as being smart or talented based on which group one belongs to. Negative stereotypes focus on the bad characteristics and may lead to prejudice and discrimination.

Stigma

A stigma refers to the idea that a person, or group of people, views someone else negatively based on that person's beliefs, behaviors, or other qualities. These qualities often differ from social and cultural norms, and can be characteristics such as religious views, money problems, sexual orientation, or even disease. Many things that are stigmas are thought to be the fault of that person and lead to the dislike or mistrust of a person because it is believed they can control it. However, mental disorders that are out of a person's control, or problems that are caused by external circumstances, can also be stigmatizing and thought to be shameful or disgraceful.

Ethnocentrism

Ethnocentrism is the idea that a specific culture or ethnic group is better than another. This often occurs when a specific individual views his or her own culture or ethnic group as superior because of his or her own biases surrounding this topic. If a person believes that they are better than others, they may judge people based on their culture and ethnicity, leading to prejudice and discrimination. There are also concepts that help explain ethnocentrism: in-groups and out-groups. An in-group is a group with which a person identifies and claims membership, while an out-group is one with which an individual does not identify. Out-groups are viewed as "others" and as threats to the in-group's superiority. An example of this would be a person who identifies as Christian and views other religions as inferior to his own. Because this person believes that he is right about religious topics and thinks that Christianity is the best religion, he may treat people from other religions with contempt and view other religions as morally wrong.

Cultural Relativism

Cultural relativism is the idea that all cultures and ethnicities are equal and that no group is better than another. This is the opposite of ethnocentrism and proposes that no culture is at the center of the universe, nor one more morally correct than another. In this view, people don't discriminate against others based on language, religion, race, or other cultural differences, and instead embrace the idea that these differences do not pertain to morality or truth.

Self-Fulfilling Prophecy

Self-fulfilling prophecy is a way in which a person's behavior is shaped by the way people see them. If a person is viewed negatively, people may treat them in a way that reinforces this view and causes that person to behave in a way that confirms this negative view. An example of this would be a teacher who thinks that a student is a troublemaker based on either a stereotype, or unconscious bias that the teacher holds. Due to his or her opinion, the teacher treats the student as a troublemaker by expecting the student to misbehave, getting mad at the student for minor mishaps, or paying more attention to this student than the others. This treatment is likely to elicit bad behavior, and because of this, the student may misbehave more and more, thereby confirming the original view of the teacher.

Stereotype Threat

A stereotype threat is the idea that a person's awareness of a stereotype about his or her own race, gender, or other characteristic may cause anxiety and fear of confirming this stereotype. This anxiety and fear may also negatively influence one's ability to perform well on certain tasks, putting the individual at risk for confirming the stereotype simply by being defensive or worried about it. An example of this would be the stereotype that females have poor mathematical skills. If a girl wants to disprove this stereotype, it may cause her anxiety about her performance. Because of this anxiety, when the girl takes a math test, she may not perform very well, and confirm the stereotype she was so worried about in the first place.

Types of Status in Relation to Social Interaction

A person's status describes where that individual fits into society. Two types of status describe this position in society, and they interact with one another to determine this position. Achieved status is one that is earned by different accomplishments and events. Examples of this type of status would be getting an education, getting married, or getting a job. Within this status, there are different levels, such as income, fame, or social status. The second type of status is known as ascribed status. Ascribed status is something an individual is born with and they inherit through birth. Examples of this would be gender, race, sexuality, or socioeconomic status.

Role Conflict and Role Strain

A social role is something that an individual is assigned or chooses to be a part of, and it is defined by a set of rules and normative behaviors. As a member of society, each individual has a role based on lifestyle, occupation, or relationship. When a person has trouble following the rules and responsibilities of her role, this is known as role strain. An individual may, for instance, feel that her role of being a leader of a group is too much of a responsibility and she doesn't have enough time to fulfill this role. An individual may also have two different roles that she must adhere to. When these different roles interfere with one another, this is known as role conflict. If an individual is a mother, for example, but also has a full-time job, she may feel conflicted when she has to choose between going to a meeting and taking her child to a school event.

Role Exit

Social roles are helpful in understanding one's position in the world and how he or she is expected to behave. However, when a role is too demanding or conflicts with another, a person may choose to give up a role. This concept is known as role exit. An example of this would be a father who feels conflicted in his role as a father and as a full-time employee. He may decide that, because one role is more important, or because he no longer wants to adhere to a certain role, he must exit one of his roles. By choosing to be a stay-at-home dad and quitting his job, the father may decide to exit his role of being a full-time employee.

Primary and Secondary Groups

Throughout the lifespan, a person may fit into many different groups based on their social interactions and environment. There are two main types of groups that explain the differences in these relationships, called primary and secondary groups. Primary groups are groups in which a person has a long-term relationship and/or interaction with the members of the group. These groups spend significant amounts of time together and interact over lengthy spans of time. Examples of primary groups would be a person's immediate family, core group of friends, or spouse and children. Secondary groups are more temporary and don't spend as much time with one another. These groups have a specific purpose and are not as deep or personal. Examples of these groups are a person's classmates, coworkers, or a client in a professional setting.

In-Group and out-Group

Individuals often perceive the world according to the groups they fit into. These groups can be based on characteristics such as gender, race, sexual orientation, or other cultural differences. People often view the world based on in-groups and out-groups as well. An in-group is one with which the individual identifies in which he feels that he belongs. An out-group is a group that the individual does not feel as though he belongs to, and he may hold different opinions or prejudices towards this group.

Group Sizes

A person may identify with various types of groups. Different sizes of groups may influence the relationship or help to strengthen the bonds between the group members. A dyad is a group that is made up of two individuals. These groups may be very close and connected, such as a husband and wife, or father and son, but they may also be less interpersonal, such as a doctor and patient, or a salesman and a customer. Another type of group size is a triad. This type of group has three members. An example of a triad would be two parents and a child, or a single parent and two children.

Networks

People have many different methods of interacting with others, and one way of doing this is through the use of networks. Networks are made up of connections between different individuals and groups of people. These networks can be made of connections based on culture, environment, interests, and various other ties that connect people socially. The structure of most societies is based on these networks and help people interact with one another. The terms used for the different aspects of networks are nodes and ties. Nodes are the individuals or groups that exist in a larger group. These nodes are connected to one another via ties, and these ties can either be weak or strong. Weak ties connect individuals who are not as close personally, and can be used to expand one's network. Stronger ties help connect people and create close, personal bonds with one another. The negative aspect of stronger ties, however, is that these connections help connect people of similar interests and backgrounds, creating less diversity, which may impede creative endeavors.

Formal Organization

Organizations are a social structure in which people are connected through a professional association and work together to achieve a common goal. These organizations are a singular unit that has its own culture and structure to help the members accomplish their goals. Within these organizations exist methods of containing this structure and holding members responsible for their actions. This can be through the use of committees or judicial entities, and it is also through the use of a hierarchical system to maintain order. Formal organizations are a type of organization made of less personal connections and the individuals serve a specific purpose of the group. Examples of these formal organizations are government departments, public or private universities, healthcare networks, or private companies.

Ideal Bureaucracy

An ideal bureaucracy is one that successfully carries out the responsibilities of the government through the use of government officials. These officials are not elected representatives, but they make decisions for the system of government they serve. An ideal bureaucracy consists of a hierarchical authoritative system with promotions based on merit or achievement. This system is efficient, impersonal, and effectively divided in order to accomplish the goals set forth by the system. Explicit rules concern behavior, goals, and methods for accomplishing these goals.

Perspectives on Bureaucracy

Bureaucracy can be approached in a variety of methods in order to achieve success. One such perspective is known as the iron law of oligarchy. In this theory, it is believed that there will inevitably be a tendency for individuals in elite positions to rule the government. These systems start out as democratic, with elected officials, and grow further and further away from this concept, turning towards a system controlled by a selected number of individuals. Another perspective on bureaucracy is that of McDonaldization. This concept refers to the McDonald's-type fast food restaurants and the efficiency of such businesses. McDonaldization is the idea that it would be easy and efficient to use these business structures as a guideline for bureaucracy and strive for more efficiency, more predictability and standardization, and the ability to calculate and control behaviors and productivity.

Role of Gender in the Expression and Detection of Emotion

Expressing and detecting emotions can differ due to multiple variables, including gender. Gender plays a significant role in this process through an individual expressing emotion, but also in the detection of that emotion based on that individual as well as the observer. Masculine individuals are more likely to exhibit aggressive and forceful emotions, while femininity is related to gentle and expressive emotions. Because of these gender-based expectations, this may cause an individual to express emotions based on his or her gender. For instance, boys are expected to be tough and are less likely to cry or exhibit any signs of weakness, while girls are supposed to be "lady-like" and not behave aggressively. It is also thought to be easier for females to detect emotion because of their tendency to express more emotions than males.

Role of Culture in the Expression and Detection of Emotion

Some cultures express emotion differently and are able to detect different emotions more easily. In societies that are more individualistic (Western countries), individuals are more likely to express emotions, such as pride or jealousy, because these are emotions focused on the individual as opposed to the rest of society. In addition, individualist countries may encourage the expression of emotions more than in other societies, allowing people to feel more comfortable expressing these emotions. In collectivist cultures (countries in Asia or Africa), individuals may be more likely to express feelings based on group dynamics, such as shame or friendliness, because these emotions are felt in relation to society. In these collectivist countries, people may also be less likely to express personal emotions because of the effect it may have on those around them. Detecting emotions also varies based on cultures, as culture may influence which emotions an individual pays attention to, such as the idea that Americans may be more likely to detect the emotion of another individual easily, but someone from Japanese culture may be more likely to detect the emotions of background figures or other group members more easily.

Impression Management in Relation to Presentation of Self

Individuals are likely to present themselves in such a way that purposefully influences those they interact with. How a person dresses, what they say, how they say it, and how a person acts are all ways in which people present themselves to others according to the way they wish to be seen. For instance, a doctor may want to dress professionally and wear a lab coat in order to demand respect and authority with his or her patients. If a person wants to be seen as friendly and sociable, he or she may decide to speak to strangers or pretend to like something that the other person likes in order to achieve this goal.

Front Stage and Back Stage Self

The concept of a frontstage self and a backstage self is a dramaturgical approach to describe how people interact with one another in society. This approach uses theater as a metaphor for explaining how people present themselves. The frontstage self is one in which the individual knows people will be watching and "performs" for these people. He or she follows rules for how to act in society and performs in a way that fulfills the expectations of the observer. The backstage self is when the individual is able to behave in a way that aligns with his or her true self and doesn't have to perform for others. This is when the individual is by him or herself and can regroup and prepare for the next "performance."

Verbal and Nonverbal Communication

People are able to communicate their emotions and feelings to others though various methods. Verbal communication, in addition to nonverbal communication, work to express thoughts and emotions in order for an individual to be better understood by his or her peers. Verbal communication consists of words and language that are spoken to others, or written down in order to convey a message. This type of communication can be in person, over the phone, through media outlets, or in a written note. Nonverbal communication can consist of facial expressions, body language, and other methods of conveying information without directly expressing it. For instance, someone may initiate eye contact with another person in order to send a message to that person. Crying, gesturing, or emoting in other ways also uses nonverbal communication to interact with others. Verbal and nonverbal communication can work together or even contradict one another, and they also both may be misinterpreted if the meaning is unclear.

Animal Signals and Communication

Animals can communicate with one another in similar ways as humans, in that they may use sounds to express themselves as well as body language and physical touch. However, animals may also communicate in additional methods that better convey their meaning. Some animals sing to one another during mating rituals, while others use auditory methods of displaying aggression and hostility. Physical touch and body language, such as cuddling or baring teeth, also work to convey messages to other animals. In addition to these methods, visual displays of information, such as size, shape, color, facial expression, and movement, also help to signal signs of danger, food sources, or different emotions. Animals also emit different chemical odors in various methods to communicate; pheromones and urine are two ways that this occurs. Animals not only interact with others within their own species, but also other animals in order to convey warnings or deception. For instance, some insects disguise themselves through different colors and symbols on their bodies in order to avoid being attacked by predators.

Attraction

Individuals behave differently in social situations due to various factors. One of these factors is attraction. Attraction is defined as feeling positively about a person based on different characteristics. Physical attraction occurs when someone views another as visually appealing, while sexual attraction refers to being aroused sexually by another. Attraction can also be the result of personality traits and behaviors, along with shared interests and other similarities. Being attracted to another person may establish relationships and continue into loving feelings when this attraction is strong. How much a person is attracted to another can be based on the physical traits, personality, and/or sexual attraction, but proximity and continued interaction also contribute to this. Being exposed to another is, in itself, often enough to develop attraction and the longer and more consistent this exposure, the more likely a relationship is able to form.

Aggression

Aggression is one way in which individuals may behave in certain social situations. The purpose of aggression is to harm another person either physically or emotionally, but it also may be an expression of anger or fear, as well as an intimidation technique to assert dominance. Different types of aggression may be exhibited within social interactions: indirect, direct, emotional, and instrumental. Indirect and direct aggression is a person's intent to harm someone; direct refers to the interaction being face-to-face, while indirect is not. Emotional aggression is a result of feelings of anger and the intent to hurt someone is not necessarily present. Instrumental aggression serves the purpose of achieving an objective that is not considered aggressive in nature. All these different types of aggression share the characteristic of wanting to hurt another individual, though the method or emotion behind the behavior may vary.

Attachment

Attachment refers to the idea that two (or more) people are connected emotionally and often is described in reference to parent-child interactions. In this type of attachment, the relationship is said to develop during the first 2 years of a child's life. This was studied by Harry Harlow through the parent-child relationships of monkeys. This psychologist found that the relationship between a mother and her infant is very important to the survival of the infant. However, he also found that this relationship was not based solely on necessities such as food and water, but instead based on the comfort and warmth from the mother. In John Bowlby's attachment theory, there are different forms of attachment for young children: secure, avoidant, ambivalent, and disorganized. Secure attachment is what should be strived for and is considered normal; in this bond, the child trusts the parent and prefers him or her to strangers. Avoidant attachment refers to a child who doesn't share a unique bond with the parent due to the uncaring nature of the mother or father, and the child is likely to treat the parent as he or she would another stranger. Ambivalent attachment occurs when a child has an inconsistent parent and doesn't trust the parent to return when he or she leaves. The child is often upset when this happens and cannot be comforted upon the parent's return. Lastly, disorganized attachment is when a child is abused by the parent and behaves unpredictably whether the parent is there or not.

Altruism

Altruism is the idea that a person will help another despite this assistance possibly impeding upon his or her life. Another term for this concept is selflessness, as it refers to the idea that the individual doesn't think about him or herself before helping someone else. This type of behavior is not something that the individual feels obligated to do; instead the motivation comes from the person's desire to help someone else. Evolutionarily, altruism is sometimes explained by the desire to indirectly help oneself through the continuation of his or her genes. For instance, it is more likely for a person to help someone who is biologically related to them, as opposed to someone who does not share their genes. It is also likely for a person to benefit indirectly from altruistic behavior through the idea that if a person helps someone else, that other person may return the favor in the future.

Social Support

Social support can be defined as the emotional or physical assistance and/or reinforcement of individuals within one's social network. This can include friends, family, coworkers, or anyone else who offers support. Often this support is in reaction to an individual experiencing a difficult situation or crisis when he or she needs the help and comfort of those around him or her. This social support is useful in times of need in order to reduce stress and frustration concerning the situation. Types of social support include emotional, instrumental, and informational. Emotional support is a way that the individual feels included or important to the people in his or her life, as well as within society as a whole. Emotional support may come in the form of listening or simply just spending time with the individual. Instrumental support is when a tangible form of assistance is provided, such as money, physical assistance, or food. Informational support is when someone in a person's social network offers advice or information pertinent to the situation at hand in order to problem solve.

Foraging Behavior

Certain behaviors in animals can be explained through biology, including foraging behavior. Foraging behavior is the act of looking for food in order to eat and survive. Different animals may do this in different ways, but the purpose is the same: to survive and reproduce. Some of these behaviors may include foraging alone or within a group, using sticks or other tools, or storing food for the future. The main goal of these foraging behaviors is to allow the animal to gather and eat the most amount of nutrients with the least amount of effort. Variables also influence an animal's ability to forage, including how they learn, genetics, the presence of predators, or parasites that may be lurking in food sources. Animals work to decrease the risks to foraging, such as avoiding parasites and predators, in order to increase their chance of survival.

Mating Behavior and Mate Choice in Animals

One way in which animals strive to keep their own species alive is by mating. They may do this by mating with a single animal or they may have multiple partners. In addition, animals may also differ in how they select their mates. This may vary based on species or even gender. Some species prefer to mate with any partner they are able, known as random mating, while others prefer those with similar characteristics, known as assortative mating. However, when assortative mating occurs, this may lead to increased instances of inbreeding, which may negatively influence later generations. There is also the concept of non-assortative mating, which is when animals with different characteristics mate with one another. Non-assortative and random mating lead to more diversity and don't have as many limitations or consequences as assortative mating. It has also been found that females are more particular about the mate that they choose and it is said that the females look for more superior characteristics such as genetics or survival when choosing a male to mate with. Males on the other hand may not be as simple: there is controversy surrounding how males choose mates, and it is said that they often are more particular when there is more diversity within potential mating pools.

Game Theory

Game theory is the idea that one can use mathematics to better understand how decisions are made. This theory explains that every decision has a ratio of the costs and benefits, and the decision with the best ratio is the one that is chosen. When this is applied to animal behavior, it allows for the ability to describe how animals are able to survive and reproduce. This is done by analyzing the offspring as a benefit, or signal of better fitness. When a species has an increase in offspring while other species have less in comparison, this is a sign of fitness. Game theory helps humans to better analyze and understand choices of optimal behavior and to see how changes occur.

Inclusive Fitness

Altruism is the idea that an individual will voluntarily help another individual, even if it comes at the expense of their own livelihood. This is often a characteristic of people who are selfless, but with humans, this may also lead to positive feelings that help drive this personality trait. With animals, on the other hand, altruism can be described evolutionarily; animals are likely to participate in altruism because they expect tangible and beneficial results from such behavior. For instance, a mother bear will protect her young in order to carry on her own genes, or may help another bear in the expectation of reciprocity. This phenomenon is known as inclusive fitness, also defined as altruistic behavior that indirectly benefits an animal by helping to increase its chances of survival in terms of itself or its kin. In other words, the selfless behavior is detrimental to the animal's own fitness, but benefits the fitness of the other. In this sense, the animals share this fitness in order to indirectly improve survival and reproduction.

Discrimination

Individual Versus Institutional Discrimination

Discrimination is the act of treating a group of people (or single person) differently due to characteristics such as ability, age, religion, race, gender, or sexual orientation. When a singular person participates in discriminatory behavior, this is known as individual discrimination. This can occur when the person behaves differently towards a person on the basis of one of these traits, and treats them in an undesirable manner. Discrimination can also happen at an institutional level, also known as institutional discrimination, and it occurs when a system put in place by the government or organization inherently treats people differently based on the qualities they possess that were previously mentioned. This leads to biased views and actions towards these groups by others, and how visible this discrimination is can range from blatant abuse to subtle differences in access to various opportunities. Examples of this might be a person of color being refused admission to a university or refusal of a marriage license due to sexual orientation.

Relationship Between Prejudice and Discrimination

Prejudice can be defined as having a negative or unwarranted attitude towards another person or group of people based on qualities these groups possess, such as race, religion, sexual orientation, social class, or age. This differs from discrimination, as discrimination is the act of behaving differently towards these people based on the group they belong to. Although these concepts differ (one is an attitude and the other is behavior) each can lead to the other in a cyclical relationship. If a person has prejudicial views towards individuals of a different group, he or she may behave in a way that reflects this attitude. On the other hand, if discrimination occurs through either governmental institutions or through chance by an individual, this may lead to negative views about a group of people. Discrimination can also occur through the behavior of others; if the individuals in one's social group discriminate towards people of a different group, this may lead that person to also act in this manner, possibly leading to his or her own prejudices being formed.

Power, Prestige, and Class

Being in a position of power gives a person control over the lives of others. Having this power can contribute to treating others differently and creating a larger gap between those in power and the rest of society. Individuals with power are able to use this power in order to make the world work in a way that favors people in majority groups, leaving marginalized populations to become increasingly less powerful and more separated from those in power. Having prestige, or a good reputation, is also a way that influences discrimination. People with more education or more achievements are given more opportunities, leaving those with less prestige to become more marginalized and have less ability to overcome this discrimination. Social and economic class also impact discrimination, as those with more money and higher social status are able to get what they want more easily than those with a lower status. This causes people in high classes to treat others in a more negative manner, discriminating against people simply because of their social status.

Social Structure and Demographics

Microsociology and Macrosociology

In sociology, there are two different main fields of study when it comes to understanding social structures: microsociology and macrosociology. Both of these concentrations are important to understanding social behavior and motivation, but they are quite different in terms of how this topic is studied. Microsociology is the study of the individual social interactions, while macrosociology is the study of the larger social systems and structures such as governments and organizations. While microsociology focuses on personal values, beliefs, and behaviors, macrosociology focuses on shared cultures, languages, and social roles. An example that illustrates this difference is the impact of socioeconomic status on behavior. At the individual level, microsociology would be focused on how a person is treated based on this status. If the person is of a lower socioeconomic status, microsociology would look at the patterns of behavior and beliefs of those who interact with this individual. Macrosociology would, instead, look to the institutional level and evaluate the differences in policies and cultural norms that influence socioeconomic status.

Functionalism

Within societies, there are structures in place that can be studied and explained. This is known as functionalism. Functionalism is a theory developed by Emile Durkheim in order to describe the structure of society and how it functions. This theory holds that society is complex but each part contributes to the whole by working together and creating unity; when one part of society fails, this leads to unwanted change and chaos. Functionalism works because there is harmony and understanding between the different parts of society, which creates a united social structure. However, this theory doesn't acknowledge the negative consequences that conformity can produce and ignores the individuals of the society in terms of activism and social justice.

Conflict Theory

Conflict theory is an idea put forth by Karl Marx that explains how conflict within a society arises through the competition of resources, both economically and socially. Because different groups of society maintain different levels of wealth or power, there is inherently conflict between these social groups. There is a lack of harmony between these groups of people and the control of society is maintained by those in power. This leads to the exploitation and discrimination of those with less power and of lower social or economic classes. Although there are discrepancies in benefit and a lack of mutual aid, this unequal distribution of power is also theorized to be the reason social order is possible. Because of the vast amounts of control these groups of power have, there is more ability to keep order and control unwanted behavior.

Symbolic Interactionism and Social Constructionism

Symbolic interactionism is the idea that groups of people interact using symbols to convey meaning. Different groups of people have different interpretations of these symbols, however, and people act on these symbols based on their interpretations. For instance, one culture may view a gesture positively, while another views it negatively. In America, holding up two fingers is a way to convey peace, while in England, this is an offensive gesture. Social constructionism is the idea that meaning comes from the constructs set forth in a society. These constructs can be perceived as reality, or even questioned by people within the society, which creates an ongoing and fluctuating reality that is both subjective and objective. An example of a social construct is money. Pieces of metal and paper may not literally have value, but people place value on these objects, creating a socially constructed method of currency. There are two main types of social constructionism: weak and strong. Weak social constructionism is when facts are the basis for reality, while strong social constructionism relies on language and behaviors.

Exchange Theory and Rational Choice Theory

Exchange theory and rational choice theory are part of a concept known as exchange-rational choice. Exchange theory is the idea that exchanges of goods and/or services create relationships and these relationships explain social change and stability. In this theory, both sides of the exchange benefit from this negotiation, driven by a process of costs and rewards to each party. Rational choice theory, or rational action theory, explains that the choices and exchanges a person makes work through a process of minimizing costs and maximizing rewards. The decision that the individual makes is based on this idea, allowing him or her to make the most rational choice.

Feminist Theory

Feminist theory is a concept that describes the roles and rights of women in society. This theory examines the inequality of the genders based on ideas such as gender roles and objectification, as well as systemic sexism within government organizations. Feminist theory has various forms that have developed throughout history and range from liberal feminism to radical and Marxist feminism. Each type examines a different facet of the gender divisions such as gender characteristics, inequalities, oppression, and structural persecution.

Education, Hidden Curriculum, Teacher Expectancy, and Educational Segregation and Stratification

Education is a social institution that revolves around learning and acquiring knowledge of a broad range of topics. In the United States, this institution is divided into different levels of education that an individual may move through during his or her lifespan. The system includes early childhood education such as preschool and kindergarten, primary school, secondary school, college or university, and graduate school. During these levels, the schools impose curriculums that are believed to help the child succeed later in life. However, there is a concept known as hidden curriculums which are topics that are not explicitly taught, and are instead implied or mistakenly communicated. For instance, the relationships between a teacher and his or her students may dictate how the students are expected to act. If the teacher reacts negatively to lots of questions, the students may think that asking questions is bad, leading to a continuation of this behavior later in life. This also relates to the idea of teacher expectancy; if a teacher expects a child to behave a certain way, this may inadvertently influence his or her behavior towards the child, resulting in the child behaving in a way that confirms the teacher's expectations. Lastly, educational segregation and stratification refers to the differences in quality of education in various regions and schools because of the financial aspects of that area. Namely, if a school is underprivileged, the students will not have a worthwhile education.

Family Structure and Forms of Kinship

A family is a social group that is connected through marriage and ancestral relationships. There are various forms of families, but the main structure of a family includes parents, grandparents, siblings, children, spouses, and extensions of these relationships. Primary kins are related directly, through connections such as spouses, children, and siblings. Secondary kins are separated by one family member. Examples of these are grandparents, aunts, and uncles. For instance, your mother's sister is separated from you by one family member: your mother. Tertiary kins are separated by two relatives. A common example of a tertiary kin is a cousin. This would be your mother's sister's children, for example, separating you and your cousin by both your mother and your aunt.

Family structures may differ in many ways. Adoption, divorce, family death, families with same-sex parents, or families with step-parents are all different forms of relationships that occur. Within these structures are concepts such as marriage and divorce that tie families together. Marriage is a legal concept that allows individuals to be connected through the law. This is often helpful in healthcare decisions, as married individuals are able to make these decisions or are named next-of-kin when one person in the marriage is ill or passes away. In the instance of divorce, these marriages are terminated and the individuals are able to separate these responsibilities and legal ties. A divorce may also allow the individuals to move forward and marry again, thereby creating step-parents to any children involved in the previous marriage.

Violence Within Families

An important concept when discussing families is violence within these relationships. Members of a family may report abuse from other members of the family, such as spouses, children, parents, or members of the extended family. This violence can come from any member of the family and target any other member, regardless of age or gender. This violence may not always be in the form of physical abuse, with some abuse being emotional or sexual. Common examples describe a male family member abusing younger children or a female spouse; however, female family members are also known to be abusive at times. In addition, elder abuse is also a form of family violence, with children extorting or physically abusing older parents and relatives.

Religiosity and Religious Organizations

Religion is a significant aspect of society and can influence these societies in many ways. How religious a person is can be referred to as his or her religiosity, which helps to explain how a person views the world, their sense of purpose, and the concept of a higher power. Different types of religious organizations include churches, sects, cults, and denominations. Churches are a structured, stable, and government-aligned organization that teach its members about specific religious beliefs. These beliefs can be from religions such as Judaism, Christianity, Islam, or Hinduism, but there are also many others. Denominations are independent branches of a religion, but still recognized by that church. Sects are organizations that have broken off from the church's teachings in order to promote a version of that religion that is more in line with traditional belief systems. Cults are also organizations that have broken from the church, but instead of upholding traditional teachings, cults are considered to teach innovative and new beliefs and are often led by an individual who is enigmatic and confident.

Relationship Between Religion and Social Change

Religion can play an important role in society, especially in reference to social change. Social change and religion influence one another and together have an impact on society as a whole. Modernization is an example of this as a vehicle of social change. Modernization refers to the concept that as society learns and creates new technology, that society becomes more modern. This transition and/or continuous process of change can also lead to a change in beliefs and in turn can impact religious views. In some cases, this can lead to religion having a reduced impact on people, known as secularization. This concept explains how religion becomes less important in societies, influencing how people learn to view the world and their own purpose in this world. Fundamentalism is also a way in which religion and social change are related. This concept refers to the process of religious teaching becoming more traditional or literal in terms of interpretations of religious texts. This fundamentalism may be in response to social change, but also may lead to social revolution in order to bring religion back to the forefront of society.

Power and Authority in Government and Economy

Power and authority are two of the ways in which a government is able to function in society. Governments make and enforce the rules of this society for the purpose of maintaining order, which gives the government a significant amount of power. This power is maintained by money and systemic measures put in place to govern the people of a society. With threats of punishment and conformity of the members of a society, this power is kept intact. In other words, in order for the government to maintain its status quo, the individuals of the society must accept the authority of this structure and follow the rules set forth. If the government lost its ability to follow through with threats when laws are broken, or if many people fight against this authority, the government has the potential to be overthrown and cease to function as intended.

Economic and Political Systems

While the government creates and enforces the rules of a society, the economy refers to how the people of a society are able to get the things they need, such as money and goods. Different systems can be utilized to impact both government and the economy simultaneously. In other words, certain methods of governing influence the economic systems that bolster society. The two main systems are known as capitalism and socialism. Capitalism is a concept that describes how privately owned companies produce and distribute resources in order to make a profit. This type of system is self-sufficient and relies solely on consumers in order to prosper. Socialism on the other hand is a system where these resources are produced and distributed through the government and are not owned by a sole company or individual. These goods are owned by the government and regulated as such in order to evenly distribute the resources to society. A system known as mixed-economy uses a combination of capitalism and socialism to regulate and distribute resources in order to support the economy.

Division of Labor

Division of labor refers to the idea that each individual in a society contributes to society in a different manner. For instance, one person is trained in farming, while another practices medicine. These two individuals are experts in their respective fields, but may not know anything about the other person's field of work. These two people work together and provide services for one another (the doctor treats the farmer's illnesses, while the farmer provides food to the doctor) and benefit from the other person's knowledge. This division of labor allows individuals to become experts in a single topic and be able to live a full life, without knowing everything from each different field of work. If the doctor was instead required to farm his own crops, build his own house, and make his own clothes, he wouldn't need the farmer, or anyone else, but he also may not be efficient or even skilled at any of these different trades. The division of labor allows for more efficiency and expertise within a society.

Medicalization and the Sick Role

Medicalization is the process of classifying human conditions as treatable illnesses. These conditions are seen as separate from the individual and can be studied in order to develop treatments for such conditions. For instance, if a person is sick, he will go to the doctor who will diagnose him with an infection. The doctor then prescribes the patient antibiotics in order to get rid of the infection. Within this process of medicalization is also something called the "sick role." Someone who is sick is thought to have the right to disengage from his or her normal social roles because he or she is not at fault for such an illness. The person is also expected to try to get better by seeing a doctor or taking medicine. However, medicalization is also common for psychological conditions that are more difficult to deal with. A person with depression may be prescribed antidepressants, but this may not address the underlying cause of the depression. By medicalizing mental illness, patients may not be given the proper counseling or care required to help them, and because they are classified as sick, a person with depression who does not get better on medication may be told that she is not fulfilling the obligations of the sick role by trying to get better. This person may in turn be blamed for her illness or stigmatized, which may lead to her not wanting to be classified as sick.

Illness Experience and Delivery of Health Care

When a person is sick, he or she has something called the "illness experience." The illness experience is the process of experiencing an illness and going through certain steps in order to get better. An example would be if Joe were experiencing stomach pain. First, he would have the pain symptom, and then he would label himself as sick, taking on the sick role. Once he labeled himself as sick, Joe would go to a doctor seeking treatment for his illness. While at the doctor, Joe would develop a relationship with the doctor, where the doctor would help relieve Joe of his stomach pain. This might include performing surgery, prescribing medication, or advising Joe to stay away from certain foods or activities. After this Joe would follow the doctor's instructions and begin to recover from his illness. Within this illness experience is the healthcare system. Delivery of health care involves a primary care doctor who helps the patient or refers him or her to a specialist in order to better treat the illness. Different types of medical staff help in this process, including doctors (who diagnose and treat the illness), nurses (who monitor the patient and administer treatments), and emergency responders (who care for the patient on the way to the hospital).

Social Epidemiology of Health and Medicine

Epidemiology refers to the study of illnesses by understanding how many people are affected, who develops the disease, and how to control the disease. Disparities and social factors also impact illnesses, which are studied through social epidemiology. This branch of medicine determines how society influences the health of a population and how to better control the disease based on this information. For instance, people with poor living conditions and lower socioeconomic status may be more prone to disease, or develop specific diseases because of where they fit into society.

Elements of Culture

Culture has influence on many aspects of life and society, but it is also somewhat difficult to define. Culture is a wide-reaching concept that encompasses many different elements in order to better explain collective groups of people. The elements involved in culture include language, customs, rituals, social patterns, organization, religion, artistic expression, government, economy, and values. These elements differ between cultures and influence how the individuals who identify with a certain culture behave, speak, think, and feel about a vast number of topics. In addition, these different elements fit into two separate categories: material and symbolic culture. Material culture refers to physical or concrete elements of society such as clothing, buildings, or technology. Symbolic culture is more elusive and refers to the elements of culture that are not visible or well-defined, such as language, values, and traditions.

Culture Lag and Culture Shock

Culture lag refers to the idea that different forms of culture change over time while other forms of culture are slower to adjust to these changes. The two main forms of culture in this theory are material and non-material, or symbolic, culture. This concept states that material culture, such as clothing, technology, and other physical types of culture, are the first to change over time, while non-material culture, such as religion, values, and traditions, are slow to follow suit. Culture shock is the idea that a person is surprised by the differences in different cultures when being exposed to a new culture. For instance, if a person comes from a small, quiet town where everyone knows each other, that person may experience culture shock when she moves to a big city, such as New York.

Assimilation and Multiculturalism

When a person moves to a new city or experiences a new culture, he may have to integrate and learn how to live in a manner consistent with this culture. This is known as assimilation. An example would be if a person moves to a new country and learns the language, engages in that country's traditions and rituals, and learns to how interact with the citizens of that country. If the person was unable to do these things, he may have trouble assimilating to the new culture. Some people and places, however, do not have just one culture, and instead have a melting pot of different traditions, languages, and beliefs. This is known as multiculturalism. New York is a great example of multiculturalism with the many different people living there who come from all over the world.

Subcultures and Countercultures

Within larger cultures often exist smaller cultures known as subcultures. These subcultures are distinct from the larger culture and add to the variety and complexity of a society. Some of these subcultures may develop through sociological changes and advancements, while others fade after a period of time. These subcultures include variation in style of clothing, music, traditions, and other beliefs and behaviors. Examples of subcultures can include emo or gothic cultures, or even religious traditions such as wearing a hijab in an American society. Some subcultures are vastly different from the predominant culture and may oppose this way of life; these are known as countercultures. Countercultures are forms of subcultures that don't fit into the mainstream society and don't share the values of this society. An example of a counterculture would be in the 1960s when American hippies were prevalent. This group of people opposed the government, listened to different music, and created their own communities apart from the American mainstream culture.

Mass Media and Popular Culture

Popular culture is the mainstream and predominant culture within a society. This can refer to the types of fashion, music, or activities associated with a culture that are common at a certain point in time. This culture is widely accepted, but also can be criticized by others who don't participate in the popular culture. In addition, popular culture is often greatly influenced by mass media. Mass media refers to the abundant and various forms of media that work together to inform the public. These forms of mass media include movies, television, newspapers, radio, websites, and more. By reporting on a specific cultural phenomenon, these forms of mass media broadcast the ideas of a culture to make it more popular and widespread.

Relationship Between Evolution and Human Culture

Evolution can influence culture, but it can also be a product of this culture. Culture is a way in which each generation can pass information and traditions to future generations. Society has also evolved over time and the cultures of such societies can depend on this evolution. For instance, when societies are smaller, they may be community oriented, with each member helping the others and contributing where they are needed most. This type of culture is dominant because it is necessary for survival in a society so small. However, with evolution of technology and society as a whole, this culture may need to change in order to work for the majority of the population. Developing currency and trade may be necessary in this case, and warfare may emerge through this evolution, altering the dominant culture. These are ways in which evolution influences culture, but culture may also impact evolution through new technologies and resources. With technological advances, a society may need to evolve to accommodate these changes. In addition, humans have evolved as a result of cultural changes by needing less body hair and less muscle mass than previous generations.

Transmission and Diffusion

Culture is important to different groups of people and, as such, people feel that it is necessary to distribute and communicate these cultures to others. This can happen in one of two ways: transmission and diffusion. Transmission is the process of passing cultural beliefs and traditions to future generations from parents to their children, who pass it to their own children. Culture can also be disseminated to people in other parts of the world. This is known as diffusion. When a society wishes to educate or enlighten others about their own culture, they may travel to other parts of the world or otherwise distribute these ideas and ways of living to others as they see fit. This diffusion may help to advance other societies in a positive way, but may also be detrimental and displace the cultures and well-being of other societies.

Aging and Age Cohorts

As people age, they experience different life events and new challenges, often directly associated with aging. These challenges that result from aging can include retirement, lack of independence, and a reliance on government assistance. This is significant because the aging community must put their faith in the younger generations to pay into social security or take care of them as they become more dependent on others. Imbedded in this ongoing relationship between the elderly and the younger generations is the concept of age cohorts. Cohorts are groups of people who experience similar life events and experiences at the same time due to their age. For instance, Millennials and Baby Boomers are two examples of popular age cohorts discussed in the media. Millennials include those who were born after the year 1980, while Baby Boomers were born following World War II. Baby Boomers are now between the ages of 50 and 70 years old and are a very large population due to the increased birth rate after the war. This means that Baby Boomers are going to be in need of substantial assistance from Millennials in future years, making the process of aging socially significant.

Gender

The concept of gender is derived from the idea that being a certain biological sex dictates how a person feels or behaves. Because individuals are characterized as either male or female at birth due to their anatomical features, gender is considered a binary construct as well. However, because biological sex is difficult to determine directly from appearance, there is a reliance on physical or behavioral attributes that are deemed either masculine or feminine and correspond respectively with male and female genders. For instance, long hair, makeup, and skirts are considered feminine characteristics, and therefore attributed to females. This binary description of males versus females also results in gender segregation, such as separate bathrooms or sports teams.

Race and Ethnicity

Each individual has a complex heritage and may have their ancestry traced all over the world. However, many people may not identify with these various cultures, and instead identify with a select few. These cultures that a person identifies with are known as his or her ethnicity. Some of these ethnicities are associated with different physical characteristics, leading others to classify people based on these appearances. This physical appearance is known as a person's race. Race is a socially constructed concept that allows individuals to be grouped together based on this appearance and may or may not align with one's ethnicity.

Racialization and Racial Formation

Racialization is the process of assigning a person a racial identity. This racial identity may or may not be consistent with a person's own ethnicity or identity, and is often stereotyped or generalized. Racialization may also lead to discrimination or even preferential treatment in certain situations. In job settings and education, certain races are given privileges while others are forced to exert extra effort in order to be given the same opportunities. Racial formation is the idea that race is not a concrete or stable concept and can change as societies and individuals evolve. This means that race is a social construct that helps society justify discriminatory behavior and how people of different races interact with one another.

Immigration

Immigration is the process of a person moving to a new country and can be a result of various situational factors. A person may immigrate to a country for personal reasons such as family or relationships, for education, or for economic reasons, such as better jobs or better working conditions. Immigration refers to people who are coming to a specific country to which they are not native and it may involve learning how to adapt to a new culture and society. In this process it is also possible that individuals will, over time, lose their connections to their native culture and identity by assimilating to the new country. In the United States, immigration has increased in recent years, with many people coming from Mexico, the Caribbean, or India.

Intersections of Race and Ethnicity

Due to the differing definitions of race and ethnicity, these two concepts can overlap or be separate entities. Race is often separated into 6 categories: white, black, Asian, Hispanic/Latino, Native American, or Pacific Islander. However, a person can fit into more than one of these categories based on their family's racial identities. In addition, ethnicity refers to both country of origin and family heritage, which means that this can either be separate from or combined with one's racial identity. For instance, a person who is white could have different ethnicities such as American, English, or German, while a person who is black may have grown up in England, and identify with that particular ethnicity.

Sexual Orientation

One demographic variable that is often difficult to ascertain is sexual orientation. Many research questions either do not address this topic or are unable to fully capture the complexity of one's sexual orientation. However, three categories of sexual orientation are most commonly referred to:

heterosexual, homosexual, or bisexual. Heterosexual refers to someone being attracted to individuals of the opposite sex, homosexual refers to one who is attracted to same-sex individuals, and bisexual refers to someone who is attracted to people of either sex.

Theories of Demographic Change

The two main theories regarding demographic change are Malthusian theory and demographic transition. Malthusian theory is the idea that the population of a society will grow exponentially over time and, eventually, the world will not be able to sustain the number of people with the available resources. This theory explains that there are different types of checks that help to alleviate this excessive population growth: positive checks and preventative checks. Positive checks are phenomena such as war, famine, or disease that bring the population down through death. Preventative checks are measures that are put in place to prevent overpopulation such as taxation and contraceptives. Demographic transition, on the other hand, explains that birth rates and death rates fluctuate based on societal transitions and development. This theory outlines four stages of transition: pre-industrial age (where birth rates and death rates are both high), urbanization or industrialization (where technology improvements help to decrease the death rate), the mature industrial age (where birth rates decrease due to increased access to contraception), and post-industrial age (when population is high, but the birth and death rates are both low).

Population Growth and Decline

Population growth refers to the idea that the birth rate of a population is higher than that of its death rate, while population decline refers to when the death rate is higher than the birth rate. These rates are likely to fluctuate over time, but there are also ways in which researchers are able to estimate and visualize these rates. Population projections help to estimate the future population based on current data, while population pyramids allow individuals to see the differences in certain populations. When these pyramids are larger at the bottom, this shows population growth, but when it is larger at the top of the pyramid, this displays population decline. In addition, these pyramids are able to show differences in gender by representing gender on the sides of the pyramid. If there is a skew to either side of the pyramid, this represents a discrepancy in gender within a population.

Fertility and Mortality Rates

Fertility refers to the ability to have children and there are gender differences with this fertility. Men, for instance are able to reproduce throughout the lifespan, while women are only fertile from puberty to menopause. Fertility rates are calculated as the number of children for each parental unit. Mortality rates, on the other hand, refer to how frequent death is in a certain population. For instance, females tend to have lower mortality rates than males, while babies who were just born have a higher mortality rate, but this rate decreases as time passes. Certain patterns also exist within fertility and mortality rates for different countries. For instance, countries that are more developed have lower fertility and mortality rates, while the opposite is true of underdeveloped countries.

Push and Pull Factors in Migration

The term migration refers to the relocation of a person or group of people to a new city or country. The reasons people choose to migrate are often known as push and pull factors. Push factors are the reasons a person leaves a place of residence, such as bad living conditions or poor work opportunities. Pull factors are the reasons that a person wants to go to a specific place, such as a better job, relationships, or other positive factors. Migration also is analyzed through positive and negative values of net migration, referring to the rates of people leaving or coming into an area. When these values are positive, this means more people are coming in than are leaving, while the opposite is true of negative values of net migration. Migration may be temporary or permanent depending on the reasons for migrating to a new place, and these reasons can differ based on money, personal relationships, or environmental factors.

Social Movements

Social movements are started when a group of people joins together to support a specific cause that relates to their political or social values. These movements can be very small or extremely large and may vary in terms of formality. Many movements are based on the idea of relative deprivation, which refers to the concept that individuals compare their own situations to those in our immediate vicinity, as opposed to people across the world. This means that, in fighting for certain rights, individuals are less concerned with someone's rights in another country, and more concerned with how they compare to the person down the street from them. Some movements are proactive and seek to promote specific change, such as the civil rights movements and animal rights movements. Reactive movements, on the other hand, are social movements that are fighting back against changes; anti-war movements, for instance, are reactive. Different organizations, such as civil rights organizations or animal rights organizations, also help to enable these movements and provide opportunities for activism. Advertising, creating new organizations, or participating in protests are examples of various movement strategies and tactics that help bring recognition and support to social movements.

Globalization

Globalization is the process of interacting with and incorporating different countries through trade, technology, information, and migration. Advancements in technology allow globalization to occur more easily and help to facilitate the economic interdependence of different countries as well as the ability to communicate rapidly with individuals around the world. Globalization has been touted as a positive asset to many countries, with advancements in underdeveloped countries as well as a growing worldwide economy; however, there are also criticisms of globalization. These criticisms include arguments that globalization leads to colonialism and the disenfranchisement of indigenous peoples. Globalization is also believed to create larger gaps in inequality and force the cultural assimilation of populations that may not benefit from these changes. These inequalities and cultural disadvantages have triggered social changes as well as civil unrest and terrorism, which threaten political and economic stability.

Urbanization, Industrialization, and Urban Growth

When large numbers of people move into densely populated cities from rural areas, it is known as urbanization. This process can be driven by multiple factors, including social and economic changes, such as jobs, housing, or transportation. Many of these changes are a result of modernization or industrialization, meaning more jobs in large cities creates a demand for a localized workforce. This process then results in urban growth and increases in migration to urban areas, but these changes also influence industrialization as well. For instance, as urbanization occurs, the cost of living also increases, resulting in changes in economy and living situations.

Suburbanization and Urban Decline

Although job availability and social changes lead to urbanization, this process also leads to an increased cost of living and a higher demand for more affordable housing options. Due to these reasons, and the availability of better technology and transportation, suburbanization is likely to occur in response to urbanization. Suburbanization is the process of more people moving outside of the city to suburban areas in order to avoid crime and other undesirable city living conditions. Suburbanization also may lead to urban decline due to the abandonment of certain urban areas.

These areas then experience high unemployment rates, poverty and a decline in the physical environment of the city.

Gentrification and Urban Renewal

When city areas experience urban decline, those areas are less populated and often are inhabited by people in poverty. This can sometimes result in selling large amounts of property in the area to wealthy individuals. This process is known as gentrification. Gentrification often leads to wealthy individuals raising rent prices or property values, which displaces those poorer individuals who are unable to afford better housing. Many times, gentrification also leads to urban renewal. Urban renewal, otherwise known as urban regeneration or revitalization, is the process of redeveloping those previously poor areas of cities and cleaning them up in order to make the areas more appealing or attractive.

Social Inequality

Residential Segregation

Residential segregation is the idea that different groups of people are separated into different residential neighborhoods in an area. These different groups can be based on wealth, race, or other demographics. Often, this occurs through the availability of housing and the segregation is maintained because of the inability or undesirability of relocation. This can create less desirable outcomes for marginalized groups of people, such as poor living conditions, high crime rates, or lower performing school systems. In the United States, the most segregated groups are minorities, with black Americans at the top of this list and Hispanic Americans second. These segregations are found most often in the larger urban areas, such as Los Angeles and New York. In addition, income is also known to be a factor in residential segregation, and most of these low-income individuals are also minorities.

Environmental Justice in Terms of Location and Exposure to Health Risks

Due to residential segregation, there are many discrepancies in the availability of resources in different neighborhoods. In less wealthy communities, segregation is sustained because rent is cheaper due to undesirable living conditions. For instance, there is often more pollution, higher crime, and/or less health care available in poor neighborhoods in comparison to wealthy neighborhoods. Because individuals in these areas are less financially able to relocate to a safer area, they are exposed to more health risks and are less able to get the care they need to manage these risks. Due to the increased health risks, there are social movements committed to demanding equitable distribution of health care and fewer environmental risks to people residing in poor neighborhoods.

Social Class and Socioeconomic Status

A person's finances and economic status have a great deal of importance in society. Living situation, wealth, and job status are just a few factors that are influential in society and that combine to explain a person's social class and socioeconomic status. Social class refers to where someone came from; someone who grew up in poverty would have low social class. Socioeconomic status refers to a person's current situation; a person who won the lottery would have high socioeconomic status while a person who went bankrupt would have a lower status. A person's social class will be constant, but may contribute to socioeconomic status. On the other hand, someone's status may constantly fluctuate and can change quickly. Being aware of your own social class and the current issues at hand in this class is known as class consciousness. However, if you are only aware of your own situation and believe that you are representative of an entire class, this is known as false consciousness.

Cultural Capital and Social Capital

Although financial and economic means are significant factors in achieving a higher socioeconomic status, there are also social and cultural factors that influence this as well. Cultural capital refers to the idea that cultural factors, such as education, physical appearance, or language, influence how easily a person is able to get a job or move up in society. Social capital is similar, but instead of cultural factors, it explains how social factors contribute to socioeconomic status. Social factors may include family and friends, networking abilities, location, or other relationships and connections.

Social Reproduction

Social reproduction is a concept that describes how people inherit their parents' social class, including social inequalities or privileges. For instance, a child born into a poor family will likely also experience the negative effects of being poor and may also grow up and continue to live in poverty. This works through factors such as living situation, race, ethnicity, finances, and health risks. The same child that was born into a poor family may have grown up in a poor neighborhood with no access to a quality education and have no friends with high social class. The lack of opportunities and connections will likely make it difficult for this child throughout life and he or she may never be able to overcome those difficulties without significant help.

Power, Privilege, and Prestige

Power, privilege and prestige are factors that influence a person's abilities to accomplish greater goals and having one or more of these things makes it easier to achieve a higher socioeconomic status. Power is the idea that a person has influence or control over another person and can manipulate them in a way that benefits him or herself. Privilege refers to the benefits and advantages that a person gains based on who they are or which group they are associated with. Prestige is also known as a person's reputation. This prestige influences how other people feel about a particular individual and is associated with more respect and admiration based on how an individual is perceived.

Intersectionality

is a concept that describes the various social categories that a person fits into. Having more than one marginalized identity, such as being black, being gay, or being female, is studied through intersectionality and this idea helps explain the complexity of a person's experience based on these various identities. For instance, a black person and a gay person may experience very different things throughout their lifetime in terms of discrimination and prejudice, but a person who is both black and gay may experience these things more intensely or in a different way.

Socioeconomic Gradient in Health

Although people from all different backgrounds, social classes, races, or genders are in need of health care, there are inequities that exist within the healthcare system. One of the main inconsistencies is in regard to socioeconomic status. There are many more people who are in need of health care or who don't have access to quality health care who are lower in socioeconomic status than those who are financially secure. This concept is known as the socioeconomic gradient because there is a spectrum of social classes and the health disparities among these classes are significant. Not only does this occur among the various social classes of the United States, but countries with a lower socioeconomic status also have poorer health care than more wealthy countries.

Global Inequalities

Inequalities in health care, education, and other social and cultural factors impact not just individuals or groups of people but also entire countries. Developed countries have better access to resources and are able to create more opportunities for the citizens of those countries than underdeveloped nations. Because of the power and resources available to the more developed countries in the world, these countries are able to take shortcuts and treat less developed countries unfairly, especially when it comes to trade agreements and practices. These unfair practices then create large disparities in the economies of these various countries and lead to poorer living conditions for the citizens of underdeveloped countries.

Social Mobility

Social mobility refers to the idea that a person can move up or down in terms of socioeconomic status. This can happen in a variety of ways, including generationally, individually, and through achievement. Intergenerational mobility is when the socioeconomic status of a child is different than his or her parents; the child either was able to move farther up the social ladder than his or her parents, or he or she fell below them for some reason. An individual may also move between socioeconomic classes throughout his or her lifetime; this is known as intragenerational mobility. These changes can also be ether vertical or horizontal. Vertical mobility is when a person moves up or down in terms of socioeconomic status, while horizontal mobility is when a person moves within the same socioeconomic status; getting a new job in the same social class would be an example of horizontal mobility. Lastly, a person experiences social mobility because of meritocracy. Meritocracy refers to the idea that a person's mobility or success is based on his or her achievements and talents, as opposed to privilege or prejudice.

Poverty

Poverty is a term that means a person is very poor and financially inferior. However, there are different ways in which poverty can be explained. Relative poverty, for instance, refers to a person who is poor when compared to others in his or her society. This type of poverty means that the person is unable to afford a lifestyle consistent with those around them. This is, however, different than absolute poverty, which refers to a person who is unable to afford to meet his or her basic needs, such as food and shelter, due to an insufficient income. In addition to these poverty definitions regarding how much money a person makes, social exclusion is also a contributing factor to a person being unable to afford a basic lifestyle. This concept of social exclusion refers to when a person's access to opportunities, resources, or basic rights is obstructed, despite other groups being able to access the same resources without difficulties.

Disparities in Health in Relation to Class, Gender, and Race

Although people from all different backgrounds may suffer from the same health issues, certain health problems are more common in certain populations. For instance, people in lower social classes are more likely to experience negative health concerns than people in higher classes. Certain minorities, especially those living in less populated areas, are also more prone to HIV/AIDS, heart disease, diabetes, or other diseases than white individuals. White people, on the other hand, are more likely to develop skin cancer or cystic fibrosis. Women are more likely than men to develop chronic, but non–life-threatening diseases, while men are more likely to develop serious, life-threatening illnesses or die at a younger age.

Disparities in Health Care in Relation to Class, Gender, and Race

Healthcare access, although becoming more accessible to marginalized populations, is still insufficient and unequal among these communities. People living in poverty and in poor neighborhoods are likely to be more exposed to health risks, and yet unable to afford quality health care. These populations are also less likely to have insurance, so they may be overwhelmed by enormous medical bills when they are inevitably admitted to a hospital. This is similar to some people of minority races, such as blacks and Hispanics, who are also unable to access quality health care. In addition, many minority individuals may fear discrimination and refuse to seek help, and the same is true for people who are not heterosexual. Women and men also differ in terms of health care; women are shown to be more likely to see a doctor when experiencing a health concern than men. However, women are also more likely to be responsible for a child, and when they are forced to choose between their own health care and their children's, this negatively impacts their well-being, either financially, mentally, or physically.

Critical Analysis and Reasoning Skills

The Verbal Reasoning Test consists of reading selections each followed by a series of questions. There will be several passages on the Verbal Reasoning section of the MCAT, and you can spend a little over eight minutes per passage and still finish within the time limit.

Reading Comprehension

Important Skills

One of the most important skills in reading comprehension is the identification of **topics** and **main ideas.** There is a subtle difference between these two features. The topic is the subject of a text, or what the text is about. The main idea, on the other hand, is the most important point being made by the author. The topic is usually expressed in a few words at the most, while the main idea often needs a full sentence to be completely defined. As an example, a short passage might have the topic of penguins and the main idea *Penguins are different from other birds in many ways.* In most nonfiction writing, the topic and the main idea will be stated directly, often in a sentence at the very beginning or end of the text. When being tested on an understanding of the author's topic, the reader can quickly *skim* the passage for the general idea, stopping to read only the first sentence of each paragraph. A paragraph's first sentence is often (but not always) the main topic sentence, and it gives you a summary of the content of the paragraph. However, there are cases in which the reader must figure out an unstated topic or main idea. In these instances, the student must read every sentence of the text, and try to come up with an overarching idea that is supported by each of those sentences.

Review Video: Topics and Main Ideas
Visit mometrix.com/academy and enter code: 407801

While the main idea is the overall premise of a story, **supporting details** provide evidence and backing for the main point. In order to show that a main idea is correct, or valid, the author needs to add details that prove their point. All texts contain details, but they are only classified as supporting details when they serve to reinforce some larger point. Supporting details are most commonly found in informative and persuasive texts. In some cases, they will be clearly indicated with words like *for example* or *for instance*, or they will be enumerated with words like *first, second*, and *last.* However, they may not be indicated with special words. As a reader, it is important to consider whether the author's supporting details really back up his or her main point. Supporting details can be factual and correct but still not relevant to the author's point. Conversely, supporting details can seem pertinent but be ineffective because they are based on opinion or assertions that cannot be proven.

An example of a main idea is: "Giraffes live in the Serengeti of Africa." A supporting detail about giraffes could be: "A giraffe uses its long neck to reach twigs and leaves on trees." The main idea gives the general idea that the text is about giraffes. The supporting detail gives a specific fact about how the giraffes eat.

Review Video: Supporting Details
Visit mometrix.com/academy and enter code: 396297

As opposed to a main idea, themes are seldom expressed directly in a text, so they can be difficult to identify. A **theme** is an issue, an idea, or a question raised by the text. For instance, a theme of William Shakespeare's *Hamlet* is indecision, as the title character explores his own psyche and the results of his failure to make bold choices. A great work of literature may have many themes, and the reader is justified in identifying any for which he or she can find support. One common characteristic of themes is that they raise more questions than they answer. In a good piece of fiction, the author is not always trying to convince the reader, but is instead trying to elevate the reader's perspective and encourage him to consider the themes more deeply. When reading, one can identify themes by constantly asking what general issues the text is addressing. A good way to evaluate an author's approach to a theme is to begin reading with a question in mind (for example, how does this text approach the theme of love?) and then look for evidence in the text that addresses that question.

Review Video: Theme
Visit mometrix.com/academy and enter code: 732074

Purposes for Writing

In order to be an effective reader, one must pay attention to the author's **position** and purpose. Even those texts that seem objective and impartial, like textbooks, have some sort of position and bias. Readers need to take these positions into account when considering the author's message. When an author uses emotional language or clearly favors one side of an argument, his position is clear. However, the author's position may be evident not only in what he writes, but in what he doesn't write. For this reason, it is sometimes necessary to review some other texts on the same topic in order to develop a view of the author's position. If this is not possible, then it may be useful to acquire a little background personal information about the author. When the only source of information is the text, however, the reader should look for language and argumentation that seems to indicate a particular stance on the subject.

Review Video: Author's Position
Visit mometrix.com/academy and enter code: 827954

Identifying the **purpose** of an author is usually easier than identifying her position. In most cases, the author has no interest in hiding his or her purpose. A text that is meant to entertain, for instance, should be obviously written to please the reader. Most narratives, or stories, are written to entertain, though they may also inform or persuade. Informative texts are easy to identify as well. The most difficult purpose of a text to identify is persuasion, because the author has an interest in making this purpose hard to detect. When a person knows that the author is trying to convince him, he is automatically more wary and skeptical of the argument. For this reason, persuasive texts often try to establish an entertaining tone, hoping to amuse the reader into agreement, or an informative tone, hoping to create an appearance of authority and objectivity.

Review Video: Purpose
Visit mometrix.com/academy and enter code: 511819

An author's purpose is often evident in the organization of the text. For instance, if the text has headings and subheadings, if key terms are in bold, and if the author makes his main idea clear from the beginning, then the likely purpose of the text is to inform. If the author begins by making a claim and then makes various arguments to support that claim, the purpose is probably to persuade. If the author is telling a story, or is more interested in holding the attention of the reader than in making a particular point or delivering information, then his purpose is most likely to entertain. As a reader, it is best to judge an author on how well he accomplishes his purpose. In other words, it is not entirely fair to complain that a textbook is boring: if the text is clear and easy to understand, then the author has done his job. Similarly, a storyteller should not be judged too harshly for getting some facts wrong, so long as he is able to give pleasure to the reader.

The author's purpose for writing will affect his writing style and the response of the reader. In a **persuasive essay**, the author is attempting to change the reader's mind or convince him of something he did not believe previously. There are several identifying characteristics of persuasive writing. One is opinion presented as fact. When an author attempts to persuade the reader, he often presents his or her opinions as if they were fact. A reader must be on guard for statements that sound factual but which cannot be subjected to research, observation, or experiment. Another characteristic of persuasive writing is emotional language. An author will often try to play on the reader's emotion by appealing to his sympathy or sense of morality. When an author uses colorful or evocative language with the intent of arousing the reader's passions, it is likely that he is attempting to persuade. Finally, in many cases a persuasive text will give an unfair explanation of opposing positions, if these positions are mentioned at all.

An **informative text** is written to educate and enlighten the reader. Informative texts are almost always nonfiction, and are rarely structured as a story. The intention of an informative text is to deliver information in the most comprehensible way possible, so the structure of the text is likely to be very clear. In an informative text, the thesis statement is often in the first sentence. The author may use some colorful language, but is likely to put more emphasis on clarity and precision. Informative essays do not typically appeal to the emotions. They often contain facts and figures, and rarely include the opinion of the author. Sometimes a persuasive essay can resemble an informative essay, especially if the author maintains an even tone and presents his or her views as if they were established fact.

Review Video: Informative Text
Visit mometrix.com/academy and enter code: 924964

The success or failure of an author's intent to **entertain** is determined by those who read the author's work. Entertaining texts may be either fiction or nonfiction, and they may describe real or imagined people, places, and events. Entertaining texts are often narratives, or stories. A text that is written to entertain is likely to contain colorful language that engages the imagination and the emotions. Such writing often features a great deal of figurative language, which typically enlivens its subject matter with images and analogies. Though an entertaining text is not usually written to persuade or inform, it may accomplish both of these tasks. An entertaining text may appeal to the reader's emotions and cause him or her to think differently about a particular subject. In any case, entertaining texts tend to showcase the personality of the author more so than do other types of writing.

When an author intends to **express feelings,** she may use colorful and evocative language. An author may write emotionally for any number of reasons. Sometimes, the author will do so because she is describing a personal situation of great pain or happiness. Sometimes an author is attempting to persuade the reader, and so will use emotion to stir up the passions. It can be easy to identify this kind of expression when the writer uses phrases like *I felt* and *I sense*. However, sometimes the author will simply describe feelings without introducing them. As a reader, it is important to recognize when an author is expressing emotion, and not to become overwhelmed by sympathy or passion. A reader should maintain some detachment so that he or she can still evaluate the strength of the author's argument or the quality of the writing.

Review Video: Express Feelings
Visit mometrix.com/academy and enter code: 759390

In a sense, almost all writing is descriptive, insofar as it seeks to describe events, ideas, or people to the reader. Some texts, however, are primarily concerned with **description**. A descriptive text focuses on a particular subject, and attempts to depict it in a way that will be clear to the reader. Descriptive texts contain many adjectives and adverbs, words that give shades of meaning and create a more detailed mental picture for the reader. A descriptive text fails when it is unclear or vague to the reader. On the other hand, however, a descriptive text that compiles too much detail can be boring and overwhelming to the reader. A descriptive text will certainly be informative, and it may be persuasive and entertaining as well. Descriptive writing is a challenge for the author, but when it is done well, it can be fun to read.

Writing Devices

Authors will use different stylistic and writing devices to make their meaning more clearly understood. One of those devices is comparison and contrast. When an author describes the ways in which two things are alike, he or she is **comparing** them. When the author describes the ways in which two things are different, he or she is **contrasting** them. The "compare and contrast" essay is one of the most common forms in nonfiction. It is often signaled with certain words: a comparison may be indicated with such words as *both, same, like, too,* and *as well*; while a contrast may be indicated by words like *but, however, on the other hand, instead,* and *yet*. Of course, comparisons and contrasts may be implicit without using any such signaling language. A single sentence may both compare and contrast. Consider the sentence *Brian and Sheila love ice cream, but Brian prefers vanilla and Sheila prefers strawberry*. In one sentence, the author has described both a similarity (love of ice cream) and a difference (favorite flavor).

One of the most common text structures is **cause and effect**. A cause is an act or event that makes something happen, and an effect is the thing that happens as a result of that cause. A cause-and-effect relationship is not always explicit, but there are some words in English that signal causality, such as *since, because,* and *as a result*. As an example, consider the sentence *Because the sky was clear, Ron did not bring an umbrella*. The cause is the clear sky, and the effect is that Ron did not bring an umbrella. However, sometimes the cause-and-effect relationship will not be clearly noted. For instance, the sentence *He was late and missed the meeting* does not contain any signaling words, but it still contains a cause (he was late) and an effect (he missed the meeting). It is possible for a single cause to have multiple effects, or for a single effect to have multiple causes. Also, an effect can in turn be the cause of another effect, in what is known as a cause-and-effect chain.

Review Video: Rhetorical Strategy of Cause-and-Effect Analysis
Visit mometrix.com/academy and enter code: 725944

Authors often use analogies to add meaning to the text. An **analogy** is a comparison of two things. The words in the analogy are connected by a certain, often undetermined relationship. Look at this analogy: moo is to cow as quack is to duck. This analogy compares the sound that a cow makes with the sound that a duck makes. Even if the word 'quack' was not given, one could figure out it is the correct word to complete the analogy based on the relationship between the words 'moo' and 'cow'. Some common relationships for analogies include synonyms, antonyms, part to whole, definition, and actor to action.

Another element that impacts a text is the author's point of view. The **point of view** of a text is the perspective from which it is told. The author will always have a point of view about a story before he draws up a plot line. The author will know what events they want to take place, how they want the characters to interact, and how the story will resolve. An author will also have an opinion on the topic, or series of events, which is presented in the story, based on their own prior experience and beliefs.

The two main points of view that authors use are first person and third person. If the narrator of the story is also the main character, or *protagonist*, the text is written in first-person point of view. In first person, the author writes with the word *I.* Third-person point of view is probably the most common point of view that authors use. Using third person, authors refer to each character using the words *he* or *she.* In third-person omniscient, the narrator is not a character in the story and tells the story of all of the characters at the same time.

Review Video: Point of View
Visit mometrix.com/academy and enter code: 383336

A good writer will use **transitional words** and phrases to guide the reader through the text. You are no doubt familiar with the common transitions, though you may never have considered how they operate. Some transitional phrases (*after, before, during, in the middle of*) give information about time. Some indicate that an example is about to be given (*for example, in fact, for instance*). Writers use them to compare (*also, likewise*) and contrast (*however, but, yet*). Transitional words and phrases can suggest addition (*and, also, furthermore, moreover*) and logical relationships (*if, then, therefore, as a result, since*). Finally, transitional words and phrases can demarcate the steps in a process (*first, second, last*). You should incorporate transitional words and phrases where they will orient your reader and illuminate the structure of your composition.

Review Video: Transitional Words and Phrases
Visit mometrix.com/academy and enter code: 197796

Types of Passages

A **narrative** passage is a story. Narratives can be fiction or nonfiction. However, there are a few elements that a text must have in order to be classified as a narrative. To begin with, the text must have a plot. That is, it must describe a series of events. If it is a good narrative, these events will be interesting and emotionally engaging to the reader. A narrative also has characters. These could be people, animals, or even inanimate objects, so long as they participate in the plot. A narrative passage often contains figurative language, which is meant to stimulate the imagination of the reader by making comparisons and observations. A metaphor, which is a description of one thing in terms of another, is a common piece of figurative language. *The moon was a frosty snowball* is an example of a metaphor: it is obviously untrue in the literal sense, but it suggests a certain mood for the reader. Narratives often proceed in a clear sequence, but they do not need to do so.

An **expository** passage aims to inform and enlighten the reader. It is nonfiction and usually centers around a simple, easily defined topic. Since the goal of exposition is to teach, such a passage should be as clear as possible. It is common for an expository passage to contain helpful organizing words, like *first, next, for example,* and *therefore.* These words keep the reader oriented in the text. Although expository passages do not need to feature colorful language and artful writing, they are often more effective when they do. For a reader, the challenge of expository passages is to maintain steady attention. Expository passages are not always about subjects in which a reader will naturally be interested, and the writer is often more concerned with clarity and comprehensibility than with engaging the reader. For this reason, many expository passages are dull. Making notes is a good way to maintain focus when reading an expository passage.

Review Video: Narratives
Visit mometrix.com/academy and enter code: 280100

A **technical** passage is written to describe a complex object or process. Technical writing is common in medical and technological fields, in which complicated mathematical, scientific, and engineering ideas need to be explained simply and clearly. To ease comprehension, a technical passage usually proceeds in a very logical order. Technical passages often have clear headings and subheadings, which are used to keep the reader oriented in the text. It is also common for these passages to break sections up with numbers or letters. Many technical passages look more like an outline than a piece of prose. The amount of jargon or difficult vocabulary will vary in a technical passage depending on the intended audience. As much as possible, technical passages try to avoid language that the reader will have to research in order to understand the message. Of course, it is not always possible to avoid jargon.

Review Video: A Technical Passage
Visit mometrix.com/academy and enter code: 478923

A **persuasive** passage is meant to change the reader's mind or lead her into agreement with the author. The persuasive intent may be obvious, or it may be quite difficult to discern. In some cases, a persuasive passage will be indistinguishable from an informative passage: it will make an assertion and offer supporting details. However, a persuasive passage is more likely to make claims based on opinion and to appeal to the reader's emotions. Persuasive passages may not describe alternate positions and, when they do, they often display significant bias. It may be clear that a persuasive passage is giving the author's viewpoint, or the passage may adopt a seemingly objective tone. A persuasive passage is successful if it can make a convincing argument and win the trust of the reader.

Review Video: Persuasive Text and Bias
Visit mometrix.com/academy and enter code: 479856

A persuasive essay will likely focus on one central argument, but it may make many smaller claims along the way. These are subordinate arguments with which the reader must agree if he or she is going to agree with the central argument. The central argument will only be as strong as the subordinate claims. These claims should be rooted in fact and observation, rather than subjective judgment. The best persuasive essays provide enough supporting detail to justify claims without overwhelming the reader.

Remember that a fact must be susceptible to independent verification: that is, it must be something the reader could confirm. Also, statistics are only effective when they take into account possible objections. For instance, a statistic on the number of foreclosed houses would only be useful if it was taken over a defined interval and in a defined area. Most readers are wary of statistics, because they are so often misleading. If possible, a persuasive essay should always include references so that the reader can obtain more information. Of course, this means that the writer's accuracy and fairness may be judged by the inquiring reader.

Review Video: Persuasive Essay
Visit mometrix.com/academy and enter code: 621428

Opinions are formed by emotion as well as reason, and persuasive writers often appeal to the feelings of the reader. Although readers should always be skeptical of this technique, it is often used in a proper and ethical manner. For instance, there are many subjects that have an obvious emotional component, and therefore cannot be completely treated without an appeal to the emotions. Consider an article on drunk driving: it makes sense to include some specific examples that will alarm or sadden the reader. After all, drunk driving often has serious and tragic consequences. Emotional appeals are not appropriate, however, when they attempt to mislead the reader. For instance, in political advertisements it is common to emphasize the patriotism of the preferred candidate, because this will encourage the audience to link their own positive feelings about the country with their opinion of the candidate. However, these ads often imply that the other candidate is unpatriotic, which in most cases is far from the truth. Another common and improper emotional appeal is the use of loaded language, as for instance referring to an avidly religious person as a "fanatic" or a passionate environmentalist as a "tree hugger." These terms introduce an emotional component that detracts from the argument.

History and Culture

Historical context has a profound influence on literature: the events, knowledge base, and assumptions of an author's time color every aspect of his or her work. Sometimes, authors hold opinions and use language that would be considered inappropriate or immoral in a modern setting, but that was acceptable in the author's time. As a reader, one should consider how the historical context influenced a work and also how today's opinions and ideas shape the way modern readers read the works of the past. For instance, in most societies of the past, women were treated as second-class citizens. An author who wrote in 18th-century England might sound sexist to modern readers, even if that author was relatively feminist in his time. Readers should not have to excuse the faulty assumptions and prejudices of the past, but they should appreciate that a person's thoughts and words are, in part, a result of the time and culture in which they live or lived, and it is perhaps unfair to expect writers to avoid all of the errors of their times.

Even a brief study of world literature suggests that writers from vastly different cultures address similar themes. For instance, works like the *Odyssey* and *Hamlet* both tackle the individual's battle for self-control and independence. In every culture, authors address themes of personal growth and the struggle for maturity. Another universal theme is the conflict between the individual and society. In works as culturally disparate as *Native Son*, the *Aeneid*, and *1984*, authors dramatize how people struggle to maintain their personalities and dignity in large, sometimes oppressive groups. Finally, many cultures have versions of the hero's (or heroine's) journey, in which an adventurous person must overcome many obstacles in order to gain greater knowledge, power, and perspective. Some famous works that treat this theme are the *Epic of Gilgamesh*, Dante's *Divine Comedy*, and *Don Quixote*.

Authors from different genres (for instance poetry, drama, novel, short story) and cultures may address similar themes, but they often do so quite differently. For instance, poets are likely to address subject matter obliquely, through the use of images and allusions. In a play, on the other hand, the author is more likely to dramatize themes by using characters to express opposing viewpoints. This disparity is known as a dialectical approach. In a novel, the author does not need to express themes directly; rather, they can be illustrated through events and actions. Different movements and styles become popular in different regions. For example, in Greece and England, authors tend to use more irony. In the 1950s Latin American authors popularized the use of unusual and surreal events to show themes about real life in the genre of magical realism. Japanese authors use the well-established poetic form of the haiku to organize their treatment of common themes.

RESPONDING TO LITERATURE

When reading good literature, the reader is moved to engage actively in the text. One part of being an active reader involves making predictions. A **prediction** is a guess about what will happen next. Readers are constantly making predictions based on what they have read and what they already know. Consider the following sentence: *Staring at the computer screen in shock, Kim blindly reached over for the brimming glass of water on the shelf to her side.* The sentence suggests that Kim is agitated and that she is not looking at the glass she is going to pick up, so a reader might predict that she is going to knock the glass over. Of course, not every prediction will be accurate: perhaps Kim will pick the glass up cleanly. Nevertheless, the author has certainly created the expectation that the water might be spilled. Predictions are always subject to revision as the reader acquires more information.

Review Video: Predictions
Visit mometrix.com/academy and enter code: 437248

Test-taking tip: To respond to questions requiring future predictions, the student's answers should be based on evidence of past or present behavior.

Readers are often required to understand text that claims and suggests ideas without stating them directly. An **inference** is a piece of information that is implied but not written outright by the author. For instance, consider the following sentence: *Mark made more money that week than he had in the previous year.* From this sentence, the reader can infer that Mark either has not made much money in the previous year or made a great deal of money that week. Often, a reader can use information he or she already knows to make inferences. Take as an example the sentence *When his coffee arrived, he looked around the table for the silver cup.* Many people know that cream is typically served in a silver cup, so using their own base of knowledge they can infer that the subject of this sentence takes his coffee with cream. Making inferences requires concentration, attention, and practice.

Review Video: Inference
Visit mometrix.com/academy and enter code: 379203

Test-taking tip: While being tested on his ability to make correct inferences, the student must look for contextual clues. An answer can be *right* but not *correct*. The contextual clues will help you find the answer that is the best answer out of the given choices. Understand the context in which a phrase is stated. When asked for the implied meaning of a statement made in the passage, the student should immediately locate the statement and read the context in which it was made. Also, look for an answer choice that has a similar phrase to the statement in question.

A reader must be able to identify a text's **sequence**, or the order in which things happen. Often, and especially when the sequence is very important to the author, it is indicated with signal words like *first*, *then*, *next*, and *last*. However, sometimes a sequence is merely implied and must be noted by the reader. Consider the sentence *He walked in the front door and switched on the hall lamp*. Clearly, the man did not turn the lamp on before he walked in the door, so the implied sequence is that he first walked in the door and then turned on the lamp. Texts do not always proceed in an orderly sequence from first to last: sometimes, they begin at the end and then start over at the beginning. As a reader, it can be useful to make brief notes to clarify the sequence.

Review Video: Sequence
Visit mometrix.com/academy and enter code: 489027

In addition to inferring and predicting things about the text, the reader must often **draw conclusions** about the information he has read. When asked for a *conclusion* that may be drawn, look for critical "hedge" phrases, such as *likely, may, can, will often*, among many others. When you are being tested on this knowledge, remember that question writers insert these hedge phrases to cover every possibility. Often an answer will be wrong simply because it leaves no room for exception. Extreme positive or negative answers (such as always, never, etc.) are usually not correct. The reader should not use any outside knowledge that is not gathered from the reading passage to answer the related questions. Correct answers can be derived straight from the reading passage.

Critical Thinking Skills

Opinions, Facts, & Fallacies

Critical thinking skills are mastered through understanding various types of writing and the different purposes that authors have for writing the way they do. Every author writes for a purpose. Understanding that purpose, and how they accomplish their goal, will allow you to critique the writing and determine whether or not you agree with their conclusions.

Readers must always be conscious of the distinction between fact and opinion. A **fact** can be subjected to analysis and can be either proved or disproved. An **opinion**, on the other hand, is the author's personal feeling, which may not be alterable by research, evidence, or argument. If the author writes that the distance from New York to Boston is about two hundred miles, he is stating a fact. But if he writes that New York is too crowded, then he is giving an opinion, because there is no objective standard for overpopulation. An opinion may be indicated by words like *believe, think*, or *feel*. Also, an opinion may be supported by facts: for instance, the author might give the population density of New York as a reason for why it is overcrowded. An opinion supported by fact tends to be more convincing. When authors support their opinions with other opinions, the reader is unlikely to be moved.

Facts should be presented to the reader from reliable sources. An opinion is what the author thinks about a given topic. An opinion is not common knowledge or proven by expert sources, but it is information that the author believes and wants the reader to consider. To distinguish between fact and opinion, a reader needs to look at the type of source that is presenting information, what information backs-up a claim, and whether or not the author may be motivated to have a certain point of view on a given topic.

For example, if a panel of scientists has conducted multiple studies on the effectiveness of taking a certain vitamin, the results are more likely to be factual than if a company selling a vitamin claims that taking the vitamin can produce positive effects. The company is motivated to sell its product, while the scientists are using the scientific method to prove a theory. If the author uses words such as "I think...", the statement is an opinion.

Review Video: Fact or Opinion
Visit mometrix.com/academy and enter code: 870899

In their attempt to persuade, writers often make mistakes in their thinking patterns and writing choices. It is important to understand these so you can make an informed decision. Every author has a point of view, but when an author ignores reasonable counterarguments or distorts opposing viewpoints, she is demonstrating a **bias**. A bias is evident whenever the author is unfair or inaccurate in his or her presentation. Bias may be intentional or unintentional, but it should always alert the reader to be skeptical of the argument being made. It should be noted that a biased author may still be correct. However, the author will be correct in spite of her bias, not because of it. A **stereotype** is like a bias, except that it is specifically applied to a group or place. Stereotyping is considered to be particularly abhorrent because it promotes negative generalizations about people. Many people are familiar with some of the hateful stereotypes of certain ethnic, religious, and cultural groups. Readers should be very wary of authors who stereotype. These faulty assumptions typically reveal the author's ignorance and lack of curiosity.

Review Video: Bias and Stereotype
Visit mometrix.com/academy and enter code: 644829

Sometimes, authors will **appeal to the reader's emotion** in an attempt to persuade or to distract the reader from the weakness of the argument. For instance, the author may try to inspire the pity of the reader by delivering a heart-rending story. An author also might use the bandwagon approach, in which he suggests that his opinion is correct because it is held by the majority. Some authors resort to name-calling, in which insults and harsh words are delivered to the opponent in an attempt to distract. In advertising, a common appeal is the testimonial, in which a famous person endorses a product. Of course, the fact that a celebrity likes something should not really mean anything to the reader. These and other emotional appeals are usually evidence of poor reasoning and a weak argument.

Review Video: Appeal to Emotion
Visit mometrix.com/academy and enter code: 163442

Certain *logical fallacies* are frequent in writing. A logical fallacy is a failure of reasoning. As a reader, it is important to recognize logical fallacies, because they diminish the value of the author's message. The four most common logical fallacies in writing are the false analogy, circular reasoning, false dichotomy, and overgeneralization. In a **false analogy**, the author suggests that two things are similar, when in fact they are different. This fallacy is often committed when the author is attempting to convince the reader that something unknown is like something relatively familiar. The author takes advantage of the reader's ignorance to make this false comparison.

One example might be the following statement: *Failing to tip a waitress is like stealing money out of somebody's wallet.* Of course, failing to tip is very rude, especially when the service has been good, but people are not arrested for failing to tip as they would for stealing money from a wallet. To compare stingy diners with thieves is a false analogy.

Review Video: False Analogy
Visit mometrix.com/academy and enter code: 865045

Circular reasoning is one of the more difficult logical fallacies to identify, because it is typically hidden behind dense language and complicated sentences. Reasoning is described as circular when it offers no support for assertions other than restating them in different words. Put another way, a circular argument refers to itself as evidence of truth. A simple example of circular argument is when a person uses a word to define itself, such as saying *Niceness is the state of being nice*. If the reader does not know what *nice* means, then this definition will not be very useful. In a text, circular reasoning is usually more complex. For instance, an author might say *Poverty is a problem for society because it creates trouble for people throughout the community*. It is redundant to say that poverty is a problem because it creates trouble. When an author engages in circular reasoning, it is often because he or she has not fully thought out the argument, or cannot come up with any legitimate justifications.

Review Video: Circular Reasoning
Visit mometrix.com/academy and enter code: 398925

One of the most common logical fallacies is the **false dichotomy**, in which the author creates an artificial sense that there are only two possible alternatives in a situation. This fallacy is common when the author has an agenda and wants to give the impression that his view is the only sensible one. A false dichotomy has the effect of limiting the reader's options and imagination. An example of a false dichotomy is the statement *You need to go to the party with me, otherwise you'll just be bored at home*. The speaker suggests that the only other possibility besides being at the party is being bored at home. But this is not true, as it is perfectly possible to be entertained at home, or even to go somewhere other than the party. Readers should always be wary of the false dichotomy: when an author limits the alternatives, it is always wise to ask whether his argument valid.

Review Video: False Dichotomy
Visit mometrix.com/academy and enter code: 484397

Overgeneralization is a logical fallacy in which the author makes a claim that is so broad it cannot be proved or disproved. In most cases, overgeneralization occurs when the author wants to create an illusion of authority, or when he is using sensational language to sway the opinion of the reader. For instance, in the sentence *Everybody knows that she is a terrible teacher*, the author makes an assumption that cannot really be believed.

This kind of statement is made when the author wants to create the illusion of consensus when none actually exists: it may be that most people have a negative view of the teacher, but to say that *everybody* feels that way is an exaggeration. When a reader spots overgeneralization, she should become skeptical about the argument that is being made, because an author will often try to hide a weak or unsupported assertion behind authoritative language.

Review Video: Overgeneralization
Visit mometrix.com/academy and enter code: 367357

Two other types of logical fallacies are **slippery slope** arguments and **hasty generalizations**. In a slippery slope argument, the author says that if something happens, it automatically means that something else will happen as a result, even though this may not be true. (i.e., just because you study hard does not mean you are going to ace the test). "Hasty generalization" is drawing a conclusion too early, without finishing analyzing the details of the argument. Writers of persuasive texts often use these techniques because they are very effective. In order to **identify logical fallacies**, readers need to read carefully and ask questions as they read. Thinking critically means not taking everything at face value. Readers need to critically evaluate an author's argument to make sure that the logic used is sound.

Organization of the Text

The way a text is organized can help the reader to understand more clearly the author's intent and his conclusions. There are various ways to organize a text, and each one has its own purposes and uses. Some nonfiction texts are organized to **present a problem** followed by a solution. In this type of text, it is common for the problem to be explained before the solution is offered. In some cases, as when the problem is well known, the solution may be briefly introduced at the beginning. The entire passage may focus on the solution, and the problem will be referenced only occasionally. Some texts will outline multiple solutions to a problem, leaving the reader to choose among them. If the author has an interest or an allegiance to one solution, he may fail to mention or may describe inaccurately some of the other solutions. Readers should be careful of the author's agenda when reading a problem-solution text. Only by understanding the author's point of view and interests can one develop a proper judgment of the proposed solution.

Authors need to organize information logically so the reader can follow it and locate information within the text. Two common organizational structures are cause and effect and chronological order. When using **chronological order**, the author presents information in the order that it happened. For example, biographies are written in chronological order; the subject's birth and childhood are presented first, followed by their adult life, and lastly by the events leading up to the person's death.

In **cause and effect**, an author presents one thing that makes something else happen. For example, if one were to go to bed very late, they would be tired. The cause is going to bed late, with the effect of being tired the next day.

It can be tricky to identify the cause-and-effect relationships in a text, but there are a few ways to approach this task. To begin with, these relationships are often signaled with certain terms. When an author uses words like *because*, *since*, *in order*, and *so*, she is likely describing a cause-and-effect relationship. Consider the sentence, "He called her because he needed the homework." This is a simple causal relationship, in which the cause was his need for the homework and the effect was his phone call. Not all cause-and-effect relationships are marked in this way, however. Consider the sentences, "He called her. He needed the homework." When the cause-and-effect relationship is not indicated with a keyword, it can be discovered by asking why something happened. He called her: why? The answer is in the next sentence: He needed the homework.

Persuasive essays, in which an author tries to make a convincing argument and change the reader's mind, usually include cause-and-effect relationships. However, these relationships should not always be taken at face value. An author frequently will assume a cause or take an effect for granted. To read a persuasive essay effectively, one needs to judge the cause-and-effect relationships the author is presenting. For instance, imagine an author wrote the following: "The parking deck has been unprofitable because people would prefer to ride their bikes." The relationship is clear: the cause is that people prefer to ride their bikes, and the effect is that the parking deck has been unprofitable. However, a reader should consider whether this argument is conclusive. Perhaps there are other reasons for the failure of the parking deck: a down economy, excessive fees, etc. Too often, authors present causal relationships as if they are fact rather than opinion. Readers should be on the alert for these dubious claims.

Thinking critically about ideas and conclusions can seem like a daunting task. One way to make it easier is to understand the basic elements of ideas and writing techniques. Looking at the way different ideas relate to each other can be a good way for the reader to begin his analysis. For instance, sometimes writers will write about two different ideas that are in opposition to each other. The analysis of these opposing ideas is known as **contrast**. Contrast is often marred by the author's obvious partiality to one of the ideas. A discerning reader will be put off by an author who does not engage in a fair fight. In an analysis of opposing ideas, both ideas should be presented in their clearest and most reasonable terms. If the author does prefer a side, he should avoid indicating this preference with pejorative language. An analysis of opposing ideas should proceed through the major differences point by point, with a full explanation of each side's view. For instance, in an analysis of capitalism and communism, it would be important to outline each side's view on labor, markets, prices, personal responsibility, etc. It would be less effective to describe the theory of communism and then explain how capitalism has thrived in the West. An analysis of opposing views should present each side in the same manner.

Many texts follow the **compare-and-contrast** model, in which the similarities and differences between two ideas or things are explored. Analysis of the similarities between ideas is called comparison. In order for a comparison to work, the author must place the ideas or things in an equivalent structure. That is, the author must present the ideas in the same way. Imagine an author wanted to show the similarities between cricket and baseball. The correct way to do so would be to summarize the equipment and rules for each game. It would be incorrect to summarize the equipment of cricket and then lay out the history of baseball, since this would make it impossible for the reader to see the similarities. It is perhaps too obvious to say that an analysis of similar ideas should emphasize the similarities. Of course, the author should take care to include any differences that must be mentioned. Often, these small differences will only reinforce the more general similarity.

Drawing Conclusions

Authors should have a clear purpose in mind while writing. Especially when reading informational texts, it is important to understand the logical conclusion of the author's ideas. **Identifying this logical conclusion** can help the reader understand whether he agrees with the writer or not. Identifying a logical conclusion is much like making an inference: it requires the reader to combine the information given by the text with what he already knows to make a supportable assertion. If a passage is written well, then the conclusion should be obvious even when it is unstated. If the author intends the reader to draw a certain conclusion, then all of his argumentation and detail should be leading toward it.

One way to approach the task of drawing conclusions is to make brief notes of all the points made by the author. When these are arranged on paper, they may clarify the logical conclusion. Another way to approach conclusions is to consider whether the reasoning of the author raises any pertinent questions. Sometimes it will be possible to draw several conclusions from a passage, and on occasion these will be conclusions that were never imagined by the author. It is essential, however, that these conclusions be supported directly by the text.

Review Video: Identifying Logical Conclusions
Visit mometrix.com/academy and enter code: 281653

The term **text evidence** refers to information that supports a main point or points in a story, and can help lead the reader to a conclusion. Information used as *text evidence* is precise, descriptive, and factual. A main point is often followed by supporting details that provide evidence to back-up a claim. For example, a story may include the claim that winter occurs during opposite months in the Northern and Southern hemispheres. *Text evidence* based on this claim may include countries where winter occurs in opposite months, along with reasons that winter occurs at different times of the year in separate hemispheres (due to the tilt of the Earth as it rotates around the sun).

Readers interpret text and respond to it in a number of ways. Using textual support helps defend your response or interpretation because it roots your thinking in the text. You are interpreting based on information in the text and not simply your own ideas. When crafting a response, look for important quotes and details from the text to help bolster your argument. If you are writing about a character's personality trait, for example, use details from the text to show that the character acted in such a way. You can also include statistics and facts from a nonfiction text to strengthen your response. For example, instead of writing, "A lot of people use cell phones," use statistics to provide the exact number. This strengthens your argument because it is more precise.

Review Video: Text Evidence
Visit mometrix.com/academy and enter code: 486236

The text used to support an argument can be the argument's downfall if it is not credible. A text is **credible**, or believable, when the author is knowledgeable and objective, or unbiased. The author's motivations for writing the text play a critical role in determining the credibility of the text and must be evaluated when assessing that credibility. The author's motives should be for the dissemination of information. The purpose of the text should be to inform or describe, not to persuade. When an author writes a persuasive text, he has the motivation that the reader will do what they want. The extent of the author's knowledge of the topic and their motivation must be evaluated when assessing the credibility of a text. Reports written about the Ozone layer by an environmental scientist and a hairdresser will have a different level of credibility.

Review Video: Credible
Visit mometrix.com/academy and enter code: 827257

After determining your own opinion and evaluating the credibility of your supporting text, it is sometimes necessary to communicate your ideas and findings to others. When **writing a response to a text**, it is important to use elements of the text to support your assertion or defend your position. Using supporting evidence from the text strengthens the argument because the reader can see how in depth the writer read the original piece and based their response on the details and facts within that text. Elements of text that can be used in a response include: facts, details, statistics, and direct quotations from the text. When writing a response, one must make sure they indicate which information comes from the original text and then base their discussion, argument, or defense around this information.

A reader should always be drawing conclusions from the text. Sometimes conclusions are implied from written information, and other times the information is **stated directly** within the passage. It is always more comfortable to draw conclusions from information stated within a passage, rather than to draw them from mere implications. At times an author may provide some information and then describe a counterargument. The reader should be alert for direct statements that are subsequently rejected or weakened by the author. The reader should always read the entire passage before drawing conclusions. Many readers are trained to expect the author's conclusions at either the beginning or the end of the passage, but many texts do not adhere to this format.

Drawing conclusions from information implied within a passage requires confidence on the part of the reader. **Implications** are things the author does not state directly, but which can be assumed based on what the author does say. For instance, consider the following simple passage: "I stepped outside and opened my umbrella. By the time I got to work, the cuffs of my pants were soaked." The author never states that it is raining, but this fact is clearly implied. Conclusions based on implication must be well supported by the text. In order to draw a solid conclusion, a reader should have multiple pieces of evidence, or, if he only has one, must be assured that there is no other possible explanation than his conclusion. A good reader will be able to draw many conclusions from information implied by the text, which enriches the reading experience considerably.

As an aid to drawing conclusions, the reader should be adept at **outlining** the information contained in the passage; an effective outline will reveal the structure of the passage, and will lead to solid conclusions. An effective outline will have a title that refers to the basic subject of the text, though it need not recapitulate the main idea. In most outlines, the main idea will be the first major section. It will have each major idea of the passage established as the head of a category.

For instance, the most common outline format calls for the main ideas of the passage to be indicated with Roman numerals. In an effective outline of this kind, each of the main ideas will be represented by a Roman numeral and none of the Roman numerals will designate minor details or secondary ideas.

Moreover, all supporting ideas and details should be placed in the appropriate place on the outline. An outline does not need to include every detail listed in the text, but it should feature all of those that are central to the argument or message. Each of these details should be listed under the appropriate main idea.

It is also helpful to **summarize** the information you have read in a paragraph or passage format. This process is similar to creating an effective outline. To begin with, a summary should accurately define the main idea of the passage, though it does not need to explain this main idea in exhaustive detail. It should continue by laying out the most important supporting details or arguments from the passage. All of the significant supporting details should be included, and none of the details included should be irrelevant or insignificant. Also, the summary should accurately report all of these details. Too often, the desire for brevity in a summary leads to the sacrifice of clarity or veracity. Summaries are often difficult to read, because they omit all of the graceful language, digressions, and asides that distinguish great writing. However, if the summary is effective, it should contain much the same message as the original text.

Paraphrasing is another method the reader can use to aid in comprehension. When paraphrasing, one puts what they have read into their own words, rephrasing what the author has written to make it their own, to "translate" all of what the author says to their own words, including as many details as they can.

MCAT Practice Test

Biological and Biochemical Foundations

QUESTION SET 1

The sodium-potassium adenosine triphosphatase (Na+/K+ ATPase) enzyme maintains a resting potential of –70 mV across a neuronal cell membrane. A complex 3D structure, Na+/K+ ATPase is encoded by several genes. Powered by adenosine triphosphate (ATP) and consuming between 15% and 25% of a typical human cell's energy, the enzymatic pump is fundamental in maintaining the body's homeostasis.

It is the pump's hyperpolarization of the neuronal membrane that results in a brief refractory period during which the cell cannot be depolarized.

Researchers have extracted a portion of the cell membrane containing the Na+/K+ ATPase and treated the tissues with an acidic solution. They measured the latency before another action potential with the following results:

Solution	Action potential latency
0.02% solution	2 msec
0.04% solution	1.88 msec
0.07% solution	0.75 msec

1. What is the approximate charge of the membrane potential during the refractory period?

a. –65 mV
b. 25 mV
c. 180 mV
d. –75 mV

2. How do the characteristics of the phospholipid bilayer of the cell impact the movement of Na+ and K+?

a. Sodium and potassium are both highly charged cations. They cannot easily diffuse through the phospholipid bilayer, and thus they require active transport to move against a concentration gradient.
b. Sodium and potassium are both small ions, and they can thus diffuse through the phospholipid bilayer according to the concentration gradient, but they require an ATP-powered pump to overcome the concentration gradient.
c. The phospholipid bilayer contains phosphate molecules, which can interact with and bind to Na+ and K+.
d. The phospholipid bilayer of a nonneuronal cell does not have Na+/K+ ATPase because nonneuronal cells do not carry an action potential.

3. What factors may change the behavior of enzymatic proteins?

a. Temperature, diffusion, pH, and an attached molecule at the binding site
b. Hydrogen concentration, water, and pH
c. Temperature, hydrogen concentration, and an attached molecule at the binding site
d. Temperature, pH, and concentration gradient

4. How does the solution applied in this experiment alter the activity of the pump?

a. The solution deactivates some of the pumps, prolonging the refractory period.
b. The solution deactivates some of the pumps, reducing the latency.
c. The solution prolongs the activity of some of the pumps, prolonging the latency.
d. The solution prolongs the activity of some of the pumps, reducing the refractory period.

5. How does the refractory period after an action potential affect a neuronal cell's ability to preserve the integrity of the action potential?

a. The action potential cannot move in a reverse direction due to the latency produced by the refractory period.
b. The latency protects the cell membrane from injury, which could be caused by excessive concentrations of sodium.
c. The latency allows for a response from the target organ prior to initiation of another action potential.
d. The latency of the action potential prevents the neuron from becoming overstimulated, and it prevents overconsumption of neurotransmitters at the synapse.

6. How could an experimental design using any of these solutions determine the relative density of Na+/K+ ATPase-activated pumps between two different types of cells?

a. Both cell types should be treated with 0.02% and 0.04% solution. The cell type with the greatest drop in latency is the cell type with the greater density of Na+/K+ ATPase-activated proton pumps.
b. Both cell types should be treated with 0.04% and 0.07% solution. The cell type with the smallest drop in latency is the cell type with the greater density of Na+/K+ ATPase-activated proton pumps.
c. Both cell types should be treated with all three solutions to determine which cell types showed the biggest change in latency because that would be the cell type with the greater density of Na+/K+ ATPase-activated proton pumps.
d. Both cell types should be treated with the 0.07% solution. The cell type showing a longer latency upon treatment with the 0.07% solution is likely the cell type with the lower density of Na+/K+ ATPase-activated proton pumps.

Question Set 2

During mitosis, deoxyribonucleic acid (DNA) replication produces a copy of the genetic information encoded in the DNA molecule. Given the specialized differentiation of eukaryotic cells, portions of the DNA molecule may be intermittently activated in some cells, but not in other cells.

A nucleotide base pair substitution mutation has been incidentally identified in a series of DNA analyses performed on a population that has a known hereditary genetic disorder that impairs T-cell function. The locus of the genetic abnormality that causes the T-cell dysfunction has not yet been established. The phenotypic effects of the incidentally located mutation have not yet been determined, if there are any.

Preliminary findings of 1000 subjects and 10,000 controls

T-cell function impairment		Presence of base pair mutation
Controls	0.001%	0%
Group 1	0.5%	2.01%
Group 2	0.67%	1.52%
Group 3	0.78%	1.67%

7. How may a substitution mutation occur and yet not produce a change in the protein that it encodes?

a. The DNA molecule is a double helix, and therefore the complementary strand can compensate for a mutation in one strand.
b. Due to the redundancy of the genetic code, a substitution mutation can code for the identical "correct" amino acid in a protein, and consequently it might not affect the protein structure.
c. A eukaryotic cell is diploid, and by definition it contains two copies of every gene. The homologous copy that does not have a mutation should code for the correct protein.
d. An abnormal protein would not be able to function, and it would most likely be destroyed by phagocytes.

8. During cell division, how could a DNA replication error resulting in a base pair substitution being repaired?

a. During transcription, several enzymes, such as ribonucleic acid (RNA) polymerase, interact with the DNA molecule to ensure accuracy.
b. When cell division occurs, segregation of homologous chromosomes ensures that the correct number of chromosomes ends up in each cell.
c. It cannot be repaired. If a mutation has already occurred, every copy of the gene will be faithfully copied with the mutation through the process of semiconservative replication.
d. DNA polymerase and the associated enzymes essentially "double-check" a replicated DNA strand to correct an error during the replication process.

9. How are the base pair mutation and the T-cell dysfunction in the above DNA analysis functionally related?

a. It appears that the base pair mutation improves with worsened T-cell function.
b. It appears that the base pair mutation is unrestrained, in part, by T-cell dysfunction. This is likely due to the role T-cells play in protecting the body against precancerous cells with DNA mutation.
c. They are not directly functionally related. The increased presence of the base pair mutation in the population with T-cell dysfunction does not suggest a functional relationship.
d. The base pair mutation may be in a locus that encodes T-cells.

10. Could the nucleotide base pair substitution and the base hereditary T-cell dysfunction share linkage?

a. Given the marked increase in T-cell dysfunction in the population with base pair mutation, that is a likely possibility.
b. It is unlikely given that the base pair mutation was an incidental finding.
c. They cannot be linked on the same gene because the incidence of T-cell dysfunction is not equal to the incidence of base pair mutation.
d. The loci of the two genes must be located near each other to establish linkage. Because T-cell function is being compared to a mutation, it cannot be established whether the conditions are located on the same gene.

11. How may RNA polymerase affect the outcome of the mutation during transcription?

a. RNA polymerase may correct the mutation during transcription, analogously to the way that DNA polymerase may aid in repairing a mutation.
b. RNA polymerase aids in building the mRNA molecule, which should faithfully copy the code on the DNA template, maintaining the code determined by the mutation.
c. RNA polymerase may form transfer RNA (tRNA) molecules that match amino acids to the messenger RNA (mRNA) strand during transcription.
d. RNA polymerase allows the rRNA molecules to join a stream of abnormal mRNA molecules to amino acids, which may exaggerate the effects of the mutation.

12. How may a DNA base pair substitution during meiosis affect the longevity of the mutation?

a. The mutation may continue to affect the individual for the duration of his or her life, depending on its impact on the resulting protein.
b. The mutation will only affect half of the divided cells due to the segregation of homologous chromosomes during cell division during meiosis and thus will only be partially expressed in the individual.
c. The mutation will only affect one-fourth of the divided cells due to the segregation of homologous chromosomes during cell division during meiosis. Because the resulting cells are only haploid cells, the consequences will be less significant.
d. The mutation will affect only germ cells, and thus it may be carried to the offspring, but it will not affect the individual in whom the mutation occurred.

Question Set 3

Glucose 6-phosphate dehydrogenase (G6PD) deficiency is a condition in which the G6PD enzyme is deficient. This enzyme is necessary for the metabolism of certain medications such as sulfa medications and some foods such as fava beans. Symptoms include life-threatening hemolysis shortly after the ingestion of food or medication that requires G6PD for proper metabolism. Currently, there is a blood test available that can measure the presence and quantity of G6PD, but there is not a reliable genetic test for the condition. This is an X-linked recessive disorder.

A pregnant woman, Stephanie, has a family history of G6PD deficiency, but she does not have G6PD deficiency. Stephanie's father does not have the condition, and Stephanie has male cousins on her mother's side of the family who have G6PD deficiency.

13. How can one determine with certainty and without a genetic test if Stephanie is a carrier?

a. Measure Stephanie's G6PD level.
b. Perform a fetal ultrasound.
c. In the absence of a genetic test, there is no way to know for certain whether Stephanie is a carrier for the condition unless she gives birth to a son who has the condition.
d. Give her fava beans or sulfa medications and observe the reaction.

14. How would an X-linked gene be expressed as codominance in an individual's phenotype?

a. If a female carries a nucleotide sequence on her X-chromosome that is homozygous to the nucleotide sequence on her other X-chromosome in the corresponding locus, she will express a codominant phenotype.
b. If a female carries a heterozygous nucleotide sequence for a genome on the corresponding loci of both of her X-chromosomes, her phenotype will express characteristics encoded by both genomes if both sequences code for proteins that may exist and function in each other's presence.
c. If a male carries a gene on his X-chromosome that is homozygous to the gene on his Y-chromosome, he will express codominance.
d. If a male carries a heterozygous nucleotide sequence for a genome on his X-chromosome and his Y-chromosome, his phenotype will express characteristics encoded by both genomes if both sequences code for proteins that may exist and function in each other's presence.

15. If you were to learn that G6PD deficiency is more prevalent among populations that are exposed to malaria, how would you distinguish between an evolutionarily adaptive protection against malaria and a link between sickle-cell disease and G6PD deficiency?

a. Because sickle-cell disease is also more prevalent among populations that are exposed to malaria, and because they are both X-linked conditions affecting red blood cells, they are linked by the X-chromosome.
b. One would have to assess how frequently the two disorders occur together and separately and compare that with how frequently sickle-cell disease occurs with and separately from other disorders that occur with the same frequency as G6PD deficiency in this population.
c. One would have to assess the frequency with which both diseases are present in the population versus the frequency with which both genetic alterations are present in the population to determine whether the genetic correspondence is equivalent to the disease correspondence.
d. One would have to expose red blood cells of individuals with G6PD enzyme and individuals without G6PD enzyme to malaria to determine whether it is, in fact the malaria that contributed to the prevalence among the population or whether it is a genetic link.

16. How could the proteins encoded by a recessive genome differ from the proteins encoded by a dominant genome?

a. The genome of a dominant gene codes for products that essentially cancel out the effect of the products encoded by a recessive gene on the same locus of a homologous chromosome.
b. The proteins encoded by a recessive genome are shorter and more easily denature than proteins encoded by dominant genes on the same locus of a homologous chromosome.
c. The proteins encoded by a recessive genome are generally not produced in the presence of a dominant gene on the same locus of a homologous chromosome.
d. The genome of a dominant gene activates transcription and translation more effectively than the genome of a recessive gene.

17. How could the development of immunization against malaria affect the prevalence of G6PD deficiency?

a. Because G6PD deficiency has been found to provide partial immunity against malaria, immunization against malaria would be expected to reduce the incidence of G6PD over several generations in regions with a high exposure to malaria.
b. Because G6PD deficiency is present in the population in regions with a high exposure to malaria, the evolutionary adaptation has already occurred and is unlikely to change.
c. Because G6PD deficiency is a hemolytic disease, an immunization against malaria would protect individuals with G6PD deficiency from the hemolytic effects of malaria and allow the disease to become more prevalent in the population.
d. Because G6PD deficiency only provides partial protection against malaria, an immunization against malaria may or may not affect the prevalence of G6PD deficiency in the population. The prevalence would depend, most importantly, on the mortality of the G6PD itself.

18. How could administration of G6PD enzyme determine whether the triggers for the hemolytic reaction include sulfa medications and fava beans and whether there are other triggers?

a. Administration of the enzyme could be given whenever a hemolytic reaction occurs.
b. Administration of the enzyme could be given at random intervals to determine the intensity of hemolytic reactions to various exposures.
c. Administration of the enzyme could be withheld in order to determine the source of the hemolytic reactions.
d. Administration of the enzyme could be given when there is exposure to sulfa medications or fava beans, but not during other times, to evaluate whether a hemolytic reaction occurs in the absence of these exposures.

Question Set 4

Carbohydrates and proteins provide the body with four calories per gram, whereas fats provide the body with nine calories per gram.

Glucose, a simple carbohydrate molecule, enters the Krebs cycle after glycolysis yields only two ATP molecules, pyruvate and acetyl coenzyme A (acetyl-CoA). The reduced form of nicotinamide adenine dinucleotide (NADH) and flavin adenine dinucleotide (FADH2) formed in both glycolysis and the Krebs cycle subsequently enter the electron transport chain.

Complex polysaccharide carbohydrates take longer for the body to digest, absorb, and metabolize than simple monosaccharide carbohydrates.

Fatty acids are broken down to acetyl CoA, which is used in the Krebs cycle, and NADH and FADH2, which enter the electron transport chain.

Saturated fatty acids differ from unsaturated fatty acids in several ways. Saturated fatty acids are less likely to become rancid. Yet, researchers have noted an association with heart disease that makes saturated fatty acids somewhat less desirable. The causative link between saturated fatty acids and heart disease is not completely understood.

19. What chemical differences between monosaccharides and polysaccharides explains their differences in metabolism?

a. Polysaccharides are larger molecules containing more subunits than monosaccharides, and therefore they take longer for enzymes to break down to small molecules for absorption.
b. Polysaccharides are larger molecules containing more subunits than monosaccharides and therefore they contain more electron bonds, which produce more energy per gram.
c. Polysaccharides are molecules with a more complex chemical configuration, and thus they enter the Krebs cycle after an initial modification, similar to the initial step of fatty acid metabolism.
d. Polysaccharides must be broken down into small glucose subunits prior to glycolysis, and therefore it takes longer for the body to metabolize polysaccharides than monosaccharides, but they yield the same number of calories per gram.

20. How do the differences between unsaturated fatty acids and saturated fatty acids contribute to the increased tendency of unsaturated fatty acids to become rancid?

a. Fatty acids with only single bonds are more stable and less likely to interact with other molecules in the environment, which could cause them to change their chemical structure and become rancid.
b. Saturated fatty acids are completely saturated with electrons and therefore they are not as easily disrupted.
c. Unsaturated fatty acids are more likely to be liquid at room temperature, so they can more quickly reach a boiling point, making them unstable molecules.
d. Unsaturated fatty acids can have a trans configuration, and trans fats are more unstable molecules that have a higher tendency to become rancid.

21. How should unsaturated fatty acids and saturated fatty acids compare in energy yield?

a. They should yield nine calories per kilogram. This number is primarily based on the number of bonds, which are equivalent in saturated and unsaturated fatty acids.
b. They should yield nine calories per kilogram, which is based on the number of single bonds. There are more single bonds in saturated than in unsaturated fats, so there is a slight difference in caloric yield, with saturated fats yielding more calories than unsaturated fats.
c. They should yield nine calories per kilogram, with some slight differences based on the relative stability. Because saturated fats are more stable molecules, they are more difficult to digest and absorb, and, because they contain some indigestible portions, they yield slightly fewer calories than unsaturated fats, which are easier to digest and absorb.
d. It depends on the size and shape of the molecule and how many bonds are present.

22. How do the calories produced from glycolysis compare to the calories produced in the Krebs cycle and the electron transport chain?

a. There are fewer calories produced from glycolysis than from either the Krebs cycle or from the electron transport chain.
b. The net calories produced in glycolysis are equivalent to the net calories produced in the Krebs cycle, but fewer than those produced in the electron transport chain.
c. The net calories produced in glycolysis are greater than the calories produced during the Krebs cycle, but fewer than those produced in the electron transport chain.
d. The net calories produced in glycolysis are fewer than the calories produced in the Krebs cycle, but more than those produced in the electron transport chain.

23. If you were to design an experiment to better understand why there is a stronger causative relationship between saturated fatty acids and heart disease than between unsaturated fatty acids and heart disease, which of the following would you need to control?

a. The polyunsaturated fat content versus monounsaturated fat content consumed.
b. The number of total calories consumed by research subjects.
c. The baseline heart condition of subjects participating in the experiment, to avoid confounding bias.
d. The number of calories of fat consumed, to ensure that the relationship is not based on the slightly higher calorie yield of saturated fats.

24. How does oxygen affect metabolism?

a. Oxygen is required for metabolism glucose.
b. Oxygen can allow for the production of more ATP molecules in each step of the metabolic process, including glycolysis, the Krebs cycle, and the electron transport chain.
c. Oxygen makes metabolism more efficient because glycolysis, which does not require oxygen, produces a low energy yield.
d. Oxygen can accept hydrogen atoms at the end of the electron transport chain, yielding a rich supply of ATP.

Question Set 5

When blood flow to human tissue is interrupted, the lack of sufficient blood supply is called ischemia. If ischemia is not restored quickly, the affected tissue may undergo a process called infarction, which involves a series of chemical changes that damage the tissue.

The lack of blood supply results in lack of oxygen, and thus lactic acidosis. Mitochondrial dysfunction results.

Microscopic examination and chemical analysis of ischemic cells reveal membrane degeneration, excessive calcium (Ca+) inside the cell, and free radical formation, accompanied by a reactive inflammation and free fatty acid formation.

A research experiment is designed to evaluate the response of infarcted tissue to intra-arterial administration of an antioxidant. Preliminary results demonstrate that follow-up evaluation of tissue exposed to intra-arterial antioxidant injection resulted, on average, in a smaller area of infarcted tissue after seven days when compared to controls without exposure to the antioxidant. It was noted that 70% of the patients who demonstrated smaller areas of infarction also had a notable decease in edema of the ischemic tissue lasting about 6 to 10 hours after injection.

25. What is a possible explanation for the relationship among antioxidant injection, edema, and tissue damage?

a. Antioxidants produce anti-infarction biochemical reactions that decrease the size of the infarct.
b. Antioxidants decrease tissue damage by decreasing edema.
c. The prevention of tissue damage may be produced by a combination of the effect of decreased edema and the injection of antioxidants.
d. Increased blood flow causes paradoxical tissue damage due to ischemia.

26. How would mitochondrial dysfunction contribute to calcium influx?

a. Active transport, which maintains Ca+ concentrations inside and outside the cell, requires ATP, which is produced by the mitochondria.
b. Mitochondrial membranes contain Ca+, and thus degeneration of mitochondrial membranes leaks Ca+ into the cell's cytoplasm.
c. The mitochondria are the site of ATP production. ATP is required to maintain Ca+ movement against the concentration gradient.
d. The lack of oxygen results in metabolic acidosis, and the ionic shift permits Ca+ into the cell.

27. How could lactic acid production and free fatty acid formation contribute to organelle dysfunction?

a. The acidity of these molecular products, when uncorrected, alters the cell's pH beyond that which the cell can compensate for. Organelles, containing proteins, denature as a result.
b. Lactic acid production and free fatty acid formation function like free radicals, altering the structure of the molecular components of the organelles.
c. Lactic acids and free fatty acids crowd the organelles within the cells, preventing them from communicating with each other in the cytoplasm.
d. Lactic acids and free fatty acids are hydrophobic and thus can enter the membranes of the organelles, disrupting their function.

28. Why does a lack of blood supply cause lactic acidosis?

a. Organelle membranes are composed of hydrophilic lactic acid, which is released during organelle apoptosis.
b. Without inadequate oxygen, cell metabolism formation must follow an alternate pathway, which uses the pyruvate produced in glycolysis and produces lactic acid as a by-product.
c. Lactic acidosis provides quick bursts of energy, which the cell needs to counteract the effects of infarction.
d. Lactic acidosis is the result of lactic acid production because lactose is a sugar that can provide energy. It is present in dairy products.

29. Why does membrane degeneration contribute to inflammation?

a. The infarcted cell membrane becomes infected by microorganisms already present in the body, as evidenced by the presence of bacteria on microscopic examination of infarcted tissue.
b. Inflammatory cells are a component of the edematous fluid present during infarction.
c. The white blood cells that are present in inflammation are generally a normal component of the body and are no longer contained, due to membrane degeneration, and they are able to leak down the concentration gradient.
d. The cell becomes altered and the body attempts to repair itself and "clean up" debris produced by cellular degeneration.

30. What is the difference between membrane leakiness and capillary leakiness?

a. The leaky membrane of the capillary can allow cells to leak out, whereas the membrane of the leaky cell can allow fluid to leak out.
b. Membrane leakiness is a consequence of degeneration of the cell membrane and dysfunction of membrane protein channels and pumps, whereas capillary leakiness results in edema due to capillary permeability.
c. Membrane leakiness is the result of degeneration of the phospholipid bilayer of the cell, whereas capillary leakiness is the cause of degeneration of the phospholipid bilayer.
d. Membrane leakiness causes edema, whereas capillary leakiness causes inflammation.

Question Set 6

Regulatory proteins and hormones direct embryogenesis. Germ cells originate in the embryo during the second trimester. Later, gametogenesis occurs.

The development of epithelial tissue and neuronal tissue from the common ectodermal precursor occurs in the first month after fertilization, and then cells continue to differentiate.

The mesoderm forms the heart and muscles during the first month, and the heart begins to function within the first four weeks after fertilization. Complete pulmonary function is not established until later in gestation.

31. How are genetic disorders different from developmental disorders?

a. Genetic disorders are physical conditions, whereas developmental disorders are more complex disorders involving emotional and cognitive processing.
b. Genetic disorders are caused by an inherited trait encoded on the DNA, whereas developmental disorders are caused by DNA damage due to environmental factors during embryogenesis.
c. Genetic disorders are caused by alterations in the gene, whereas developmental disorders are caused by alterations in cellular differentiation.
d. Developmental disorders may be caused by genetic alterations or by environmental causes or by unknown causes and include a diverse group of conditions characterized by physical, speech, emotional, or cognitive dysfunction.

32. How would nondisjunction affect the chromosome number of a gamete?

a. Nondisjunction would result in a gamete that does not have exactly 23 chromosomes.
b. Nondisjunction would result in a gamete that does not have exactly one of each chromosome.
c. Nondisjunction causes either one more or one fewer than the correct number of chromosomes in the resulting gamete.
d. Nondisjunction would cause nonhomologous chromosomes to be present in the gamete when there should not be.

33. If a researcher wanted to determine whether embryonic stem cells could differentiate into cells for therapeutic use, how could he or she improve the chances of success?

a. Use cells from the ectoderm to replace ectodermal tissue, from the endoderm to replace endodermal tissue, or from the mesoderm to replace mesodermal tissue to improve the chances of proper differentiation.
b. Use a matched-type donor to minimize the chances of transplant rejection.
c. Use stem cells from the embryonic bone marrow.
d. Use cells from the gamete because they have not yet differentiated.

34. How would prematurity of about six weeks affect oxygenation?

a. Pulmonary surfactant is not well developed at this stage, and thus the baby would not have the ability to expand the lungs, leading to poor oxygenation.
b. The skeletal muscles are not well developed at this stage, and thus inspiration would be impaired, leading to poor oxygenation.
c. The heart is not well developed at this stage, and thus the baby would not be able to circulate oxygen to the tissue.
d. The hemoglobin molecule is not well developed at this stage, and thus the baby would not be able to carry enough oxygen through the blood.

35. How do germ layers differ from germ cells?

a. Germ cells are produced during gametogenesis, whereas germ layers are produced after fertilization.
b. Germ cells are diploid cells that are precursors to gametes, whereas germ layers are composed of differentiating diploid cells.
c. Germ layers are different parts of the germ cells.
d. Germ cells are haploid, whereas germ layers are diploid.

36. How does the chromosome number of the germ cell chromosome produce the resulting chromosome number of a gamete?

a. A germ cell is haploid and matures into a haploid gamete.
b. A germ cell is diploid and divides to become two haploid gametes.
c. A germ cell is diploid, doubles, and then divides into four haploid gametes.
d. A germ cell is haploid, doubles, and then divides into two haploid gametes.

Question Set 7

Several organisms can invade the human body and cause what is classified as an infection. However, there are vast differences between such infective agents as bacteria, fungi, parasites, viruses, and prions.

37. Which of the following contain diploid genetic material?

a. Parasites
b. Bacteria
c. Prions
d. Viruses

38. How can a virus evade an immune response?

a. A retrovirus can invade immune cells.
b. It is too small to be detected.
c. It can hide inside a cell.
d. It can mimic a cell.

39. How does a bacterial cell reproduce?

a. Binary fission
b. Conjugation
c. Sexual reproduction
d. Insertion of genetic material into the host genome

40. How does a retrovirus differ from a virus?

a. A retrovirus infects a host cell by inserting genetic material, whereas a virus invades the cell wall.
b. A retrovirus causes cancer, whereas a virus causes disease.
c. A retrovirus is an old virus.
d. A retrovirus genome is composed of RNA, and a viral genome is composed of DNA.

41. What are the structural components of the bacterial cell?

a. Cell wall and nucleus
b. Cell membrane, cell wall, and nucleoid
c. Cytoplasm, nucleus, and nucleoid
d. Cytoplasm, cell wall, and nucleus

Question Set 8

The endocrine and nervous systems interact with each other in several ways.

The hypothalamus, located in the brain, sends messages to the anterior pituitary gland via the hypothalamo-hypophyseal portal system and to the posterior pituitary gland via the hypothalamo-hypophyseal tract. Adrenocorticotropic hormone (ACTH) is released by the anterior pituitary gland and sent via the circulation to the adrenal medulla, which produces neurotransmitters that regulate the autonomic nervous system.

Myelinated axons of the somatic nervous system release acetylcholine, a neurotransmitter that binds to skeletal muscles.

42. How may demyelination of the central nervous system (CNS) affect acetylcholine release from the peripheral nerves?

a. Demyelination of the CNS would impact the CNS response to peripheral nerve stimulation and thus would not affect acetylcholine release at the neuromuscular junction because that event occurs prior to the stimulus from the peripheral nerve entering the spinal cord.
b. When demyelination of the CNS occurs, it can slow down the signal in the nerves, slowing down and decreasing the amount of acetylcholine released by the peripheral nerves.
c. When demyelination of CNS tissue occurs, demyelinated neurons in the brain and/or spinal cord might not transmit an action potential, and thus they might not send messages to the peripheral nerves, which means that acetylcholine will not be released.
d. Demyelination of the CNS does not affect acetylcholine release from the peripheral nervous system (PNS) because the CNS consists of the brain and spinal cord, whereas the PNS consists of nerves.

43. How does communication differ among the hypothalamus and the anterior and posterior pituitary glands?

a. The posterior pituitary gland receives electrical signals from the hypothalamus, triggering the production of hormones, whereas the anterior pituitary gland receives hormones from the hypothalamus directly through the blood.
b. Communication between the hypothalamus and the anterior pituitary gland is via the blood, whereas communication between the hypothalamus and the posterior pituitary gland is via the axons.
c. Communication between the hypothalamus and the anterior pituitary gland is regulated by negative feedback, whereas communication between the hypothalamus and the posterior pituitary gland is regulated by negative feedback and positive feedback, due to the production of oxytocin.
d. The hypothalamus communicates with the posterior pituitary gland by inhibiting hormone production and with the anterior pituitary gland by stimulating hormone production.

44. How may negative feedback mechanisms regulate the autonomic nervous system in the setting of a hyperactive pituitary tumor?

a. A hyperactive pituitary tumor may be expected to produce excessive adrenocorticotropic hormone (ACTH), and thus negative feedback due to overstimulation of the autonomic nervous system would reach the hypothalamus as well as the pituitary gland and the adrenal medulla, which would in turn decrease the release of ACTH from the anterior pituitary gland and epinephrine from the adrenal medulla.
b. Negative feedback mechanisms would decrease stimulation of the hypothalamus, which would produce the desired effect on the anterior pituitary gland, effectively maintaining regulation of the autonomic nervous system.
c. Negative feedback mechanisms would inhibit release of hormones that stimulate the sympathetic nervous system so that the parasympathetic nervous system can function properly.
d. A hyperactive pituitary tumor would be expected to produce and release excessive ACTH, so the negative feedback mechanisms would decrease epinephrine production by the adrenal medulla and desensitize the adrenal medulla to the excessive ACTH.

45. If researchers examined a series of CNS specimens to evaluate the rate of serotonin reuptake, how would they measure the effect of additional serotonin on the rate of serotonin reuptake?

a. Researchers would measure the difference between serotonin levels in the controls and the experimental group treated with serotonin immediately after the serotonin has had its desired effects and at several intervals after that.
b. Researchers would measure the quantity of serotonin in controls versus the experimental group treated with serotonin at intervals after the treatment to determine the rate of uptake.
c. Researchers would measure the concentration of serotonin in experimental groups treated with several different concentrations of additional serotonin.
d. Researchers would measure the concentration of serotonin in controls versus the experimental group treated with additional serotonin prior to the experiment and at several intervals after the treatment to determine the rate of reuptake.

46. How do neuroglia differ from neurons in terms of oncologic potential?

a. Neuroglia are supportive cells and thus do not have oncologic potential, whereas neurons, which are highly functioning and are more likely to be affected by toxins and free radicals, have greater oncologic potential.
b. Neuroglia are more prone to retrovirus exposure due to the selective blood-brain barrier protection of neurons, and thus they have greater oncologic potential than do neurons.
c. Neuroglial cells are better able to repair themselves, and they also have a higher oncologic potential than do neurons.
d. Neuroglia are not myelinated, whereas neurons are myelinated, and thus the exposure of neurons to carcinogens is reduced in comparison to neuroglia.

47. How would the optic nerves be impacted by a hypofunctioning adrenal medullary gland?

a. A hypofunctioning adrenal medullary gland would result in compensatory overstimulation of the hypothalamus, which would in turn overstimulate the anterior pituitary gland to release ACTH. The enlargement of the pituitary gland would produce pressure on the optic nerves.
b. A hypofunctioning adrenal medullary gland would directly stimulate activity of the pituitary gland and would result in enlargement of the pituitary gland, putting pressure on the optic nerves.
c. A hypofunctioning adrenal medullary gland would result in inconsistent overstimulation of the pituitary gland, and thus the gland would become intermittently enlarged, periodically putting pressure on the optic nerves.
d. A hypofunctioning adrenal medullary gland would result in inconsistent overstimulation of the hypothalamus and the pituitary gland, but this would not result in enlargement of the pituitary gland and thus not affect the optic nerves.

Question Set 9

Chronic anemia and acute anemia both elicit compensatory mechanisms that maintain homeostasis.

Data from a sample of patients who suffered from chronic anemia, a sample of patients who experienced acute anemia due to traumatic bleeding, and a sample of patients with a normal red blood cell (RBC) count were collected. Using a control baseline of 1 for all values, averages of the relative heart rates, erythropoietin (EPO) levels, blood pressure measurements, and respiratory rates were plotted.

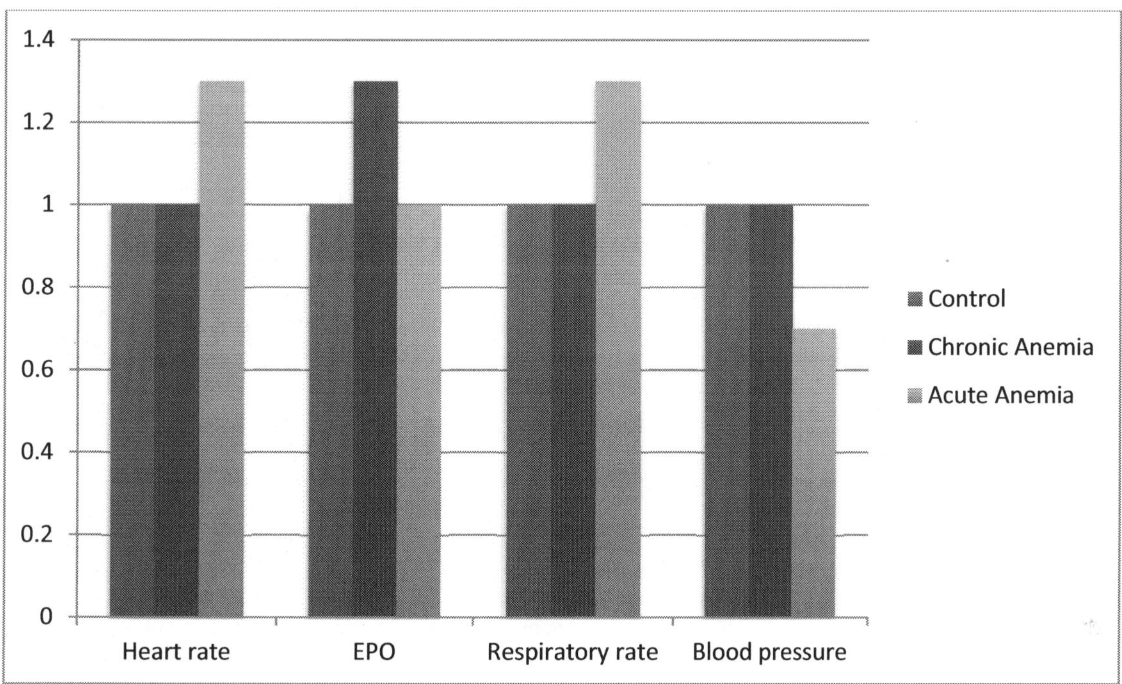

48. Why does the acute anemia in this sample cause a change in heart rate?

a. Acute anemia results in volume deficit and O2 deficit due to the loss of RBCs and hemoglobin.
b. Acute anemia causes lactic acidosis due to conversion to an anaerobic metabolic pathway.
c. Acute anemia results in CO2 buildup, which triggers adjustment of the heart rate produced by the sinoatrial (SA) node in the heart, driven by the medulla in the brainstem.
d. Hemoglobin breakdown, a characteristic of hemolytic anemia, results in lower oxygen-carrying capacity.

49. Which factors are most likely to control erythropoietin levels?

a. Volume loss as blood flows through the kidneys.
b. Oxygen concentration in the blood as it flows through the kidneys.
c. Urine output of the kidneys.
d. Stem cell activity in the bone marrow.

50. What factor controls blood pressure on acute anemia?

a. Vasospasm
b. Arterial regulation
c. RBC concentration
d. Venous regulation

51. How do carbon dioxide levels affect respiration?

a. When carbon dioxide concentrations change, the adrenal medulla adjusts the respiratory rate and volume by sending hormones to adjust the width of the bronchi.
b. When the carbon dioxide concentration changes, it acts directly on the alveoli, allowing them to expand or contract as necessary.
c. When carbon dioxide concentrations change, the medulla in the brainstem adjusts the respiratory rate and volume.
d. When the carbon dioxide concentration changes, receptors on the respiratory muscles adjust the rate and force of inspiration and expiration.

52. How would an agglutination reaction to a blood transfusion affect erythropoietin in the first few minutes?

a. An agglutination reaction would stimulate erythropoietin production in the kidneys.
b. An agglutination reaction would stimulate an attenuated response to erythropoietin in bone marrow.
c. An agglutination reaction would inhibit the release of erythropoietin due to stimulation of the sympathetic nervous system.
d. An agglutination reaction would maintain the level of erythropoietin within the first few minutes.

53. How would you evaluate the kidneys' response to chronic anemia?

a. Measure the blood pressure and the erythropoietin production in comparison to controls.
b. Measure the erythropoietin production and the urine content in comparison to controls.
c. Measure the urine volume and the erythropoietin level in comparison to controls.
d. Measure the blood pressure and the antidiuretic hormone in comparison to controls.

Discrete Questions

54. Fetal exposure to excessive quantities of vitamin A, a fat-soluble vitamin, such as the quantities present in some prescription-strength oral acne treatments, have been associated with neural tube defects. Folate deficiency has also been associated with neural tube defects. What would you conclude about folate in the developing fetus?

a. An adequate supply of folate is important prior to and within the first month of gestation to decrease the risk of neural tube defects.
b. An adequate supply of folate is necessary during the first month of gestation to prevent neural tube defects.
c. Folate must be fat soluble, and it is necessary during the first month of gestation to prevent neural tube defects.
d. Folate intake during pregnancy drives the development of the epidermal tissue of the fetus.

55. How does egg cell morphology differ from that of a sperm cell?

a. An egg cell has a larger cytoplasm and more mitochondria than a sperm cell.
b. An egg cell contains an X chromosome, and a sperm cell contains a Y chromosome.
c. An egg cell has a nucleus, whereas a sperm cell does not.
d. A sperm cell may be used as a donor in reproductive technology, but an egg cell cannot.

56. Antigens on the surface of pathogens provoke an immune response due to action mediated by

a. lymphocytes
b. leukocytes
c. antibodies produced by B lymphocytes and other leukocytes
d. antibodies and erythrocytes

57. How do the cell junctions between epithelial cells affect the communication between neighboring cells?

a. Gap junctions allow a space between neighboring cells, preventing direct contact between neighboring cells, whereas tight junctions form a barrier to prevent fluid from entering between the cells.
b. Tight junctions firmly attach neighboring cells, decreasing flexibility while increasing strength.
c. Adhering junctions connect cells to each other to form a barrier against fluid entering between the cells.
d. Gap junctions connect the cytoplasm between cells, allowing material to flow from one cell to another.

58. If an experiment were designed to determine the conditions that promote gluconeogenesis, which tissue would be studied?

a. The mitochondria, because gluconeogenesis occurs in the mitochondria of a eukaryotic cell using amino acids.
b. The slow muscle fibers, because they are rich in mitochondria and may convert to alternate energy pathways such as aerobic respiration.
c. The liver because the liver is one of the cell types in which gluconeogenesis occurs in the mitochondria, using amino acids.
d. Adipose tissue because fat cells undergo oxidation to enter the Krebs cycle and the electron transport chain in order to provide the body with energy in the form of ATP.

59. How does a proto-oncogene relate to an oncogene?

a. A proto-oncogene promotes proliferation of an oncogene.
b. A proto-oncogene is a normal gene. But if it undergoes a mutation, a proto-oncogene can become an oncogene.
c. A proto-oncogene is a protein encoded by an oncogene.
d. An oncogene codes for a mutation that can inhibit apoptosis, whereas a proto-oncogene codes for a mutation that affects mitosis.

Chemical and Physical Foundations

PASSAGE 1

Read the paragraphs below and answer questions 1-5.

Analysis of a protein or food sample for amino acid composition can be critically important in evaluating its nutritive value. Amino Acid Analysis provides this information by hydrolyzing proteins into individual amino acids, separating them chromatographically, and quantitating them. Many different methods are used for these steps, and understanding the properties of proteins and individual amino acids is important in evaluating potential new methods of analysis.

Among the amino acids detected in a particular analysis are those with the properties shown in Table 1.

Table 1. Properties of selected amino acids

Amino Acid	Solubility in water (mol/kg at 25°C)	pKa1	pKa2	pKa R group	Specific Rotation $[\alpha]_D^{25}$
L-Alanine	1.9	2.34	9.69	--	+1.8
L-Lysine	1.7	2.18	8.95	10.53	+13.5
L-Valine	0.50	2.29	9.72	--	+5.6
L-Leucine	0.17	2.36	9.60	--	-11.0
L-Tryptophan	0.065	2.38	9.39	--	-33.7
Unknown	0.060	2.19	9.67	4.25	+12.0

One of the most common ways to separate amino acids is by ion exchange chromatography. A typical amino acid analysis involves using a cation exchange resin consisting of beads of polystyrene sulfonate in a chromatographic column. In this method, the sulfonate groups on the beads are loaded with sodium ions prior to analysis. The fluid containing the amino acids passes down the column, over the beads, and exits at the bottom. Based on properties like those shown in Table 1, some of the amino acids adhere to the beads more strongly. The strongly bound amino acids travel more slowly down the column and the amino acids separate based on their relative adherence to the beads.

1. The peptide below has four labeled bonds. Which of these bonds break during hydrolysis if subjected to 6 M HCl at 110°C for 24 hours?

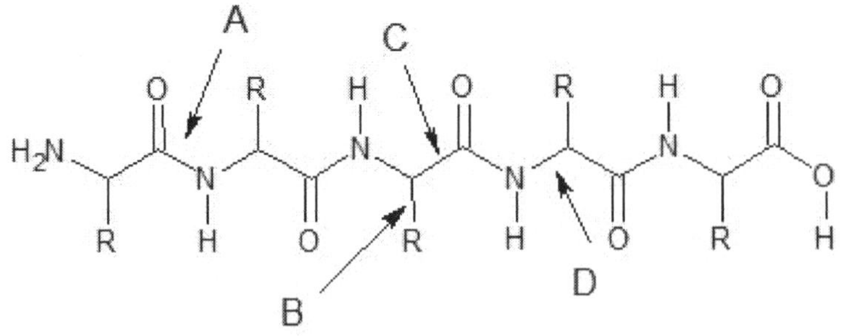

a. Bond A
b. Bond B
c. Bond C
d. Bond D

2. Based on the properties listed in Table 1, the identity of the amino acid labeled as Unknown is most likely to be which of the following?

a. L-Phenylalanine
b. L-Glycine
c. L-Cysteine
d. L-Glutamic Acid

3. When the amino acids listed in Table 1 separate by ion exchange chromatography using a cation exchange resin, which of the amino acids is most likely to elute last from the column?

a. L-Lysine
b. L-Valine
c. L-Tryptophan
d. The amino acid labeled unknown

4. Which of the following is a correct representation of the structure of L-alanine (which is also correctly known as (S)-Alanine)?

a. 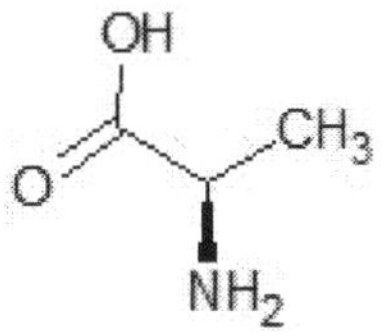 OH, O, CH_3, NH_2
b. 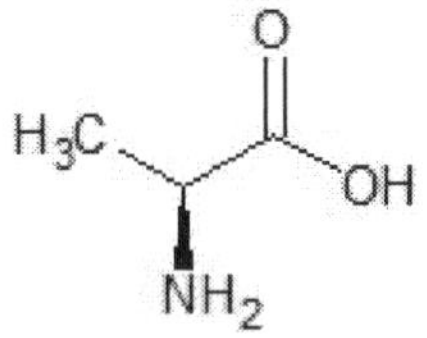 O, H_3C, OH, NH_2
c. 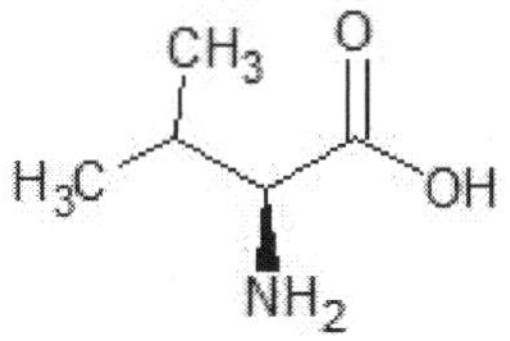 CH_3, O, H_3C, OH, NH_2
d. 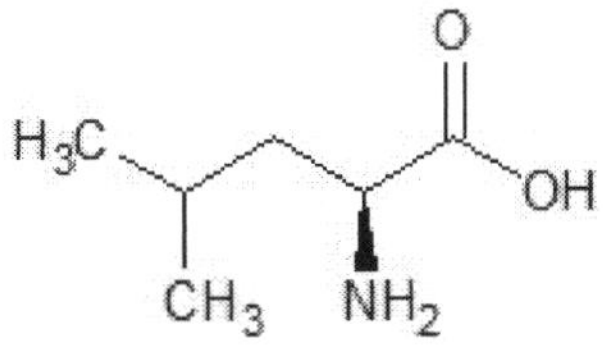 O, H_3C, OH, CH_3, NH_2

5. Assume that a fluid used in an ion exchange separation of amino acids has a pH of 5. Which of the amino acids in Table 1 provides the most buffering capacity at that pH?

a. L-Alanine
b. L-Lysine
c. L-Leucine
d. The amino acid labeled unknown

Passage 2

Read the paragraphs below and answer questions 6-10.

Many of the properties of molecules depend on their shapes. In some cases, such as for nitrogen-containing molecules, the oxidation states of the atoms in the molecule control the shape. Nitrogen can form stable compounds with oxidation states on nitrogen ranging from -3 to +5.

Lewis dot structures and the VSEPR (valence shell electron repulsion) theory can predict the shapes of many compounds. Shown below is the Lewis structure of ammonia, where the nitrogen atom has an oxidation state of -3.

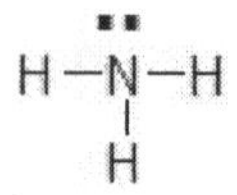

H–N–H
|
H

Since there are four regions of paired electrons around the nitrogen atom, we can predict those four regions will spread out as far from one another as possible, resulting in a tetrahedral shape, as shown below.

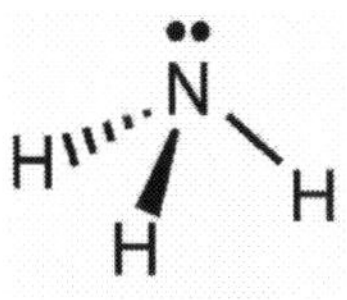

N
H H H

Similar analyses for other nitrogen compounds give the results shown in Table 2.

Table 2. Properties of nitrogen molecules			
Molecule	**Formula**	**Oxidation state of N**	**Shape**
Ammonia	NH3	-3	trigonal pyramidal
Hydrazine	N2H4	-2	trigonal pyramidal at N
Azide ion	N_3^-	-1/3	linear
Dinitrogen	N2	0	--
Nitrous oxide	N2O	+1	linear
Nitric oxide	NO	+2	--
Nitrite ion	NO_2^-	+3	bent
Nitrogen dioxide	NO2	+4	bent
Nitrate ion	NO_3^-	+5	trigonal planar

6. How many valence electrons are there in the Lewis dot structure for nitrate ion?

a. 5
b. 8
c. 23
d. 24

7. What is the formal charge on the nitrogen atom in the Lewis structure of the nitrite ion?

a. -1
b. 0
c. +1
d. +3

8. Using the information in Table 2, which of the following molecules ALL have a dipole moment?

a. Ammonia, nitrous oxide, and nitrogen dioxide
b. Ammonia, nitric oxide, nitrogen dioxide
c. Nitrous oxide, nitric oxide, nitrogen dioxide
d. Ammonia, dinitrogen, nitrous oxide

9. There are several resonance structures for the azide ion. Which is the major contributor to the actual ion structure?

a. $N{\equiv}N^{+}{-}N^{2-}$
b. $N{=}N{-}N^{-}$
c. $N^{-}{=}N^{+}{=}N^{-}$
d. $N{=}N{=}N^{-}$

10. One nitrite ion and one azide ion can react with each other in acid (using 2 H+) so that all of the nitrogen atoms change their oxidation state. The products of this reaction are one dinitrogen molecule and which other compound(s)?

a. Nitric oxide
b. Nitric oxide and water
c. Nitrous oxide
d. Nitrous oxide and water

PASSAGE 3

Read the paragraphs below and answer questions 11-15.

32P-labeled phosphate has numerous uses in both biomedical research and in clinical patient therapy. One use is as a palliative treatment for patients with painful bone metastasis. Bone takes up the phosphate and it delivers its radiation locally. The standard method of production involves bombardment of 32S with neutrons. The sulfur takes on a neutron and simultaneously ejects a proton to become 32P.

Direct neutron capture by 31P allows a manufacturing process with improved product purity and less radioactive waste. In that process, red phosphorus was bombarded with neutrons at a rate of 8×1013 neutrons/(cm2·s) for 60 days. The final step involves conversion of the product into sodium phosphate and addition to sterile vials for injection. Table 3 shows the results.

Table 3. Properties of 32P-phosphate made by direct neutron capture	
Property	**Result**
Radioactive half-life	14.29 days
Specific Activity	6.2±0.4 mCi/mg
Radionuclide purity	>99.9%
Radiopurity with respect to phosphate	~99%
Activity per dose	10–15 mCi
pH	7.4
Type of decay	Beta
Energy released	1.709 MeV

11. Adding phosphate to a solution containing calcium can result in a precipitate. This precipitate most likely has which stoichiometry?

a. CaPO3
b. CaPO4
c. Ca2(PO4)3
d. Ca3(PO4)2

12. An extended in vivo experiment involves studying the distribution and excretion of injected 32P-phosphate in mice using the product manufactured by direct neutron capture with 31P. The entire experiment lasts for 43 days. Compared to the radioactivity of the initial phosphate dosed to the animals, how much of the initial radioactivity remained when the experiment ends?

a. 100%
b. 87.6%
c. 12.4%
d. 1.24%

13. An extended in vivo experiment involves studying the distribution and excretion of injected 32P-phosphate mice. Samples from each day of the 43-day experiment were stored in a -80°C freezer until analysis on day 54. Which of the following attributes of the storage conditions affects the total radioactivity of each sample?

a. pH in the sample before freezing
b. Temperature in the freezer
c. Calcium concentration in the sample before freezing
d. The storage conditions will not influence radioactivity

14. When 32P decays, the product is which of the following?

a. $^{32}_{16}S$
b. $^{32}_{16}S^{+}$
c. $^{32}_{14}Si$
d. $^{32}_{14}Si^{-}$

15. Graphite is an important material in the construction of nuclear reactors. One drawback is the production of radioactive 14C in the graphite by direct neutron capture, causing the material to become a long-term waste disposal problem. Which of the following materials in the graphite is the most likely atom to capture of a single neutron and become 14C?

a. $^{13}_{7}N$
b. $^{12}_{6}C$
c. $^{13}_{6}C$
d. $^{14}_{5}N$

PASSAGE 4

Read the paragraphs below and answer questions 16-20.

Bilirubin is a waste product that the body produces as it breaks down hemoglobin, and excessive bilirubin in the body can be an indicator of disease. Bilirubin is colored, and this absorption of light can be used both as a way to detect bilirubin in blood samples, and as a way to therapeutically treat excessive bilirubin in the body. Shown below is the structure of bilirubin:

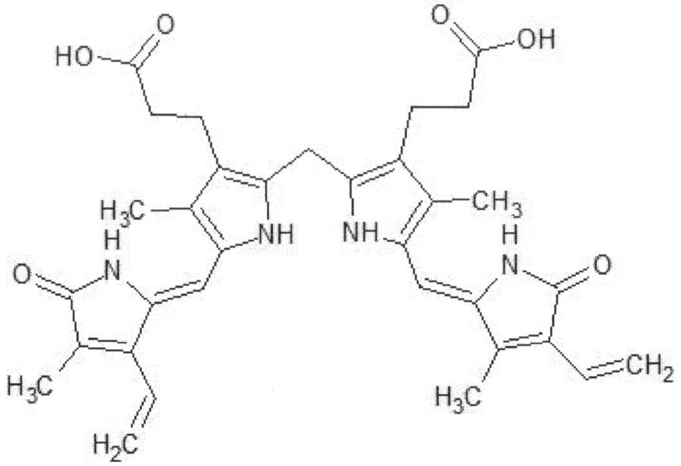

HO O OH O H_3C H N NH NH CH_3 H N O O H_3C H_2C H_3C CH_2

Hemoglobin 02 can interfere with the absorbance measurements used to measure bilirubin because they both absorb light in the range from 360 to 500 nm (see Table 4). In order to subtract the contribution of hemoglobin to absorbance of bilirubin in a measurement at 457 nm, the hemoglobin concentration is first determined by measuring absorbance at 582 nm, where the bilirubin does not absorb. The expected absorbance of the hemoglobin at 457 nm is then calculated and subtracted from the actual measurement at 457 nm to get the absorbance due to bilirubin alone.

Using this method allows bilirubin in the sera of newborns with levels of 100-400 μM to be measured to within a few percent despite the potential presence of up to 25 g/L of hemoglobin 02 (390 μM of the tetramer).

Table 4. Optical Properties of bilirubin and hemoglobin 02		
Compound	**Molar Absorption Coefficient at 457 nm (M-1cm-1)**	**Molar Absorption Coefficient at457 nm (M-1cm-1)**
Bilirubin	48,907	17
Hemoglobin 02	48,496	43,304

16. The light used to detect bilirubin in the passage is which color?

a. Red
b. Yellow
c. Green
d. Blue

17. What is the energy of the photons used to detect bilirubin in the passage? The following constants may be useful: speed of light in vacuum = 3.00×108 m/s; Faraday constant =96 485.3 C/mole; Planck's constant = 4.1 ×10−15 eV/s

a. 0.27 eV
b. 2.07 eV
c. 2.7 eV
d. 27 eV

18. The transmittance of a particular bilirubin sample is 0.85 in a cuvette with a path length of 1 cm. If analysis of the same sample takes place in a cuvette with a path length of 3 cm, what will the transmittance be?

a. 0.39
b. 0.55
c. 0.61
d. 0.85

19. What is the expected absorbance of a 1.0 μM bilirubin standard at 457 nm in a cuvette with a path length of 2 cm?

a. 0.010
b. 0.050
c. 0.10
d. 0.50

20. Which of the following structures made by modifying bilirubin would not absorb visible light?

a.

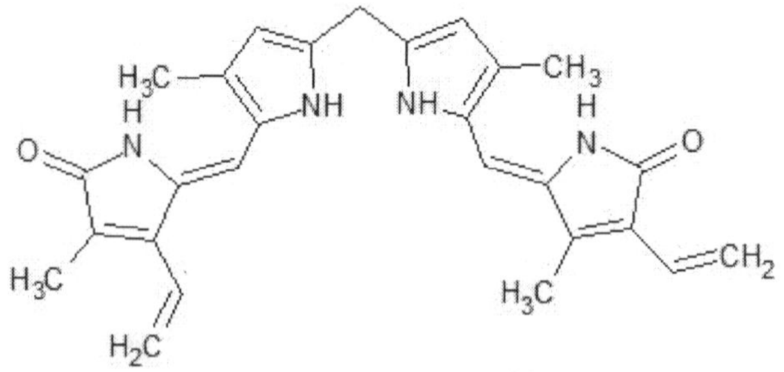

b.

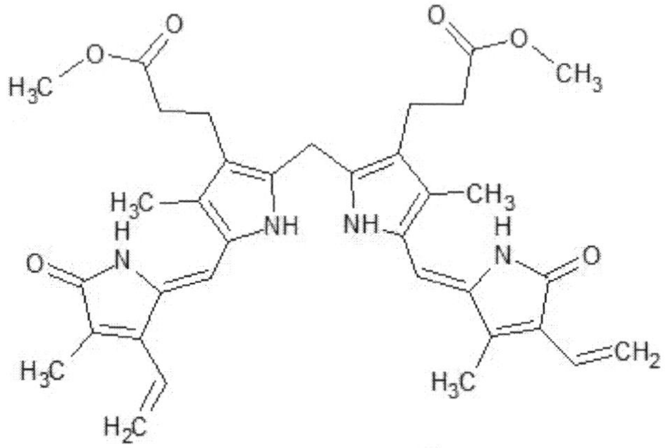

c.

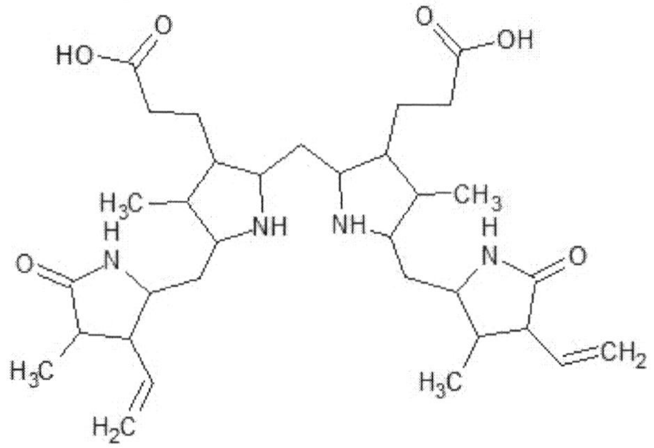

d.

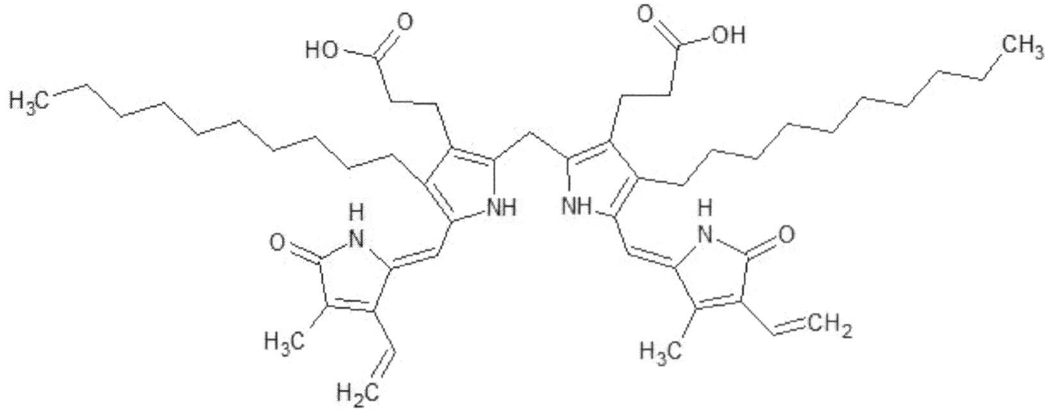

PASSAGE 5

Read the paragraphs below and answer questions 21-25.

One of the important impacts of the burning of fossil fuels and the elevation of the carbon dioxide concentration in the atmosphere relates to the impact of this additional carbon dioxide on the oceans. In order to study this effect, Pat begins a series of experiments to understand how carbon dioxide influences the solubility of calcium carbonate in the ocean. The shells and skeletons of many organisms, such as clams and corals, are made of calcium carbonate, and its solubility may have an impact on their ability to survive.

The solubility of calcium carbonate is governed by the solubility product constant Ksp

Ksp = [Ca2+][CO32-]

Carbon dioxide can affect this relationship by dissolving into the water as carbonic acid:

CO2 + H2O ←→ H2CO3

The concentration of carbonate required in the Ksp relates to the pH through the acid/base properties of carbonic acid, bicarbonate and carbonate:

$H_2CO_3 \leftrightarrow HCO_3^- + H^+$ pKa1

$HCO_3^- \leftrightarrow CO_3^{2-} + H^+$ pKa2

where pKa1 and pKa2 are the pKa values for carbonic acid and bicarbonate, respectively. Table 1 shows the pKa values for these two reactions in seawater as a function of temperature:

Table 5. pKa values for carbonic acid and bicarbonate in seawater as a function of temperature		
Temperature (°C)	**pKa1**	**pKa2**
5	6.05	9.28
15	5.94	9.09
25	5.85	8.92
35	5.76	8.75

21. Knowing the pKa values from Table 5 and that the pH of ordinary seawater is approximately 8.2, what form of dissolved carbon dioxide predominates in the ocean at 25°C?

a. Carbonic Acid
b. Bicarbonate
c. Carbonate
d. Not enough information is given

22. Starting with a mixture of solid calcium carbonate in equilibrium with seawater, Pat adds enough solid sodium carbonate to double the carbonate concentration. She then waits until a new equilibrium is established. Which of the following is the best description of the resulting mixture?

a. Compared to the starting mixture, the dissolved calcium concentration rose
b. Compared to the starting mixture, the dissolved calcium concentration dropped
c. Compared to the starting mixture, the dissolved calcium concentration remained the same
d. Some of the solid calcium carbonate dissolved

23. Starting with a mixture of solid calcium carbonate in equilibrium with seawater, Pat adds enough solid calcium carbonate to double the amount of undissolved calcium carbonate in the mixture. She then waits until a new equilibrium is established. Which of the following is the best description of the resulting solution?

a. There is no change in the dissolved concentration of calcium or carbonate
b. The dissolved calcium rises and the dissolved carbonate falls
c. The dissolved calcium falls and the dissolved carbonate rises
d. Both the dissolved calcium and the dissolved carbonate rise

24. Pat knows that adding carbon dioxide to seawater will lower the pH, and to study the system she starts by studying the addition of a strong acid, hydrochloric acid, to seawater. She starts with seawater at pH 8.2 and adds 1 M hydrochloric acid until the pH reaches 7.8. Compared to the solution she started with, which of the following statements is true for the final solution, based on the known pKa values?

a. The carbonate concentration rose and the carbonic acid concentration fell
b. The carbonate concentration fell and the carbonic acid concentration rose
c. Both the carbonate and carbonic acid concentrations fell
d. Both the carbonate and carbonic acid concentrations rose

25. Pat is also worried about the effect of a rise in the ocean temperature on the potential solubility of calcium carbonate. She initially considers just the effect of temperature on the pKa values in Table 1, and how those impact the concentration of carbonate in the ocean. In considering a rise in temperature from 25°C to 30°C, what happens to the concentration of carbonate in seawater?

a. As the temperature rises, bicarbonate becomes a stronger acid, so carbonate rises
b. As the temperature rises, bicarbonate becomes a weaker acid, so carbonate rises
c. As the temperature rises, bicarbonate becomes a stronger acid, so carbonate falls
d. As the temperature rises, bicarbonate becomes a weaker acid, so carbonate falls

PASSAGE 6

Read the paragraphs below and answer questions 26-30.

The human knee joint forms a complex connection between the femur and the tibia. It is subjected to considerable forces, both when standing still and when in motion. These forces can eventually damage the knee and cause considerable pain and disability. Table 6 shows the measured forces on the knee for a variety of activities, as well as the flex angle of the knee during those activities. The forces on the knee vary with the body weight of the individual, so the forces shown in Table 6 are normalized for these differences.

Table 6. Flex angle and compressive force on the knee		
Activity	**Knee Flex Angle (°)**	**Normalized Peak Compressive Force on Knee (times body weight)***
Cycling	60-100	1.2
Walking	15	3.0
Stairs	60	3.8
Stairs	45	4.3
Squat-rise	140	5.0
Squat-down	140	5.6
*Calculated from peak force divided by (body mass times acceleration due to gravity (9.8 m/s2))		

Since the forces acting on the knee joint are a function of body mass, a study in obese individuals demonstrated the effect of body mass reduction on these forces. Table 7 shows the changes in body mass and BMI over the course of this study.

Table 7. Weight loss during study		
Parameter	**Baseline Values (kg ± SEM)**	**After Weight Loss (kg/m2 ± SEM)**
Body Mass	93.2 ± 1.3	90.8 ± 1.4
Body Mass Index	34.0 ± 0.4	33.0 ± 0.4

After adjusting each patient for baseline body mass, the reduction in peak compressive force on the knee while walking was found to be statistically significant ($P = 0.002$). Each 1 kg reduction in body mass was associated with a 40.6 N (1.4%) reduction in compressive force.

26. A woman with a body mass of 55 kg is standing up straight and not moving. Assuming the mass of each leg below her knee is 2.5 kg, what is the vertical force acting on each knee joint?

a. 245 N
b. 270 N
c. 490 N
d. 539 N

27. A woman with a body mass of 55 kg is walking with a knee flex angle of 15°. What is the peak compressive force on her knee?

a. 81 N
b. 539 N
c. 1617 N
d. 3593 N

28. Based on the data in the passage, a woman who loses body mass from 55 to 53 kg would have peak compressive forces on her knee while walking change in what way compared to before the weight loss?

a. Increase by 1.4%
b. Increase by 2.8%
c. Decrease by 1.4%
d. Decrease by 2.8%

29. A 65 kg woman descends twelve stairs with a total height of 3 m. She uses a 45°-knee flex angle. What is the decrease in her gravitational potential energy from descending the stairs?

a. 195 J
b. 819 J
c. 1911 J
d. 8217 J

30. At the end of a cycling test to evaluate knee joint force, the cyclists stopped rapidly. How much energy is required to stop a 70 kg man on a 5 kg bicycle, both of which are travelling 8 m/s?

a. 280 J
b. 560 J
c. 2240 J
d. 2400 J

PASSAGE 7

Read the paragraphs below and answer questions 31-35.

The physical properties of molecules are very dependent on their molecular shapes and sizes. Alcohols, for example, form a series where the trends of physical properties with size and shape can be clearly seen (Table 8). Boiling point, heat capacity, and the enthalpy of vaporization all rise substantially as the molecular weight increases.

Likewise, these properties vary significantly for different shapes of alcohols, as seen by comparing the two isomers of propanol and the three isomers of butanol. In the case of the butanols in the table, tert-butanol has the highest heat capacity, but the lowest boiling point and enthalpy of vaporization.

Table 8. Physical properties of alcohols

Alcohol	Boiling Point (°C)	ΔvapH° (kJ/mol)	Heat Capacity (liquid; J/mol·°C; at 25 °C)
methanol	65	38	81
ethanol	78	42	112
n-propanol	97	47	144
2-propanol	82	45	89
n-butanol	118	52	177
sec-butanol	100	48	198
tert-butanol	82	46	215
n-pentanol	138	57	208
n-hexanol	158	61	240

31. The boiling point, heat of vaporization, and heat capacity of n-hexanol are all considerably higher than the same properties of methanol. The reason that best explains that result is:

a. n-Hexanol is more effective at hydrogen bonding because it has a higher molecular weight than methanol.
b. n-Hexanol is more effective at hydrogen bonding because of its longer alkyl chain than methanol.
c. n-Hexanol is more effective at London dispersion interactions because it has a higher surface area than methanol.
d. n-Hexanol is more effective at ionic interactions because it has more carbon atoms than methanol.

32. How much energy is required to raise 23 grams of liquid ethanol at 72°C to its boiling point?

a. 138 J
b. 336 J
c. 672 J
d. 1120 J

33. How much energy is required to convert 64 grams of liquid methanol to vapor at the same temperature?

a. 19 J
b. 38 J
c. 76 J
d. 76,000 J

34. What is the minimum increase in entropy required for the vaporization of hexanol to be spontaneous at 25°C?

a. 178 J/(mole · K)
b. 53.2 J/(mole · K)
c. 24.0 J/(mole · K)
d. 1.58 J/(mole · K)

35. Which if the following is NOT an isomer of tert-butanol (boiling point = 82°C)?

a. diethyl ether (boiling point = 35°C)
b. 2-methoxypropane (boiling point = 39°C)
c. 2-methyl-1-propanol (boiling point = 108°C)
d. 3-methyl-1-butanol (boiling point = 131°C)

PASSAGE 8

Read the paragraphs below and answer questions 36-40.

The need for artificial devices for surgical replacement of damaged arteries is significant, but the demands put on the devices provide a difficult challenge for engineers. Evaluation of prototypes consisting of polymer tubing of various diameters is the first step toward developing such products.

John devised two different types of devices. One is rigid and retains its dimensions regardless of the internal pressure. The second type can expand slightly as the internal pressure increases, just as natural arteries can. For both types, testing involves a variety of different diameter tubes.

Table 9 shows some of his early testing of the flow rate of water through fixed lengths of tubing. The elastic tubing samples showed slightly higher flow rates than the rigid tubing of the same internal diameter. Using this data, John can evaluate whether the elastic tubing is expanding in a useful way compared to the rigid tubing, and whether either can do the job required.

Table 9. Evaluation of tubing as artificial arteries

Sample	Inner Diameter (mm)	Elastic	Rigid	Flow Rate (mL/min)*
A	10	No	Yes	160
B	8	No	Yes	65
C	4	No	Yes	4.1
D	1	No	Yes	0.02
E	10	Yes	No	187
F	8	Yes	No	77
G	4	Yes	No	4.8
H	1	Yes	No	0.02

*Measured with a pressure of 110 mm Hg at the proximal end and open to the air at the distal end.

36. Which of the following represents the best ranking of the relative blood pressure in the different parts of the circulatory system?

a. veins > venules > capillaries > arterioles > arteries
b. arterioles > arteries > capillaries > veins > venules
c. arteries > arterioles > capillaries > venules > veins
d. arteries > capillaries > arterioles > venules > veins

37. Which of the following is the primary benefit provided by the elasticity of natural arteries?

a. The minimum diastolic blood pressure is lower
b. Blood continues to flow between beats of the heart
c. Oxygen more readily diffuses from the arteries
d. The walls of the arteries can be thinner than veins

38. In the initial calibration of the device to measure the flow rate through the artificial arteries, a scientist attaches a pressure gauge to the distal end of each tube. With the pressure gauge attached, the pump is turned on, but there is no flow because the gauge blocks the fluid. Which expression best describes the pressure at the end of Sample C compared the pressure at the end of Sample A?

a. Sample C shows 25% of the pressure of Sample A
b. Sample C shows 400% of the pressure of Sample A
c. Sample C shows 2.6% of the pressure of Sample A
d. Both show the same pressure

39. If the pressure of the pump used to drive the flow of the test fluid is increased from 110 mm Hg to 160 mm Hg, the flow from Sample B is most likely to be which of the following?

a. 95 mL/min
b. 85 mL/min
c. 75 mL/min
d. 65 mL/min

40. Repeating the experiments in Table 9 with whole blood instead of water gives different results. Using a whole blood sample that has viscosity four times that of water, what is the expected flow rate of whole blood through Sample G with a starting pressure of 110 mm Hg?

a. 1.2 mL/min
b. 1.6 mL/min
c. 2.4 mL/min
d. 4.8 mL/min

PASSAGE 9

Read the paragraphs below and answer questions 41-45.

When carbon dioxide dissolves in biological solutions such as blood, it equilibrates with a number of different forms, including unhydrated carbon dioxide, carbonic acid, bicarbonate, and carbonate. The hydration of carbon dioxide and the dehydration of carbonic acid are each relatively slow, with half-lives of 18 and 0.05 seconds, respectively (Table 10).

Table 10. Reaction constants for the hydration and dehydration of carbon dioxide in water at 25°C (pH 7)

Reaction	Uncatalyzed hydration constant, k (s-1) at 25°C	Uncatalyzed hydration half-life (s) at 25°C	Uncatalyzed dehydration constant k(s-1) at 25°C	Uncatalyzed dehydration half-life (s) at 25°C
CO2 + H2O → H2CO3	0.0375	18	--	--
H2CO3 → CO2 + H2O	--	--	13.7	0.05

These conversion rates are too slow for a variety of biological processes, and many organisms employ enzymes to speed the process. Many isozymes of carbonic anhydrase catalyze both the hydration and dehydration reactions to speed processes such as excretion of carbon dioxide from the lungs.

Judy believes she has isolated a new isozyme of carbonic anhydrase from mouse tissue. She measures some of its attributes in catalyzing the hydration of carbon dioxide (Table 11). She also modifies certain amino acids in the enzyme to see how altering them affects catalysis and whether they are critical for functionality (Table 11).

Table 11. Attributes of modified versions of carbonic anhydrase to catalyze the hydration of carbon dioxide in water at 25°C (pH 7)

Enzyme Modification	Km (mM)	(Kcat; s-1)	Kcat/Km (M-1s-1)
Native	4.0	2 × 105	5 × 107
1	4.2	3 × 105	7 × 107
2	4.8	1.5 × 105	3 × 107
3	56.1	3 × 104	5 × 105
4	2.9	2 × 103	7 × 105
5	13.1	1 × 105	8 × 106

Judy also studies the effect of the glaucoma drug acetazolamide on the activity of these enzymes since it is known to affect the activity of other isozymes of carbonic anhydrase (Table 12).

Table 12. Attributes of modified versions of carbonic anhydrase in presence of acetazolamide (5 μM) in water at 25°C (pH 7)

Enzyme Modification	Km (mM)	(Kcat; s-1)	Kcat/Km (M-1s-1)
Native	26	2 × 105	8 × 106
1	40	3 × 105	8 × 106
2	4.8	1.5 × 105	3 × 107
3	160	3 × 104	2 × 105
4	12	2 × 103	2 × 105
5	56	1 × 105	2 × 106

41. A Lineweaver-Burk plot used by Judy to determine Km is a plot of which of the following parameters?

a. 1/vo vs 1/[S]
b. 1/Vmax vs 1/[S]
c. 1/vo vs 1/Km
d. 1/Km vs 1/Vmax

42. Which modified enzyme has the highest affinity for carbon dioxide in water at 25°C (pH 7)?

a. Modification 1
b. Modification 3
c. Modification 4
d. Modification 5

43. Which modified enzyme is able to convert carbon dioxide to carbonic acid the fastest under conditions of saturating carbon dioxide concentrations?

a. Native Enzyme
b. Modification 1
c. Modification 4
d. Modification 5

44. Based on the data in the passage, acetazolamide is which of the following?

a. A noncompetitive inhibitor of Native Enzyme
b. A competitive inhibitor of the Native Enzyme
c. A mixed inhibitor of the Native Enzyme
d. Not an inhibitor of the Native Enzyme

45. Based on the data in the passage, if Modified Enzyme 3 is tested for activity in the presence of 10 μM acetazolamide, which result is most likely?

a. Km = 450 mM
b. Km = 160 mM
c. Km = 56 mM
d. Km = 23 mM

Discrete Questions

46. The electrical energy (W) stored in the membrane potential of a living cell can be modelled as a parallel plate capacitor. If the thickness of the cell membrane doubles and the charge on each side remains the same, what is the change in the stored energy in this model?

a. no change to W
b. increases to $2W$
c. decreases to $\frac{W}{2}$
d. decreases to $\frac{W}{\sqrt{2}}$

47. Which of the following glass optics in air is a diverging lens?

a. 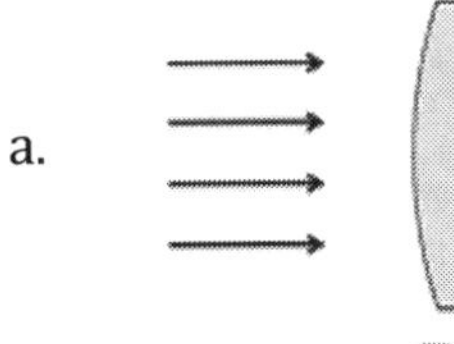

b. 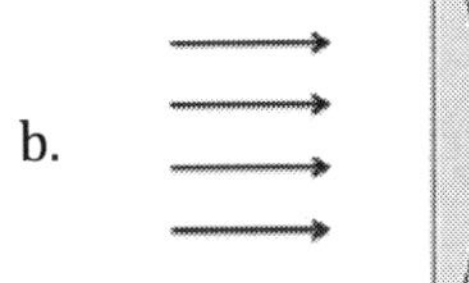

c. 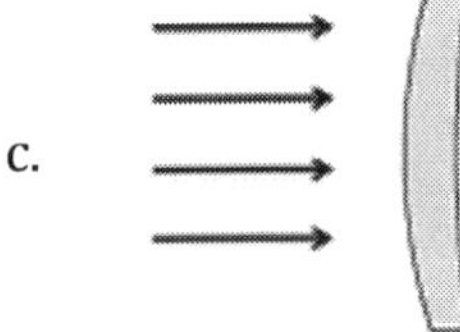

d. 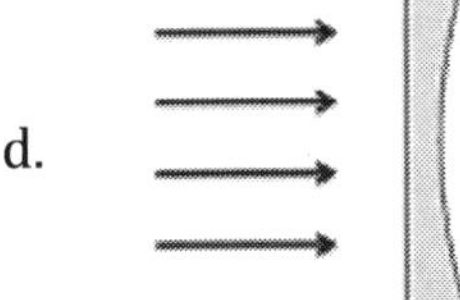

48. Which of the following chemicals is NOT produced and consumed in part of the standard tricarboxylic acid cycle?

a. Succinate
b. Oxalate
c. Fumarate
d. Malate

49. Fish living in arctic waters have a variety of adaptations to function in such a cold environment. One of these is to increase their membrane fluidity at lower temperatures, relative to temperate fish. Which of the following 22-carbon fatty acids would contribute most to increased fluidity of a cell membrane at low temperature?

a. CH3(CH2)20CO2H
b. all-cis-CH3(CH2)4CH=CHCH2CH=CH(CH2)11CO2H
c. all-cis-CH3CH2CH=CHCH2CH=CHCH2CH=CHCH2CH=CHCH2CH=CHCH2CH=CHCH2CH2CO2H
d. all-trans-CH3CH2CH=CHCH2CH=CHCH2CH=CHCH2CH=CHCH2CH=CHCH2CH=CHCH2CH2CO2H

50. A protein at its isoelectric point has which of the following attributes?

a. It moves in an electric field at a rate proportional to its molecular weight.
b. It has no net electric charge.
c. Its solubility is at a maximum.
d. It contains no charged functional groups.

51. Bacteria have a cell membrane to help provide physical protection to the cell. The rigid structural framework of the cell wall is composed of which materials?

a. polysaccharide chains covalently crosslinked with peptide chains
b. polysaccharide chains ionically crosslinked with peptide chains
c. proteins crosslinked with hyaluronic acid
d. hyaluronic acid crosslinked with N-acetylneuraminic acid

52. Messenger RNA in a mammal has which of the following attributes?

a. It is single stranded
b. It is double stranded
c. It is synthesized in the ribosome
d. It contains two phosphate groups per nucleotide

53. Which of the following is the correct structure of pyrimidine?

a. 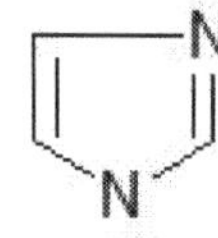

b. 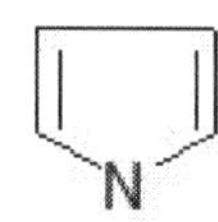

c. 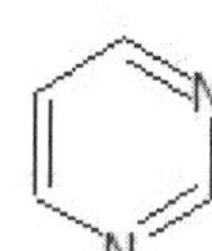

d. 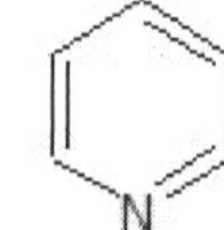

54. Where does protein translation takes place in a eukaryote?

a. on ribosomes in the nucleus
b. on ribosomes in the cytoplasm
c. on the mRNA in the nucleus
d. on the DNA in the cytoplasm

55. Which of the following reactions shows a keto-enol tautomeric pair?

a.

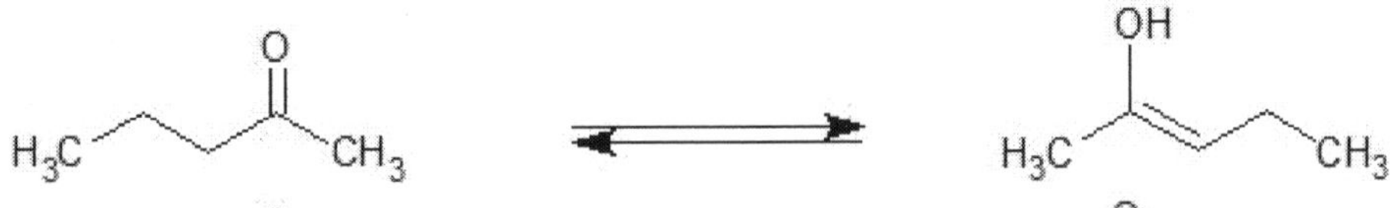

b.

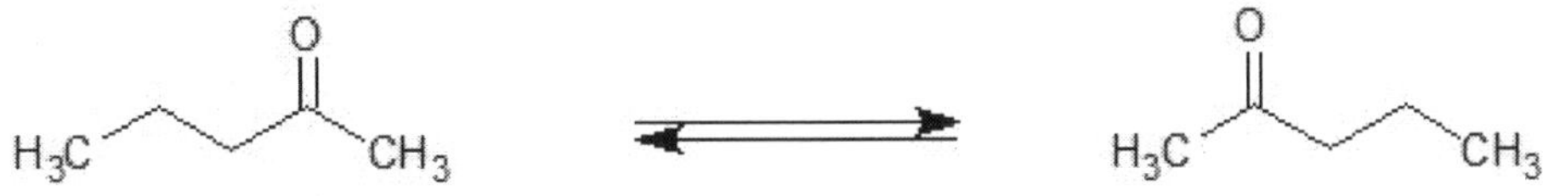

c.

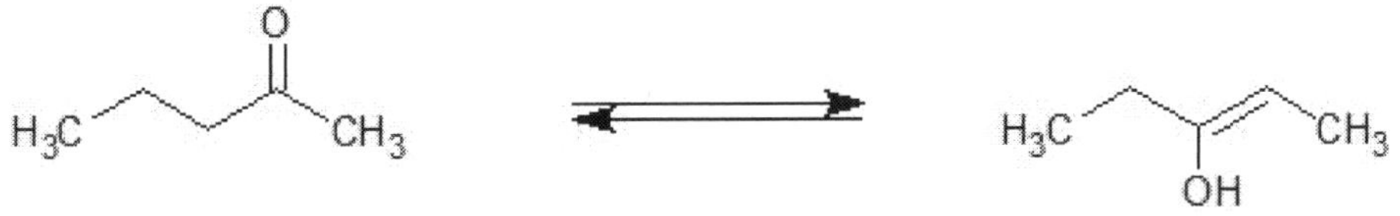

d.

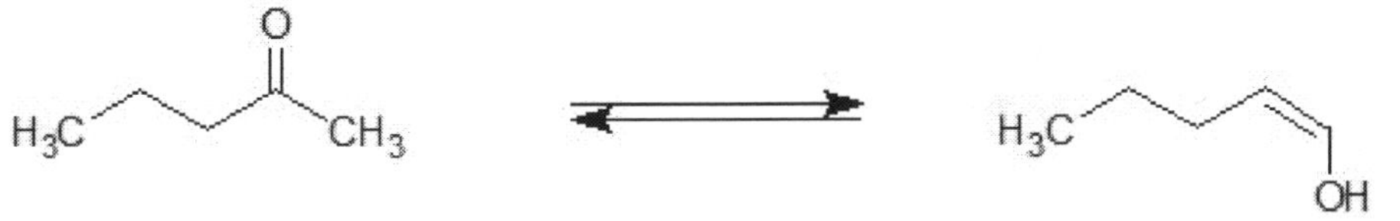

56. Which of the following structures does NOT represent a mechanistic step in the acid-catalyzed hydrolysis of methyl acetate?

a.

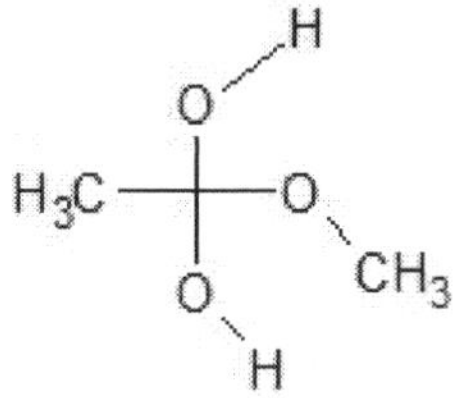

b.

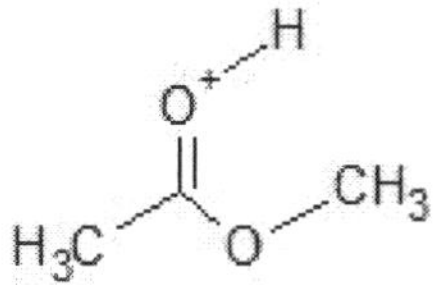

c.

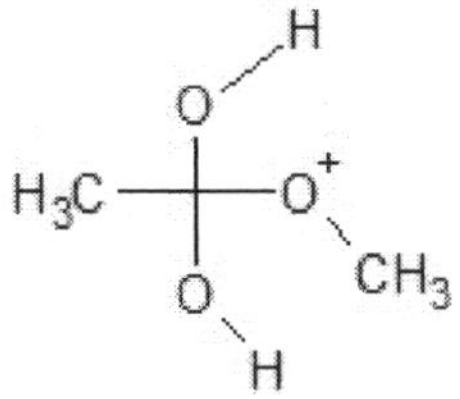

d.

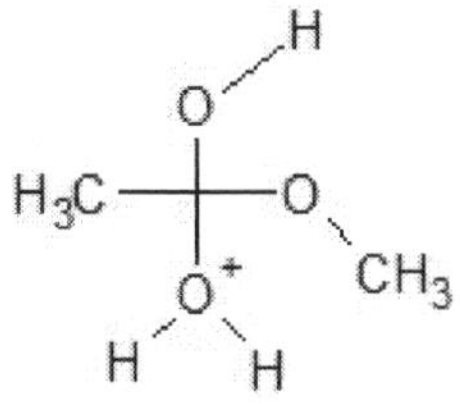

57. Isocitrate dehydrogenase catalyzes the following reaction in the tricarboxylic acid cycle:

isocitrate + NAD+ → α-ketoglutarate + CO_2 + NADH + H+

Which of the following half reactions correctly represent this reaction?

a. isocitrate → α-ketoglutarate + CO_2 + 2H+ + 2e-
NAD+ + 2H+ + 2e- → NADH
b. isocitrate → α-ketoglutarate + CO_2 + 2H+ + 2e-
NADH + H+ + 2e- → NAD+
c. isocitrate → α-ketoglutarate + CO_2 + 2H+ + 2e-
NAD+ + H+ + 2e- → NADH
d. isocitrate → α-ketoglutarate + CO_2 + H+ + 2e-
NAD+ + H+ + 2e- → NADH

58. Which of the following Fischer projections represents the aldohexose D-glucose?

a.
O
H — OH
H — OH
H — OH
OH

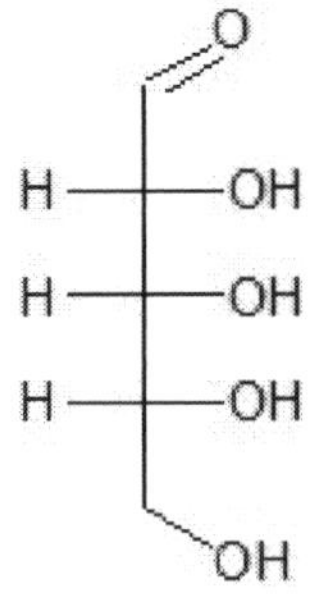

b.
OH
=O
HO — H
H — OH
H — OH
OH

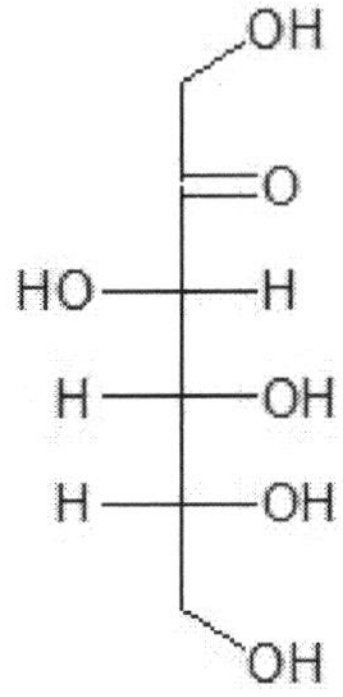

c.
O
H — OH
HO — H
H — OH
OH

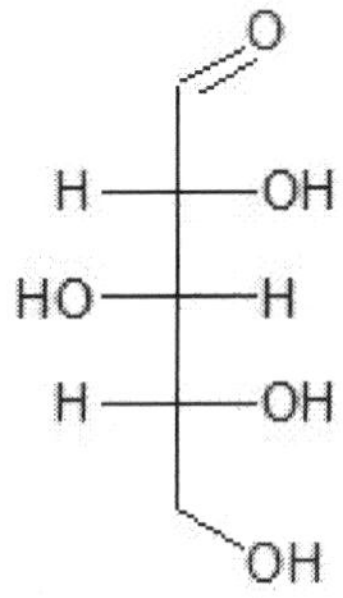

d.
O
H — OH
HO — H
H — OH
H — OH
OH

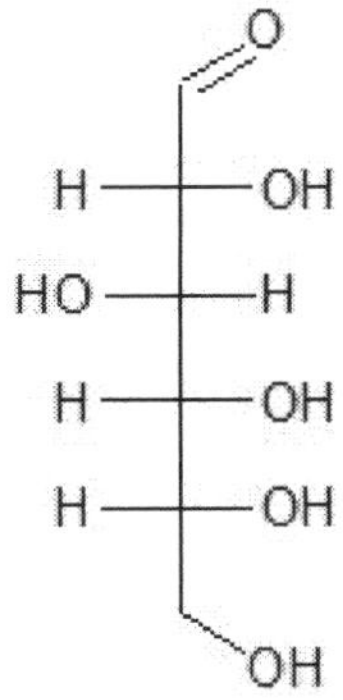

59. Which of the following pairs of chemicals are most completely separated by simple batch distillation?

a. CH3CH2CH3 and CH3CH2CH2F
b. CH3CH2CH3 and CH3CH2CH2Cl
c. CH3CH2CH3 and CH3CH2CH2Br
d. CH3CH2CH3 and CH3CH2CH2I

Psychological, Social, and Biological Foundations

Passage 1

A retrospective research study evaluated more than 2,400 employees from three different companies to determine the risk factors for leaves of absence from work due to psychiatric ailments. Questionnaires including queries about childhood events were distributed to participants who were selected at random. Survey respondents' answers were compared to their work attendance records. Documented absences from work for psychiatric ailments were divided into the five categories listed below. Employees who had at least one documented leave of absence for a psychiatric ailment lasting for at least one day and individuals who did not have a documented leave of absence for a psychiatric ailment were included in the study. The study was designed to determine whether there was a link between childhood experiences and the development of behavioral and psychiatric disorders during adulthood. The study evaluated male and female participants aged 20–55. The data, which are reported as average days absent from work during a one-year period, are shown below.

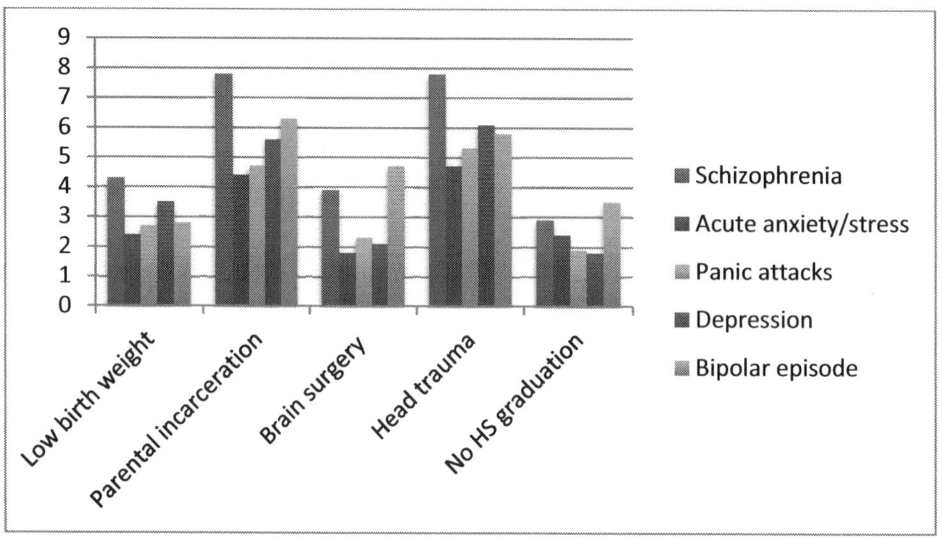

Low birth weight was considered birth weight below the 10% percentile.

Parental incarceration prior to age 18 of the study participant.

History of brain surgery prior to age 18.

History of head trauma hospitalization not requiring surgery prior to age 18.

High school graduation versus no high school graduation.

1. How could you explain the stronger relationship between head trauma and work absences than between brain surgery and work absences?

a. Mood disorders and psychiatric disorders are often amplified by emotional events and therefore are often triggered by posttraumatic stress after head trauma, whereas surgery produces neurological changes such as weakness due to structural abnormalities.
b. Disruptions in the central nervous system (CNS) blood-brain barrier and electrophysiological alterations in the brain that persist after head trauma cause persistent symptoms that are difficult to manage, whereas symptoms that occur after brain surgery are more often manageable with medications.
c. Brain surgery is a therapeutic procedure that repairs disease, whereas head trauma causes disease.
d. Brain surgery is usually asymmetric, and psychiatric ailments and mood disorders are caused by symmetric deficits.

2. Why would schizophrenia appear to be the most common cause of work absence in this study if mood disorders such as depression are more prevalent in the population?

a. If a person has a mood disorder, the work setting is found to be therapeutic, and therefore individuals with mood disorders are less likely to take time off from work.
b. Schizophrenia is, in fact, more common than mood disorders, but due to the social stigma, it is not as well recognized.
c. Mood disorders are not severe enough to require affected individuals to take time off from work.
d. Schizophrenia is the most likely of these diagnoses to precipitate exacerbations severe enough to necessitate medical treatment or hospitalization.

3. How does bipolar disorder compare to depression and schizophrenia?

a. Bipolar disorder and depression are both mood disorders that are not associated with alterations in perception of reality, whereas schizophrenia is manifested by paranoid delusions and altered perception of reality, not mood alterations.
b. Although bipolar disorder is manifested by extreme mood alterations, it is more likely to present with clinical characteristics that resemble schizophrenia, such as agitation and paranoia, than with predominantly depressive symptoms.
c. Bipolar disorder produces a combination of contrasting symptoms, which requires a combination of medications that affect behavior of different neurotransmitters, whereas depression and schizophrenia often vary in symptom severity over time and require medication adjustment, but they are generally treated with medications that target a more limited group of neurotransmitters.
d. Bipolar disorder is associated with relapses and remission, and thus individuals can take a medication "vacation," whereas depression and schizophrenia require constant therapy for symptomatic control.

4. How would you expect acute anxiety to affect attitudes toward missing work?

a. People with acute anxiety and stress have normal brain structure and function, and thus most likely call off work only when there is a real threat in the work setting.
b. Those with acute anxiety are most often afraid to call off work for fear of being fired, and thus they are expected to go to work even during times of illness.
c. Acute anxiety makes the prospect of missing work and the prospect of going to work both threatening options, and thus individuals with acute anxiety view the notion of missing work as an added source of anxiety.
d. People who are anxious are usually overachievers and transfer a sense of anxiety and drive to others around them, and thus they would be more likely to be angry with others for missing work, while forgiving themselves under the same circumstances.

5. How can social cognitive theory explain a difference in calling in sick between individuals of differing income levels?

a. Individuals observe behavior and consequences among peers and learn through the outcomes of peers who hold an equivalent position and status whether it would be favorable or not to call in sick in that particular work environment.
b. Those with lower income levels want to even the playing field by calling in sick, thus "compensating" for lower hourly pay by decreasing the number of hours worked.
c. Social peer group acceptance determines whether individuals call in sick, and thus those at a lower income level strive to imitate the actions of those at the higher income level.
d. Calling in sick at work is based on cognitive criteria that encompass the safety of coworkers, and thus social cognitive theory suggests that individuals with a greater sense of responsibility will take action to ensure that the work is done and to ensure the safety and health of the peer group.

PASSAGE 2

Social dynamics of migrant populations may appear to be different than nonmigrant social groups at first glance. Many members of immigrant populations look to peers within their immigrant group, and particularly to influential members of the peer groups, as anchors by which they can interpret the values of the new society in light of the established values of the baseline society from which they came from and more closely identify with. The older an individual is when moving to a new setting, the more he holds the values of his original environment and the more he craves approval from peers of his native land than approval from peers of his new setting. In fact, dominant peers within an immigrant community may be so influential as to establish new social norms that they safely combine selected values of the adopted region with unalterable values of the original setting. It is through a process of subconscious and conscious exploration driven in large part by the most esteemed members of the migrant peer group that new social norms are established.

This makes the local media, which is often a binding force among inhabitants of a region, less important to immigrant communities. The media in such situations is viewed through a lens that may be different from that which is intended. However, even among indigenous social groups, local dynamics play a role in establishing social norms.

An experiment designed to evaluate conformity evaluated college students who were registered for a year-long seminar. Students' attire was noted at every class session, which met twice per week. Graduate student leaders were instructed to dress in a professional manner in order to assess whether the college students altered their attire. At the first session, 90% of the college students wore blue jeans, leggings, or shorts. Within the first month, 40% of the college students wore pants or skirts that were similar in style to the graduate students' attire, and by the last month, 70% of the college students wore pants or skirts similar in style to the graduate students' attire.

6. How does social control result in sanctions that affect college students who dress more casually than the expected standards in a seminar and sanctions that affect guests at a party attended exclusively by immigrants from the same region?

a. Students may be excluded from opportunities to answer questions in class or lead group activities, whereas guests at a social event may be excluded from peer group conversations and further invitations if the unwritten rules of behavior are not followed.
b. Students will receive low grades due to evaluators' perception that the students don't care about the material, whereas guests at a party will find themselves victims of peer group gossip as peers attempt to understand or explain nonconforming behaviors or styles of dress.
c. Students will be marginalized by peers who do not want to be associated with a negative image, whereas other guests at a party would want to avoid being seen with nonconforming guests to avoid being regarded with low status.
d. Students would work harder in the course due to a subjective personal inference that they are not ready for the level of rigor, and guests at a party would try harder to find ways to fit in with the majority of the group at the next party.

7. How would group polarization affect the actions of students who choose not to dress in more formal attire during the seminar?

a. Students who dress in less formal attire would attempt other ways to compensate, such as showing up on time or answering questions during class.
d. The students who dress in less formal attire would view themselves as less suited for the course and thus would study more for the seminar and achieve better test grades than those who do not.
c. Students who dress in less formal attire for the seminar would try to undermine peers who also dress in less formal attire in order to achieve some sense of power.
d. Students would exaggerate their casual dress style to show solidarity and rejection of the formal attire and the unwritten code associated with it.

8. Group hysteria is acceptable in one setting but not in another. What would inhibit an individual from participating in events involving group hysteria if his previous group did not accept group hysteria but his adopted group does?

a. Social control
b. Peer pressure
c. Deindividuation
d. Deviance

9. How would the prospective power of sanctions play a role in compelling dominant individuals in a small ethnic group to follow norms?

a. Dominant characters do not feel the need to follow norms because they are more likely to set the norms, and thus they can more easily choose how to blend characteristics of both cultures, often to their own preference.
b. Dominant characters do not have to follow social norms because they decide who is in the in group and who is in the out group, and thus they are not concerned about sanctions, whereas most members of the social group are concerned about sanctions.
c. Some dominant members may be acutely fearful of sanctions and thus driven to follow norms, whereas some nondominant members may be less invested in the group, and thus they are less fearful of sanctions resulting from neglecting norms.
d. Dominant characters rely on the acceptance of their lower status peers for self-esteem and social interaction, and thus they are likely to follow social norms as faithfully as less dominant individuals in the group, but with an emphasis on maintaining an appearance of less effort, and often they must be the first to "try on" social norms of the adopted culture in order to maintain unwritten status as leaders.

10. Which of the following is a method by which individuals can protect themselves against anomie?

a. Construct laws to prevent chaos.
b. Maintain a connection with a group or society to avoid the alienation that can occur from social stigma.
c. Work to ensure that expected norms are relaxed to avoid a sense of lack of acceptance from the prevailing group.
d. Uphold a strong moral compass to avoid falling into a disoriented state personally and socially.

11. Conscious awareness of and adaptations to the various standards expected in diverse settings is a personal characteristic of many individuals. How would awareness of differing agents of socialization protect an individual from the mental anguish of ostracism?

a. Awareness of the differing agents of socialization can help an individual objectively defend himself against unfair or biased reasons for ostracism so that he does not suffer from the anguish of ostracism.
b. Awareness of differing agents of socialization can build empathy, which prevents an individual from being ostracized and thus from experiencing the emotional pain of ostracism.
c. Awareness of differing agents of socialization among different populations allows an individual to combine elements of one community's social norms with that of another, essentially gaining a better rounded social ability than other members of the community.
d. Awareness of the differing agents of socialization allows an individual to understand that socialization and norms are not set as universal, which can protect an individual from the emotional turmoil of rejection.

Passage 3

Associative learning is generally achieved with little, if any, effort. However, our understanding of the volitional ability to harness associative learning has allowed therapists to use learning methods to help people manage acquired and inborn emotional deficits in empathy. A group of stroke survivors was assessed for their ability to identify emotions by watching videos. Two other groups, a group of age-matched individuals with Asperger's and a group of age-matched controls, were also evaluated.

The three groups participated in a yearlong longitudinal study, which involved watching five different three-minute videos. After watching one minute of each video, participants were asked to identify the emotions of the people in the video, and after watching two additional minutes of the video, participants were provided with accurate labels of the emotions represented in the videos. Tests were repeated every two months. The same video was never repeated so that participants would avoid memorizing the answers. The scores are shown below.

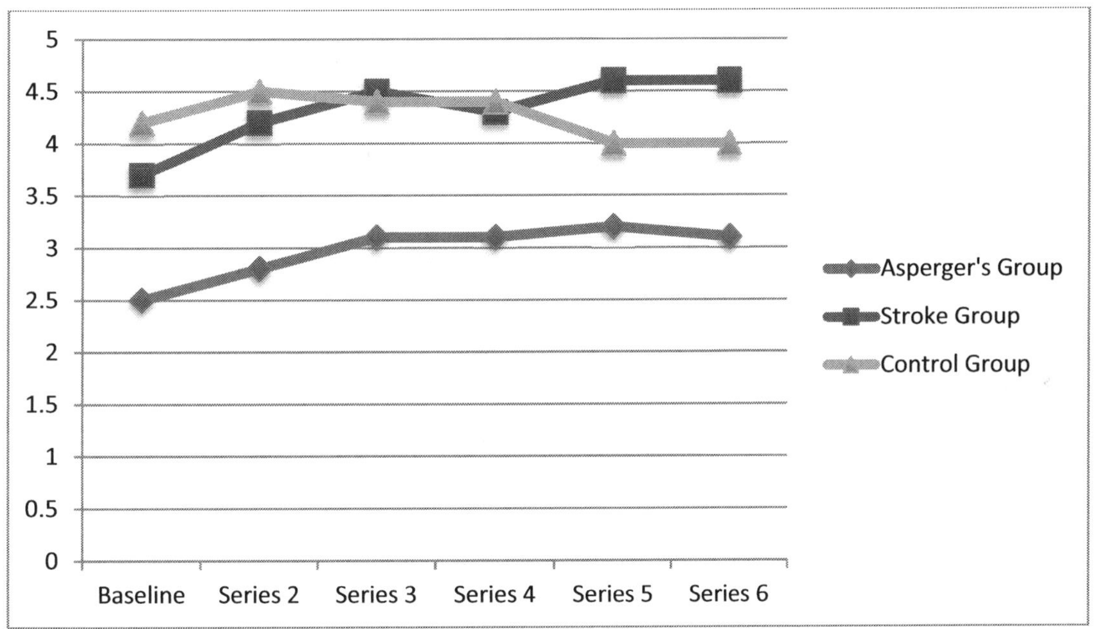

12. How would you explain the finding that the stroke group improved more than the Asperger's group?

a. The stroke group has had more real-life experiences that included positive reinforcement for correctly identifying emotions, which is a motivating factor in learning this skill, whereas the Asperger's group has not had as many real-life experiences or motivation to build on.

b. The stroke group had visual problems but not deficits in emotional perception, and thus they were more easily able to work on relearning how to recognize visual cues, whereas the Asperger's group had a more difficult task of learning how to recognize emotional cues.

c. The Asperger's group doesn't place a strong emphasis on social interaction, whereas the stroke group is invested in improving social skills to regain past abilities.

d. The Asperger's group has a deficit that is present from birth, and thus it has a severe lack of activity in certain areas of the cerebral cortex, whereas the stroke group is more disposed to the reparative effects of neuroplasticity.

13. What is the most likely explanation for the decreased score in the control group?

a. Prolonged exposure
b. Extinction
c. Habituation
d. Dishabituation

14. Using operant conditioning, which type of reinforcement schedule is most consistent with real-life application of this skill?

a. Fixed-ratio schedule
b. Fixed-interval schedule
c. Variable-interval schedule
d. Variable-ratio schedule

15. Which group would you expect to have a higher recruitment of mirror neurons in learning the correct responses?

a. The Asperger's group
b. The control group
c. The stroke group
d. All groups are expected to be equal.

16. One of the participants who had a particularly low score to begin with did not improve at all during the yearlong study. Interestingly, videos of his participation demonstrated that his own face reflected the expressions of the actors in the videos he was watching. According to classical conditioning, what does his own facial response represent?

a. The conditioned stimulus
b. The conditioned response
c. The unconditioned stimulus
d. The unconditioned response

Passage 4

The degree to which an individual believes he can control external events is determined by a combination of personal nature, environmental influences, and personal experiences that modify beliefs about the consequences of personal action. An individual's overall sense of control over his environment is generally overarching throughout most aspects of his life. Yet, an individual may have a greater or diminished sense of control over certain aspects of his life in comparison to his overall baseline sense of control.

An experiment endeavored to observe waiters' sense of control over their environment. The experiment also attempted to modify waiters' sense of control over their environment and, finally, to teach them how much control they had over their environment through the results of the experiment.

New waiters in a restaurant who were still in the training phase were divided into two groups for the experiment. One group of trainees was told that guests of the restaurant were particularly generous with tips, whereas the control group of waiter trainees was not given any verbal or nonverbal signal regarding the tipping tendencies of guests. The guests were not aware of the experiment.

At the end of the six-hour shift, the waiters were asked their subjective opinions about the tips and were asked to report the numbers. The waiters who had been previously told that guests of the restaurant were generous tippers tended to describe guests as generous, whereas the control group, who had not been provided with any persuasive messages, described the tips as average. The waiters who had been told that guests were generous received tips that were, on average, 30% higher in total than the other group.

17. What concept explains the difference in tips?

a. Self-fulfilling prophecy
b. Stereotyping
c. Prestige
d. Stigma

18. How could the owners use this experimental information to motivate staff to avoid stereotyping guests?

a. Give the guests instruction on how to act in ways that are opposite to stereotypes.
b. Explain the experiment to demonstrate to the staff that guests show appreciation for good treatment.
c. Give the staff a financial incentive for treating all guests equally.
d. Present information and examples of ways that guests behave in ways that counteract and reverse stereotypes.

19. After comparing the tips, a waiter with a strong internal locus of control would be expected to relate to a waiter who did not receive a tip in which of the following ways?

a. With an attitude that encourages self-control in dealing with disappointment.
b. With benevolence and charity.
c. With concern for the victim's self-esteem more than concern for the victim's short-term finances.
d. With blame for causing his own misfortune.

20. Which of the following would be expected to drive modifications in the control group's behavior as they serve customers throughout the six-hour shift?

a. Positive reinforcement, in which the waiters receive good tips and thus are motivated to provide high-quality service in order to continue receiving good tips.
b. Negative reinforcement, in which the waiters initially receive poor tips and are motivated to provide better service so as to receive higher tips.
c. Punishment, in which the waiters are reprimanded by their supervisor if they receive a poor tip and admonished to provide better service.
d. All three of these are expected to play a role in the modification of behavior during the shift.

21. How can instructors in the experiment use the peripheral route described in the elaboration likelihood model to persuade waiters that customers who order alcohol are more or less trustworthy than customers who do not order alcohol?

a. Instructors can stimulate the visual pathways of the waiters' peripheral nervous systems by showing them different-colored drink menus to trigger a psychological color response associated with trustworthiness.
b. Instructors can state that the non-alcohol-drinking group is trustworthy and omit mentioning the other group to raise questions about the group's trustworthiness
c. Instructors can remind a waiter of a feature present in a third group of individuals who the waiter believes to be untrustworthy, where that same feature is also present in the alcohol-drinking group.
d. Instructors can elaborate on peripheral details of the situation that are not necessarily relevant to trustworthiness to build an additive effect of peripheral details that are difficult to ignore and that outweigh the core features related to generosity.

Passage 5

Children of one or more emotionally unstable parents experience a great deal of stress, which can be expressed in a variety of ways. Multiple factors, including the condition of the parents' marriage, the degree of parental emotional instability, and parental attitudes toward and interactions with the children play roles in how the child senses and reacts to the parental emotional and behavioral turmoil.

A pediatric hospital screens for child abuse and childhood stress by asking pediatric patients to fill out nonmandatory surveys in the waiting room prior to their appointments.

Survey questions include the following:

- How good are you at taking care of yourself?
- Do you ever worry that your parent will not be able to take care of you anymore before you graduate from high school?
- Do you think that your parents are able to take care of you as well as, better than, or worse than other kids' parents?
- Do you ever have to take care of your parents?
- Some open-ended questions include the following:
    - What have you learned from your parents?
    - What does one of your parents do that you want to learn how to do?
    - What compliment does your mother give you?
    - What compliment does your father give you?
    - What compliment from someone who is not in your family most surprised you?
    - What word best describes you?

Approximately 60% of the patients filled out the forms. Children who were younger than six years old often asked parents for help in filling out the forms. Approximately 40% of the parents refused to have their children complete the forms. It was noted that patients who had a high copay were three times more likely to refuse to fill out the forms than patients who had a low copay or no copay.

22. Which of the following factors would cause a child to avoid answers that reflect negatively on his parents?

a. Role strain and role conflict
b. Altruism and deindividuation
c. Fear of role exit
d. Obedience and role conflict

23. Why would a child try to alter a parent's back-stage self to match the parent's front-stage self?

a. The parent's front-stage self is more desirable for the child.
b. This is a child's attempt at impression management.
c. In order to blend better with others.
d. To avoid social stigma.

24. Given the disparity in compliance rates based on the level of copay, what is the most valid conclusion that can be drawn regarding the parents' response with regard to the survey?

a. Those who had a low or no copay were more concerned with obedience toward their health-care providers.
b. Those who had a higher copay behaved with higher sense of power and authority.
c. Those who had a higher copay were more likely to have privacy concerns.
d. Those who had a low or no copay were not as busy and had more time to complete the survey.

25. If a child's answer regarding a word that best describes her is based on a compliment that she receives regarding a particular trait, what influence is at play in forming her identity formation?

a. Low self-esteem
b. Looking-glass self
c. Self-fulfilling prophecy
d. Impression management

26. If a child answers that he wants to learn something from his parent, but upon learning the skill he is ridiculed by his peers, how would he most likely view his parent's lesson based on this external response?

a. With rejection
b. With sympathy
c. With mistrust
d. With craving for acceptance

PASSAGE 6

Globalization is an inevitable result of affluence, education, and technology. Views about religion are susceptible to the influences of globalization. The way that patients view health care has historically been shaped by parochial values, but this view is becoming more influenced by attitudes and outcomes in geographically distant lands. International medicine includes international medical education, medical missions, and medical tourism. These costly enterprises are heavily swayed by the availability of and sources of funding.

An international medical care experience scholarship for medical students is funded by an organization dedicated to promoting young women's education (YWE) for the longitudinal purpose of reducing infant mortality and domestic abuse. Scholarship recipients will see patients in a local clinic. Recipients will also maintain contact with young female patients by sending them reminders to enroll in school, encouragement to study for exams, and requests to report whether they have passed each year of school

Electronic medical records (EMRs) are also being implemented in the region, and although they are being funded and set up by a different organization, the YWE program has made plans to allow scholarship benefactors to use the EMR system for input and gathering patient information during medical visits in the local clinic.

Medical student scholarship applicants are asked several questions during the interview including the following questions: "How important is it to respect the religion of tribes and regions?" and "What do you define as a cult versus a religion?"

27. How could a hidden curriculum influence which applicants are granted the scholarships?

a. The scholarship benefactors may want students to teach religion classes to villagers, despite the fact that it is not stated as one of the responsibilities in the program description.
b. The scholarship benefactors may want to select students who are of the same religion as members of the YWE program to make working together easier.
c. The scholarship benefactors may be irreligious and believe that all religions are cults and thus select applicants who feel the same way.
d. The scholarship benefactors may have a biased opinion of religion and use the program to indoctrinate students in their viewpoint on religion, even though it is not the stated objective.

28. How would the medicalization of domestic abuse affect treatment of domestic abuse survivors in the region where this medical project is taking place?

a. It would cause the burden of care to fall solely on physicians.
b. It would eliminate the gender stigma of men who are victims of domestic abuse.
c. It would result in increased funding and attention being devoted to addressing the issue.
d. It would become tolerated as a medical condition rather than viewed as the fault of the perpetrator, and thus it may become socially acceptable.

29. According to the concept of symbolic interactionism, how would you expect a medical student's interaction with a patient in another culture to proceed if the patient reminds the student of a friend who betrayed her trust?

a. She would be expected to try to ignore the reminder of the betrayal by adopting an intentionally cheerful attitude around the patient.
b. She would be expected to subconsciously attempt to repair her feelings regarding the broken relationship through her interactions with the patient.
c. She would be expected treat the patient with mistrust based on the patient's similarities with the betraying friend.
d. She would not be expected to have any response because symbolic interactionism describes a strictly voluntary response.

30. When electronic medical records (EMRs) are implemented in the region described in this example, there will be a lag in the seamless adoption of the EMR system. How does culture lag explain the relative similarities in adoption rates of EMRs among developing and developed nations despite the profound material differences?

a. Developed nations lag behind in EMR technology because they do not have a large enough workforce to construct the technology, so it is easier for developing nations to catch up with EMR despite material disadvantages.
b. Both developing and developed nations take time to adopt newly available technology, so a nation that lacks the material resources can implement EMR almost as quickly a nation with material resources because the people in both cultures spend time learning how to use the technology before it becomes widely available and practical for use.
c. The technology lags behind the culture in developed nations due to resistance because of the innate efficiency of the health-care workforce in developed countries, so the end result is that a system such as EMR is adopted at the same rate in developed and developing nations.
d. The technology pulls the developing nations forward so that people can learn how to use technology as well as the people in developed countries.

31. How would a woman who was chronically deprived of power and independence in the population being served by the YWE program view a meritocratic environment, as compared to another woman who was unable to attain recognition in such an environment due to lack of effort?

a. The woman without power and the woman who failed despite having had opportunities would each disapprove of a meritocracy because neither was able to achieve recognition.
b. The woman without power positively views a system of meritocracy because she believes it would have allowed her to achieve recognition, whereas the woman who failed craves a different system in which she would be shielded from failure.
c. The woman without power appreciates the meritocracy because she can enjoy experiences through mirror neurons, whereas the woman who failed cannot do so.
d. It depends on each person's individual experiences and alliances and well as his or her social position and empathy.

Passage 7

The prison population is largely supported by public funds. Health care is provided to prisoners through public funds, and therefore reduction of disease-related complications is expected to reduce the cost of maintaining the health of prisoners. This population has unique demographic characteristics and a different distribution of health conditions than the general population.

Persistent pain, refractory to pain medication, was noted in a cost-control analysis of prisoner health costs. Attempts to decrease costs by using generic medications were found to be ineffective after a six-month trial. A different approach was then adopted. This approach was to determine the etiology of pain and treat the underlying cause.

A preliminary subset of prison patients with refractory neuropathic pain was selected. A retrospective chart review conducted using the medical records of a prisoner population and the medical records of controls sought to evaluate the etiology of neuropathic pain, a condition associated with a variety of etiologies.

The results are found in the chart below.

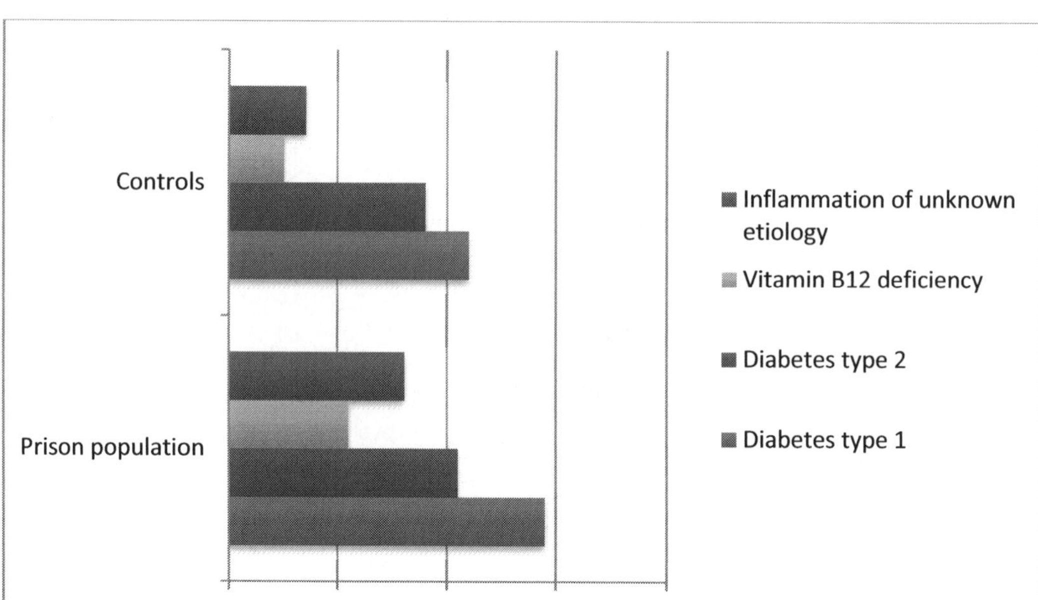

32. What could explain the relatively higher incidence of inflammation of unknown etiology in the prison population compared to the other diagnoses?

a. Inflammation of unknown etiology noted at higher rates in the charts of the prison population is indicative of diminished access to care, which results in reduced accuracy of diagnoses of etiology and reduced treatment of inflammatory conditions.
b. Inflammation is a finding in the central nervous system tissue of individuals with drug abuse and with psychiatric diagnosis, both of which increase the risk of criminal behavior.
c. The prison setting exposes people to infections that trigger difficult-to-diagnose inflammatory conditions.
d. People with inflammation are excluded from the general population and therefore have to turn to criminal behavior.

33. Why would type 1 diabetes be so much more common in the prison population?

a. People with type 1 diabetes are marginalized in society and thus more likely to unfairly end up in prison.
b. Prisoners can't get the necessary insulin, and therefore they are more likely to have persistent type 1 diabetes.
c. It is not likely more common, but rather it is a more common cause of neuropathy due to lack of access to health care and lack of compliance.
d. Poor parenting started in utero causing low birth weight, and also the same poor parenting led to criminal behavior.

34. Would treatment with vitamin B12 pills or vitamin B12 injections for remission of neuropathic pain simultaneously be effective in preventing dementia in the prison population?

a. Both treatments would only be effective in preventing dementia among individuals who have a vitamin B12 level in the low range, but not among individuals who have adequate levels of vitamin B12.
b. Vitamin B12 pills would not be effective in prevention of dementia due to ineffective absorption through the stomach, but vitamin B12 injections would be effective in preventing dementia.
c. Neither treatment would help in preventing dementia because individuals who suffer from vitamin B12 deficiency-related neuropathy are not necessarily susceptible to vitamin B12 deficiency-related neuropathy.
d. Either treatment would be effective in preventing the development of dementia caused by vitamin B12 deficiency.

35. Why would an individual in this study population fear effective treatment of neuropathy?

a. Once treatment is achieved, medical attention will decrease in frequency, and thus attention and interaction with supportive health-care staff will diminish.
b. Pain medications for neuropathic pain offer pleasant side effects, and thus they are desirable.
c. If the neuropathy is effectively treated, health reimbursements would decrease, making it difficult to obtain supplemental income and health coverage.
d. Effective treatment of neuropathy requires diagnosis using small needles and electrical shocks.

Passage 8

Balance impairment results from several neurological conditions. Balance relies on integration among the senses, including vision, hearing, and proprioceptive touch. Consciousness-altering drugs disrupt balance through several different mechanisms that can last while a drug is in its active chemical form and even after the body metabolizes and eliminates the drug from its system through the residual physiologic action of metabolites or prolonged receptor activity. The mechanisms by which a psychoactive compound can cause addiction are distinct from the mechanisms by which a psychoactive compound diminishes balance. A study using blood analysis to measure the concentration of metabolic by-products of a psychoactive drug as well as physiological parameters such as pulse and blood pressure was performed on volunteers who were given the drug in a low-dose oral form for the study. Measurements were taken 30 minutes after drug use. Approximately half of the participants were users of the drug, whereas half had not previously used the drug. Users varied in their frequency and amounts of drug use. Results of the measured parameters are below.

Objective measures of balance:

- Romberg rated 1–10 (where 10 is perfect)
- Toes walking rated 1–10 (where 10 is perfect)
- Standing on one foot rated 1–10 (where 10 is perfect)

	Blood Pressure	**Pulse**	**Metabolite 1**	**Metabolite 2**	**Romberg**	**Toe Walking**	**Balance on One Foot**
Drug Users	129/89	102	0.67%	0.89%	6.1	5.9	6.23
Non-Drug Users	137/92	116	0.42%	0.92%	6.4	5.78	6.56

36. Why did the drug user group have a lower blood pressure and pulse than the nonuser group and a higher concentration of metabolite 1?

a. The drug users had a higher level of metabolite 1 because they already had some metabolites in their bodies prior to the experiment. This made additional drug intake inconsequential.
b. The drug users experienced altered metabolism of the compound due to repeated exposure to the drug. The drug users also experienced a diminished physiological response to the drug compared to the non-drug users.
c. The drug users became addicted to the drug because they needed it to manage blood pressure. Thus, the drug users were primed to have lower blood pressure and pulse rate in response to the drug.
d. The drug users' ability to properly metabolize the chemical is enhanced by frequent use. The drug users had better baseline health to begin with, and thus they have lower blood pressure and pulse than the non-drug users.

37. How can a psychogenic drug affect immediate responses to visual and auditory threats if it doesn't cause objective vision or hearing deficits?

a. The response time to visual and auditory threats is slowed because psychoactive drugs affect the processing and integration of sensory information as well as the speed of the responses.
b. Psychoactive drugs make threats appear to be nonthreatening, and thus they slow the individual's perception that a response is needed.
c. The person's vision and hearing slowly deteriorate with the use of psychoactive drugs over the long term, but the effect is subclinical, and therefore it is not diagnosed.
d. Addiction is a by-product of the use of psychoactive drugs, and addiction alters conscientiousness.

38. Why would some individuals view perceived socially threatening situations as less threatening with the use of consciousness-altering drugs than without the use of consciousness altering drugs?

a. Sensory adaptation
b. Diminished self-awareness
c. Overconfidence
d. Memory decay

39. How does memory affect an individual's physiological response to a consciousness-altering drug?

a. Memory of impaired consciousness helps an individual consciously resist the effects of a consciousness-altering drug in order to adapt behavior to stay safe and avoid an excessive physiological response to the drug.
b. Memory of the previous experience with the drug elicits a degree of neurotransmitter release ahead of time.
c. Memory does not affect a person's physiologic response.
d. Sensory memory allows an individual to recall previous experiences and restimulate sensory receptors.

PASSAGE 9

The circadian rhythm is driven by the pineal gland in the brain. Some individuals are more sensitive to disruptions in their circadian rhythm than are others.

A study of shift workers attempted to determine whether their disrupted circadian rhythms could be adjusted with meditation. Participants were selected from a company that operates on a 24-hour basis. There was a reported high turnover, reported as a four-year average span on the job. However, some employees were working at the company on a shift basis for up to 25 years. Newer workers may have been new to shift work, or they may have had jobs entailing shift work prior to this employment. Participants were selected at random among this company's employee population who performed shift work.

Workers were asked to participate in meditation sessions two times per week. Twelve hours after work shifts were completed, phone text questions were sent out, asking participants to rate their levels of fatigue and stress on a scale of 1–10. Objective weights were measured and reported at weekly intervals.

The nonintervention shift workers, on average, rated their stress at the following levels:

- levels of 6.2 after 3 weeks
- levels of 5.9 after 6 weeks
- levels of 6.7 after 9 weeks
- levels of 6.6 after 12 weeks

The intervention shift workers, on average, rated their stress at the following levels:

- levels of 6.3 after 3 weeks
- levels of 4.7 after 6 weeks
- levels of 3.3 after 9 weeks
- levels of 3.4 after 12 weeks

The weight-gain chart is below.

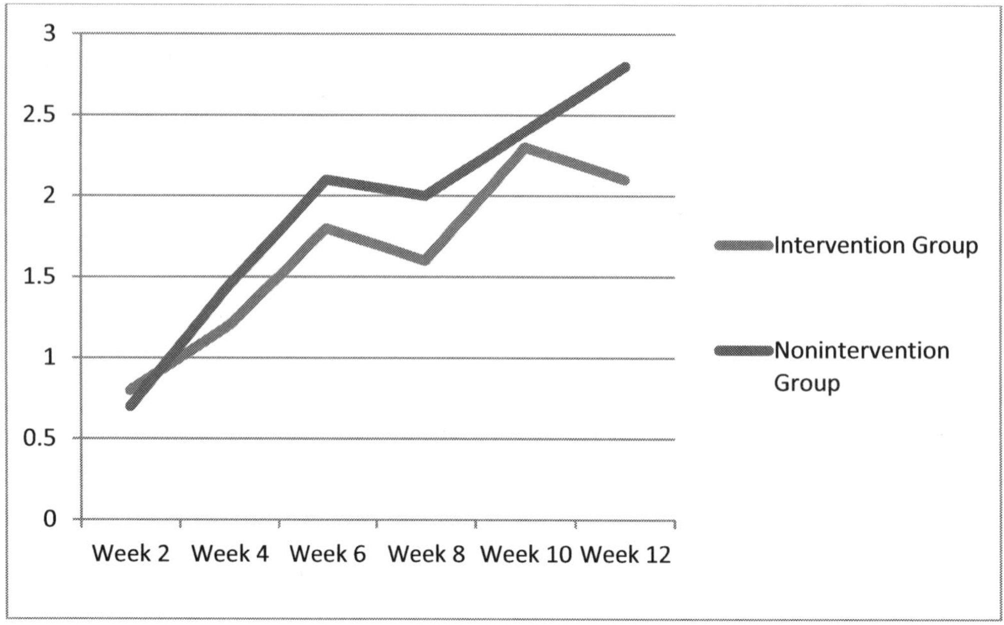

40. How did disruption of the circadian rhythm affect weight gain?

a. As a result of being awake during the night on some days and during the day on other days, participants were not able to maintain a steady diet.
b. When the circadian rhythm is interrupted, there is usually a lack of exercise combined with increased sleep, so individuals don't have the opportunity to burn calories.
c. Study participants' meal cycles were disrupted, causing fluctuations in metabolism as well as hunger and overeating.
d. Seasonal affective disorder (SAD) resulted from lack of regular exposure to sunlight. SAD causes depressive symptoms associated with overeating.

41. How did participants' reports of their fatigue and stress levels reflect their sleep–wake cycle adjustments with meditation?

a. Individuals learned to become more alert through meditation.
b. Meditation helped participants undergo adjustments of the sleep–wake cycle, including a shorter lag prior to the first rapid eye movement (REM) period.
c. Long-term potentiation elicited with the aid of meditation helped in learning adaptations after long-term sleep variations.
d. Neural plasticity is encouraged by meditation, and this mobilized neurons to readjust the sleep–wake cycle.

42. How would study participants' problem-solving responses be affected by lack of sleep?

a. Selective attention is more pronounced because of a decreased ability to focus.
b. Problem solving depends on intelligence, so it is not impaired.
c. Selective attention and divided attention are impaired by lack of sleep.
d. Brainstem-controlled reflexes are severely impaired by lack of sleep.

43. If a participant experienced a catastrophic event during the later weeks of the study, how would her stress self-rating compare to an individual who had an anxiety disorder?

a. The participant who experienced situational stress would rate her stress level as low because she understands that her experience is the result of a situation, whereas the participant with an anxiety disorder would rate her stress level as high because she experiences physiologic anxiety.
b. The participant who has experienced a catastrophic event would rate her stress level as especially high during the period in which she is experiencing the effects of stress, whereas the participant with an anxiety disorder would rate her stress as high due to the stress of participating in the study itself.
c. The participant who has an anxiety disorder would rate her stress as high throughout the study, whereas the participant with acute stress would experience a protective effect against stress as a result of the study.
d. The participant with a catastrophic event would rate her stress level with a number that deviated from her usual stress rating during the weeks in which she is experiencing the effects of the situational stress, whereas the participant with an anxiety disorder would have a relatively consistent self-rated stress level.

44. Which of the following is the LEAST valid conclusion that could be drawn from the apparent stabilization of average stress levels in week nine and beyond in the intervention group and the nonintervention group?

a. The intervention achieved its maximum effectiveness after only nine weeks and should not be expected to further positively impact the stress of participants.
b. The apparent stabilization observed in the responses of the nonintervention group is the result of simple random variation.
c. Members of the nonintervention group observed the lower stress levels in members of the intervention group, and their stress levels increased to a steady higher level as a result of envy.
d. After several surveys, members of both groups developed a learned response to the questions and consistently reported the same responses.

Discrete Questions

45. Population-based studies demonstrate an increased predisposition for schizophrenia in individuals who have Parkinson's disease and in their family members. How can you explain these findings?

a. Dopamine is the common factor in these disorders, and thus medications for one disorder may trigger the other disorder.
b. Genetic loci for both disorders are proximate to each other, and thus, unaffected family members of Parkinson's patients may experience schizophrenia.
c. Environmental factors predispose to both disorders, and families often share environmental situations.
d. The average age of onset of schizophrenia is in the early twenties, whereas the average age of onset of Parkinson's disease is later, so it is difficult to do an accurate study on siblings.

46. If an individual is requested to fill out a brief anonymous survey sent by mass email, what social factor is most likely to prevent the individual from responding?

a. Peer pressure
b. Positive reinforcement
c. Bystander effect
d. Social norms

47. Why would a person revert to a habit of blaming others for his unhappiness after having discontinued that habit for several years?

a. Instinctive drift
b. Because new issues causing unhappiness arise
c. Because his original theory that others are responsible is proven correct
d. Extinction

48. How does the limbic system control an individual's response to human faces?

a. The occipital lobe allows detailed perception of faces.
b. The amygdala is a portion of the limbic system that assesses faces for traits such as trustworthiness.
c. The hippocampus is a portion of the limbic system that aids in remembering names based on facial recognition.
d. The temporal lobe is activated in the process of recognizing faces.

49. How does Korsakoff's syndrome affect an individual's ability to function independently?

a. It causes emotional lability manifest by unexplained crying episodes.
b. It causes vision loss.
c. It causes amnesia.
d. It causes thiamine deficiency.

50. How does emotional stress impact the endocrine system and the autonomic nervous system?

a. Serotonin is increased, whereas epinephrine is decreased in response to emotional stress.
b. Cortisol is decreased, and epinephrine and norepinephrine are increased as a result of emotional stress.
c. Acetylcholine and cortisol are increased, whereas epinephrine and norepinephrine are decreased in response to emotional stress.
d. Epinephrine, norepinephrine, and cortisol are increased as a result of emotional stress.

51. How can the genetic versus environmental etiology of behavioral traits be differentiated based on metabolic brain imaging studies?

a. Metabolic brain imaging studies cannot differentiate between genetic and environmental etiologies because if a metabolic variation is noted, it is a phenotypic trait not a genotypic trait.
b. Environmental factors should not alter the physiological function of the brain, and thus, metabolic brain imaging studies are an effective means of identifying genetic behavioral traits.
c. Metabolic brain imaging studies determine the functional activity of different regions of the brain and thus can help in identifying subclinical pathology in unaffected relatives of affected individuals, potentially establishing a genetic etiology.
d. If metabolic changes can be triggered by environmental stimuli, then it is more likely that the trait is environmental in etiology rather than genetic.

52. How may ascribed status in a primary group affect a person's dedication to the secondary group?

a. The person who has low ascribed status in the primary group rejects the primary group in favor of the secondary group.
b. The person who has a higher ascribed status in the primary group is dedicated to promoting the primary group's status within the secondary group.
c. It is difficult to counteract or change ascribed status, which can motivate an individual to be more devoted to the secondary group and to work harder on earning achieved status in the secondary group.
d. The person who has a higher ascribed status in the primary group rejects the secondary group for fear of not attaining the same status.

53. How does attribution error explain a professor's attitude toward a student arriving late to class versus the professor's attitude when she, herself, arrives late to class?

a. The professor gives herself permission to start class upon her own arrival, whereas she is disappointed that the student did not try hard enough to please her.
b. The professor acknowledges that she may arrive late to class due to external factors such as traffic but attributes the student's tardiness as the result of a personal deficit or negligence.
c. The professor would be upset when she arrives late to class because this compromises class time, whereas she views the student's late arrival as an issue that only penalizes the student.
d. The professor would view the student's tardiness as disruptive to the whole class, whereas she views her own tardiness as inconsequential because she does not produce an interruption when she arrives late, but rather, a delay.

54. How could a teenager's primary group function to lower her self-esteem while the secondary group raises her self-esteem?

a. The primary group assigns ascribed status, whereas the secondary group assigns achieved status, which is more important to a teenager and thus raises her self-esteem.
b. The secondary group's opinion is more important to the teenager because the secondary group is composed of peers, whereas the primary group is her family. Thus, the secondary group has the power to raise the teenager's self-esteem even if the primary group lowers it.
c. The primary group provides direct feedback, whereas the secondary group provides indirect feedback. Thus, because indirect feedback is not as insulting, the primary group lowers the self-esteem and the secondary group raises it.
d. Whether the status is achieved or ascribed, in this example, the status given to the teenager is self-confidence building in the secondary group and devaluing in the primary group.

55. How does perception of an acceptable family structure change within a culture?

a. Diffusion is the passive sharing and transfer of cultural norms and values, and thus perception is affected by watching surroundings.
b. Transmission is the method by which a culture alters its routines.
c. Assimilation describes blending into a new culture, and thus those who assimilate must accept different family structures within the new community.
d. Multiculturalism describes the integration of different cultures within a geographic region, including what each culture considers an acceptable or normal family structure.

56. How would racialization affect attitudes toward the evaluation and treatment of infertility in a patient who is part of a population typically associated with high birth rates?

a. The patient and the doctor are more likely to see the problem as a serious problem due to the deviance from the typical rates of fertility associated with the patient's race.
b. The doctor is more objective, whereas the patient is more concerned about social exclusion.
c. The patient would consider the problem within the context of being a medical issue, whereas the doctor's attitude is colored by prejudice.
d. The patient and the doctor would make inaccurate judgments based on ethnic and racial stereotypes.

57. In light of the fertility problem noted in the previous question, how would the theory of intersectionality influence the doctor-patient relationship and the patient's marriage?

a. The patient thinks the doctor and the spouse can't understand the experience.
b. The intersection of cultures between the couple's experience is more helpful for the doctor than that of the patient alone.
c. The intersection of cultures allows the doctor to work with the patient to create a better therapeutic plan that the patient will comply with.
d. The intersection of male and female experiences causes conflict in the context of infertility.

58. Pheromones are chemicals that can be detected by other organisms of the same species. Most scientific knowledge about pheromones comes from studies of animal species, not humans. However, evidence suggests that humans also release and respond to pheromones. Why are pheromones associated with both sexual attraction and aggression?

a. The physiological response varies depending on the gender of the person releasing the pheromones and the gender of the recipient.
b. The physiological response varies depending on the intention of the person releasing the pheromone.
c. Pheromones encompass a variety of chemicals, and not all recipients have active pheromone receptors at a given time.
d. The physiological response depends on how many people are present because the concentration gradient of the chemical pheromone disseminates among many individuals, altering the type of group response.

59. A physician has a high population of teenage patients who come to him for medical care. He notes that some teens drive themselves to clinic appointments, whereas others come in with their parents. The physician reports that the teen patients who drive themselves tend to have better recoveries. However, a chart review reveals that the recoveries are equivalent between both groups, with equal incidence of complications. Furthermore, the chart review also reveals that the majority of the teenagers who are driven by their parents come from a neighborhood of a different socioeconomic level than the majority of the teenagers who drive themselves. How would you explain the doctor's faulty conclusion?

a. Belief perseverance
b. Poor recall
c. Self-fulfilling prophecy
d. Labeling theory

Critical Analysis and Reasoning Skills

PASSAGE 1

It is mathematics, not art, which clearly drives trends in fashion, design, and music. The true mathematical genius can calculate what the populace is prepared to accept as the color, material, or style that represents modernity. The mastermind of quantitative statistical analysis can then sell his manufactured productions to the masses, masking his algorithmic talents as an intangible artistic gift.

Artists, by nature, are inspired to creativity through emotion. These sensitive passions may deliver original art, but the depth of artistry will not produce that which the general public is prepared to accept or to incorporate into daily life.

The evolution of trends in color, melodies, and material follows principles based on what the eye and the mind interpret as new. Yet, there is more than originality that drives public approval of fashion. While the new may appear to be new, it must never be too different from the old, or else the populace will reject it as too strange.

Thus, any successful designer must be, above all else, a brilliant mathematician. He must consciously compute patterns in shades of color and material that others can only appreciate on a subliminal level. The changes brought about by fashion must convince the consumer that he is forward thinking, while subconsciously comforting him at the same time. The designer must be intentionally aware of the consumer's boredom with available products around him, while allowing the consumer to cling to the features that he needs on a deep emotional level.

It is the fashion critic who exists in the middle of this relationship between the designer and the consumer. The critic, who lives a dedicated, reflective love of design, is more prone to boredom by what is currently available than the consumer. Thus, he is likely to reject the creation of the highly mathematical designer, and instead be drawn to the creations of the true artist. The consumer, only frivolously interested in fashion as an amusement rather than as a deeply meaningful symbol of himself, often rejects the opinions of the critic as eccentric, impractical, and outlandish.

Thus, there is a wide disconnect between the critic and the consumer. In the meantime, the mathematical, systematic designer continues to please the wide audience, to the dismay of the critic and the artist. The true artist, however, may enjoy lavish praise from the critic. However, if he remains true to himself, he cannot overcome his lack of appeal to the consumer who is not obsessed with art and fashion.

A true artist has a signature that is independent of current fashion. The mathematician knows that too much change can be unsettling for the consumer and takes caution to avoid disturbing the peace of the consumer's existence, convincing him that his taste is a sign of his extraordinariness, when in reality, that which he believes to be his own individual preference is so predictable that it can be charted on a graph.

What, then, is the true artist to do? Should he learn the methodical rules as a student of the designer? Or should he continue to attempt to astonish the audience with his own brand of magic, hoping that when he finally reaches the pinnacle of popular recognition, his works will crush the limited scope of math and science?

1. According to the passage, what is the central difference between a designer and an artist?

a. The designer intends for mass production, while the artist does not intend to mass-produce his creations.
b. The designer bases his work on his assessment of what will be accepted, while the artist creates through emotion.
c. The designer has had a high level of formal education, while the artist is self-taught.
d. The designer is wealthier than the artist.

2. Suppose that an artist were to receive a negative review from a respected art critic. According to the passage, how would the artist react?

a. The artist would publicly condemn the critic as unsophisticated.
b. The artist would try to improve his work to please the critic.
c. The artist would stay true to his signature style, choosing to retain his creativity despite lack of praise.
d. The artist would become a student of the designer.

3. According to the passage, a successful designer must be a "brilliant mathematician." What does the author mean by the phrase "brilliant mathematician"?

a. Someone who is so advanced in mathematical skills that he can deceive others.
b. A person who has reached a very advanced level in sophisticated models of math and who is able to do calculations without the aid of a calculator.
c. A person who is brilliant in all areas of academics, as math is an inclusive indicator of academic abilities.
d. A person who is able to take mathematical principles and apply them to design.

4. Based on the premise of the passage, how would a commercially successful musician react to a negative review from a respected music critic?

a. He would not be very concerned because his goal is to achieve popularity and recognition among the populace, not music critics.
b. He would reformulate his approach to better tailor to the tastes of the music critic who can sway the public.
c. He would shower the music critic with gifts to win his approval.
d. He would attempt to gain favor with different music critics so they can give him valuable insight into the tastes of the public.

5. According to the passage, what is one choice the artist has in overcoming his inability to achieve popular acceptance?

a. He can learn to be more like the commercially successful designer.
b. He can accept his station in life as a starving artist.
c. He can try to gain acceptance and praise from art critics.
d. He can try to become better at mathematics than anyone else, in order to squash his competition.

6. Suppose the author is a buyer for a large commercial fashion retailer. Based on the premise of the passage, how would you describe the likely relationship between the author and the commercial designer?

a. They are generally loyal business partners who share the same objective of reaching a wide popular consumer base.
b. They are competitors, each trying to outdo the other.
c. They are generally business partners, but the commercial designer attempts to appeal to many buyers, while the buyer shops around among many commercial artists.
d. The author wants to entice artists to leave their trade and become commercial designers.

Passage 2

The Meeting of St. Anthony and St. Paul, a painting by Sassetta, lies in the National Gallery of Art in Washington D.C.

Like many of his contemporaries, Sassetta often used religious events and symbolism in his work. The image, which was painted on wood, relays a sense of warmth and comfort provided by the use of easy, rounded brush strokes; soft colors; and a soothing backdrop. The scene depicts several characters, including a busy gardener. The two men for whom the painting is named stand at the opening of a wide and welcoming cave. As St. Anthony and St. Paul greet each other, they bend towards each other ever so slightly, appearing to be shorter than the mouth of the cave. The cave itself is presented as a spacious underground tunnel, arcing from below, as a miniature hill above it forms a softly curved walkway for casual passersby. The sand, the trees, and the grass surrounding the cave from all directions are lush, soft, and full of life. The area bordering the cave appears to be a hilly community, populated with villagers.

The painting surely would inspire a visitor to seek solace and peace in the area around the famed cave, located in the depths of Egypt's hot and mountainous desert.

However, the entry of the cave itself is not nearly as generous, nor is the immediate environment bursting with greenery, as it appears to be in the painting. In fact, in reality, one cannot help but wonder how St. Anthony managed to discover the short, narrow opening of the cave that blends inconspicuously with the mountain in which it is nestled. Deeply embedded in dense rock, there is almost no loose sand to be found. Above the cave there is no walkway—only the hard, jagged, steep mountain that would be challenging, if not dangerous, to climb for anyone but a seasoned mountain climber. Even more bewildering, the walk up to the cave, which is located about a quarter of the way up the mountain, is only made possible because of the man-made, irregularly-shaped steps extending from the bottom of the mountain up to the cave, which must have been painstakingly paved.

Surely the Italian artist must not have travelled to Egypt to visit the mountain itself. Yet he knew of the mountain and the cave. He must have learned the details of the setting through stories that passed through many fervent storytellers before finally reaching his ears.

The cave itself can only be accessed through a short opening, followed by a constricted, elongated entrance that unexpectedly widens after at least 40 steps, at which point a soft, illuminating sunlight fills the sizeable cave that is large enough to hold at least 10 adults comfortably. The coolness inside the cave is mild, unlike the blistering heat immediately outside. However, because the atrium is so narrow as to be deceiving, one wonders why someone unfamiliar with the inside would venture past the tight entryway.

Perhaps Sassetta did know such details about the inside of the cave. Could it be that his warm portrayal was an attempt to represent the inside of the cave, rather than revealing the misleading exterior?

7. According to the passage, how does the painting of the mountain's landscape diverge from the landscape of the mountain itself?

a. The colors are soft in the painting, but the colors of the mountain are harsh in reality.
b. The painting conveys a sense of warmth, while the mountain is cold.
c. The painting presents the mountain as green and full of life, while in reality it is rocky and jagged.
d. The painting suggests that the mountain is small, while in reality it is quite large.

8. Suppose the author of this passage encountered a wild animal inside the cave. What would the author conclude about Sassetta's knowledge of the cave?

a. Sassetta had never personally visited the mountain or the cave, and thus had an inaccurate idea about the setting, which was reflected in his painting.
b. Sassetta was aware of the wild animal, but was hiding the truth about the harsh reality of the cave because he wanted his painting to be calm and serene.
c. Sassetta had lived in the cave and had been able to survive despite the brutal environment.
d. Sassetta visited the cave, but did not encounter a wild animal, and thus did not portray an animal in the painting.

9. How does the author explain a discrepancy between the artistic representation of a setting and the setting itself?

a. The alterations in climate modify the topography of the land over time.
b. Sassetta's research into the details of the environment was flawed due to political partiality.
c. The artist was commissioned to produce a painting of historical and religious relevance, so he used names of well-known Christian saints to elevate the status of his painting.
d. The artist's purpose was to portray the feelings evoked by the site, rather than the physical features.

10. Based on the passage, why did the author venture past the atrium of the cave if it was so unwelcoming?

a. He was adventurous and he went to the locale to challenge himself.
b. He was convinced that there must be a tunnel leading to the exit from the cave.
c. He wanted to create a painting of the inside of the cave.
d. He was, in some way, familiar with the inside of the cave.

11. If the artist had not used religious representation in this painting, instead painting anonymous people and naming the painting Peace, how would this have affected the identification of the cave?

a. The cave would have seemed less peaceful without the religious representation and fewer people would be interested in locating it.
b. Without some historic context or narrative provided by the artist, there would have been no reason to believe the actual location existed.
c. Geographic characteristics and clues found in the painting would have been used to guide a seeker to the mountain and the cave.
d. The author would have had to research the artist's life to determine where the mountain and cave were to be found.

12. Was the author alone on the journey to St. Anthony's cave?

a. Yes, the author was alone, searching for the mountain he saw in a painting and found it in Egypt.
b. No, the author was likely with at least one guide, given the difficulty in climbing the mountain and finding the location of the cave.
c. No, the author was accompanied by at least 10 adults.
d. Yes, the author was probably alone because he did not mention other travelers.

Passage 3

In 1926, esteemed Spanish architect Antonio Gaudi was struck by a moving tram. Seriously injured, he was transported to a hospital. He had no identifying information and was thus given the medical treatment considered appropriate for a pauper. His condition deteriorated. After some time, a chaplain recognized him as the famous, highly respected Antonio Gaudi. Despite the hospital's fervent efforts it was too late for the prominent architect to benefit from the best medical treatment available, and he died shortly afterwards.

This true story seems almost as it were made up to prove a point about healthcare policy. Fairness, mercy and justice are all central tenets in the formulation of healthcare policy in developed countries.

Whether a physician delivers care to a pauper or to an esteemed pillar of the nation itself, healthcare decisions are based on a number of complex factors. The most obvious element of medical care is determining the best treatment option. Yet, even this choice is not always a simple or straightforward judgment that can be boiled down to a basic checklist. Minimally divergent scientific studies and discrepancies in clinical research data that differ by only a few percentage points can arbitrarily alter the favored options made available for millions of patients.

The tale of Antonio Gaudi seems to indicate that the better medical options for his injuries were clear. The ability of the patient to pay for the care appears to be a central component of the outcome in this situation. However, there are always other, more subtle factors at play when it comes to choosing among the available alternatives in medical treatment.

For instance, the value of a person to the people around him and to society may play a role in the quality of healthcare delivered. How many people are expected to mourn the loss of an unknown pauper? This is an ethical question that may seem disgusting to many of us.

Another important factor at play in healthcare delivery is whether the patient will put in the effort to maintain his health after the professional care is delivered. For example, will he keep his surgical wounds clean? Will he take his medication? Will he follow dietary instructions? Imagine the heartbreak of the medical team who worked for hours to save the life of a patient only to learn that he indulged himself in harmful recreational drugs before his wounds had healed.

Yet current healthcare policy is in a tug of war between the rights of the Antonio Gaudis of the world and the rights of the pauper. For society to pay for the pauper who cannot pay for himself, society must have either an abundance of extra resources or a sense of responsibility towards the anonymous pauper. The monetary value of a person who cannot pay for his own healthcare is an issue that cannot be resolved in any dignified way. A true case of mistaken identity illustrates the grey area of healthcare rights and responsibilities like no fact-filled political debate or rambling health policy book can. What if the mistaken identity were reversed? What if the pauper was the doppelganger of a famous person?

13. Suppose healthcare policies were debated between two political opponents, how would a political candidate appeal to the broadest voter base?

a. The candidate would discuss a detailed policy proposal to be transparent to voters.
b. The candidate would discuss generalities that favor the majority of the voters based on their socioeconomic status, salaries, and benefits.
c. The candidate would display a sense of fairness to the most disadvantaged members of society.
d. The candidate would remind voters that their situation is better than that of citizens in most other countries.

14. Based on the passage, how is "best medical care" defined?

a. Best medical care is determined by scientific studies and clinical research data.
b. Best medical care is arbitrarily determined based on the study authors who push their data as superior to other data.
c. Best medical care is defined based on widely divergent results which produce data that clearly demarcate the ideal treatment options for all patients.
d. There is no accurate definition of best medical care, as it is assigned completely arbitrarily.

15. The passage asks, "How many people are expected to mourn the loss of an unknown pauper?" Why is this question described as disgusting?

a. The question is described as disgusting because it suggests the presence of a degenerative, unsightly disease.
b. The question is described as disgusting because it raises the point that few people will mourn the loss of a pauper.
c. The question is described as disgusting because it suggests that if few people would mourn the loss of a paper, the hospital might not exert great effort in saving his life.
d. The question is described as disgusting because it suggests that there is a grey area in health policy.

16. When the passage brings up the point that some patients may not put in the effort to maintain health after professional care is delivered, who is the author concerned about?

a. The author seems concerned that some patients might not receive proper instruction in self-care after release from the hospital.
b. The author is concerned that the public is forced to pay for the healthcare of a person who might not follow through with necessary self-care.
c. The author is concerned about the few loved ones who will mourn the loss of the pauper.
d. The author is concerned about the medical staff who will exert a great amount of effort, only to have it go to waste when some patients do not put in the effort to care for themselves.

17. Suppose the story at the beginning of the passage described an infamous, unrecognized escaped convict. Based on the premise of this passage, how would the monetary value of the person's life be determined?

a. The monetary value of an escaped convict's life would be less than that of a pauper or of a famous architect who could pay for his own care.
b. The monetary value of a criminal is equal to that of a pauper or a famous architect.
c. It depends on whether society has an abundance of resources.
d. The monetary value of a person's life cannot be resolved in any dignified way.

18. What does the author imply about fact-filled political debates and rambling books?

a. They may or may not be accurate, but they do not get at the crux of the dilemmas in health policy the way this true story does.
b. They are valuable, but they are biased due to partisanship and political motives.
c. They may be inaccurate because of statistical error and inconsistency in healthcare costs.
d. They are unfair to people who cannot pay for their own healthcare.

PASSAGE 4

A number of well-conducted surveys suggest that ageism is emerging as a legitimate obstacle in the workplace. Mature workers increasingly report an alarming lack of job security as well as age-related barriers to finding jobs once the need arises. Despondent and anxious, the outcry has become impossible to ignore for many growing companies that flourish on competitiveness, but do not want to stand accused of discrimination. Yet, at the same time, an abundance of salary data reports point to a trend of superior compensation associated with seniority, even among experienced workers who change jobs. There must be an explanation for this disparity.

The answer could lie in a tendency of the work environment to operate in a "survival of the fittest" mode. Seasoned workers who have proven themselves valuable in the workplace may indeed enjoy generous promotions in position and salary. Yet, given the job insecurity reported by older workers, it appears that age alone does not guarantee promotions, salary advances, or even basic contract renewal.

Perhaps older workers who are frustrated in their job searches are being unrealistic, expecting offers of leadership positions better suited to their high-performing peers. A more practical option could involve pursuing jobs that demand fewer responsibilities, offer less prestige, and provide lower rates of reimbursement. On the other hand, such entry-level positions may not be open to experienced workers who are humble enough or desperate enough to seek them.

Perhaps the older workers who feel a sense of job insecurity are not actually inferior workers, but might, in fact, be honest citizens who found themselves victims of bullying, bias, or dishonesty at the hands of their former peers and supervisors. Perhaps older workers who consider themselves at a disadvantage in the professional world display a poor work ethic, behave with entitlement, or rest on their laurels.

The professional world is not solely based on performance. Some may suffer due to poor social skills, unattractive appearance, or naïveté. Jobs that provide generous compensation packages are generally few and far between, as the workplace hierarchy is pyramidal. Fewer administrators are needed to manage and direct many mid-level employees. Is it realistic, then, to assume that all workers who started in the same position with the same qualifications will go on to enjoy a slice of the best piece of pie? Yet, is it fair for older workers to be discarded as outdated and unskilled simply because they are average? Those who want to continue to do the same tasks for many years, resisting new technology, may eventually find themselves vulnerable to a bitter reality.

So, whose responsibility is it to keep stale workers up to date? Should workplace leaders employ paternalistic attitudes, holding their unmotivated workers' hands in the scary waters of newness? Or should the workplace employ only the fittest, regardless of the cost? Both approaches are susceptible to inducing a degree of bitterness—either on the part of the below-average worker who is shed by his innovative employer or on the part of his coworkers who must pick up the slack while he passively and peacefully grows deep roots in the company.

19. The passage asks, "Should the workplace employ only the fittest, regardless of the cost?" What is the meaning of "cost" in this phrase?

a. "Cost" taken here means the overall cost to the company in productivity, as better workers may cost more and thus may decrease the company's profit.
b. "Cost" is taken to mean the cost of producing bitterness among aging employees who are shed because they are not the fittest.
c. "Cost" taken here means that, when the workplace is hierarchical, those at the bottom may suffer from a sense of discouragement as a consequence of remaining at a deferential role.
d. "Cost" taken here means that, when a company employs only the fittest, it may stand accused of discrimination.

20. The author wavers in attempting to explain why a senior worker may be at a disadvantage in the workplace. Why do you think the author is so ambiguous?

a. The author has been accused of discrimination and would like to avoid another such incident.
b. The author wishes to fire one or more underperforming senior employees, but is unsure whether the employees have a poor work ethic, or suffer from setbacks to good job performance due to issues such as workplace bullying.
c. The author is upset that aging workers suffer from job insecurity, but wants to present a balanced point of view.
d. The author is an indecisive individual, which is precisely the problem with average workers.

21. Suppose young workers were complaining of discrimination in the workplace. How would that change the premise of the passage?

a. The author would definitely feel that young workers have no right to complain because they have many years ahead of them to earn and save money.
b. There would not be such a concern about a responsibility towards young workers because they have not invested years learning the skills needed for the company and the industry as a whole.
c. The author may feel a responsibility towards helping young workers develop to their potential.
d. The passage would likely have a tone of urgency regarding possible accusations of discrimination, as younger people are more vocal regarding their rights.

22. What does the passage suggest about older workers who are leaders and presumably receive high levels of monetary compensation?

a. They are high performers who achieve recognition either through hard work or through intimidation and bullying.
b. They made it to the top of the workplace pyramid, but no one can really pinpoint why.
c. They are completely secure in their jobs and they do not fear unemployment.
d. They have chosen to give entry-level positions to young people, rather than to senior workers, in an attempt to mentor new leaders.

23. If you were to learn that the vast majority of older workers who have been laid off were mothers who requested part-time work hours after having received excellent company-created performance reviews, how would that affect the author's concern about discrimination?

a. The author would be rightly concerned about discrimination charges, given that good performance reviews bolster a laid off worker's sense of unfairness.
b. The author would be able to resist discrimination charges because part-time work hours are inherently less valuable to a company.
c. The author would be able to support the layoffs because of issues related to tardiness and lack of technology know-how.
d. The author would have to redefine the qualities of a valuable worker to avoid discrimination charges.

24. Suppose that computers and robots took over most laborious workplace tasks. Would jobs that provide generous compensation packages remain few and far between?

a. No, because everyone would become a supervisor to the computers and robots.
b. There would be many jobs that provide generous compensation, but they would be available at outside companies.
c. Yes, these jobs would remain scarce because few leaders are needed to supervise computers and robots, which do not take responsibility for high-level decisions.
d. Few people would need to work, so they would have more time to become entrepreneurs.

Passage 5

Objective testing of children's academic and reasoning abilities has become highly valued in public schools. Students' performance benchmarks are used in combination with each individual student's year-to-year improvement to provide objective criteria with which to evaluate school and teacher effectiveness, which is then used as a financial incentive.

Yet, all educators and parents know that standardized measures obtained through multiple choice examinations provide only a limited view of educational gains.

The problem lies in the excessive classroom time devoted to standardized testing. This time does not serve in any way to provide students with educational enhancement, but rather steals from learning opportunities. Even more than divesting valuable time, the ensuing exhaustion that results from sitting for lengthy examinations leaves students less equipped to benefit from any remaining constructive instruction during the remainder of the school day.

On the other hand, non-curriculum-based activities such as recess, field trips, and school assemblies enhance students' abilities to absorb concepts and to exercise creativity.

The rigid requirements imposed by hours and hours of in-school testing create a tenuous situation in which emergency school cancellation becomes particularly damaging to students because, while a number of school days are forsaken, the total number of hours devoted to standardized testing remains inflexible, disproportionally affecting instructional classroom time in school.

Some schools' academic functioning is undoubtedly poor. Students in a percentage of school districts lag behind in basic skills such as reading, math, writing, and reasoning. The harmful long-term effects of such deficiencies cannot be understated. Yet, implementing required testing in all school districts to identify the few that underperform seems a monumentally wasteful way of identifying and managing educational shortcomings.

Perhaps a better method would include devoting time and energy to providing additional instruction in the schools that repeatedly underperform on widely-used exams such as the SAT and ACT. Or perhaps, online courses designed to reteach lagging skills can make the time spent on this matter more productive than consuming classroom time with testing that does not serve to educate the majority of the students. Surely, with today's technology, computer programs can be used to identify benchmark skills and, subsequently, to teach students at a gradual and personalized pace.

In fact, if testing must remain a part of schooling, then computerized tests coupled with supplementary activities should be required of all students. Those who lag behind would be directed to math and reading problems that help them learn the skills necessary to reach appropriate targets, while those who test ahead of grade level can be given the opportunity to practice with problems that challenge them and make them even better academically.

Most importantly, the classroom itself is a valuable place for all students. Do the high academic achievers have nothing to learn from those who perform at lower levels in math? Could not the lower scholastic achievers be gifted socially? Standardized testing misses the societal value of schools completely. School children benefit from being with their peers in the school setting more than they benefit from the academic instruction provided by the schools.

25. The passage states that "all parents and educators know that objective measures provide a limited view of educational gains." What data is used to support this statement?

a. It is obvious that this statement is true, so no data is needed.
b. Parents and educators have reported these facts through personal narratives to the author.
c. No data is provided to support this statement. It is the author's opinion.
d. No data is provided to support this statement, thus it is false.

26. Suppose the author is a teacher at a school in which students generally perform in the 60th percentile on standardized tests and her students performed in the 88th percentile, well above the school's average. How would that inform your interpretation of the author's purpose?

a. The teacher is showing off her superior teaching skills, and is thus drawing attention to testing results.
b. This teacher feels competent in teaching the basics and wants to have more freedom in teaching.
c. The teacher wants to show other teachers how to improve their students' objective scores.
d. The teacher would like to defend her school from being penalized for low test scores.

27. According to the passage, what is the biggest problem with testing?

a. It consumes time and energy from learning in the classroom.
b. It does not provide accurate insight into children's educational ability.
c. It does not examine social skills.
d. It does not inherently provide a means to repair lagging skills.

28. The passage says that "perhaps online courses to reteach lagging skills can make the time spent on this matter more productive..." What do the words "this matter" refer to?

a. Over-testing of school children, which results in wasted time and exhaustion.
b. The problem of underperforming schools and students who lag behind their peers in some academic skills.
c. The inability to teach students that lag behind.
d. The fact that students who have to do homework on worksheets do not get immediate feedback on their answers.

29. Suppose the author were asked about the value of student diversity. What do you think the answer would be?

a. The author most likely values student diversity because it allows students to learn more about culture and art, reinforcing the material learned in the classroom.
b. The author most likely does not value student diversity because it can be overwhelming, possibly preventing teachers from being able to teach academics at a uniform level.
c. The author likely does not think that student diversity is necessarily good or bad for students.
d. The author likely values student diversity because interaction with students who are different teaches school children social skills.

30. The author states that, "school children benefit from being with their peers..." Which of the following statements is most likely to accurately represent the author's view about teachers' interactions with school children?

a. Schoolteachers should spend more time focusing on group activities instead of the curriculum.
b. Schoolteachers should have students share their test scores with each other as a way to promote healthy competition.
c. Schoolteachers come from varied backgrounds and thus can teach children about different cultures using maps and projects.
d. Schoolteachers have different personalities, and exposure to these different personalities allows students to learn how to navigate the social world.

Passage 6

It is only now with the minimally requisite impartiality that economists and historians can begin to piece together the meaning behind the economic disaster that grew, in part, out of the proliferation of subprime mortgage rates in the 1990s. Articles and books already abound on the subject, but most are colored by too much self-interest, political partisanship, special interests, and even emotions stemming from personal consequences of the events.

The economic atmosphere of the 1990s appeared to be unparalleled to many of those living it. Low interest rates coupled with the promise of economic growth, property appreciation, and unquestioned rising incomes set the stage for speculation in the housing market and the business world alike. Globalization also provided a seemingly sage explanation for the acceptance of unprecedented expansion, even for those who were skeptical of the ability of domestic economic growth to provide enough support to justify the disproportionate optimism characteristic of those years.

However, it seems that the notions of creative destruction and capitalism as a perfect self-regulating system may have delivered the ultimate weakness in preventing the corruption that was part of the eventual collapse of economic growth.

It was an environment that seemed one in which everyone could profit, leaving behind any traditional sense that for one to win, someone else must lose. The principle of unrestricted inflation itself suggests a profit for all, as inflation promised, sometimes with validity and sometimes erroneously, to feed the income of many. Yet, reality proves that the price paid by the consumer must be finally acknowledged as a net loss for the consumer. The denial that insists that the consumer benefits to such a degree from inflation—either directly in wages or through investments that seamlessly filter to everyone—asserts that the consumer can forever remain unscathed by increasing costs of goods and services.

The irony of this flawed supposition is that, while it rewards innovation in a classically capitalist system, it craves rewards for those who took no part in innovation at all. Congratulating itself, this high-flying yet benevolent economy fails to see itself as the untruthful Ponzi scheme that it really is.

The supposition that, even if profits are temporarily exaggerated, they will buffer any future plateau, was, unfortunately, also flawed. And those who suffered from great losses were not necessarily responsible for the faulty reasoning that led to an inescapable trap, as they simply accepted employment and bought shelter as is necessary to live.

It may have been a strange sense of responsibility carried by some at the top of the economic ladder that necessitated a degree of belief that wealth was being shared. Yet many who found themselves in the same position chose instead to abuse the freedom that leadership provided them, surreptitiously deceiving those who trusted them without any regard for the future.

How then, can elected officials prevent themselves from being blinded to corruption when they are able to relish and take responsibility for the achievement of the good outcomes they so fervently work towards? Are not economic prosperity and creativity the goal of a society? How can lawmakers prevent themselves from savoring noble outcomes, instead persistently probing for hidden problems?

31. What role did globalization play in the economic disaster described in the passage?

a. It provided a backdrop for economic growth that would not have been sustained domestically.
b. It provided a rational explanation for skeptics of unprecedented expansion.
c. It created a situation in which global growth could allow everyone to be a winner.
d. It created an environment of extremes, allowing some nations to experience generous growth, while others quietly suffered.

32. How could a belief in capitalism as a perfect self-regulating system fail to prevent corruption?

a. It allowed for unchecked dishonesty to occur because of the unwarranted dependence on capitalism as a self-regulating system.
b. It causes dishonesty because it rewards inequalities in income, as opposed to a socialist system, which does not incentivize disparities in output.
c. It allows oppression of those who are not financially creative.
d. It does not provide a setting that allows for laws that limit the effects of subprime mortgages.

33. Who does the author believe to be most responsible for the economic disaster of the 1990s?

a. The lawmakers because they did not notice deceptive practices.
b. The unreasonably optimistic business leaders.
c. Those who unwisely invested their assets in speculative ventures.
d. Those who corrupted the economy by deceitful practices.

34. Suppose that lawmakers who had noticed the corruption and wanted to prevent economic disaster had been forcibly prevented from doing so by lawmakers who were financially influenced by corrupt businesspeople. How would the author most likely describe lawmakers?

a. The author would describe lawmakers as a group without enough background in economics.
b. The author would describe lawmakers as put into office by equally corrupt voters.
c. The author would describe them as a heterogeneous group of varied interests and ethics.
d. The author would describe the lawmakers as cynical and always looking for problems.

35. How does guilt play a role in the economic disaster described in the passage?

a. Guilt prevents some business leaders from acting in a corrupt manner.
b. Guilt forces some business leaders to share wealth.
c. Guilt forces lawmakers to look the other way, not wanting to believe that anyone could be culpable of corruption.
d. Guilt allows some business leaders to pat themselves on the back for creating a system that they believe is beneficial for everyone.

Passage 7

Thomas Mann's 1929 novella, Mario and the Magician, skillfully uses familiar elements of the human psyche to establish for the reader the manner and techniques that a government has at its disposal to manipulate its population. Yet, while some believe the ending of the story to be an exhibition of liberty, it is not reassuring that one of the victims of the brutal magician ends his torment by killing the tyrant.

The story most certainly had the impact on the audience that was originally intended by the author at the time it was written, and it is because of this that he was relegated to exile. But after the fascist era ended, the anecdote depicts a disturbing tale because the use of human interaction as a tool for symbolism underscores one of the many weaknesses of human character.

Indeed, political submission is often acknowledged as inescapable, even today. However, the toleration of personal indignities is more alarming in today's world, reflecting feebleness in self-determination that is viewed as more dishonorable and less understandable that it was at the time of the novella.

The advances in the science of psychology have made a weak sense of dignity something to be ashamed of. In fact, those who suffer from biologically based debilitating psychiatric illness may suffer less reproach than those who simply display an ineffectuality of disposition, passivity, or a subordinate personality.

Fiction of the past may be grounded on an acceptance as normal of personality traits that are seen as reprehensible in a western view of the world that rewards self-assurance above all other elements of one's personality. Indeed, a lack of self-confidence is often seen as a product of bad mothering in the same way that biochemical psychiatric disorders were seen as a consequence of bad mothering in years past, prior to modern scientific discoveries.

Timeless fiction speaks to a deep place in human consciousness that transcends culture and time. The manner in which we appreciate most fiction is based largely on cultural norms, which differ among societies and generations, deeming most fiction only transiently relevant.

For Mario to resort to destroying the cruel villain assumes that he does not have the power to resist the villain, to coexist with the villain, or to dominate him. It clearly communicates that the only way Mario and his fellow victims can escape the treacherous magician is to eliminate him from the world completely. A more sophisticated approach would be more useful to the modern reader. The simplistic murder by any of one of the magician's victims, or even by the hero of the story himself, just emphasizes how the magician is so easily able to hypnotize all of his victims, to their dismay.

The political analogy aside, the conviction in the innate human ability to overcome tyrannical domination or any form of hypnosis is noteworthy in the sense that it is not a timeless principle. Thus, politically symbolic fiction, in general, is not as likely to enjoy timeless appeal as other types of fiction because it relies on basic creeds of society to illustrate its point, tenets that may be so outdated at a later era as to alter the message as it was originally intended.

36. According to the premise of this passage, can a fictional story be timeless in appeal?

a. It cannot, because the basic societal values change so much over time as to make central points not relatable.
b. Only if the author of the fictional story has better insight into the deep-seated and unchangeable traits of human nature than the author discussed in this passage.
c. A fictional story can have timeless appeal if it does not rely on tenets that become so outdated as to lose resonance with the reader.
d. A fictional story can have timeless appeal, but not necessarily across all cultures.

37. Did the story of Mario and the Magician achieve the objectives of its author?

a. Yes, he made his message clear to the audience as evidenced by his exile.
b. He had many messages and it is unclear whether they were well received.
c. He was not viewed as a political leader or a revolutionary, but rather was exiled. This indicates that he failed in his objective.
d. Given that Thomas Mann is a well-known author, it appears that he achieved recognition, which is likely his most important objective.

38. Suppose Thomas Mann's father was a high-ranking official in the rising fascist government. How would this affect the psychological interpretation of the story?

a. The story would have been less dangerous for Thomas Mann because his father would have pardoned him.
b. The hero's actions would have to be interpreted in light of a son's rebellion against his father.
c. The story would be viewed as Thomas Mann's complaint that his father did not appoint him to a high rank in the government.
d. The story would have to be reinterpreted as a support for fascism, given a son's loyalty to his father.

39. How has the science of psychology affected those with a weakness of character?

a. It has made them stronger and better able to overcome their character weaknesses.
b. It has provided a biological explanation for weakness of character.
c. It has freed them from the oppression of bad mothering.
d. It has made weakness of character something to be ashamed of.

40. How is political submission viewed in the world today, as suggested by the passage?

a. It is a product of weak self-determination.
b. It may be inescapable at times.
c. It is prevalent when there is an absence of political fiction and symbolism in political fiction.
d. It is inevitable.

41. How might the author have preferred the story of Mario and the Magician to end?

a. The author would have liked to see a less extreme solution, possibly to help him model a solution to a problem that he is dealing with.
b. The author would have preferred to see the group of victims joining together to destroy the oppressor, for a more unified solution.
c. The author would have liked to see the magician submitting to the victims and apologizing.
d. The author would have preferred a different ending because the murder in this story was too violent.

Passage 8

Sustainable energy is innately equipped with ample features that make it attractive to consumers. The public, generally conscientious, but with understandably limited power over energy sourcing and pricing, favors the idea of clean energy. A sustainable stock of energy allows for thoughtful preservation, rather than consumption of the environment due to the renewability of natural and non-consumable resources. A minimal need for the use of contamination-prone production techniques that have a tendency to produce damaging effects such as air and water pollution makes sustainable energy desirable.

However, many who are responsible for providing energy comprehend the inherent difficulty that is one of the realities of harnessing and preserving some forms of the abundant and readily available springs of sustainable energy, such as solar power and wind energy, obtained, for instance, through the use of innocuous windmills. They argue that barring powerful incentives (or disincentives) and revolutionary methods of stabilizing energy in a reservoir-like form, the current mechanisms of producing and consuming sustainable energy have already neared their peak capacity for applied use.

However, the problems with the dominant energy sources and our dependence on heavy energy consumption are not going to go away, but instead are likely to worsen if left unchecked. Efforts to curb worldwide energy use have not been a priority for any reputable faction. Thus, sustainable energy offers a reasonable path to forge as we look for solutions.

Investment in sustainable energy is one mechanism that consumers have the power to use to encourage the research and development of sustainable energy by putting actual dollars and self-interest into the process.

Legislation and advocacy are other steps that the consumer can use to encourage the development of sustainable energy, but these steps require a reasonable amount of time, energy, money, and research into the substance of the science as well as the sociological repercussions.

Investments in sustainable energy sources can serve to provide a solid and reliable approach for consumers to benefit from the inevitable future developments in engineering. Surely, a broad-based investment methodology can help secure a buffer against policy, business, and technological variants in this area. Given the budding potential, coupled with the demand for sustainable energy, it is unlikely to be a risky investment or a short-term trend in emerging technology.

Different types of renewable energy include wind energy, solar energy, wave-generated energy, plant produced energy, and others. Some of these technologies are likely to be developed further by existing energy suppliers while emerging energy suppliers may also enter the industry. When research is the primary goal, it is likely that competing companies will have similar interests in terms of political lobby. It is only after the profitability of sustainable energy becomes undeniable that competing profit centers will battle, limiting profit margin and essentially creating an environment in which the science can progress, but the business becomes complex. Such a scenario is unlikely to disrupt an investor's plans in the near future, or even in the next 20-30 years. However, before this danger materializes, forewarnings will abound, easily providing notice to consumer-investors to safely divest.

42. How would the author explain a significant investment loss to a client who invested in sustainable energy years ago?

a. The author would likely explain the loss as a consequence of a lack of financial responsibility among energy producing companies.
b. The author would likely explain the loss by stating that sustainable energy was not financially profitable in the past, but that it will be in the future.
c. The author believes that risky investments are unwise, and would advise the client to steer clear of making the same mistake again.
d. The author believes that investments must have inherent value beyond simple numbers, and thus would say that the investment was beneficial to the community as a whole, even if it was not beneficial to the individual.

43. Based on the passage, why is sustainable energy attractive to consumers?

a. Sustainable energy is more efficient than other forms of energy.
b. Sustainable energy is naturally produced and thus less costly.
c. Sustainable energy is a product of nature, and thus does not involve the same amounts of chemicals that may harm the environment.
d. Sustainable energy does not get old or expire, thus requiring disposal, which can harm the environment.

44. How may legislation alter the use of sustainable energy?

a. Legislation can disincentivize energy sources that produce pollution to the environment.
b. Legislation can require companies to consume less energy in their operations.
c. Legislation can protect the consumer from the effects of pollution by providing individual consumers with more choices regarding their energy suppliers.
d. Legislation can provide consumers with more transparent information regarding sustainable energy and other energy sources so that consumers can make informed choices.

45. Why is the author interested in telling the reader about sustainable energy?

a. The author is a proponent of clean energy due to concerns about the environment.
b. The author is starting a new company and wants to raise funds for his company.
c. The author is appealing to investors to convince them to invest in diversified sustainable energy funds.
d. The author has a strong interest in educating the reader about the benefits of sustainable energy.

46. How may existing energy suppliers interact with emerging energy suppliers in the field of sustainable energy?

a. They may partner with each other in the areas of research and development, at least early in the process.
b. They may not compete with each other in the areas of research and development.
c. They may join forces to overcome legislative barriers to distribution.
d. They may leave each other alone while they focus on gaining footing in the areas of research and development.

47. What is the scientific barrier to the proliferation of the use of sustainable energy?

a. It is difficult to extract energy from sustainable sources.
b. It is difficult to preserve extracted energy from sustainable sources.
c. It is not practical to use energy obtained from sustainable sources.
d. Sustainable sources are already at their peak because nature cannot make more sustainable material.

PASSAGE 9

The interaction between humans and animals encompasses a range of vital relationships. Animals may assist as part of a laboring workforce, as beloved human companions and as food sources. A respect for the gentle creatures as well as the wild beasts of nature is an essential part of preserving these varied bonds, which often depend on one another. Even when animals are raised for the ultimate purpose of the sustenance of humans or other living creatures, the maintenance of animals' dignity during their lives plays a large role in a farmer's awareness. Yet, the unique connection between man and animal in situations when animals pose a threat to man must incorporate a special reverence for life itself.

The fascinating and true account of Jim Corbett's commissions to exterminate threatening man-eating tigers identified in human inhabited communities in the early 1900s illuminates the balance between human safety and a guarded admiration for the animal kingdom.

Man-Eaters of Kumaon, authored by Jim Corbett, is widely recognized as historically accurate in its details. A conservationist and a military officer, he was called upon at times by the British government to hunt rare man-eating tigers that were jeopardizing the lives of clans in Indian villages.

One of the most fascinating ventures in the book is the precarious story of a Bengal tiger given the name Thak. She was a tiger who had previously survived an unexplained gunshot wound. By the time she was recognized by the British government, she was notorious as a man-eating tigress who terrorized villages while she dwelled in a region populated with Indians and where the British government had plans to dispatch hundreds of workers for a construction project. Interestingly, Jim Corbett, having already succeeded at hunting assignments directed at several other man-eating tigers, grew to understand the habits of tigers. He explained Thak's unusual man-eating practice, not characteristic of most tigers, to her desperation during a period of possible incapacity for a time after having been shot and badly wounded. It is unclear when or why she had been targeted and by whom, but this explanation postulated by an experienced tiger expert suggests a rapidly evolving impact of the human population on the survival behaviors of animals. While man-eating may have been a survival skill that served to save her at a desperate time, it has certainly served its short-lived value, and later operated to resolve her unavoidable fate.

The interaction between the tiger and her hunter was complex. She became suspicious, growing cautious and deliberately eluding usual tiger hunting techniques, perhaps because she had been shot before, and thus was already schooled in the possibility that sudden, unexpected threats unfamiliar to the wild could overwhelm her at any time. Yet, despite her intelligence, she still succumbed to her instinctive needs for nourishment and breeding. Boisterously calling for a mate, she was caught by the hunter who was able to draw her closer with a loud response, finally killing her and leaving the village safe again. Planned construction began, without the threat of tigers.

This was Jim Corbett's last tiger hunt. After this experience, he became a photographer of tigers, with the objective of capturing their majesty in their natural habitat.

48. How does the passage depict the astuteness of the tiger?

a. It was typical of a tiger in survival mode.
b. Unusually sharp, and able to detect and elude human hunters.
c. She was primitive, because she succumbed to innate needs that resulted in her discovery and death.
d. Her intelligence was inferior to that of the hunter, who was able to shoot her.

49. Why does respect for the tiger play a role in the hunt?

a. The method of hunting the tiger should be humane, as an injury can result in more pain and agony for the tiger than killing it.
b. Respect is not relevant because the tiger is not being raised as a pet.
c. The best means of showing respect would be to capture the tiger and place her elsewhere.
d. Respect for the tiger in this instance prevents the further killing of tigers.

50. How does evolution, as discussed in the case of Thak, play a role in producing man-eating tigers?

a. The principle of survival of the fittest can make a trait such as man-eating more prevalent.
b. Over time, the abundance or lack of prey can cause an ecosystem to favor man-eating behavior among predators.
c. Mutations in the genes of tigers can create a man-eating tendency.
d. Impactful events can cause a behavioral change in predators due to adaptation.

51. How would the intimate knowledge of tiger habits that made Corbett an expert tiger hunter translate into his new profession of photographing tigers?

a. It would help him locate tigers while they are mating.
b. It would help him recognize when a tiger is hungry so it can be fed, posing less danger to the photographer.
c. It would help him interpret a tiger's movements, sounds, and smell to know whether it is safe to photograph.
d. It would help him to capture close-up still photos after befriending the tiger.

52. Suppose that Thak had given birth to a baby tiger one week before her death at the hands of the hunter, and this tiger later grew up to be a man-eating tiger like its mother. What impact would this have on Corbett's theory of why Thak was a man-eating tiger?

a. It would indicate that the man-eating trait was probably environmental rather than learned.
b. It would support the possibility that Thak was genetically predisposed to eating humans.
c. It would have little impact on the theory about Thak, since her offspring's behavior can be explained by having learned the behavior from its mother.
d. It would imply that Thak's memories of being hunted by humans were passed down to her offspring.

53. Suppose the man-eating tiger, Thak, had killed the hunter rather than being killed by him. How would the author likely describe the hunter's techniques?

a. The techniques were suitable for hunting tigers in the past, but species evolve to counter hunters' techniques over time.
b. The techniques were too reliant on the hunter's personal experiences, rather than on scientifically proven methods.
c. The techniques were effective for many tigers, but were not sophisticated enough for a tiger that had been previously survived being shot.
d. The techniques could not have been improved upon, given that this hunter was the preeminent tiger hunter of the time.

Answer Key and Explanations

Biological and Biochemical Foundations

Question Set 1

1. D: Hyperpolarization means a more extreme difference in electrical charge than the –70-millivolt (mV) baseline. A charge of –75 mV is more negative than a charge of –70 mV, and thus a membrane with –75 mV is hyperpolarized.

A charge of –65 mV is closer to zero than –70 mV, and thus it would not be hyperpolarized. A charge of 25 mV is also closer to zero than a charge of –70 mV, and thus it would also not be hyperpolarized. A charge of 180 mV is farther away from zero than –70 mV, and it could be defined as hyperpolarized. However, given that the refractory period produced by the pump's hyperpolarization is brief, the charge of the membrane could not be so far from the resting potential of –70 mV. Given that the hyperpolarization is an overcorrection of the action potential, it could not result in a positive charge, but it would be expected to result in a more negative charge than the –70 mV resting potential of the cell membrane.

2. A: Sodium and potassium are highly charged positive ions and are not lipid soluble. Therefore, they need a protein channel or an enzymatic protein to move across the hydrophobic portion of the plasma membrane.

Sodium and potassium are both small ions that can diffuse across some membranes, but because they are hydrophilic, they cannot diffuse across the fatty cell membrane. The phosphate present in the phospholipid bilayer is tightly bound to fatty acids and therefore cannot interact with Na+ and K+. A neuronal cell contains more Na+/K+ ATPase in its cell membrane than other cells of the body. But most cells contain Na+/K+ ATPase embedded in their cell membranes because it is used as a means to drive active transport.

3. C: The temperature can alter the 3D shape and, thus, the behavior of an enzymatic protein by altering the covalent bonds due to changes in electron movement. The hydrogen concentration, often fluctuating with pH, but also fluctuating in the presence of water molecules, can also alter the 3D shape of a protein because hydrogen is a very reactive atom due to its single electron in the outer shell. A molecule that attaches to the binding site of an enzymatic protein can alter the protein's structure and function.

Diffusion is not a factor in altering enzymatic protein shape or behavior. Water and pH both determine the hydrogen concentration, so answer B is redundant and does not include temperature, a very important determinant of the behavior of enzymatic proteins. Answer D is not correct because the concentration gradient can change the availability of a substrate, but it does not change the behavior of a protein.

4. B: Under normal circumstances, one of the effects of the pumps is to produce latency while returning the membrane to its resting potential. The more concentrated solution in this experiment made the latency shorter, and thus it must have deactivated some of the pumps, producing a reduced latency time period.

The solution did not prolong the refractory period. The length of the refractory period is directly correlated with the latency because it is the refractory period that makes it impossible for the

NA+/K+ ATPase to resume activity. If the solution worked to prolong the activity of some pumps, then the latency would have been longer with the more concentrated solutions, particularly with the 0.07% solution.

5. A: Because of the refractory period, an action potential cannot stimulate a membrane that has already been stimulated within the refractory period, and thus an action potential cannot move in the reverse direction,

Excessive concentrations of sodium could potentially damage the cell, but the latency period does not remove sodium from the cell; instead, it is the result of a slight change in the membrane's charge due to the movement of sodium. The refractory period is often believed to have some relationship with the target organ or with the synapse, but it does not. A different pathway could potentially stimulate the target organ again. Similarly, the synapse may receive a signal from a different source, and thus it is not mandatorily protected by the refractory period, which takes place at some distance.

6. D: The 0.07% solution had the most dramatic effect on the cells in this experiment. It would be expected that the cell with a lower Na+/K+ ATPase-activated proton pumps at baseline would have a more dramatically reduced action produced by deactivation of the pumps and, consequently, a shorter latency.

The greatest drop in latency between the two less-concentrated solutions would not necessarily clarify which cell has a higher density of pumps. The difference in latency between the two higher concentrations of solution, while more effective in deactivating the pumps than the lower concentration, would not necessarily deactivate the pumps of greater density more or less than the pumps of lower density, and it would be unreliable to interpret the data that way. Similarly, the relative change in latency upon exposure to all three solutions would not reveal which cell has a higher or lower density of Na+/K+ ATPase-activated proton pump.

Question Set 2

7. B: The genetic code is redundant. There are 64 codons and only 20 amino acids used in protein formation. Because of this redundancy, often a substitution mutation has no effect on the protein product.

The complementary strand in a DNA molecule must follow the base pairing rules. If a mutation of any sort affects one strand, it automatically must affect the other. The homologous copy of a DNA molecule may or may not be able to compensate or correct for a mutation — depending on whether the homologous, nonmutated DNA molecule codes for a dominant or nondominant gene. An abnormal protein product encoded by a faulty DNA molecule might be destroyed by the body's immune system, but, depending on its ultimate function, it may wreak havoc on the body, causing mild to serious problems.

8. D: Enzymes such as DNA polymerase can work to correct an error during DNA replication, which is an important part of cell division.

Cell division does not involve transcription. Transcription is the process by which a single-stranded mRNA molecule is produced based on a DNA template. DNA replication is the process by which a double-stranded DNA molecule is produced based on a DNA template. Segregation of homologous chromosomes occurs during cell division in meiosis to ensure one copy of each gene, rather than during the replication process, which is part of mitosis. A substitution mutation can be repaired when it occurs, and this is the role of some of the enzymes that are involved in the DNA replication process.

9. C: There is a weak association between the two conditions. However, it does not appear to be a functional relationship, because there is not a direct increase in T-cell impairment with base pair mutation.

The base pair mutation does not improve with worsened T-cell function because there is only one data point of improvement between group 1 and group 2. But there is an increase in base pair mutation between the control group and group 1 as with between group 2 and group 3. T-cell function plays a role in protecting the body against precancerous cells, but in this situation, it does not appear that T-cell dysfunction is the reason for the mutation because of the fact the controls had some T-cell dysfunction without base pair mutation. More importantly, there was also a decrease in base pair mutation between groups 1 and 2 despite the increase in T-cell dysfunction. The fact that the base pair mutation is more prevalent than the T-cell dysfunction does not support the answer that the base pair mutation causes the T-cell function impairment.

10. A: The dramatic increase in the presence of base pair mutation in the experimental group suggests an association between the two conditions. However, there does not appear to be a causative effect or a functional relationship, based on the pattern of the results. Genetic linkage would be the most likely explanation for the difference between the control group and the experimental group.

The fact that the base pair mutation was an incidental finding speaks to whether the genotypic mutation results in a phenotypic change, which it might not, as discussed in question (1). Linkage between two genes does not necessarily have to result in a 1:1 correlation or a direct, linear relationship. The loci of the two genes must, indeed, be located near each other to establish linkage. However, comparing function to genetics in this instance does not preclude a nearby location. In fact, in many instances, an observation such as this is the hint or clue in locating a genetic abnormality on a gene.

11. B: During transcription, enzymes involved in producing a messenger RNA (mRNA) molecule work to make a faithful copy of the nucleotides encoded on the DNA molecule, even if it is faulty.

RNA polymerase will not correct a substitution mutation or any mutation during transcription, because a mutation is part of the DNA molecule. When transfer RNA (tRNA) molecules match amino acids to mRNA molecules, this puts the abnormal code into "action." But this step is a part of translation, not transcription. The rRNA does play a role in joining tRNA and amino acids with mRNA molecules during translation, not transcription. But the consequences of this step will maintain the effects of the mutation, not decrease or increase it.

12. D: Meiosis results in the production of germ cells. A mutation during meiosis affects the offspring, but not the individual in whom the mutation occurred.

The mutation will not affect the individual at all, regardless of whether the impact on the protein encoded for is negligible, mild, or serious. The mutation will affect all of the haploid daughter cells produced during meiosis, because it would occur during DNA replication and prior to segregation and reductional division.

Question Set 3

13. C: Given that her father is not affected by this X-linked recessive disorder, her carrier status can only be determined retrospectively if she has a son who has G6PD deficiency.

Stephanie's G6PD levels are expected to be normal or near normal even if she is a carrier. This disorder is a metabolic disorder and does not manifest anatomically; thus, it would not be detectable by ultrasound. Exposing her to the offending agents may or may not produce a hemolytic reaction in the fetus – but such a trigger could be dangerous and is thus neither a safe nor a reliable way to check for her carrier status.

14. B: An X-linked gene can be expressed as codominance if the heterozygous homologous X-chromosomes both have genomic sequences encoding proteins that can be expressed simultaneously, essentially producing a blend of characteristics.

If the homologous genes on the X-chromosomes are homozygous, then the phenotype expressed will be either homozygous dominant or homozygous recessive, but not codominant. The genes on the Y-chromosome do not correspond to the genes on the X-chromosome, and thus there is no opportunity for codominance.

15. B: To determine linkage, one would have to evaluate whether the two disorders occur together at a rate higher than expected based on their individual rate in the population. Similarly, the reverse statistical analysis would yield similarly useful information: assessing how frequently G6PD deficiency occurs with and separately from other disorders that occur with the same frequency as sickle-cell disease in this population.

The fact that both genomes are located on the X-chromosome does not imply linkage. Linkage occurs when genes on the same chromosome are located at nearby loci, decreasing the chances of crossing over. The genetic prevalence versus the phenotypic occurrence would not help in determining whether malaria resistance was an evolutionary advantage for individuals with G6PD unless this data were compared with data from generations ago. Whether the RBCs have a hemolytic response to malaria exposure can help in assessing how malaria affects RBCs with and without G6PD enzyme, but not whether there could have been any linkage with sickle-cell disease or whether the response of the RBCs was, in fact, an evolutionary advantage.

16. A: The genomes of a dominant and recessive gene both work independently of one another to produce products. This explains the phenomenon of codominance. However, the products of a dominant gene are expressed, whereas the products of a recessive gene are not, mainly because the products of a dominant gene cancel out the expression or behavior of the products of a recessive gene.

The proteins encoded by either recessive or dominant genes may be long or short, small or large. Products of recessive genes are not expressed less due to denaturing of proteins, but rather because of some type of interaction with or effect of products produced by dominant genes. A dominant gene's products may "turn off" the genetic transcription of a recessive gene, but the presence of the dominant gene itself would not turn off transcription. RNA assembly of nucleotides encoded by a dominant genome is not more effective or more powerful for dominant genes than for recessive genes.

17. D: G6PD deficiency provides partial protection against malaria, and therefore a vaccine that protects against malaria may affect the incidence of G6PD deficiency in the population after some generations, but it might not if the mortality of the enzyme deficiency itself is high.

Answer A is too simplistic for a real population. Although adaptation most likely has already occurred to a degree, that does not preclude further adaptation within the population if the circumstances change due to a vaccination. An immunization would protect individuals from the hemolytic effects of malaria, but there are other triggers for hemolysis in G6PD-deficiency-affected individuals than malaria. Additionally, malaria produces hemolysis among those without G6PD deficiency, so an immunization would not preferentially aid those with the deficiency.

18. C: If the enzyme replacement were completely withheld, this would be the most effective way to determine the triggers of hemolysis. Of course, it would be unethical to willingly expose patients to potential triggers of hemolysis and withhold the enzyme.

The enzyme itself could not correct a hemolytic reaction in progress, but rather the absence of the enzyme causes a hemolytic reaction in response to certain triggers. Administration at random intervals would not differentiate between various triggers. Answer D would not establish whether sulfa medications and fava beans trigger hemolytic reactions because the enzyme would potentially prevent the hemolytic reaction. But this method could identify other triggers.

Question Set 4

19. D: Polysaccharides are metabolized in the same manner as monosaccharides, but they must first be digested and absorbed, as well as broken down into smaller subunits prior to entry into glycolysis, prolonging the metabolic process, but yielding the same energy per gram.

Polysaccharides are indeed larger and take longer to digest and absorb. But it is important to understand that there is a difference between digestion, which is breaking down the bolus into small molecules for absorption, and metabolism, which involves energy production. Polysaccharides are, indeed, larger than monosaccharides, and they do contain more calories than monosaccharides, but they contain the same number of calories per gram. Polysaccharides are directly broken down into simple glucose molecules and enter glycolysis, unlike fatty acids, which undergo a different initial step of oxidation prior to entering glycolysis.

20. A: Saturated fatty acids only have single bonds, and this molecular configuration is more stable than unsaturated fatty acids, which have double bonds and may be destabilized by molecules in the environment.

Saturated fatty acids are completely saturated with hydrogen atoms, not with electrons, which are subatomic structures of hydrogen atoms. Unsaturated fatty acids are more likely to be liquid at room temperature and to reach a boiling point faster than saturated fatty acids, but it is not this feature that makes them more likely to become rancid. Unsaturated fatty acids can have a trans configuration, but a trans configuration is not associated with greater molecular instability. Unsaturated fatty acids with a cis or with a trans configuration have a greater tendency to become rancid than saturated fatty acids.

21. B: It is the number of single bonds in a molecule that yields energy. Saturated fatty acids have more single bonds than unsaturated fatty acids and thus contain slightly more calories per gram.

The number of calories is based on the number of single bonds and double bonds. But two single bonds yield more calories than one double bond, which means that despite the equivalent number of bonds, the caloric count per gram is slightly higher in saturated fats. Some molecules are more difficult to absorb. Starches, for example, which are complex carbohydrates, may contain indigestible portions that are not absorbed and thus do not yield calories. This feature does not analogously apply to fatty acids. Unsaturated fats contain fewer calories per gram than saturated fats due to the lack of double bonds within saturated fat molecules, regardless of the size or total number of bonds per molecule. The size of the molecule and the number of bonds affects the mass and thus the weight. Calories are considered per gram, which takes into account the size and number of bonds.

22. B: Glycolysis consumes 2 ATP molecules and produces a gross yield of 4, which is a net yield of 2 ATP molecules. The Krebs cycle yields 2 ATP molecules, whereas the electron transport chain yields 32 ATP molecules.

23. D: Because saturated fats contain slightly more calories than unsaturated fats, such an experiment would require control of caloric intake to differentiate the effects of saturated fat versus unsaturated fat, independent of calories.

If the experiment were designed to determine the difference between saturated versus unsaturated fatty acids in the context of heart disease, adding another variable, which is the measure of polyunsaturated fat, would not directly help answer the question. The numbers of total calories consumed by research subjects can affect the development of heart disease, but this would not help to differentiate the effects of saturated versus unsaturated fats. Preexisting heart disease can certainly alter the results, but it wouldn't alter the difference between saturated fat versus unsaturated fat.

24. C: Oxygen allows metabolism to produce more ATP per glucose molecule than the ATP produced in glycolysis alone, which does not require oxygen. Because the Krebs cycle and electron transport chain together produce 34 ATP molecules, oxygen makes metabolism more efficient.

Oxygen is not required for the metabolism of glucose, although the metabolism is less efficient in the absence of oxygen. Oxygen is not required for glycolysis, and thus it is not part of every step in the metabolic process. It is the electrons in the electron transport chain that result in the rich supply of ATP, not hydrogen.

Question Set 5

25. C: The experimental results do not demonstrate or prove that the antioxidant is responsible for the decrease in edema or that edema is the cause of tissue damage. However, because patients exposed to the antioxidant had a smaller area of infarcted tissue, it appears that the antioxidant has a beneficial effect. Most, but not all, of the patients with smaller areas of infarct also had decreased edema, suggesting that edema may also play a role. This suggests that some type of combination of the presence of edema and antioxidants was at play when decreased tissue damage was observed.

There was no measured relationship to blood flow. It is unclear exactly why the antioxidant-injected samples showed deceased damage, and it is a leap to suggest that the antioxidants themselves produce chemicals or biochemical reactions that decreased the size of the infarct or the edema.

26. C: Most of the cell's ATP production occurs in the mitochondria. The Ca^+ concentration is maintained by active transport, which requires ATP. Ca^+ leaks into the ischemic cell due to passive transport when ATP is inadequate to overcome the concentration gradient.

Active transport does maintain the Ca^+ concentration, but ATP is produced in the mitochondria, not by the mitochondria, which is an important distinction. Mitochondrial membranes contain Ca^+, but mitochondrial dysfunction occurs prior to mitochondrial degeneration, and the calcium influx is largely a consequence of mitochondrial dysfunction. The lack of adequate oxygen forces the cell to rely in lactic acidosis, which can cause ionic shifts. But this is not the driving force behind the calcium influx.

27. A: In small quantities, lactic acids and free fatty acids are tolerable due to the cell's ability to buffer mild pH changes. However, in an ischemic setting, the cell cannot correct the pH changes, and thus the proteins that form the structural and functional components of the organelles begin to denature.

Lactic acids and free fatty acids are acidic, meaning that they contribute hydrogen atoms to the environment, whereas free radicals are deficient in electrons. Although the volume of acidic molecules within the cell is not beneficial for the organelles, their pH is their most harmful characteristic and thus the most immediately damaging consequence. Free fatty acids are hydrophobic and thus may be able to pass through organelle membranes, but they cause organelle dysfunction from outside the organelle in the cytoplasm as well.

28. B: A cell relies on anaerobic respiration when aerobic respiration, which depends on oxygen, cannot provide the necessary substrates for the Krebs cycle and the electron transport chain. The by-product of anaerobic respiration is lactic acid.

Lactic acidosis is the product of lactic acid production during infarction, not the consequence of a molecule already present in the cell, the organelles, or the membranes. Lactic acid is a by-product of anaerobic respiration, which provides energy, but the lactic acid itself does not provide energy. Lactate is a sugar present in dairy products, whereas lactose is an enzyme that breaks down lactate. Lactic acid is a by-product of anaerobic metabolism. Although the three molecules have similarities in structure and name, and they can be easily confused, they are not the same.

29. D: As the tissue becomes damaged and the cells become altered, inflammatory white blood cells arrive to remove debris and to repair damaged tissue.

There have been microorganisms noted in and around infarcted tissue, and the presence of subclinical infection has been imputed as a possible contributor to ischemia, but not directly to the fast damage of infarction that occurs as a result of ischemia. The inflammatory cells are a component of edematous fluid that is present during infarct, but this does not explain how membrane degeneration contributes to inflammation because the inflammation is more likely a response to the membrane degeneration. The white blood cells that arrive so quickly during the inflammatory response to ischemia are likely already present in the body moments prior to the ischemic event; however, they arrive to the site of damage as a result of cytokines and other modulators, rather than due to passive transport driven by the concentration gradient.

30. B: The physical degeneration of the phospholipid bilayer of the membrane, as well as the dysfunction of protein channels and pumps, allows ions and other molecules to leak into or out of the cell, driven by the concentration gradient. Capillary leakiness is the result of separation of the endothelial cells that line the capillaries, which can allow fluid and cells, including inflammatory cells, to leak into or out of the capillary.

The membrane of the capillary, if it becomes pathologically permeable, would allow fluid and cells to leak in or out. The membrane of the cell would allow fluid and ions into or out of the cell if it becomes leaky. Membrane leakiness both contributes to and results from degeneration of the phospholipid bilayer, whereas capillary leakiness results from separation of the endothelial cells that line the capillaries. Membrane leakiness and capillary leakiness both contribute to edema and inflammation by allowing fluid, white blood cells, and other molecules to flood the site.

Question Set 6

31. D: Developmental disorders may have a number of possible etiologies, including alterations of the genome or environmental causes. Developmental disorders may begin prior to fertilization, due to alterations in the gamete, during embryogenesis, or even after birth.

Genetic disorders as well as developmental disorders may both include physical conditions, defects in emotional processing, or cognitive disorders. Genetic disorders involve alterations in the DNA nucleotide sequence and can be produced before, during, or after embryogenesis as a result of inherited DNA alterations, environmentally triggered DNA alterations, or spontaneously occurring DNA alterations.

32. B: Nondisjunction is the imperfect separation of homologous chromosomes during meiosis and results in a gamete that does not have one of each chromosome from a homologous pair.

Nondisjunction may result in a chromosome number other than 23, but nondisjunction may result in a chromosome number of 23 if a different nonhomologous chromosome replaces one chromosome. Most of the time, nondisjunction results in 22 or 24 chromosomes in a haploid gamete, but this is not necessarily the case because nondisjunction might result in replacement of one chromosome with a nonhomologous chromosome or it may result in more than one missing or more than one extra chromosome.

33. A: Using one of these germ layers to replace the type of cell that originates from the corresponding type of germ layer maximizes the potential for proper differentiation.

A matched-type donor may minimize rejection, but this would not improve the chances for proper differentiation. Bone marrow stem cells would have already progressed beyond the embryonic stage of ectoderm, mesoderm, and endoderm, making them less likely to differentiate into the target cell type. Gametes are unfertilized and are therefore haploid, so they are not able to replace diploid cells.

34. A: Pulmonary surfactant develops late in gestation, and therefore prematurity can result in respiratory distress syndrome, which occurs because the alveoli may collapse when pulmonary surfactant is deficient, leading to poor oxygenation.

The skeletal muscles are not the factor limiting oxygenation when premature birth occurs at this stage of fetal development. The heart function and hemoglobin are both adequate because respiratory support for premature babies born at this stage of fetal development provides adequate oxygen to the body.

35. B: Germ cells are diploid cells that will later undergo meiosis to produce haploid gametes, whereas germ layers are composed of diploid cells. The ectoderm, mesoderm, and endoderm are the differentiating germ layers of the embryo.

Germ cells are not produced during gametogenesis. Gametes are produced during gametogenesis. Germ layers are produced after fertilization. Germ layers are not parts of germ cells. Germ cells are diploid, as are the cells of germ layers. These terms sound similar, and thus they can be confusing.

36. C: A germ cell is a diploid cell produced during embryogenesis. After birth, during puberty or adulthood, oogenesis and spermatogenesis produces gametes, which are haploid cells. A germ cell replicates its chromosomes and produces four daughter gametes, each with a haploid chromosome number.

A germ cell does not mature into a gamete, but, rather, it undergoes a more complex process of gametogenesis. A germ cell does not simply divide to produce two gametes. A germ cell is diploid.

Question Set 7

37. A: A parasite can be haploid or diploid and may go through phases of diploid or haploid genomic number.

Bacteria and viruses are haploid, whereas prions do not contain genetic material.

38. C: A virus may invade a cell and evade an immune response by essential hiding inside the cell so that leucocytes may not identify the virus. Sometimes the virus alters the host cell so that the cellular immune system is activated.

A retrovirus can invade immune cells, as is the case with the human immunodeficiency virus (HIV), but other viruses that selectively invade cells that are not part of the immune system may evade an immunologic response as well. So, deactivating the immune system is not the only mechanism a virus uses to avoid identification and destruction by immune cells. And not all viruses infect immune cells. A virus is small, and this aids in its evasion of the immune system by allowing it to enter inside a cell, but it is not too small to be detected by the immune system. A virus does not typically mimic a cell, but instead it enters the cell and uses the cell's genetic tools to make new copies of itself.

39. A: Binary fission is the process by which bacteria grow and replicate their DNA and then divide.

Conjugation is a method of transferring genetic material between bacteria, and it may be a part of the bacterial reproduction process. Bacteria do not reproduce by sexual reproduction. A virus inserts its genetic material into the host's genome, whereas bacteria do not.

40. D: A retrovirus genome is composed of RNA nucleotide, whereas a viral genome is composed of DNA. Both insert into the host cell and use its reproductive tools to make new viruses.

Both a retrovirus and a virus may insert genetic material into a host cell's DNA, and they can both enter the cell membrane of the host. The cell wall is present in bacterial cells but not in human cells. A retrovirus or a virus can alter a cell's DNA to cause a precancerous transformation of the host cell. A retrovirus is not an old cell, despite the sound of the name.

41. B: The bacterial cell has a cell wall; a cell membrane and cytoplasm; and a nucleoid, which holds the DNA. But a bacterial cell does not have a nucleus.

Question Set 8

42. C: Nerves that are part of the CNS often send messages to the peripheral nervous system (PNS). The somatic nerves in the PNS may then send nerve signals that ultimately release acetylcholine at the neuromuscular junction. Because an action potential is an all-or-none event, demyelination in the CNS may prevent any signal from reaching the peripheral nerve.

It is true that afferent peripheral nerves send electrical signals to the CNS, but acetylcholine, associated with nerves that stimulate skeletal muscle, is a neurotransmitter associated with efferent nerve stimulation that originates in the CNS. An action potential is an all-or-none event, and thus demyelination does not result in slowing or a diminished signal, but it results in either no effect or in a complete loss of the action potential. The CNS interacts with the PNS, and thus, depending on the exact location of demyelination, CNS problems can affect the PNS.

43. B: The hypothalamus communicates with the anterior pituitary gland through the vascular system and with the posterior pituitary gland through axon extensions. Additionally, the posterior pituitary is composed of neuronal tissue, whereas the anterior pituitary, despite its location in the brain, is not neuronal tissue.

The hypothalamus produces hormones that are sent to the posterior pituitary gland through the axons, are stored in the posterior pituitary gland, and then are released. The anterior pituitary gland makes hormones in response to chemical stimulation from the hypothalamus. Communication between the hypothalamus and both the anterior pituitary gland and posterior pituitary gland is regulated by positive and negative feedback. Negative feedback is the predominant mechanism. Oxytocin, released by the posterior pituitary gland, is associated with elements of positive feedback, but the anterior pituitary gland responds to positive feedback as well. The hypothalamus primarily stimulates hormone release or hormone production and release in both the anterior and posterior pituitary.

44. A: A hyperactive pituitary tumor may overstimulate the adrenal medulla, and thus produce negative feedback reaching several levels, including the hypothalamus and the pituitary gland, and the adrenal medulla would regulate the hormones that regulate the autonomic nervous system.

The negative feedback regulating the hypothalamus would not be the only negative feedback in place, and, alone, it would not effectively control the hyperactivity of the anterior pituitary gland. Although negative feedback would help regulate hormonal production, it is unlikely to effectively balance the activity of the sympathetic and parasympathetic divisions of the autonomic nervous system. Additionally, negative feedback generally works to decrease stimulation of hormones rather than to directly inhibit them. It is not characteristic that overproduction of ACTH would desensitize the adrenal medulla to overstimulation. Hormone regulation is most commonly controlled by negative-feedback mechanisms.

45. D: The change in concentration over time would be partially controlled by the rate of reuptake, but it would also be controlled by other mechanisms of serotonin decomposition. Taking initial measurements of concentration and following the change at several intervals would help determine the effect of additional serotonin on the rate of reuptake.

The reuptake function does not rely on a neurotransmitter having a desired effect on an end organ. Reuptake or any type of neurotransmitter deactivation is based on concentration, not quantity. The results of the experiment comparing different concentrations of serotonin treatment would not provide as much value as comparing a treated group to a control group because a baseline value is necessary to establish the normal rate of reuptake.

46. C: Neuroglial cells are better able to repair themselves than are neurons, and possibly because of their increased capacity for cell division over a person's lifespan, they may undergo alterations that could lead to cancer.

Neuroglia are indeed supportive cells, but this characteristic does not preclude cancer potential. Neurons are not more likely to experience toxin, free-radical, or retrovirus exposure than do neuroglia due to their functional status. The blood-brain barrier protects the CNS, including the neurons and the neuroglial cells, and thus retroviruses, which can cause oncologic changes, are not preferential to neuroglia or neurons. Both neuroglia and neurons are myelinated, but some neuroglial cells provide myelin for the neurons. Myelin is not protective against cancer-causing materials. Myelin insulates neuronal tissue to maintain the action potential.

47. D: A hypofunctioning adrenal medulla would result in inconsistent compensatory stimulation of the hypothalamus and pituitary gland rather than a steady overstimulation. But the compensatory response of the pituitary would not cause a benign or malignant enlargement of the pituitary gland, and thus it would not affect the optic nerves.

Pituitary enlargement would produce pressure on the optic nerves, but overstimulation by negative feedback mechanisms should not cause enlargement of the pituitary gland. The thyroid gland is the gland typically associated with enlargement in response to hypofunction, hyperfunction, hypothyroidism, or hyperthyroidism.

Question Set 9

48. A: The oxygen deficit that results from blood loss as well as the volume deficit stimulates a compensatory response of the heart rate.

Although a lack of oxygen may force the body to use an alternate metabolic pathway that results in lactic acidosis, this is not the driving force behind the resulting tachycardia. CO2 buildup does provide feedback to the brainstem medulla that adjusts the heart rate, but in the setting of acute anemia, it is the volume loss and oxygen deficit that elicit the heart rate adjustment. Hemolytic anemia is a type of acute anemia, but it is caused by the breakdown of red blood cells within the body, not by the volume loss experienced during traumatic bleeding.

49. B: The kidneys detect the oxygen concentration in the blood and produce erythropoietin to stimulate the bone marrow to produce erythrocytes, which are red blood cells.

The volume of fluid that passes through the kidneys is a factor in determining the urine output from the kidneys, but it does not stimulate erythropoietin production. The stem cells in the bone marrow respond to erythropoietin to increase the production of red blood cells.

50. B: Blood pressure is a measurement of arterial pressure. In the setting of acute anemia, arterial regulation adjusts in response to fluid levels, tissue needs, and oxygen concentration.

Vasospasm may occur in the setting of acute bleeding that causes tissue irritation or in the setting of acute hypertension. Red blood cell concentration is not a factor in acute anemia, but it is a factor in chronic anemia. Venous regulation is the regulation of veins, which are blood vessels. However, blood pressure is measured in arteries, not in veins.

51. C: The brainstem medulla detects carbon dioxide levels and sends hormones to adjust the size of the alveoli, the width of the bronchi, and the rate and force of inspiration by control of the respiratory muscles.

The medulla in the brainstem is different from the adrenal medulla, which is part of the adrenal gland, a gland that sits above the kidney. The kidney also has a renal medulla. Although the name "medulla" repeats in anatomy, these are distinct locations that can be easily confused.

52. D: Within the first few minutes of an agglutination reaction, the acute hemolysis would stimulate the sympathetic nervous system, but this would not have an effect on erythropoietin to correct the hemolytic anemia yet.

Eventually, if the patient survives a hemolytic reaction, the kidneys would produce erythropoietin to increase red blood cell production in the bone marrow. The response to erythropoietin would not increase or decrease due to anemia or hemolysis, and the sympathetic nervous system would not inhibit the release of erythropoietin.

53. A: The kidneys control and adjust blood pressure in response to several factors, including fluid content and fluid volume. The kidneys produce erythropoietin in response to oxygen concentration and oxygen partial pressure.

The urine content is a function of the kidneys, but the kidneys' response to blood pressure determines the fluid content in the body. The urine content depends on a number of factors, and thus it would not be a reliable measurement of the kidneys' response to chronic anemia. The urine content and volume are dependent on fluid and electrolytes. Antidiuretic hormone is produced in the anterior pituitary and acts on the kidneys, so it would not be a good indicator of the kidneys' response to chronic anemia.

Discrete Questions

54. A: The neural tube begins to develop within the first month of gestation, so a folate deficiency resulting in neural tube defects would be expected to begin having deleterious effects within or even prior to the first month of gestation.

If a vitamin deficiency increases the risk of any type of birth defect, an adequate supply of the vitamin does not necessarily prevent all of the defects from occurring because developmental problems generally have more than just one etiology. Thus, eliminating one of the causes does not necessarily eliminate all of other causes of the defect. Although vitamin A is fat soluble, one cannot infer that all vitamins impacting gestation are fat soluble because there are several routes by which nutrients can reach the fetus. Although epidermal tissue and nerve tissue are derived from a common germ layer, they diverge and thus do not necessarily rely on the same nutrients for proper differentiation.

55. A: An egg cell is larger than a sperm cell, containing a larger cytoplasm with more adenosine triphosphate (ATP)-producing mitochondria.

An egg cell is haploid, as is a sperm cell. A sperm cell may contain a Y or an X chromosome, whereas an egg cell must contain an X chromosome and cannot have a Y chromosome. Both egg cells and sperm cells have nuclei. In reproductive technology, a sperm cell or both an egg cell and a sperm cell can be isolated and used in an in vitro procedure.

56. B: Leukocytes are white blood cells. Antigens on pathogens elicit a leukocyte response. Lymphocytes are a subset of leukocytes.

B-lymphocytes make and release antibodies in response to antigens on the surface of pathogens. Other leukocytes, T-cells, do not produce or release antibodies, instead carrying out the cell-mediated immune response, which is not antibody mediated. Erythrocytes are red blood cells and do not have a major role in the body's immune response, nor do they produce antibodies.

57. D: The names of junctions between cells are often counterintuitive. Gap junctions form a channel between the cytoplasm of neighboring cells, allowing material to flow from one cell to another.

Gap junctions do not allow a space between neighboring cells, despite the name's implication. Tight junctions form a barrier to prevent fluid from passing between neighboring cells, whereas adhering junctions cement neighboring cells together. It is not adhering junctions that form a barrier to block fluid, it is tight junctions.

58. C: The liver, the kidney, and the small intestine cells can use amino acids in the process of gluconeogenesis in the mitochondria. The mitochondrion is the site for gluconeogenesis, but not all cells are capable of gluconeogenesis. The muscle fibers, particularly the slow muscle fibers, are rich in mitochondria, but muscle cells are not a site for gluconeogenesis, even when an alternate energy-producing pathway is needed. Adipose tissue stores fat molecules. The energy-producing process that uses fat molecules is not gluconeogenesis, but rather oxidation and then entry into the Krebs cycle and the electron transport chain. Gluconeogenesis uses amino acids to build carbohydrate molecules for energy.

59. B: A proto-oncogene is a normal gene that may undergo an alteration and become an oncogene. An oncogene is an abnormal gene that may cause cancer. Proto-oncogenes generally encode for cell activity related to cell death or cell division. Thus, when proto-oncogenes are altered in certain ways, cells may become cancerous.

A proto-oncogene does not promote an oncogene, although the name would make it sound so. A proto-oncogene is not a protein, although the name could be mistaken for a protein. A proto-oncogene encodes functions related to cell apoptosis and mitosis, as does an oncogene, because they are both forms of the same gene. But a proto-oncogene is normal, whereas an oncogene is abnormal.

Chemical and Physical Foundations

Passage 1

1. A: Bond A is the amide bond linking the amino acids together to form a peptide. For amino acid analysis, hydrolysis of peptide bonds with hydrochloric acid is preferred over hydrolysis with strong base because hydrochloric acid is much less likely to break any other bonds in a protein, leaving the individual amino acids largely intact.

2. D: (L-Glutamic Acid). The easiest way to recognize the correct answer is by the pKa of the R group of this amino acid. Since it has a pKa of 4.25, it must be a carboxylic acid. Of the choices given, only glutamic acid has a carboxylic acid on the R group.

3. B: (L-Lysine). This question requires understanding of how cation exchange chromatography separates amino acids based on charge, as well as recognizing the charge on amino acids based on memorization of the structures or the pKa data presented in the passage.

The protonated amine groups on the amino acids carry a positive charge. These positive charges interact most strongly with the negatively charged sulfonate groups on the ion exchange beads. If you did not know that sulfonate is negatively charged, you can deduce this fact by recognizing either that it is a cation exchange resin, or that it is preloaded with positively charged sodium ions. When the positively charged amine groups interact with the negatively charge beads, the beads slow the movement of those binding amino acids down the column.

In this example, L-Lysine, with the positively charged R group (seen from the pKa of the R group in Table 1) and the positively charged α-amino group consequently carries two positive charges, while all of the other choices only carry one positive charge (from the α-amino group). Hence, L-Lysine interacts more strongly with the negatively charged beads and is the slowest of the amino acids listed to elute from a cation exchange chromatography column.

O

H_3C OH

4. B: (NH_2). Choice (b) is the stereochemical representation of L-alanine. Incorrect answers are: (a) D-alanine, (c) L-valine, and (d) L-leucine. This question requires understanding of the structure of amino acids (by memorization), as well as stereochemistry, either by memorization, or by determination using the rules of organic chemistry for R and S enantiomers. The specific rotation values given in the passage are not, by themselves, useful in figuring out structure.

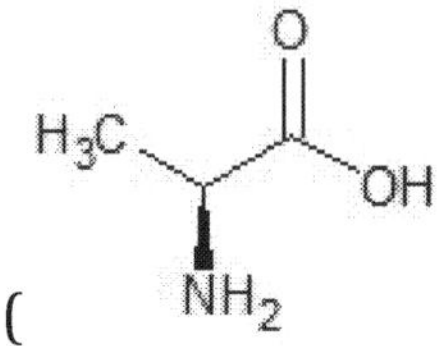

5. D: (The amino acid labeled unknown). Examination of the pKa values in Table 1 provides this answer. Buffering by an acid/base pair is strongest near the pKa of the acid. Of the amino acids available as choices, only unknown, with an R group pKa of 4.25 has a pKa near 5, so only it buffers at that pH. This fact is why most amino acids (except histidine) do not generally provide significant buffering in the physiologic range of pH 6-8.

Passage 2

6. D: (24). Each of the three oxygen atoms contributes six, nitrogen contributes five, and the negative charge contributes one additional electron.

7. B: (0). The formal charge is the difference between the charge on the valance electrons in an individual atom (such as the nitrogen atom), and the charge on the electrons assigned to it in the Lewis dot structure. Nitrogen has five valence electrons when it is an individual atom, and the Lewis dot structure of nitrite has five assigned to it (one for the single bond to oxygen, two for the double bond to the other oxygen atom, and two nonbonding electrons). Since there are five valance electrons in the individual atom and five electrons assigned to it in the nitrite ion, the formal charge is zero.

8. B: (Ammonia, nitric oxide, nitrogen dioxide). Ammonia is trigonal pyramidal with nitrogen at the vertex, so the polar bonds from the nitrogen to each of the hydrogen atoms add together to form a molecular dipole pointing up through the nitrogen atom. Nitric oxide consists of only two atoms with different electronegativity, so it has a molecular dipole pointing from the nitrogen to the oxygen atom. Nitrogen dioxide is a bent molecule, so the two polar bonds from the central nitrogen atom to the two oxygen atoms add together to give a molecular dipole pointing through the oxygen atom and away from the nitrogen atoms. Nitrous oxide is incorrect because it is a linear molecule and the contributions to the molecular dipole from each of the polar nitrogen to oxygen bonds cancel each other out. Dinitrogen is incorrect because it is a molecule consisting of two identical atoms, and so there are no polar bonds.

9. C: ($\overset{-}{N}=\overset{+}{N}=\overset{-}{N}$). Of the possible resonance structures, (c) has the fewest formal charges and hence is the dominant form. The answer (a) is a possible resonance structure for azide ion, but since it has more formal charges than (c), it is not the dominant contribution. The answers b and d are not dominant resonance structures of azide ion since they do not satisfy the octet rule around each of the nitrogen atoms.

10. D: (Nitrous oxide and water). The easiest way to solve this problem is to balance the redox reaction, starting with:

$$N_3^- + NO_2^- + 2H^+ \rightarrow N_2 + ???$$

Balancing the nitrogen atoms means the right-hand side must contain an additional two nitrogen atoms. Given the answer choices, that means either one N2O or two NO molecules.

$$N_3^- + NO_2^- + 2H^+ \rightarrow N_2 + N_2O + ???$$

or

$$N_3^- + NO_2^- + 2H^+ \rightarrow N_2 + 2NO + ???$$

Balancing oxygen atoms (two on the left implies two on the right) by adding water to the right gives a balanced reaction for the first equation (and is the correct answer):

$$N_3^- + NO_2^- + 2H^+ \rightarrow N_2 + N_2O + H_2O$$

However, the second reaction is already balanced with respect to oxygen, so must not have any water as a product:

$$N_3^- + NO_2^- + 2H^+ \rightarrow N_2 + 2NO + ???$$

Since this reaction producing nitric oxide cannot balance with respect to H and O, either with or without water added to the right-hand side, it cannot be the correct choice.

PASSAGE 3

11. D: (Ca3(PO4)2). Calcium is an alkaline earth metal that, as an ion, always carries a +2 charge. Phosphate (PO43-) carries a -3 charge. In order to achieve charge balance, there must be equal positive and negative total charges in the crystal, so there must be three calcium ions for every two phosphate ions.

12. C: (12.4%). While an exact equation can determine how much radioactivity remains as a function of time, it is easiest to estimate in this case. Forty-three days is about three half-lives (3 × 14.29 = 42.87 days). Each half-life drops the radioactivity by half. At day 0 the activity is 100%, after 1 half-life it is 50%, at 2 half-lives it is half again, or 25%, and after three half-lives it is half again, or 12.5%. The answer is 12.4% because 43 days is just a little longer than three half-lives.

13. D: (The storage conditions will not influence radioactivity). Radioactive decay rates are not dependent on temperature or the chemistry around the atom, which is why radioactive decay rates are so useful for dating old objects or tracking the movement of atoms.

14. B: ($^{32}_{16}S^{+}$). According to Table 3, 32P undergoes beta decay. Beta decay involves a neutron turning into a proton with the loss of an electron. Consequently, the nuclear charge increases by +1. When starting with phosphorus that has 15 protons, an increase of one proton turns the atom into a sulfur atom with 16 protons. Since the phosphorus atom started with no charge, and lost an electron with a negative charge, the final atom must have a positive charge.

15. C: ($^{13}_{6}C$). Capture of a neutron adds a neutron to the nucleus, and leaves the electrons and protons unchanged. Consequently, to get to $^{14}_{6}C$ by neutron capture, one has to start with a carbon atom with one less neutron.

PASSAGE 4

16. D: (Blue). The wavelength used to detect bilirubin in the passage is 457 nm. Blue light has wavelengths between about 450 nm and 495 nm.

17. C: (2.7 eV). The equation used to calculate the energy of a photon from the wavelength is E = hc/λ, where h is Planck's constant, c is the speed of light in a vacuum, and λ is the wavelength. In this case, E = (4.1 ×10−15 eV/s)(3.00 × 108 m/s)/(457 nm) = (1.2 × 10-6 eVm/s)/457 nm. In order to divide the values, first convert nm into meters. 1 nm = 1 × 10-9 m, so 457 nm = 4.57 × 10-7 m. Substituting 4.57 × 10-7 m for 457 nm in the earlier equation gives E = (1.2 × 10-6 eVm/s)/(= 4.57 × 10-7 m), which equals 2.7 eV. The Faraday constant is not required to answer this question.

18. C: (0.61). Transmittance is the fraction of light passing through the sample, T = P/P0, where T is transmittance, P0 is the incident light, and P is the light passing through the sample. The easiest way to determine this answer is to recognize that for each 1-cm that the light penetrates through the solution, 0.85 (85%) of the initial light passes through. Since the same fractional decrease is true for each of the 1-cm lengths, the transmittance is 0.85 × 0.85 × 0.85 = 0.61.

This answer can be also calculated from the Beer-Lambert Law, T = 10-εlc, where ε is the molar absorptivity, l is path length in cm, and c is the concentration. The only variable in this equation that changes is l. For the 1 cm path length, T = 10-εlc = 10-εc = 0.85. For a 3 cm path length, T = 10- εlc = 10-3εc. Separating the exponent into two parts, we get T = (10-εc)3 and substituting in 0.85 for 10-εc we get T = (0.85)3 = 0.61.

19. C: (0.10). Absorbance is defined by Beer's Law, A = εlc, where A is absorbance, ε is the molar absorptivity, l is path length, and c is the concentration. In this case, ε = 48,907 M-1cm-1, l is 2 cm, and c = 1 μM = 1 × 10-6 M. Consequently, A = (48,907 M-1cm-1)(2 cm)(1 × 10-6 M) = 0.098 which rounds to 0.10.

20 C:

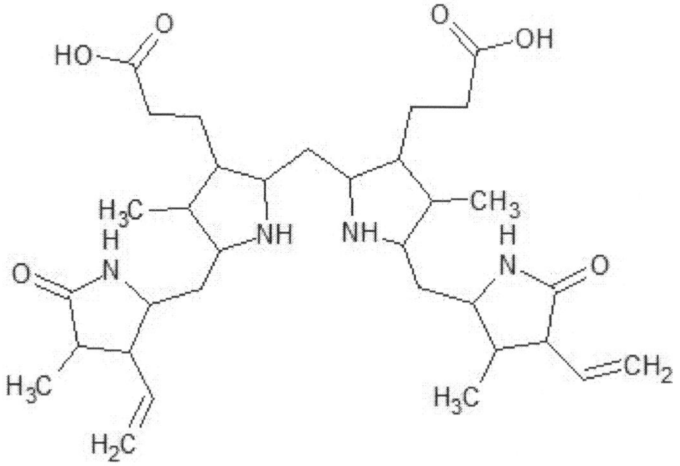

Conjugated carbon-carbon double bonds in organic compounds such as bilirubin absorb visible light. There are no conjugated double bonds remaining in structure (c), so it would not absorb visible light. Structure (a) has the two carboxyethyl moieties removed, and these structures would not eliminate the absorption of visible light by the conjugated double bonds. Structure (b) has methyl esters on the carboxylic acids, which would not significantly alter the absorption of light. Structure (d) has added two hydrocarbon moieties to the structure, which would not preclude the absorption of light by the conjugated double bonds.

PASSAGE 5

21. B: (Bicarbonate). This question focuses on understanding the meaning of acid/base chemistry, buffers, and pKa values. From the pKa value of the carbonic acid/bicarbonate buffer system

$H_2CO_3 \leftrightarrow HCO_3^- + H^+$ pKa1 = 5.85

we can see that pH 8.2 is well above the pKa (5.85), so there must be substantially more of the conjugate base, bicarbonate, than carbonic acid.

From the pKa value of the bicarbonate/carbonate buffer system

$HCO_3^- \leftrightarrow CO_3^{2-} + H^+$ pKa2 = 8.92

we can see that pH 8.2 is well below the pKa (8.92), so there must be substantially more of the conjugate acid, bicarbonate, than carbonate. Hence, the answer must be B.

22. B: (Compared to the starting mixture, the dissolved calcium concentration dropped). This question focuses on the use and meaning of a solubility product.

Ksp = [Ca2+][CO32-]

Since there is solid calcium carbonate and a solution at equilibrium, the Ksp must be equal to the solubility product constant, and any additional calcium or carbonate added to the system pushes the Ksp higher than the constant, and precipitation results. Only carbonate was added and calcium carbonate precipitated, so calcium must have declined. The sodium is unimportant to the question except as a way of delivering the carbonate.

23. A: (There is no change in the dissolved concentration of calcium or carbonate). This question focuses on the nature of a solubility product and the fact that solid materials do not enter such a calculation as they do not change their concentration.

Ksp = [Ca2+][CO32-]

The fact that there is no term for the solid material in the Ksp demonstrates that the amount of solid material present is not important to the solubility. As long as there is some solid material in contact with the solution at equilibrium, the solution is saturated (that is, all that can dissolve has dissolved). Having more or less solid material present does not change the amount that can dissolve at equilibrium, as long as there is some undissolved solid calcium carbonate.

24. B: (the carbonate concentration fell and the carbonic acid concentration rose). This question focuses on acid/base chemistry, and Le Chatelier's principle.

$H_2CO_3 \leftrightarrow HCO_3^- + H^+$ pKa1 = 5.85

$HCO_3^- \leftrightarrow CO_3^{2-} + H^+$ pKa2 = 8.92

At pH 8.2, we are below pKa2 and above pKa1. Consequently, there is both carbonate and bicarbonate (and a small amount of carbonic acid) present. On addition of a strong acid, H+, the pH drops. As that happens, Le Chatelier's principle tells us that both of the reactions shown above will push to the left: carbonate converts into bicarbonate and bicarbonate converts into carbonic acid. Consequently, carbonate declines and carbonic acid increases.

25. A: (As the temperature rises, bicarbonate becomes a stronger acid, so carbonate rises). This question involves knowing that a lower pKa implies a stronger acid, as well as the fact that a stronger acid will dissociate into H+ and it conjugate base more than a weaker acid. As the temperature rises from 25°C to 30°C, the pKa of bicarbonate drops from 8.92 to 8.75. The drop in pKa shows that it is becoming a stronger acid. As the bicarbonate becomes a stronger acid, the reaction below shifts more to the right:

$HCO_3^- \leftrightarrow CO_3^{2-} + H^+$ pKa2

Consequently, it dissociates more into H+ and carbonate, and carbonate rises.

Passage 6

26. A: (245 N). If each leg below her knees has a mass of 2.5 kg, then her total mass above her knees is 55 kg – 2 × (2.5 kg) = 50 kg. The force of gravity is 9.8 m/s2, so the gravitational force pulling down on her body from F = ma is F = 50 kg × 9.8 m/s2 = 490 kg m/s2. 1 N (Newton) = 1 kg m/s2, so the total force is 490 N. Since only half of that force is on each knee, the answer is 490/2 N = 245 N.

27. C: (1617 N). According to Table 1, a woman walking with a knee flex angle of 15° experiences a peak compressive load on her knees of three times her body weight. The force can then be calculated as 3 × 55 kg × 9.8 m/s2 = 1617 kg m/s2 = 1617 N.

28. D: (Decrease by 2.8%). According to the passage, each 1 kg loss in body weight resulted in a 1.4% decline in the peak compressive load while walking. So a 2 kg loss in body weight is associated with a 2 × 1.4% = 2.8% decline in peak compressive load.

29. C: (1911 J). Gravitational potential energy is weight times height, or mass times acceleration due to gravity times height. In this case, mass is 65 kg, acceleration due to gravity is 9.8 m/s2, and the height is 3 m. PE = 65 kg × 9.8 m/s2 × 3 m = 1911 kg m2/s2. Since 1 kg m2/s2 = 1 J (joule), the answer is 1911 J. The facts of the knee flex angle used and the number of stairs are unimportant to the question.

30. D: (2400 J). The energy required to stop the man and bicycle is the same as the kinetic energy of motion. The kinetic energy of linear motion is calculated from KE = ½ mv2. We use m = 75 kg to account for both the bicycle and the man, and m = 8 m/s. KE = ½ × 75 kg × 8 m/s × 8 m/s = 2400 kg m2/s2. Since 1 kg m2/s2 = 1 J (joule), the energy required = 2400 J.

Passage 7

31. C: (n-Hexanol is more effective at London dispersion interactions because it has a higher surface area than methanol). The positive interactions between methanol molecules and between n-hexanol molecules consists primarily of hydrogen bonding and London dispersion forces. Methanol has a higher proportion of hydrogen bonding moieties (the -OH groups) than does n-hexanol (because the hexyl chain is large and has no role in hydrogen bonding except potentially getting in the way), so methanol is more effective at hydrogen bonding (ruling out answer choices a and b). There are no ionic interactions between these uncharged molecules, so choice d is incorrect. London dispersion forces take place between molecules, including nonpolar molecules, though the interaction of instantaneous multipoles. The strength of these forces depends on the number of electrons involved and the surface area of interaction, so larger molecules tend to interact more.

32. B: (336 J). Ethanol has a molecular weight of 46 g/mole, so 23 grams is 0.5 moles. To determine the energy required to warm the ethanol to its boiling point, we use the heat capacity of 112 J/mol·°C. The rise in temperature is 72°C to 78°C, or an increase of 6°C. The energy of warming is 0.5 mol × 6°C × 112 J/mole·°C = 336 J.

33. D: Methanol has a molecular weight of 32 g/mole, so 64 grams is 2.0 moles. To determine the energy required to vaporize the methanol, we use the heat of vaporization of 38 kJ/mol. The energy required is 2 moles × 38 kJ/mol = 76 kJ, or 76,000 J.

34. A: To determine spontaneity of a phase transition, we use the free energy, ΔG. To be spontaneous, ΔG must be negative. Knowing $\Delta G = \Delta H - T\Delta S$, we can state that $\Delta H - T\Delta S < 0$. We can use ΔH from the table (53.2 kJ/mol) and T = 25°C = 298 K. Putting those values into the equation, we get 53.2 kJ/mol –298K × (ΔS) < 0. Subtracting 53.2 kJ/mol from both sides we get –298K × (ΔS) < –53.2 kJ/mole. Dividing by –298K we arrive at ΔS > 0.178 kJ/(mole · K) (note that when dividing both sides of an inequality by a negative number, the inequality switches: < becomes >), or 178 J/(mole · K) is the minimum increase in entropy.

35. D: (3-methyl-1-butanol). Isomers are compounds with the same molecular formula and different structural organization. In this case, some isomers of tert-butanol are alcohols, but others are not. The chemical formulas for a, b, and c are all the same as tert-butanol: C4H10O. The formula for choice d is C5H12O, so it is not isomeric with tert-butanol. The boiling points are not useful in answering this question.

Passage 8

36. C: (arteries > arterioles > capillaries > venules > veins). Blood pressure drops continuously as one proceeds through the circulatory system, out of the heart and back again. The order of progression through the system is consequently the answer.

37. B: (Blood continues to flow between beats of the heart). With each beat of the heart, the pressure in nearby arteries rises. The increased pressure expands these arteries. When the pressure from the heart declines, the arteries relax to their original size, squeezing out blood that continues to push through the system until the heart beats again. Choice a is wrong because the diastolic pressure rises because of arterial expansion and contraction, and would be very low without it. Choice c is wrong because oxygen does not generally leave the arteries in significant quantities. Choice d is wrong because the walls of arteries are thicker than the walls of veins.

38. D: (Both show the same pressure). The fact that there is no flow means that this is a question relating to static pressure. According to Pascal's Law, static pressure applied to any part of a fluid transmits equally to all other parts of the fluid. In this case, it transmits unchanged through the tubing regardless of diameter.

39. A: (95 mL/min). According to Poiseuille's Law, flow through a pipe is directly related to the pressure across the pipe. In this case, the pressure increases from 110 mm Hg to 160 mm Hg, which is a factor of 160/110 = 1.45. Since the flow at 110 mm Hg for Sample B was 65 mL/min, the new flow rate is 1.45 × 65 mL/min = 95 mL/min.

40. A: (1.2 mL/min). According to Poiseuille's Law, flow through a pipe is inversely related to the viscosity of the fluid. In this case, the viscosity increases by a factor of four. Since the flow at 110 mm Hg for Sample G was 4.8 mL/min, the new flow rate is 1/4 × 4.8 mL/min = 1.2 mL/min. The fact that the tubing is slightly elastic will have no significant effect on the change in the flow rate with viscosity.

PASSAGE 9

41. A: (a. 1/vo vs 1/[S]). A Lineweaver-Burk plot is a graph of 1/vo vs 1/[S], where the x-intercept is -1/Km and the slope is Km/Vmax.

42. C: (Modification 4). The Michaelis Constant, Km, is the substrate concentration at which the substrate occupies half of the active sites on the enzyme. A lower value of Km means higher binding strength since it takes less substrate in solution to occupy the active site. From Table 11, Modification 4 has the lowest Km (2.9 mM) and so has the highest binding strength.

43. B: (Modification 1). Kcat is a measure of the turnover rate of substrate in the active site of the enzyme under optimal (substrate saturation) conditions. The time required to process a single substrate is 1/Kcat. Faster conversions mean a higher Kcat, or a lower 1/Kcat. From Table 11, Modification 1 has the higher Kcat (3 × 105 s-1) and hence the fastest conversion time (1/Kcat) of 1/(3 × 105 s-1) = 3.3 × 10-6 s.

44. B: (A competitive inhibitor of the Native Enzyme). A competitive inhibitor increases the Km and leaves Kcat unchanged. A competitive inhibitor is competing with carbon dioxide for the binding site. When the inhibitor gets into the binding site, it effectively makes the carbon dioxide unable to bind and reduces the apparent binding (increasing Km). Kcat is unchanged because, by definition, Kcat is determined in a condition where there is a great surplus of the substrate (carbon dioxide) and the reaction is not substrate limited. With unlimited substrate, the active site is always occupied by substrate, regardless of whether there is an inhibitor present in solution or not. Answer (a) is wrong because for noncompetitive inhibition, Km is unchanged and Kcat is reduced. Answer (c) is wrong because for mixed inhibition, Km is increased and Kcat is reduced. Answer (d) is wrong because the Km rose, so acetazolamide is an inhibitor.

45. A: (Km = 450 mM). The easiest way to answer this question is to look at the trend between the Km of Modified Enzyme 3 in the absence of inhibitor (56.1 mM; Table 11) and the Km in the presence of 5 μM of acetazolamide (160 mM). This inhibitor at 5 μM increased the Km by a factor of two. Additional inhibitor added to reach 10 μM will further increase the Km, and the only choice higher than 160 mM is choice a (450 mM).

Discrete Questions

46. C: (decreased to W/2). Electrical energy (W) in a parallel plate capacitor is defined as W = CV2/2, where C is the capacitance and V is the voltage. Capacitance (C) of a parallel plate capacitor is defined by C= εA/d, where ε is the permeability, A is the cross-sectional area of the plates, and d is the distance separating the plates. Combining equations, we have W = εA V2/2d. Consequently, when d doubles (to 2d), the energy (W) decreases to W/2.

47. D: A diverging lens is thinner in the middle than at the edges. Only choice d is thinner in the middle. Choices a, b, and c are all thicker in the middle than at the edges and are converging lenses.

48. B: (oxalate). In part of the tricarboxylic acid cycle, succinyl-CoA → succinate → fumarate → malate → oxaloacetate, so choices a, c, and d are wrong. Oxalate is the correct choice because it is not consumed in the standard tricarboxylic acid cycle. The similarly named but different molecule, oxaloacetate, is part of the cycle but oxalate is not.

49. C: Unsaturated fatty acids (choices b, c, and d) have lower melting points and lead to more membrane fluidity than saturated fatty acids (choice a) of a similar length because the double bonds break up the packing of the chains. The more unsaturation sites (that is, the more double bonds) the lower is the melting point and the higher the membrane fluidity. In addition, cis double bonds have a larger effect on melting point and fluidity than trans double bonds because the cis bonds disrupt packing to a greater degree. Choice c is the correct answer because it has the most unsaturation and has all cis bonds.

50. B: (It has no net electric charge). The definition of the isoelectric point is the pH where the protein has no NET electric charge, but it can contain equal numbers of positive and negative charges (indicating answer d is wrong). Since the protein has no net negative charge, it does not move in an electric field (indicating a is wrong). When proteins have no net negative charge, they no longer repel each other electrically and tend to precipitate, reducing the solubility (indicating answer c is wrong).

51. A: (polysaccharide chains covalently crosslinked with peptide chains). The rigid structural framework of the cell wall is a peptidoglycan, and is composed of parallel polysaccharide chains (largely a repeating disaccharide of N-acetyl glucosamine and N-acetylmuramic acid. It is covalently crosslinked via the carboxylic acid group on the N-acetylmuramic acid. The composition of the peptide varies with the species of bacteria.

52. A: (It is single stranded). Messenger RNA is single stranded and made in the nucleus or the mitochondria in a process called transcription. RNA contains one phosphate per nucleotide.

53. C: (N N). Pyrimidine is an aromatic six-membered ring with nitrogen groups at the 1 and 3 positions. Structure a is imidazole. Structure b is pyrrole. Structure d is pyridine.

54. B: (on ribosomes in the cytoplasm). In eukaryotes, ribosomes are located in the cytoplasm, and that is where protein translation (synthesis) takes place. Prokaryotes are different, and translation can take place on ribosomes in their nuclei.

O OH

55. A: (H_3C CH_3 ⇌ H_3C CH_3). Although flipped in orientation from each other, choice a shows keto-enol tautomers. In such a pair, the double bonded oxygen becomes a hydroxyl group attached to the same carbon, and a double bond forms between the carbon of the previous carbonyl and an adjacent carbon atom. Incorrect choices c and d show the oxygen migrating to a different carbon atom, and incorrect choice b shows the same form in two different orientations with no enol form.

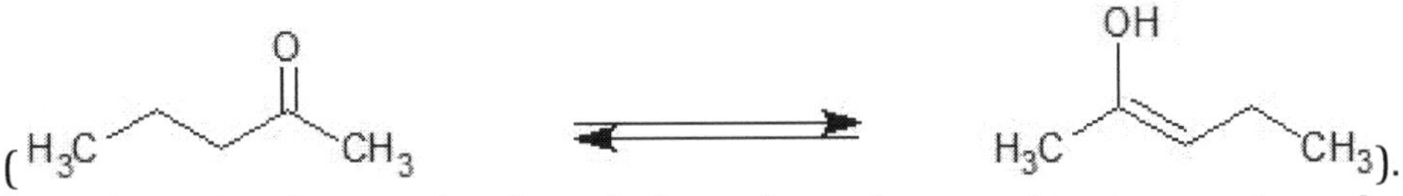

H
O
H_3C O^+
O CH_3

56. C: (H). The mechanistic steps in the acid-catalyzed hydrolysis of methyl acetate are methyl acetate → answer b → answer d → answer a → → products. Answer c shows a positive charge on an oxygen atom that has just two bonds. The only other mechanistic step in this reaction that has a positive charge on this oxygen atom also has a hydrogen atom attached to it:

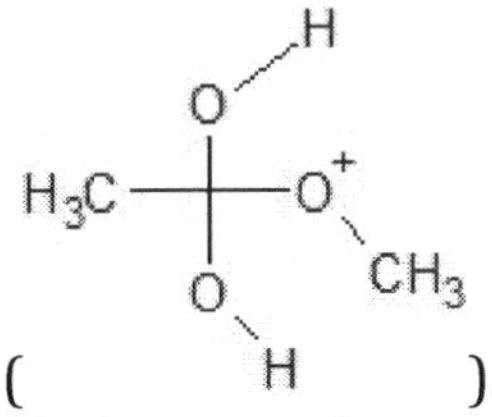

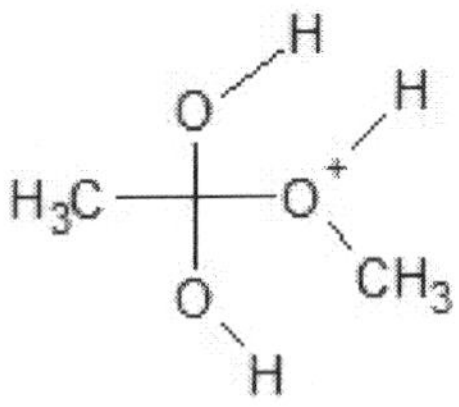

H
O H
H_3C O^+
O CH_3
H

57. C: When added together, the half reactions in choice c correctly give the full reaction. The NAD+/NADH half reaction of choice a has too many protons, and too much positive charge, on the left-hand side, and consequently is not a balanced half reaction. Choice b has NAD+ and NADH on the wrong sides of its redox half reaction to add up to the full reaction. The NAD+/NADH half reaction of choice b is also not electrically balanced. Choice d has too few protons in the isocitrate/ α-ketoglutarate half reaction, and is not electrically balanced.

58. D: The question reminds one that glucose is an aldohexose , which is an aldehyde-terminated six-carbon sugar. Choice d correctly shows glucose as a six-carbon sugar with a terminal aldehyde group. Choices a (D-ribose) and c (D-xylose) show five-carbon sugars and are clearly incorrect. Choice b (D-fructose) shows a six-carbon sugar with a ketone group at the second carbon rather than an aldehyde at the terminal carbon (hence it is a ketohexose rather than the required aldohexose), and is incorrect.

59. D: (CH3CH2CH3 and CH3CH2CH2I). Answering this question requires knowing two things. First, that separations by simple batch distillation are most complete with two compounds that differ the most in boiling point. Second, that the boiling point of homologous alkyl halides (and most other organic compounds) rises as the molecular weight rises. In this case, the boiling points are propane (–42°C), n-propyl fluoride (–3°C), n-propylchloride (47°C), n-propylbromide (71°C), and n-propyl iodide (102°C). So, the combination of propane and n-propyl iodide has the largest boiling point difference.

Psychological, Social, and Biological Foundations

PASSAGE 1

1. B: Severe head trauma, particularly that prompting hospitalization, produces defects in the function of the brain and spine blood-brain barrier, mild electroencephalogram (EEG) changes, and neurotransmitter dysfunction. Physiological changes induced by head trauma can produce and exacerbate mood disorders as well as psychiatric conditions. These symptoms are particularly challenging to manage, and many head trauma patients are living with refractory symptoms. The mood disorder symptoms that occur after brain surgery may be debilitating, but the treatment protocols are more effective and well established at this time than are the treatment protocols for severe head trauma. The psychiatric sequelae of head trauma are notably increased even when posttraumatic stress is controlled for as a factor. Brain surgery is a therapeutic procedure, but brain surgery survivors experience a higher incidence of mood disorders and psychiatric ailments than the general population. Although brain surgery is typically asymmetric, electrophysiological findings demonstrate that individuals with schizophrenia exhibit deficits in cerebral lateralization as well.

2. D: Schizophrenia is less prevalent than are mood disorders such as depression, but symptomatic episodes of schizophrenia are more likely to require intensive medical attention. Individuals with diagnosed mood disorders experience fluctuations in symptoms more often due to lack of proper medication than to social factors such as work. The work setting may alleviate some symptoms of mood disorders for some individuals but may exacerbate symptoms of mood disorders as well. Schizophrenia occurs at rates between 1% and 2% of the population, which makes it common, but not as common as mood disorders. Symptoms of mood disorders can be severe enough to prevent people from functioning and also may require intense medical treatment and/or hospitalization.

3. B: Bipolar disorder often presents with symptoms of agitation and paranoia that appear similar to symptoms of schizophrenia. In fact, the two conditions may be confused or misdiagnosed in the initial stages. Bipolar disorder is a mood disorder characterized by episodes of depression and episodes of mania. The episodes of mania are, more often than not, unsettling for the individual who has bipolar disorder. Depression is a mood disorder predominantly characterized by feelings of sadness, despair, and loss of hope. Schizophrenia is characterized by paranoid auditory delusions as well as agitation and a number of other symptoms. However, individuals with diagnoses of bipolar disorder or with diagnoses of depression may experience severely altered perceptions of reality, albeit not as frequently as individuals who suffer from schizophrenia. Individuals with schizophrenia also experience dramatic mood shifts in addition to the delusions and hallucinations that are a hallmark of schizophrenia. Bipolar disorder is, indeed, characterized by opposing symptoms, and the symptoms of schizophrenia and depression are often more homogeneous. However, surprisingly, the combination of medications required and the neurotransmitters targeted are not more complicated in the treatment of bipolar disorder than in the treatment of depression or schizophrenia. The treatments and combinations of medications required to control symptoms of depression and symptoms of schizophrenia are surprisingly complex. Depression, schizophrenia, and bipolar disorder are all disorders with a degree of symptom variation. Individuals with any of the three disorders may be able to take a medication "vacation," but overall, patients more often than not need to take medication in order to manage symptoms.

4. C: Acute anxiety can be so acute that anxiety may build over hours, days, or weeks and cause episodes when affected individuals are unable to function in the work setting due to real or perceived threats so severe that it may result in the inability to function in the work setting. However, missing work itself causes anxiety that may be out of proportion to the real repercussions of missing work. Acute anxiety can cause an individual to feel threatened when there is a minimal or even nonexistent threat. Symptoms of acute anxiety can be more severe than the fear of being reprimanded for missing work. Anxiety is not the same as determination or conscientiousness, and thus it does not necessarily have an impact on an individual's attitude toward coworkers' work attendance.

5. A: Social cognitive theory explains behavior when individuals observe others' actions and the consequences of those actions in order to determine the effects of social and interpersonal interactions. Thus, individuals observe the outcome when peers call in sick in order to determine whether it would be beneficial or detrimental. When individuals observe others calling in sick, they take into account whether there was a benefit or penalty for that action and also whether those observed are subjected to similar work conditions and policies. Social cognitive theory is about learning by observing and modeling, rather than offsetting perceived unfairness. The incentive theory of motivation explains that individuals act in certain ways to gain rewards. Although rewards such as free time or rest may be a motive for calling in sick, social cognitive theory is about absorbing information about actions, including whether those actions bring about positive rewards. Responsibility toward others is a motivating factor in behavior, but it is not typically learned through social cognitive observations, but through reasoning.

Passage 2

6. A: Sanctions are methods by which unwritten rules of social control are enforced by excluding those who do not follow norms. Sanctions in the social setting are not associated with concrete penalties such as low grades. Sanctions are mechanisms of exclusion rather than social tactics such as gossip or overt shunning. Peers may try to avoid those who do not conform for fear of being similarly excluded. This action itself is not a form of sanctions, but it is rather an action taken by those who are not in a dominant position in order to avoid the consequence of sanctions. The long-term consequences of sanctions on those who are excluded may be actions such as leaving the situation or adjustment of behaviors to fit social norms, but that is not a description of how social controls operate to produce sanctions.

7. D: Group polarization is the inclination of individuals within a group to deliberately become more like each other while they amplify the contrast in their behavior or beliefs from those of another, usually opposing, group. In this example, group polarization would likely result in a group of students who insist on a more casual style of clothes than they would have worn otherwise, in order to bond with each other while rejecting the unwritten, more formal, dress code. Group polarization would result in less formally dressed students believing that they are correct in their style of clothes, and thus they would not feel the need to "compensate" for shortcomings. The tendency of students to study more or less based on factors such as attire is more in line with the idea of a self-fulfilling prophecy than with group polarization. The undermining of fellow students who are also dressed less formally is the opposite of the solidarity expected as a result of group polarization. Students might, however, respond by undermining the more formally dressed students who belong to the other group.

8. A: Social control is a method by which individuals avoid actions that might result in some type of rejection. In this example, the rejection is unlikely to actually take place because the peer group is not present currently, only in the individual's memory. The previous peer group in this example has functioned to place strong social control even in its absence. Peer pressure may influence an individual to participate in activities he may have not otherwise joined. Deindividuation occurs when an individual becomes less self-aware within a group and takes actions he might not have done on his own. Deindividuation encourages, rather than discourages, group hysteria. Deviance is the nonconformity to social norms; it is not a driving force in avoiding group action. Deviance would describe behavior of an individual who would risk rejection by acting in a way that is likely to be rejected by the peer group.

9. C: Whether a character is dominant or not within a social group is often determined more by a person's individual temperament combined with his investment and devotion to the group than by his concern about sanctions. Dominant members of a social group may or may not be more or less affected by the prospect of social sanctions than less dominant members of the group. Dominant characters are not necessarily as independent of the need for social acceptance as the group may believe. Dominant characters do have a great deal more influence than other members of the group, but they often look to other, less influential members for subtle cues. A portion of dominant personalities is very dependent on their status and prestige, but not all of these individuals have a strong need for their established social position or place an extremely intense effort on maintaining the social hierarchy.

10. B: Anomie is the circumstance in which society lacks moral guidance. Individuals may experience a sense of alienation in this context. Therefore, an individual can shield himself from this type of isolation by maintaining an association with a group that holds a set of principles with which the individual, for the most part, agrees. Creating laws does not necessarily preserve moral standards, but rather it establishes the appearance of selected moral standards. Promoting more lenient principles or ethics may create a new sense of inclusion for some individuals, but this can easily exclude a different set of individuals at the same time, and thus it does not necessarily foster a sense of inclusive acceptance nor protect against a sense of isolation. Maintaining personal principles can help prevent a sense of ethical disorientation, but this does not prevent a feeling of isolation from a principled and ethical community.

11. D: When a person is aware of the various agents involved in socialization, he is more resistant to the negative psychological effects of social exclusion. However, even those who are knowledgeable regarding the range of social and psychological elements of behavior can be susceptible to the emotional effects of social inclusion and exclusion. An understanding of the differing agents of socialization can aid an individual in adapting to expectations and avoiding social errors that can lead to exclusion, such as deviating from norms. This understanding can help a person defend himself against formal methods of exclusion resulting from bias or unfairness. Defending oneself aids in financial or legal issues, but it does not aid in gaining social inclusion. Empathy is a beneficial trait that can prevent social ostracism in most circumstances, but it is not a result of the understanding and awareness of agents of socialization. Blending the norms of different social groups is not an effective way to gain social acceptance because some peer groups may have completely opposing ideas of standards and acceptable behavior, and they may reject the social norms of another society.

Passage 3

12. A: Learning is an ongoing process facilitated by lessons such as this experience, but it also involves improving with practice within the context of real life. The stroke group had a baseline deficit in their ability to accurately identify emotions, compared to controls, but also had a history of intact emotional recognition prior to the stroke. This aided in supplementing the ability to learn the lessons taught through the experiment. Stroke survivors experience deficits in emotional recognition independent of acquired visual deficits. The majority of individuals with Asperger's disorder would prefer to have satisfying social interactions. Neuroplasticity is a characteristic of neuronal tissue, and individuals who have Asperger's as well as stroke survivors have a degree of neuroplasticity. Neuroplasticity refers to the ability of neurons to be redirected or reprogrammed. Both groups are teachable, a trait which depends on the ability to learn, not on neuroplasticity.

13. C: Habituation is decreased response to an input. The control group initially improved in performance and then declined, likely due to diminished response or interest to the stimulus. Prolonged exposure is a type of therapy intended to diminish a negative response. Extinction occurs when a conditioned response no longer produces a positive reward and therefore diminishes. This is not the case in this experiment. Dishabituation is the renewed response to an input that ceases and then restarts again.

14. D: A variable-ratio schedule is a pattern in which reinforcement is given after a variable number of correct responses. In real-life situations, positive feedback linked to accurately identifying emotions does not occur with each success or after a set ratio of success, but, instead, at random. A fixed-ratio schedule is a pattern or reinforcement that is given after every successful task or every other successful task or another fixed ratio. This is not consistent with real life because human responses are not so predictable. A fixed-interval schedule suggests that the positive reinforcement occurs at exactly the same interval after successful completion of the task. As with a fixed-ratio schedule, this is not consistent with real life. A variable-interval schedule is a pattern of reinforcement that is given at different intervals after successfully doing the task. In this instance, positive reinforcement may occur immediately or it may occur after a prolonged period of time after correctly reading a person's emotions. Generally, accurately reading emotions, if rewarded, occurs within a reasonably consistent time frame. Thus, the variable-interval schedule is less similar to real life than the variable-ratio schedule.

15. B: The control group has the least innate deficit in neuropsychological function and is better able to learn social skills through voluntarily imitating other people.

16. D: In classical conditioning, the unconditioned response is the natural response that occurs in response to a stimulus. In this instance, the study participant imitates or reflects the emotions that he is viewing, even without being able to accurately identify the emotion itself. The conditioned response is a learned response to a stimulus, which would be a conditioned ability to correctly identify emotions. The unconditioned stimulus is the event that triggers a response, which in this instance would be the emotions viewed in the videos. The conditioned stimulus is an additional stimulus that is often associated with the unconditioned stimulus and thus evokes the same response as the unconditioned stimulus. There is no conditioned stimulus in this experiment. The names of these stimuli and responses may seem confusing.

Passage 4

17. A: A self-fulfilling prophecy describes an outcome that occurs because a prediction influences behavior that makes the outcome more likely. In this instance, the waiters who believed that guests were generous were more likely to provide service that encouraged guests to give them larger tips. Stereotyping is the use of an oversimplified belief about a subgroup of individuals. Although the waiters were told that the guests were generous tippers, there was no implication or belief that a certain subtype of guests had particular traits. Prestige describes the esteem given to an individual or group. Some of the waiters in the experimental group might have attributed prestige to the guests, but it was the behavior of the waiters and the promise of a material reward that drove the difference in tips. Stigma describes a negative attitude toward an individual, a group, or a characteristic. Stigma is associated with discrimination, not with positive behavioral modification.

18. B: After an experiment such as this one, individuals are able to effectively alter their behavior if they understand the factors that contributed to the positive outcome. Instructing guests to defy stereotypes might change the preconceived stereotypes of the waiters, but the brief interactions and possibly inconsistent "acting" of guests may shape a different set of stereotypes, even if false. Giving financial incentives can alter behavior, but may not alter beliefs. Presenting objective information that counteracts stereotypes is not as effective as real-life experiences in overcoming stereotypes.

19. D: A man with a strong internal locus of control believes that he has a great deal of influence and control over events in his life. Thus, he would have a tendency to have less compassion and to blame others for their misfortune, believing that they bear a degree of responsibility for their own bad outcomes. A strong internal locus of control is a principle held by an individual who believes that he has a significant effect on events, which is not the same as self-control. Self-control is the ability to restrain one's own behavior or emotions. Although a strong internal locus of control shifts the responsibility for external events toward the individual, it does not necessarily foster or preclude or a sense of altruism, which is a separate matter. A person with a strong locus of control may or may not value self-esteem more or less than material possessions.

20. A: This experiment initiates a virtuous cycle of positive behavior by seeding the participants with the expectation of rewards and reinforcing that behavior when they respond appropriately. Positive reinforcement adds a reward when good behavior takes place, whereas negative reinforcement removes a negative consequence when a desirable action is taken, and punishment adds a negative consequence when an undesirable action is taken. Negative reinforcement is not the absence of a reward; it is the absence of an undesirable outcome.

21. C: According to the elaboration likelihood model, the peripheral route is a weak method of persuasion that is effective when the recipient of the message has little ability, background, or interest in the subject. Thus, if the feature present in an untrustworthy person is emphasized to a waiter, he might also view the customer as untrustworthy because the customer has the same feature, even if it is irrelevant. Visual pathways are not part of the elaboration likelihood model. Omission is not a method used through the peripheral route in the elaboration likelihood model; peripherally associating two concepts is the method used. Using irrelevant or peripheral details is not a component of the elaboration likelihood model; associating these details is the main component.

PASSAGE 5

22. D: The child is dependent on the parent, and thus she is likely to obey instructions. Additionally, the child is in a role that entails allegiance toward the parents. The opposing demands of honesty in the survey and loyalty toward her parents presents an example of role conflict because honest answers may reflect poorly on the parents or might make them unhappy. Role strain is the description of a stress and pressure induced by a role, but not necessarily a conflict. Role strain is a component of some children's roles, but it is not a factor that would cause the child to avoid certain answers on the survey. Altruism is behaving in a kind and unselfish way for the benefit of others. A child might avoid answering questions that could hurt his parents out of altruism, but deindividuation, which is a loss of self-awareness in the group setting, is not a factor. Role exit is a voluntary process in which an individual leaves an undesirable role or identity. Although the child may wish for role exit and fear it at the same time, answers on the questionnaire do not have an impact on the process of role exit.

23. A: The child may see a front-stage self that the parent puts on for others and wish that the more private and authentic behavior, described as the back-stage self, was as pleasant, confident, or kind as the front-stage self. The parent's front-stage self is an attempt at impression management, whereas the back-stage self is largely unseen by everyone except those who are closest to them. An improvement of the back-stage self is not witnessed by others and thus would not help with blending in. However, children tend to believe that others' front-stage selves match their back-stage selves, while they fret and agonize over their own families' inadequate back-stage selves. Social stigma occurs when a person, group, or object is rejected. This requires recognition of undesirable qualities, which would not happen if the front-stage self were acceptable.

24. B: Those who had a higher copay felt more authority and power over the details regarding their health-care visit and thus were three times more likely to refuse to have their children fill out the survey than their counterparts who had a low copay or no copay. Parents who had a low copay did not demonstrate obedience by participating because the survey was nonmandatory. Individuals who pay a higher or lower copay do not have differences in the amount of private information shared with the health-care system. Similarly, there is no consistent relationship between how busy an individual is and how high his copay is.

25. B: The looking-glass self describes the tendency of a person's sense of self to be heavily influenced by others' perceptions and feedback. Thus, an individual who repeatedly receives a particular compliment, even if it is inconsistent with his self-view, will begin to believe that he possesses the attributes credited to him. Compliments, particularly when echoed by several individuals, raise the recipient's self-esteem. Compliments are also more likely to be accepted by an individual who already has a healthy self-esteem. A self-fulfilling prophecy is an alteration of behavior based on beliefs, rather than an alteration of the beliefs themselves. Impression management in psychology is a description of a person's conscious or subconscious control of others' perception of himself. This example is the reverse of impression management because it is an example of altered perception of self in response to others' impressions.

26. A: The child is likely to reject his parent as a role model based on the ineffectiveness of the lessons learned and the spurn of the target audience. The child is naturally more inclined toward self-preservation, and thus sympathy toward the parent is a low priority compared to the psychological wounds incurred by rejection of the parent's lesson. Although the child will reject the parent, it is not necessarily due to a feeling of mistrust because the parent may be incompetent, but this may not be due to overt disingenuousness. The child looks to the parent for modeling and for acceptance, but, upon rejection from peers, the child does not turn to the parent as a substitute for peer acceptance.

Passage 6

27. D: The benefactors of the scholarship may have biases that impact the selection of students, even unintentionally. These biases may also continue to play a role in shaping the students' experiences throughout the trip. Hidden curriculum is less directed than the example in choice A, which would be a deliberate, not a hidden, means of approaching the goal. The selection process might be biased toward students who practice or believe in the same religion as members of the scholarship organization, but this does not reflect a hidden curriculum because it would not constitute teaching the recipients of the scholarship, but rather selecting students who already have the same religion as the benefactors. The exact attitude toward religion of the interviewers or the benefactors is not entirely clear based on the questions asked during the interview.

28. C: Medicalization of a social problem can result in increased health-care funds, training, time, and attention allotted for the care and toward the prevention of the condition. Health-care funds are allotted to medical care delivered by physicians as well as to care that is delivered by other health-care providers. Medicalization of domestic violence could result in treatment of victims or perpetrators as patients with medical conditions. Medicalization of a social problem can help reduce stigma over the long run, but such a consequence requires a great deal of planning and public awareness. Medicalization of a condition is not, in itself, capable of reducing stigma. However, medicalization would not result in tolerance of violence, even if the behavior were considered to be caused by a psychological ailment of the perpetrator.

29. B: According to the concept of symbolic interactionism, individuals view others as representatives of previous experiences. This means that the student would be expected to subconsciously view the patient as a meaningful symbol of the broken friendship and thus might attempt to repair the broken relationship through her interaction with the patient. The theory of functionalism would suggest that the student view the patient through a more pragmatic lens and would approach the interaction with the goal of learning about the patient's medical condition or the goal of improving the patient's medical condition. The expectations of a student health-care provider to be completely objective is unrealistic because previous interactions, particularly emotionally consequential interactions, more often than not play a role in how we view others. Given that her experiences cause her to subconsciously link the patient with her former friendship, she might not directly understand her strong feelings of mistrust that are provoked by the patient. The concept of association is about learning, not about misplaced interpersonal judgments.

30. B: Culture lag describes the delay in practical adoption of scientific advances such as technology. The electronic medical record (EMR) is an example of a technology that has theoretical benefits as well as practical disadvantages in real-world application. Thus, while the workforce adapts, it is not relevant whether the material acquisition of resources is present or not, because seamless application of EMR tools is not instantaneous and does not coincide with the availability of the material equipment. The size of the workforce is not a limiting factor that contributes to culture lag, but rather, the learning curve is the major factor. It is true that attitudes and preexisting efficiency can limit or promote adoption of new technology, but that is not the factor in cultural lag. In some instances, technology can aid developing nations and diminish material disadvantages, but adopting new technology depends on whether people can learn the necessary skills.

31. D: A meritocracy is a system in which recognition is based on earned status, rather than ascribed status. Although either woman in this example would have reason to resent the recognition awarded to high achievers in a meritocracy, acceptance or rejection of the system itself is a product of multiple factors, including the individual's social position and empathy toward others. The woman who did not have power or independence may believe that she could have achieved recognition had she been given the opportunity, but her lack of freedom might have led her to believe that she is incapable. The woman who failed might prefer a system that doesn't bare her failures, but she might also have hope that she could have a second chance, which is a more common opportunity for people who exist in a system of meritocracy. Mirror neurons are physiological occurrences that aid people in modeling behavior, not in imaging behavior that is unlikely ever to occur.

Passage 7

32. A: Inflammation is a nonspecific finding that may be particularly difficult to diagnose. Therefore, it may be detected on diagnostic tests, but in a population with a lack of follow-up care and access to care, it is likely that the etiology may not be determined and that the treatment may not be initiated. This population is also less likely to seek out care, particularly for subtle findings such as nonspecific inflammation. Inflammatory findings are noted in central nervous system (CNS) tissue of patients with psychiatric illness and patients with drug abuse, but CNS inflammation is not of high enough quantity to increase inflammatory cells in the blood. A condition such as inflammation of unknown etiology refers to inflammation determined by blood tests or peripheral nerve/muscle biopsy, rather than inflammation noted on CNS specimens. The prison population is at a higher risk of certain infections, but fevers and other signs of infection, rather than neuropathic symptoms, would accompany the inflammation noted during infections. People with inflammatory conditions often suffer from pain, tiredness, weakness, and other symptoms, but they are not generally excluded from the general population and would not be expected to turn to crime as a result of their symptoms or disease.

33. C: Type 1 diabetes would not increase the chances of an individual going to prison due to either criminal behavior or bias in the legal/judicial system. However, this population is more likely to have neuropathy due to periods of untreated type 1 diabetes, and the results of the chart review, which assessed patients with neuropathy, show higher rates of neuropathy than in the general population, regardless of the etiology. People with medical disease are, indeed, marginalized in society. However, type 1 diabetes is not expected to increase the rates of incarceration among those who have the condition. The lack of proper diabetes treatment, which would cause an increased rate of neuropathy, most likely occurred during times when the patients were not in prison because access to a necessary medication such as insulin, as well as compliance with medications, would be better in this population when health care is provided and monitored, than when individuals at high risk of noncompliance with medical instructions are on their own. Low birth weight has been associated with later development of type 1 diabetes in the child as well as with psychiatric illness later in the life of the child. Psychiatric illness itself is correlated with incarceration, but it is unclear how much parenting quality is a factor. Low birth weight, although associated with later development of type 1 diabetes in the child, is not associated with poor parenting because there are a number of medical causes of low birth weight. Additionally, high maternal weight gain is also associated with the development of diabetes later in the life of the child.

34. C: There are several medical conditions rooted in vitamin B12 deficiency including neuropathy, dementia, spine dysfunction, and anemia. Yet, despite the common etiology, the manifestation of one disorder caused by vitamin B12 deficiency does not necessarily mean that another manifestation will develop. Dementia in this population would be expected to have a wide variety of etiologies, with vitamin B12 being only one of many. Thus, vitamin B12 pills or shots would not be expected to decrease the presence of dementia. Although vitamin B12 deficiency contributes to dementia, many individuals with dementia do not have low levels of vitamin B12 and many individuals with dementia have other etiologies. It would be more effective to treat patients based on their individual risk factors. Most of the time, vitamin B12 pills are not absorbed, and people who are vitamin B12 deficient require injections for effective treatment.

35. A: Although the prison population is often labeled with many negative attributes, the vast majority of prisoners respond well to and seek positive support such as health-care interactions. The medications that are useful for neuropathic pain management do not have pleasant or addictive side effects. Treatment for medical conditions does not provide prisoners with additional funds or health-care benefits. Often, diagnosis of neuropathy involves electromyography (EMG) and nerve conduction studies, which use needles and electric shocks. Although some patients are apprehensive, the vast majority of patients of all demographics are easily able to understand the procedure and undergo testing without fear or hesitancy.

Passage 8

36. B: The body has many responses to a psychoactive drug, including metabolism of the substance and systemic effects. According to the data, the drug users in this instance had a quicker conversion to metabolite 1 than non-drug users. Because of the body's repeated exposure to the drug, the systemic effects are less pronounced in drug users than in individuals who were not previously exposed to the drug. Metabolic by-products of a compound are unlikely to last long enough in the blood to alter measurements in the study. Addictive drugs are typically addictive because they have an impact on the reward pathway in the brain by directly acting on the central nervous system or by changing a person's physical appearance, not as a result of health effects such as hypertension control. Frequent use may stimulate the body to make metabolite 1 faster or may cause metabolite 1 to last longer. However, the metabolic alterations induced by frequent use do not necessarily mean that the body is metabolizing the drug in a way that is superior. The metabolic changes induced by frequent use could have negative effects.

37. A: Psychoactive drugs, even those that are stimulants, can affect central processing and integration of sensations and can slow the production of a response. Although some drugs that affect the central nervous system (CNS) are abused because users crave a pleasant experience attributed to the drug, there is no uniformity of pleasant responses and psychoactive drugs do not convert unpleasant threats to pleasant experiences, but instead, they diminish sensory integration and may make a person unaware of threats. Psychoactive drugs do not usually harm sensory functions. Neurons involved in memory, mood, and decision making are more often targeted by long-term damage induced by psychoactive drugs. Conscientiousness is not the same as consciousness. Although most psychoactive compounds have an effect on the level of alertness (consciousness), some drug-addicted individuals also experience changes in conscientiousness (reliability and responsibility). However, consciousness does not impact a response to sensory threats, but rather the behaviors that impact daily life.

38. B: Often, consciousness-altering substances make a person less aware of and less able to integrate sensory input such as vision and proprioception. They can also make a person less aware of subtle social cues that may seem threatening. Individuals who view social interactions as particularly threatening may be more prone to use substances that can make them less aware of their social surroundings. Sensory adaptation is the body's normal adaptation to continuous sensory input, and it does result in a person ceasing to notice a sensation, but it is not relevant to social interactions, and it is a normal neurophysiological response even in the absence of psychogenic drug use. Overconfidence results when a person miscalculates his or her own abilities. This can cause a person to miscalculate his abilities when using psychoactive drugs; however, overconfidence is an evaluation of oneself, not of the outside circumstances, and it does not necessarily require the use of drugs. Memory decay is the loss of memory over time and typically refers to factual memory, whereas social apprehension is a much more complex response that is not based on the recall of factual information.

39. B: The brain can encode the memory of previous experiences, triggering the release of some neurotransmitters in anticipation of a chemical effect. However, this response is limited. Although it is very common for individuals to believe that they can "overcome" effects of a drug due to experience, memory itself does not make a person better able to willingly resist the physiological effects of a chemical substance. Memory can have a real effect on physiologic behavior by eliciting neurologic, metabolic, or endocrine responses. This effect can be pronounced or mild. Sensory memory describes the body's ability to maintain memory of a feeling elicited by a sensory stimulus. This allows a person to remember the sensations of pain, temperature, position, etc. for a brief time even after the stimulus is removed. Repeated consciousness-altering drug use would not elicit responses based on short-term sensory memory, but rather those based on longer term, more complex memory systems.

Passage 9

40. C: The circadian rhythm is most associated with sleep, but the 24-hour cycle in response to light and dark stimuli also affects the times when we anticipate food and our bodies prepare to digest and metabolize nutrients. Additionally, disruption in eating habits contributes to weight gain or malnutrition in people who have chronic disruption of the sleep–wake cycle unless deliberate efforts are made to regulate caloric and nutritional intake. Of note, some individuals are more prone to lose weight when the sleep–wake cycle is disrupted. Wakefulness during the day after disruption of circadian rhythm is not necessarily associated with weight gain. Although individuals with a disruption in their circadian rhythm might eat if they can't fall asleep during the day, they are also prone to overeat at night. But the metabolic alterations and fatigue are more significant in causing the weight gain. Usually, individuals with circadian-rhythm disruptions do not sleep a total number of hours more than usual, although fatigue can contribute to a lack of exercise. However, depending on the type of work, a high total number of calories might be used. Seasonal affective disorder (SAD) is the name for mood dysfunction, typically depression, which results from lack of daytime sunlight. Some individuals who suffer from SAD may gain weight, but this is caused by depression or by medications used to treat depression, not by circadian-rhythm disturbance.

41. B: Individuals may have adjusted to irregular sleep patterns by involuntarily developing shorter sleep latency periods and arriving at deep stages of sleep more quickly. However, meditation only minimally affected their overall stress and fatigue levels, even after adjustment of the sleep–wake cycle. Alertness is not expected to readjust or accommodate to chronic sleep disruption, even if individuals participate in meditation. In fact, individuals may operate at a lower level of alertness with slowed responses or less sophisticated responses. Long-term potentiation describes a neural process that plays a role in memory formation, but it is not strengthened by sleep disruption. Neural plasticity describes the process by which neurons are recruited to take over functions of other neurons, or relearn functions. This occurs in situations involving compensation for brain damage, but it is not involved with restructuring the circadian rhythm. Mediation would not activate neural plasticity to overcome disruptions in the sleep–wake cycle.

42. C: Selective attention describes the ability to voluntarily focus on specific tasks or problems while ignoring distractions. Divided attention describes the ability to multitask. Both of these are impaired by sleep deprivation. Selective attention is dependent on alertness and is not an involuntary response to fatigue, and thus, choice A is incorrect. Problem solving relies partially on intelligence, but intelligence is a product of the ability to pay attention and focus, both of which are impaired with lack of sleep. Although an individual may retain the ability to problem solve even in the face of sleep deprivation, subclinical impairment is expected. Brainstem reflexes rely on synapses in the motor neurons and therefore are unlikely to be impaired by sleep deprivation.

43. D: The participant who experienced a catastrophic event during the study would experience high levels of stress that may be exacerbated by her sleep patterns. The participant who has an anxiety disorder should rate her stress consistently throughout the study. The individual who suffers from anxiety may give herself a rating that could be high or low, depending on her perception of the stress scale. However, it should be consistent. Whether either participant has any insight into the cause of her stress does not diminish the experience or the physiologic response to stress. The study itself could increase stress for a person who suffers from anxiety, but often, participating in a study provides a sense of comfort for people with anxiety due to either a placebo effect or to the idea that they are receiving attention from a health-care provider. Similarly, being part of a research study can alleviate or exacerbate the stress experienced during a situational difficulty.

44. C: There is no indication that the participants are in a position to observe any participants outside their group, and indeed it would be poor study design to allow for such. A lack of further lowering of reported stress levels may indicate that the intervention has achieved all it can in terms of reducing stress. Obviously, you would want more than a single pair of data points to confirm, but this is a distinct likelihood. The nonintervention group is not expected to have any variation at all beyond random variation, so it is perfectly valid to expect an apparent stabilization there to be random. It is also to be expected that participants will eventually tire of producing new responses and begin repeating old responses.

Discrete Questions

45. B: Although not all individuals affected by these conditions have an identified genetic trait, the genetic anomalies associated with schizophrenia and Parkinson's disease have been found near each other. Dopamine activity and dopaminergic receptors are, in fact, common factors in these disorders. Although medication for one disorder may produce symptomatic side effects of the other, these symptoms are almost always reversible with medication adjustment. Environmental factors are only minor elements for the development and risk of schizophrenia and Parkinson's disease. The average age of onset of schizophrenia is during the early twenties, and the average age of onset of Parkinson's disease is during one's sixties, but this does not preclude sibling studies.

46. C: The bystander effect is when an individual is less likely to take part in an action when he assumes that someone else in the group will take action, essentially making his action unnecessary or even redundant. Thus, if a mass email is received, an individual may consider his response inconsequential. Peer pressure is unlikely to have an effect on his decision to respond to or ignore the anonymous survey request. Positive reinforcement could motivate him to respond to the survey if he has received a beneficial result of filling out a survey in the past. Social norms do not generally come into play in the context of anonymous acts.

47. A: Instinctive drift is the tendency for animals or humans to return to natural tendencies. Once the person stops putting in effort or becomes stressed, he will have a tendency to revert back to behavior that takes less effort. New issues may arise, but if he continues with his efforts, he does not have to succumb to former habits. A habit of blaming others for misfortune or in taking responsibility for one's own difficulties is based on attitude, rather than evidence. Extinction refers to conditioned behavior that ceases after the feedback ceases. In this example, the habit is a negative habit rather than a conditioned response.

48. B: The amygdala is responsible for recognition of traits such as honesty in other people's faces. The occipital lobe is the visual center, which forms the brain's perception of vision received through the optic nerve. However, neither the optic nerve nor the occipital lobe is part of the limbic system. The hippocampus aids in recollection of emotions, not in associating facial recognition with names. The temporal lobe is essential for recognizing faces, but it is not part of the limbic system.

49. C: Korsakoff's syndrome, also referred to as Korsakoff's psychosis, manifests with antegrade and retrograde amnesia and problems with spatial planning of movements. Pseudobulbar palsy is another disorder of movement that is often associated with dementia and causes unexplained crying episodes. Vision loss is not a feature of Korsakoff's syndrome, although eye movement impairment is a feature of Wernicke's encephalopathy, which usually accompanies Korsakoff's syndrome. Korsakoff's syndrome is a result of thiamine deficiency, often seen in late-stage alcoholics. It does not cause thiamine deficiency.

50. D: The autonomic nervous system is stimulated by epinephrine and norepinephrine in response to emotional stress, whereas cortisol, which increases blood glucose levels, also increases in response to emotional stress. Stress does not have a dramatic effect on serotonin, but serotonin is typically decreased in response to stress. Acetylcholine is a neurotransmitter that controls skeletal muscles and is not dramatically altered by stress.

51. C: Metabolic imaging studies can detect subclinical symptoms, and thus, they may be useful in detecting preclinical abnormalities or similarities in brain dysfunction in relatives of individuals with psychiatric symptoms. Individuals with genotypic traits may have subclinical physiological changes that can only be detected by metabolic brain imaging studies. Environmental factors can produce alterations in the physiology and metabolism of brain activity. Both genetic and environmentally induced behavioral traits are susceptible to environmental factors, and thus, alterations in metabolism as a response to an environmental stimulus would not distinguish between environmental or genetic etiology.

52. C: Ascribed status is often more difficult to escape from, and thus, a person who feels defined by his ascribed status within his primary group might focus more of his energy and time on achieving status within the secondary group. Of importance in such instances, the primary group is more firmly established, often comprised of lifelong connections, whereas it is easier to find new secondary groups throughout life. The person with low ascribed status in the primary group might or might not reject the primary group and might or might not turn to the secondary group as a substitute for approval. Some members of a primary group seek to advocate for the whole group within the secondary group. This is often a person who has high status within the primary group, particularly if it is ascribed. But promoting the primary group is not a presumed consequence of higher ascribed status within the primary group. Some individuals who are granted ascribed elevated social status choose to isolate themselves from the secondary group in order to relish in the benefits and self-confidence provided by the primary group. But many such individuals do not reject the secondary group, instead gaining confidence in their ability to thrive within the secondary group because of the approval provided by the primary group.

53. B: Attribution error describes the professor's recognition that she arrived late as being due to external factors, contrasting with her explanation of the student's late arrival as a fault of the student. The attribution error is not the same as attribution of power, which credits outcome to a person's actions. The professor may, indeed, experience stress due to her lateness that affects class time. She may also view a student's late arrival as a disruption. However, these are not examples of attribution error.

54. D: The primary group is the close group who may have known the teenager for a longer period of time and has closer interpersonal interactions with the teenager. Usually, the teenager is more dependent on the primary group. The secondary group is a wider group of acquaintances and possibly teachers. Achieved status is earned based on the teenager's social skills, athletic abilities, or other personal talents that are appreciated and valued. Ascribed status is independent of the teenager's individual personality and is based on factors such as family position or birth order. If the secondary group views the teenager with more esteem and treats the teenager better than the primary group does, the secondary group may raise the teenager's self-esteem while the primary group simultaneously lowers the teenager's self-esteem. The primary and secondary groups might have little, if any, interaction, and they may see the teenager through completely different lenses and value systems. The primary or secondary group can assign either ascribed or achieved status to any member of the group. Depending on the situation, sometimes the primary group is more important to a teenager and sometimes the secondary group is more important. Either group can provide positive or negative feedback, either directly or indirectly, depending on established patterns of communication.

55. A: Diffusion occurs when a culture adopts norms and values of other cultures, and thus, different family structures can become accepted within a culture through the effects of diffusion from other cultures. Transmission is the passing of values within a culture through generations, and thus, it is associated with preservation of values and systems, not with change. Assimilation is the blending or adapting to a new culture by migrant individuals, and therefore, it primarily describes the process of change in behavior of the migrant individual, rather than a change in perception by either of his cultures. Multiculturalism describes acceptance of diverse cultural traditions within a nation. It is primarily associated with acceptance of distinctive cultural identities rather than with changing ideas of what is acceptable.

56. D: Racialization occurs when a particular race or ethnic community (particularly a minority group) is associated with a particular trait. When racialization occurs, the ethnic community can begin to identify itself by the stereotypes ascribed to it by the majority. In this example, the patient and the doctor are both subject to racial stereotypes regarding the emblematic fertility of the patient's community. The attitudes of the patient and of the doctor can result in viewing infertility as more serious due to the atypical occurrence within the patient's population or as less serious because it is uncommon in the patient's community. Racialization can result in the physician approaching the problem with a less objective viewpoint because the physician is human and is not immune from stereotyping patients. The patient is not invulnerable from stereotyping herself based on beliefs about her community, race, or ethnicity.

57. A: The theory of intersectionality explains that discrimination can be a product of several different layers and types of oppression combined. In this example, the patient who experiences infertility may feel that the physician cannot understand her experience, even if the physician is a female, because of the different types of discrimination that result from being a female, from being infertile, and from being of this patient's particular cultural background. Similarly, the patient would also feel that her husband couldn't have the same experience that she, as a female, has, and thus cannot understand her feelings about the medical and social situation. The theory of intersectionality is not about combining different individual's experiences, but rather about the levels of one person's unique experiences based on his or her combined sources of discrimination. The combination of cultures does not help the outcome based on the theory of intersectionality. Taking into account the combined viewpoints of men and women in the context of infertility does not exacerbate the conflict.

58. C: There are a variety of pheromones, all chemicals released by individuals and detected by other individuals through chemical receptors present in the recipient. Situations and settings provoking the release of the different pheromones vary. Responses depend on the recipient's chemical receptors, which may undergo modulation in different situations and settings. It is likely that individuals of different genders release dissimilar pheromones and possess dissimilar pheromone receptors. However, not all females in the same location are expected to respond to pheromones in the environment in exactly the same way. Similarly, not all males in the same location are expected to respond to pheromones in the environment in exactly the same way. Pheromones are released involuntarily, not voluntarily or based on intention. The concentration gradient is not dependent on the number of people because the pheromones are not likely to be "consumed" by some individuals, leaving fewer chemicals available for other individuals' pheromone receptors to bind to.

59. A: The physician has a belief that teenagers with certain characteristics are more likely to have a better recovery. The demographic and personal differences misled the physician based on his preexisting belief, and his belief still persisted despite the fact that the objective facts are not as he imagines. Poor recall should affect the physician's opinions about both sets of patients. Labeling theory occurs when individuals behave in a way that is consistent with the way society describes them. This is not an example of a self-fulfilling prophecy because the outcome was not dependent on any preexisting bias. Given the similar outcomes of both sets of patients, labeling theory is not a factor here.

Critical Analysis and Reasoning Skills

Passage 1

1. B: The designer in this passage is one who creates based on his objective assessment of what will become popular, while the artist creates based on inspiration and emotion.

The passage implies that the designer intends for his creations to be mass-produced, but it does not state that the artist does not intend for his work to be mass-produced. The passage does not indicate whether the designer or the artist has received formal education. The passage implies that the designer has more commercial success than the artist, but does not state that wealth is a central difference between the two.

2. C: According to the passage, the artist may enjoy lavish praise from the critic, but the passage does not state that the artist always enjoys such praise, or that such praise supersedes his creativity or his signature style.

The passage does not present the typical artist as publicly denouncing those who do not appreciate his work. The passage implies that the artist does not consider it an improvement to change his style to suit the tastes of others, even critics. And the passage suggests that if the artist were to consider becoming a student of the designer, he would do so to please the masses, not the critic.

3. D: According to the passage, the "brilliant mathematician" can take an idea that is not typically presented in a mathematical way, such as design, and convert it to a mathematical formula to predict what the public will accept and embrace.

The passage implies that the designer can mask his concrete, mathematical talents as an artistic gift, but not that he specifically deceives others. The passage does not imply that the "brilliant mathematician" as described here can do calculations in his head or that he is a high achiever academically.

4. A: According to the premise of this passage, the commercially successful musician works to try to tailor to the tastes of the masses, not to music critics.

He would be unlikely to change his work to please a music critic, as his goal is to please the public. According to the premise of this article, the opinion of the critic does not influence the public nor does the critic know how to or care to provide insight into popular tastes.

5. A: According to the passage, the artist has the choice of learning the methodical approach from the successful designer or continuing to work hard on his brand of magic.

Accepting his station in life is not consistent with overcoming his inability to achieve popular acceptance. Also, the passage does not imply that the artist is starving, but simply that he may not have achieved widespread commercial success. The passage does not suggest that the artist could attempt to gain acceptance and praise from art critics in order to overcome his ability to gain popular acceptance, as the critic and the masses have differing opinions. The passage does not imply that if the artist learns mathematics, his work will become more popular. Instead, the passage suggests that it is the designer's application of mathematical principles to art that makes him successful, not his knowledge of mathematics.

6. C: Based on the premise of the passage, a buyer for a retailer would choose among designs of commercial designers while commercial designers would try to sell their work to retailers.

The passage does not suggest that commercial designers are secure in their work with retailers, but rather implies that they must keep working to try to appeal to consumers. The passage does not suggest that commercial designers compete with retailers. More importantly, the passage does not suggest that anyone wants to entice artists to enter the commercial world, or that there is a shortage of designers or artists.

Passage 2

7. C: The painting portrays a mountain with grass, trees, and a gardener, implying that the florae need tending. The author says that the mountain is densely rocky and jagged.

The passage did not mention whether the colors of the mountain were similar or different than the colors in the painting. The passage also did not state that the mountain was cold, but rather that there was a blistering heat outside the coolness of the cave. The passage does not imply that the painting represents the mountain as a small mountain.

8. A: The author expects the painting to reflect an accurate portrayal of the artist's knowledge of the cave. The author expects the painting to reflect an accurate portrayal of the cave and seems surprised that the mountain is unlike the mountain in the painting. The author's initial explanation of the discrepancy is that the painter did not personally know about the reality, but instead was relying on hearsay. Thus, if the author encountered a wild animal, he would conclude that the painter was unaware of animals in the cave.

The author does not suggest that the painter was hiding the truth, but rather that he was attempting to accurately portray the feelings associated with the cave and the mountain. The author does not seem to think that the painter could have survived among wild animals, nor does the author seem to understand that the setting may have changed since the painting was created.

9. D: The author infers that the painting is the artist's best attempt to represent the mountain and the cave, but that while the feelings evoked by the cave are different from its appearance, they more accurately represent the whole experience than the mountain does.

The author does not entertain the idea that climate change could have played a role in changing the topography of the land at the site. The author does not seem to believe that the artist did research on the subject, but rather that he "learned the details through stories passed by fervent storytellers," implying a passive knowledge rather than active research. The author does not entertain the idea that the painting was commissioned or that there was a motive in adding religious symbols.

10. D: The author states that "one wonders why someone unfamiliar with the inside of the cave would venture past the entryway," implying that he must have had some familiarity with what to expect inside in order to have ventured past the entryway.

The author does not reveal a sense of adventure, nor does he seem to believe there is a passageway to the exit of the cave. The author does not suggest that he has any plans to create paintings of the area, but instead seems to have gone to the location seeking tranquility as proposed by the painting.

11. B: It would have been extremely difficult to determine whether the mountain and cave even existed without some clues about the story or the location from the artist.

The painting might have a greater impact on someone who can associate it with and cares about the events depicted in the painting, but the author describes the colors, the style of painting, and the scene as peaceful, seemingly independent of historical context. The geographic details found in the painting would be unlikely to help locate the area in the painting because the actual site was different in many key features than the site represented in the painting. Because it is unclear whether Sassetta ever personally visited the location, research on the artist's life probably would not have been useful in determining the location.

12. B: Given the author's description, it is highly unlikely that he was able to find this location alone, and likely had a guide who was familiar with the location and knew the author's mission in finding the mountain and the cave.

The author was probably not alone, and there is no reason to believe that there were 10 adults present. The author estimates that at least 10 adults could fit inside the cave, but this is presented as an estimate. The author did not mention other travelers, but this does not mean that there were no travelers. The passage gives the impression that the author was not knowledgeable enough about the climb to make it alone, but does not give enough detail to ascertain who was with the author.

Passage 3

13. B: The candidate would appeal to the majority of voters by describing a healthcare environment that improves and compliments their socioeconomic situation.

The candidate would be at a disadvantage by spelling out too many details that could potentially be criticized. Favoring the most disadvantaged may paint the candidate as kind and caring, but would not appeal to voters who want better healthcare policy for themselves. Scolding voters or pointing out that they have it better than others is likely to make a candidate appear self-righteous and unconcerned about constituents.

14. A: According the passage, best medical care is determined based on clinical studies that show only a few percentage points of advantage, but that determine the fate of millions of patients. While the passage implies that the difference between the results of scientific studies are exaggerated, the passage does not argue that best medical care is completely arbitrary, and acknowledges that it relies on scientific data.

The passage does not imply that study authors push their data as superior, or that any such action has any impact. The passage states that scientific data used to determine best medical care is minimally divergent, rather than widely divergent. The study does not imply that there is no definition of best care at all, but instead that the definition may be too standardized based on scientific results that do not support widespread standardization.

15. C: The passage asks a question and describes it as disgusting because the question implies that the hospital might not put in exceptional effort to keep someone alive if it seems that no one will notice whether he lives or dies.

The passage does not suggest that the disease itself or the appearance of the pauper is disgusting. The question does not suggest that few people will mourn the loss of a pauper, but rather supposes it as the premise in suggesting that some may not consider his life worth saving for that reason. The question does not specify that there is a grey area in health policy, but rather poses an ethical element as one of the reasons that health policy is so complicated.

16. D: The passage is sympathetic to the feelings of the medical team who may experience "heartbreak" after exerting effort on a patient who does not then take care of his health.

The author does not show any concern for the patient who might not receive proper instruction on self-care, instead implying that the patient may not follow instructions. The author seems concerned with the public's ability to pay for healthcare of those who cannot pay, but not in the context of follow up self-care. And the author does not express concern about the family of the pauper at all.

17. D: While the passage brings up the dilemma, it does not attempt to resolve the issue of how a person's value to society can be calculated.

The passage does not make a strong stand that one person's life is more valuable than another's life, nor does the passage say that they are equivalent in value. The passage says that society might pay for the healthcare of the poor if there are abundant resources, but it does not draw a link between the availability of resources and the value of a person's life.

18. A: The author is clearly impressed by the story and its ability to illustrate a central dilemma in healthcare policy in a manner superior to prepared debates and lengthy books.

The passage does not address the idea of partisanship or political motives in the healthcare policy debates, nor does it indicate that data may be inaccurate. The passage does not indicate that political debates lean towards either fairness or unfairness for people who can or who cannot pay for their own healthcare.

Passage 4

19. D: The premise of the passage is that companies cannot ignore the outcry of older workers because they may stand accused of discrimination by the discarded older workers.

The cost here does not focus on economic cost incurred by wasted wages. While bitterness among workers is mentioned as a byproduct of shedding ineffective employees, it is not mentioned in the context of direct cost to the company. Instead, the accusation of discrimination is noted as a concerning outcome. Discouragement due to remaining in a lower position is not mentioned as a negative cost to the company. Instead, it is the outcry of older workers due to job insecurity and trouble finding a job that may reflect poorly on the company.

20. B: The author conveys a sense of responsibility towards both the older workers and towards the company. The author attempts to show compassion towards the average worker, but carries some frustration regarding the worker's performance.

It does not appear that the author has been accused of discrimination, but that he sees the very real possibility of that outcome if he does not approach the problem carefully. The author does not seem to primarily come from the perspective of sympathizing with the aging workers, despite a few attempts to explain that they may be victims of unfair circumstances. A conclusion about whether the author is indecisive in general cannot be drawn from the brief passage, which has a tone of hesitancy, but can also be seen as a sense of careful thoughtfulness. There is no evidence that the author is indecisive as a general rule.

21. C: The author conveys a sense of responsibility, but doesn't know exactly how to direct it. This suggests that if it were younger workers voicing an outcry about discrimination, the author may defend himself and his company, but would also consider some attempts at remedying the situation.

The passage does not give any indication that the author would feel that any workers have "no right to complain," or that the number of remaining years of earning potential plays a role in their rights.

The passage does not state that it is because of older worker's years invested in the company that he might have to keep them on as employees. The passage does not touch on inherent differences in attitude between older and younger workers or whether one population is more vocal, and thus potentially damaging, regarding workplace discrimination.

22. A: The passage provides a few explanations for why lower-ranked senior employees may have not reached high status, including bullying, bias, and dishonestly. The passage also describes "high performing" leaders, thus implying the contrasting models for how leaders may have attained their professional status.

The passage does not suggest that no one can understand or point to why individual high earning leaders reached their position; indeed, several possible models are provided. The passage also does not jump to the conclusion that high earning older workers are secure in their jobs. Early in the passage, it is mentioned that senior-level workers earn high incomes even when they change jobs, thus opening the door to the idea that job transitions occur even among those who are paid well. The passage does not state for sure that entry level positions are not open to older workers, but instead questions whether they are available to older workers. Furthermore, the passage does not attempt to explain why the entry-level position might not be open to older workers or who could be making the decisions.

23. A: The author is very concerned about charges of unfair discrimination, and if the insecure or laid off workers had received excellent reviews, this would not bode well for the company.

The author would have a hard time defending the premise that part-time workers who received excellent performance reviews were less valuable to the company. Tardiness was not mentioned as a basis for worker insecurity, while part-time work does not necessarily go hand-in-hand with a lack of technology know-how. Redefining the qualities of a valuable worker after the fact would be problematic if performance reviews were built on criteria set by the company in the first place.

24. C: There would be only a few people needed to oversee the work of many computers and robots, which can execute workplace tasks, but cannot make decisions.

There is no reason to believe that everyone would become a supervisor or an entrepreneur. Based on the premise of the passage, many mid-level workers are not high achievers, and thus, by inference, are unlikely to be effective supervisors or entrepreneurs. The overall premise of the article is that there are few jobs, both within and outside the company, that provide generous compensation and that some of the insecure workers may not qualify for these positions, even if they change jobs.

Passage 5

25. C: The author does not support this statement with any facts, and thus it must be viewed as an opinion in the context of the passage.

The statement is not necessarily obvious, particularly because the standardized tests that the author so strongly disapproves of are so prevalent, suggesting that some qualified educators believe they have value. Of course, the prevalence of the standardized examinations neither proves nor disproves their value either. However, even if a statement appears to be obvious, it cannot be accepted as true without some evidence. There is no account in the passage that parents or teachers have reported any facts or narratives to the author that support this statement. However, even if there is no data provided to support the statement, the statement is not automatically deemed false.

26. B: The teacher most likely feels that she has achieved adequate test scores in her classroom, and wants to spend more time on enriching activities for her students.

It is highly unlikely that the teacher is trying to show off, as she carries an attitude throughout the passage that inferior test scores should be addressed, but that trying to achieve higher test scores is not as valuable as other things learned in the classroom, such as social skills. It does not seem that a score of 60th percentile, the average in her school, would be a cause for penalty that she needs to defend. The author does not seem focused on raising children's scores and seems more concerned with offering enriching activities to adequately performing students than tutoring students or other teachers in how to raise test scores.

27. A: The author states that "the problem lies in excessive time devoted to testing" and goes on to say "even more than divesting valuable time, the ensuing exhaustion… leaves students less prepared for any remaining constructive instruction."

The author does not say that testing provides inaccurate insight, but rather that it is limited in value. The author does not suggest that standardized testing of social skills would be valuable. The author suggests a means for repairing lagging skills, but does not state that this absence is the problem with standardized testing. Instead, it is proposed as a compromise if testing must remain part of schooling.

28. B: The passage acknowledges that schools that have a disproportionate number of students who lag behind in academic skills must be identified and that the problem must be managed. The passage acknowledges that lagging behind academically is harmful for students.

The passage does not suggest that online courses to reteach lagging skills would save time or free children from exhaustion due to testing, but instead proposes this idea as a way to address the academic shortcomings that may be identified by testing. The passage also does not imply that there is an inability to teach students that lag behind and it does not criticize worksheets and homework as flawed.

29. D: The author values social skills more than academic skills. The passage already states that kids who are gifted socially can be of great benefit to their peers, implying that kids learn social skills from each other. Student diversity would certainly be expected to enhance those benefits, based on the tone and attitude of the article.

The author does not seem to have an attitude that the benefits of social skills lie in enhancing academic skills. The author does not seem to believe that academic uniformity would be beneficial to students, teachers, or schools. Also, the author's attitude does not seem to be one of a person who would not have an opinion about diversity one way or the other.

30. D: Based on the ideas presented, if the author were to focus on schoolteachers' interaction with students, it would likely be in the context of students' exposure to varied schoolteachers' personalities as beneficial.

While the author values extra activities, it does not seem that the author would prefer for teachers to cut back on curriculum-based activities. The biggest complaint the author has is with excessive testing. The author values student interactions, but does not seem to think that sharing scores among students would be a beneficial student interaction, as the author does not highly value ranking by tests scores, particularly so openly. The author seems to value subjective social interactions among students, and thus, carrying over that attitude towards teachers, would be more likely to view teachers' personalities as beneficial for students rather than formal education about teachers' cultural backgrounds.

PASSAGE 6

31. B: Globalization provided a seemingly sage explanation for economic expansion. The passage says that skeptics of unprecedented economic growth embraced globalization as a reasonable explanation for a change in traditional rules of economics.

The passage does not actually state that globalization fulfilled a role in economic growth, but rather that it was attributed the role. It is implied that the credit given to globalization may have been overstated. The passage does not address any inequities that may have been avoided or that may have resulted from globalization. In fact, the passage does not address any actual economic or social consequences of globalization, only presumed effects.

32. A: Capitalism is not described as negative in this article, but instead is described as having inherent features that do not necessarily discourage or encourage corruption when left unchecked.

Capitalism is not presented as a system that encourages dishonesty or that particularly allows oppression. Capitalism is not blamed for the absence of laws that limit the effects of subprime mortgages. Instead, it is stated that the belief in capitalism as a perfect self-regulating system contributed to the problem, suggesting that some level of regulation may have been lacking.

33. D: While the passage puts blame on all of the above-mentioned entities, the root of the blame is cast on corrupt individuals.

The passage implies that lawmakers, optimistic leaders, and unwise investors all played a role in the economic crisis, primarily due to inability to act on underlying problems or inability to see underlying problems, but does not cast the lion's share of the blame on any of these individual entities.

34. C: The author has a tendency of describing consumers and businesspeople as varied in personal characteristics and knowledge, and thus would likely describe lawmakers the same way.

The author would be unlikely to make a sweeping statement that lawmakers were unprepared with an adequate financial background if the lawmakers did not all avoid addressing the problem issues. Similarly, the author would be unlikely to blame any problems caused by lawmakers on the public or the voters because the passage implies a sense of limited power in terms of the public's control over the actions of elected lawmakers. The author would not suggest that those who wanted to stop corruption were looking for trouble, because the author seems to view lawmakers as responsible for the well-being of constituents.

35. D: Guilt was noted as one if the driving forces that seems to have led some business leaders to believe that their actions were beneficial for everyone.

The passage does not imply that guilt prevented business leaders from behaving with corruption, but seems to imply that business leaders were either inherently benevolent or inherently corrupt. It is not suggested that guilt caused lawmakers to fail to detect corruption, but that satisfaction in seeing prosperity among the people played a larger role. It is not suggested that leaders truly shared wealth, but rather that they convinced themselves that they were sharing wealth.

PASSAGE 7

36. C: A fictional story can have timeless appeal if readers can still find a way to connect to it. This is more likely if the central basis of the story is not so completely outdated that the reader cannot find enjoyment in the story.

The idea that changes in societal values inescapably deem a fictional story unrelatable is untrue, as the core of the story may still appeal to audiences of a different era, even if some societal values have changed. The passage does not imply that the author of the story did not have insight, but rather that his goals were immediate. The passage does not address the fact that people of different cultures may have different values and thus divergent appreciation for fictional stories.

37. A: Thomas Mann, the author of the story, was exiled. This indicated that, at the very least, the government understood his message.

A playwright with a political message is not necessarily looking to be well received, as a playwright of an entertaining play would be. Similarly, a playwright is not a political leader and thus it is unlikely that he viewed political leadership as an objective. He received recognition due to the fact that his message was recognized and rejected by the government system that he was writing against.

38. B: The story would have to be interpreted in light of a personal relationship between father and son in addition to the political message.

The novella may be more or less dangerous for the author as well as the father, depending on the intensity of political persecution. The idea that the story's author was bitter and expressing frustration at not having a high position does not fit well with his objection and with the cruelty with which he drew the magician. The story would not work in terms of being reinterpreted in support of fascism because the magician who hypnotizes his victims was killed at the end. It would be difficult to reinterpret that aspect of the story.

39. D: Modern psychology is attributed as responsible for defining weakness of character and limited self-confidence to be viewed as reprehensible products of bad mothering.

The science of psychology does not seem to have provided a method for helping people with low self-confidence become stronger or defining a biochemical basis as an explanation for a subordinate personality. According to the passage, modern psychology has blamed bad mothering for producing weakened character without providing a solution for either the mother or the offspring.

40. B: The passage acknowledges that, while the era of fascism has ended, there are situations in which political submission is inescapable.

The passage does not imply that the subjects of political tyranny have any character traits that predispose them to that situation. The passage also does not suggest that political fiction or symbolism can serve to help free people from political submission. Similarly, while the passage acknowledges the existence of inescapable political submission, it does not go as far to say that it is inevitable.

41. A: It appears that the author is looking for a way to manage a seemingly inescapable problem, and is looking to the story as a potential model, but finding only an unreasonable solution.

The author does not express a desire to see a group action and he does not seem to imagine that the magician could be believably likely to apologize. The author is not pleased with the ending, but expresses displeasure at elements of the ending besides violence. The passage does not express a sense of disapproval of the violent act itself, just at the fact that the violent act is not practical to most situations.

Passage 8

42. B: The author would likely explain that sustainable energy had not been well developed enough to yield a profit in the past.

The author would not suggest that the companies were irresponsible, because it is these same companies that he is presumably trying to promote to the reader. The author would be unlikely to tell a client to avoid further investments in sustainable energy, and would promote the idea that they may have been risky investments in the past, but are no longer risky. The author is not suggesting that the reader put money into investments purely for social responsibility, incurring an individual financial loss for the good of the whole.

43. C: The passage says that sustainable energy has many attractive features, including less harm to the environment during production.

The passage does not suggest that sustainable energy is more efficient or less costly to society or to individuals and the passage does not address any issues regarding the life cycle or the disposal of energy.

44. A: Legislation can incentivize or disincentivize the use of different types of energy.

The tone of the passage does not support the idea that decreasing energy consumption is realistic or desirable. The pollution effects mentioned in the passage include air and water pollution, which would not differ from consumer to consumer based on individual choices in energy sources. The premise of the passage is that consumers cannot individually change their own energy source, but that an overall overhaul of the production and maintenance of sustainable energy is needed, which requires more than simple transparency allowing individual consumers to make informed choices. In fact, the passage seems to discourage consumer education into the matter, emphasizing the limited benefits.

45. C: The author mentions diversification of investments as well as safe investments and a long-term outlook. He appears to be selling an investment in a sustainable energy fund that incorporates investments in a variety of emerging and existing energy suppliers.

The author mentions the benefits of clean energy, but only briefly and without mentioning any particulars about science, health, or the environment. The author does not seem to be attracting investors into his own company, as he is not selling a specific plan, but instead remaining broad and non-specific with regard to pros and cons of the various types of sustainable energy. The author's primary goal is not in providing education to the reader regarding details about sustainable energy.

46. D: They might have similar lobbying interests during the research and development phase, and thus might not disrupt each others' lobbying progress.

However, because they are competing companies, they are unlikely to help each other in areas of research and development or in business aspects related to barriers to distribution. They would likely compete with each other in areas of research and development, as the company who can develop a patent sooner is likely to benefit financially.

47. B: It is difficult to preserve sustainable energy in a holding form for later use. This is the challenge presented in the passage.

The passage does not state or imply that it is difficult to extract sustainable energy or that sustainable energy is not practical for application. Similarly, the passage does not allude to any limitations in nature restricting the availability of adequate amounts or quantities of sustainable energy.

Passage 9

48. B: The passage states that the tiger was able to elude the hunter until she finally called out for a mate, allowing the hunter to locate her, lure her in, and finally kill her.

The passage states that the tiger was deliberately eluding usual tiger hunting techniques, suggesting that she was more intelligent than a typical tiger living through a hunt. The passage does not imply that her instincts made her less astute, simply that they sabotaged her. The passage does not say that the tiger was less intelligent than the hunter because he was able to shoot her. The hunter had a weapon, an advantage that the tiger did not have.

49. A: The method of hunting must be humane in order to prevent wounding the tiger, which can prolong the animal's suffering.

Respect is relevant in every situation between man and animal, as suggested in the first paragraph of the passage. The tiger in this story is a man-eating tiger, and thus safe capture and feeding are likely to put her human caregivers in great and possibly unpredictable danger. There is no implied link between respect for the tiger in the hunt and safety of other tigers in this community or outside it.

50. D: In the case of Thak, the evolved trait of man-eating is explained as an immediate adaptation following her injury due to her inability to hunt her usual prey.

Survival of the fittest relates to the suitability of an animal to reproduce and pass on its genes. The passage does not imply that the trait of man-eating was carried from parent to offspring or that any genetic alteration or mutation occurred. The passage does not suggest that man-eating developed as a response to environmental changes or scarcity of prey, or that it develops over a long period of time.

51. C: A knowledgeable photographer will understand from various clues whether or not it is safe to photograph a tiger.

Locating a tiger while it is mating or feeding is not necessarily the reason for a photographer to understanding a tiger's habits. It is unlikely for a photographer to befriend a tiger. While rare instances may have occurred, most photographers of wild animals do not befriend their subjects, but rather maintain caution and safety.

52. B: The tiger hunter's theory as introduced in the passage was that Thak's inability to hunt her usual prey during her injury caused her to change her habits as a means of survival. However, if it were later discovered that she gave birth to a man-eating tiger, this theory of adaptation and survival would have to be reconsidered in light of the possibility that there may have been some type of genetic predisposition.

It would not indicate an environmental cause because no other tigers in the area were reported to have adopted similar habits. The idea that Thak could have already taught her tiger to hunt humans at only one week of age is unlikely. There is no evidence to support the idea that memories can be passed down to offspring.

53. C: Even if the techniques failed to eliminate Thak, and even if the hunter was killed by the tiger, it does not change the fact that the techniques were effective in killing other tigers before Thak. According to the passage, this tiger was more challenging and sophisticated than previous tigers.

The passage does not suggest that tigers in general had evolved to be able to counter hunting techniques, but rather that this individual tiger was different. Additionally, it is suggested in the passage that this type of hunt was relatively rare. Due to the infrequency of this type of task, science related to hunting a man-eating tiger was likely non-existent, and this hunter had more knowledge and experience than anything that could have been found elsewhere. The techniques, while likely the best available, could undoubtedly have been improved upon, as such a subjective task can always improve with experience, even among the most skilled hunters.

Image Credits

LICENSED UNDER CC BY 4.0 (CREATIVECOMMONS.ORG/LICENSES/BY/4.0/)

Hexokinase: "Enzyme changing shape" by Wikimedia user Thomas Shafee (https://commons.wikimedia.org/wiki/File:Hexokinase_induced_fit.svg)

Cell Division: "Hayflick Limit" by Wikimedia user Azmistowski (https://commons.wikimedia.org/wiki/File:Hayflick_Limit_(1).svg)

Protein Synthesis: "Pre-mRNA" by Wikimedia user Nastypatty (https://commons.wikimedia.org/wiki/File:Pre-mRNA.svg)

DNA Fragments: "DNA Electrophoresis" by Wikimedia user Mckenzielower (https://commons.wikimedia.org/wiki/File:Gel_Electrophoresis.svg)

Gene Intron Exon: "Segment of eukaryotic DNA" by Wikimedia user Smedlib (https://commons.wikimedia.org/wiki/File:Gene_Intron_Exon_nb.svg)

Point Mutations: "Point mutations" by Wikimedia user Jonsta247 (https://commons.wikimedia.org/wiki/File:Point_mutations-en.png)

Genetic Drift: "Genetic Drift in Population" by OpenStax user Rice University (https://commons.wikimedia.org/wiki/File:Genetic_drift_in_a_population_Figure_19_02_02.png)

Citric Acid: "Citric Acid Cycle Graphic" by Wikimedia user Marisakastner (https://commons.wikimedia.org/wiki/File:Citric_Acid_Cycle_Graphic.jpeg)

Phospholipids: "Phospholipid Structure" by OpenStax CNX Anatomy and Physiology (https://cnx.org/contents/FPtK1zmh@8.25:fEI3C8Ot@10/Preface)

Bacteria: "Bacteria shapes" by Wikimedia user CKRobinson (https://commons.wikimedia.org/wiki/File:Bacteria_shapes_01.png)

Cell Growth: "Mitosis and Meiosis" by Wikimedia user domdomegg (https://commons.wikimedia.org/wiki/File:Three_cell_growth_types.svg)

Regulation of Gene Expression: "steroid hormone receptor" by Wikimedia user Ali Zifan (https://commons.wikimedia.org/wiki/File:Regulation_of_gene_expression_by_steroid_hormone_receptor.svg)

Gas Exchange: "Alveolus Gas Exchange" by Wikimedia user domdomegg (https://commons.wikimedia.org/wiki/File:Gas_exchange_in_the_aveolus_simple_(en).svg)

Carbonic Acid Bicarbonate Buffer System: "Buffer System Illustration" by Wikimedia user BruceBlaus (https://commons.wikimedia.org/wiki/File:Buffer_Part_1.png)

Artery: "Microscope anatomy of an artery" by Wikimedia user Stijn Ghesquiere, Drsrisenthil (https://commons.wikimedia.org/wiki/File:Microscopic_anatomy_of_an_artery.svg)

Lumen of the Small Intestine: "Diagram" by Wikimedia user BallenaBlanca (https://commons.wikimedia.org/wiki/File:Esquema_del_epitelio_del_intestino_delgado.png)

Nephrons: "Nephron Anatomy" by OpenStax CNX user OpenStax College (https://cnx.org/contents/GFy_h8cu@10.53:rZudN6XP@2/Introduction)

Glomerular Physiology: "Diagram" by Wikimedia user Tieum (https://commons.wikimedia.org/wiki/File:Glomerular_Physiology.png)

T-Tubule: "Diagram" by OpenStax CNX author OpenStax College (https://cnx.org/contents/FPtK1zmh@8.25:fEI3C8Ot@10/Preface)

Nervous Control: "Motor End Plates" by OpenStax CNX user OpenStax College (https://cnx.org/contents/FPtK1zmh@8.25:fEI3C8Ot@10/Preface)

Muscle Fiber: "Organization of Muscle Fiber" by OpenStax CNX user OpenStax College (https://cnx.org/contents/FPtK1zmh@8.25:fEI3C8Ot@10/Preface)

Licensed Under CC BY-SA 3.0 (creativecommons.org/licenses/by-sa/3.0/deed.en)

Alpha Helix: "Alpha Helix Chart" by Wikimedia user A.Jashari (https://commons.wikimedia.org/wiki/File:StrukturaSekondare.jpg)

Peptide Bond: "Polypeptide Chain" by OpenStax College (https://cnx.org/contents/FPtK1zmh@8.108:Z3NTbD77@8/Organic-Compounds-Essential-to-Human-Functioning)

Antibody: "Antibody Chart" by Wikimedia use Muntasir Alam (https://commons.wikimedia.org/wiki/File:Antibody_svg.svg)

Activation Energy: "Catalytic Reaction" by Wikimedia user Mcy jerry (https://en.wikipedia.org/wiki/File:Activation2.png)

RNA: "A More Detailed Description" by NHGRI artist Darryl Leja (http://www.accessexcellence.org/RC/VL/GG/rna2.html)

DNA: "Phosphodiester Bond of DNA" by Wikimedia user Akane700 (https://commons.wikimedia.org/wiki/File:PhosphodiesterBond_of_DNA.PNG)

Purine and Pyrimidine: "Purine and Pyrimidine Labels" by Wikimedia user Blausen (https://commons.wikimedia.org/wiki/File:Purine_and_Pyrimidine.png)

DNA: "Base Pair" by Roadnottaken at English Wikipedia (https://commons.wikimedia.org/wiki/File:AT_DNA_base_pair.png)

tRNA: "Codon-anticodon Pairing" by Wikimedia user Yikrazuul (https://commons.wikimedia.org/wiki/File:Codon-Anticodon_pairing.svg)

Wobble Pairing: "Codon-anticodon interactions" by Wikimedia user Fdardel (https://commons.wikimedia.org/wiki/File:Wobble.svg)

DNA and RNA "Complementary Base Pairing" by Flickr user Genomics Education Programme (https://www.flickr.com/photos/genomicseducation/13080698075/)

Chromatin: "DNA Condensation" by Wikimedia user Magnus Manske (https://commons.wikimedia.org/wiki/File:Chromatin_chromosome.png)

Interphase chromatin: "Pluripotent cells" by StemBook user KySha and Laurie A Boyer (https://www.stembook.org/node/585)

Eukaryotic Chromosome: "Condensed Eukaryotic Chromosome" by Zephyris at the English Language Wikipedia (https://commons.wikimedia.org/wiki/File:Condensed_Eukaryotic_Chromosome.png)

Chromosomes: "Chromosomes crossover" by Wikimedia user Abbyprovenzano (https://commons.wikimedia.org/wiki/File:Chromosomal_Crossover.svg)

Y Chromosome: "Pseudoautosomal Regions" by LibreTexts author John W. Kimball (https://bio.libretexts.org/TextMaps/Introductory_and_General_Biology/Book%3A_Biology_(Kimball)/Unit_07%3A_The_Genetic_consequences_of_Meiosis/7.6%3A_Sex_Chromosomes)

Inversion: "Inversion" by Wikimedia user The cat~commonswiki (https://commons.wikimedia.org/wiki/File:Inversion.jpg)

Mutation and Selection: "Mutation and Selection Diagram" by Wikipedia user Beyond Silence (https://en.wikipedia.org/wiki/File:643px-Explanation_of_Evolution_v2.1.PNG)

Population: "Population Bottleneck" by Wikimedia user TedE (https://commons.wikimedia.org/wiki/File:Population_bottleneck.svg)

Energy: "Exothermic Reaction" by Wikimedia user Brazosport College (https://commons.wikimedia.org/wiki/File:Exothermic_Reaction.png)

Energy: "Endothermic Reaction" by Brazosport College (https://commons.wikimedia.org/wiki/File:Endothermic_Reaction.png)

Oxidation Reduction: "Two Halves to a Redox Equation" by Wikimedia user Cameron Garnham (https://commons.wikimedia.org/wiki/File:Redox_Halves.png)

Cell Junctions: "Tight junction, gap junction, and Desmosome junction" by Wikimedia user Boumphreyfr (https://commons.wikimedia.org/wiki/File:Cell_junctions.png)

Mitochondrion Structure: "Diagram of a mitochondrion" by Wikimedia user Kelvinsong (https://commons.wikimedia.org/wiki/File:Mitochondrion_mini.svg)

Golgi Apparatus: "Golgi apparatus diagram" by Wikimedia user Kelvinsong (https://commons.wikimedia.org/wiki/File:Golgi_apparatus_(editors_version).svg)

Flagellum: "Flagellum and Cilia" by Wikimedia user L. Kohidai (https://commons.wikimedia.org/wiki/File:Flagellum-beating.png)

Centrioles: "Centrioles and Microtubules" by Wikimedia user BruceBlaus (https://commons.wikimedia.org/wiki/File:Blausen_0214_Centrioles.png)

Gram Cell: "Gram-Cell-Wall" by Graevemoore at English Wikipedia (https://commons.wikimedia.org/wiki/File:Gram-Cell-wall.svg)

Binary Fission: "Binary Fission Diagram" by Wikimedia user JWSchmidt (https://commons.wikimedia.org/wiki/File:Binary_fission.png)

Bacteria: "Bacterial Growth" by Wikimedia user M.Komorniczak (https://commons.wikimedia.org/wiki/File:Bacterial_growth_en.svg)

Conjugation: "Bacterial conjugation" by Wikimedia user Adenosine (https://commons.wikimedia.org/wiki/File:Conjugation.svg)

Phage Injection: "Diagram of how some bacteriophages infect cells" by Wikimedia user Graham Colm (https://commons.wikimedia.org/wiki/File:Phage_injecting_its_genome_into_bacterial_cell.png)

Mitosis: "Stages of Mitosis" by Wikimedia user Boumphreyfr (https://commons.wikimedia.org/wiki/File:Mitosis.png)

Centriole: "Centriole Diagram" by Wikimedia user Kelvinsong (https://commons.wikimedia.org/wiki/File:Centriole-en.svg)

Condensed Eukaryotic Chromosome: "Condensed Eukaryotic Chromosome Diagram" by Zephyris at English Wikipedia (https://commons.wikimedia.org/wiki/File:Condensed_Eukaryotic_Chromosome.png)

Microtubule: "Formation of Microtubule" by Wikimedia user Group6-3 (https://commons.wikimedia.org/wiki/File:Formation_of_Microtubule.png)

Cell Cycle: "Schematic representation of the cell cycle" by Wikimedia user Zephyris (https://commons.wikimedia.org/wiki/File:Cell_Cycle_2-2.svg)

Spermatogenesis: "Spermatogenesis Diagram" by Wikimedia user Anchor207 (https://commons.wikimedia.org/wiki/File:Spermatogenesis.svg)

Fertilization: "Fertilization Sequence" by Wikimedia user Chippolito (https://commons.wikimedia.org/wiki/File:Acrosomal_reaction_of_fertilization.PNG)

Fertilization: "Fertilization Sequence part two" by Wikimedia user Chippolito (https://commons.wikimedia.org/wiki/File:Cortical_reaction_of_fertilization.PNG)

Blastocyst: "Blastocyst Diagram" by Wikimedia user Seans Potato Business (https://commons.wikimedia.org/wiki/File:Blastocyst_English.svg)

Nervous System: "Diagram of Nervous System" by Fuzzform at English Wikipedia (https://commons.wikimedia.org/wiki/File:NSdiagram.png)

Spinal Cross Sections: "Role of Spinal Cord" by Wikimedia user Polarlys (https://commons.wikimedia.org/wiki/File:Medulla_spinalis_-_Section_-_English.svg)

Neurons: "Types of Neurons" by Wikimedia user Jonathan Haas (https://commons.wikimedia.org/wiki/File:Neurons_uni_bi_multi_pseudouni.svg)

Multielectrodes: "Recording and Stimulation" by Wikimedia user Chris 73 (https://commons.wikimedia.org/wiki/File:ActionPotential.png)

Neuroglia: "Types of Neuroglia" by Wikimedia user BruceBlaus (https://commons.wikimedia.org/wiki/File:Blausen_0870_TypesofNeuroglia.png)

G Protein-Coupled Receptor: "Adenylate cyclase" by Wikimedia user Yikrazuul (https://commons.wikimedia.org/wiki/File:Activation_protein_kinase_C.svg)

Isoprene: "Isoprene Diagram" by Wikimedia user 94peter (https://commons.wikimedia.org/wiki/File:Isoprenem.png)

Respiratory System: "Respiratory System Diagram" by Wikimedia user BruceBlaus (https://commons.wikimedia.org/wiki/File:Blausen_0770_RespiratorySystem_02.png)

Respiratory Zone: "Respiratory Zone Diagram" by Wikimedia user OpenStax College (https://commons.wikimedia.org/wiki/File:2309_The_Respiratory_Zone_esp.jpg)

Thoracic Cavity: "Inspiration and Expiration" by OpenStax CNX user OpenStax College (https://cnx.org/contents/14fb4ad7-39a1-4eee-ab6e-3ef2482e3e22@6.27)

Human Heart: "Diagram" by Wikimedia user Wapcaplet (https://commons.wikimedia.org/wiki/File:Diagram_of_the_human_heart_(cropped).svg)

Capillary: "Fenestrated Capillary" by OpenStax CNX user OpenStax College (https://cnx.org/contents/FPtK1zmh@6.27:zMTtFGyH@4/Introduction)

Blood: "Centrifuge Blood Sample" by KnuteKnudsen at English Wikipedia (https://commons.wikimedia.org/wiki/File:Blood-centrifugation-scheme.png)

Lymphatic System: "Anatomy of the Lymphatic System" by OpenStax CNX user OpenStax College (https://cnx.org/contents/FPtK1zmh@6.27:zMTtFGyH@4/Introduction)

Antibodies: "Antigens and Epitopes" by OpenStax CNX user OpenStax College (https://cnx.org/contents/UsOvmjzQ@2.8:VZU-vXBp@3/Polyclonal-and-Monoclonal-Antibody-Production)

Gastric Gland: "Diagram" by Wikimedia user Boumphreyfr (https://commons.wikimedia.org/wiki/File:Gastric_gland.png)

Pancreas: "Pancreas biliary" by Wikimedia user Boumphreyfr (https://commons.wikimedia.org/wiki/File:Pancrease_biliary1.png)

Small Intestine: "Small Intestine Anatomy" by Wikimedia user BruceBlaus (https://commons.wikimedia.org/wiki/File:Blausen_0817_SmallIntestine_Anatomy.png)

Large Intestine: "Large Intestine Anatomy" by Wikimedia user BruceBlaus (https://commons.wikimedia.org/wiki/File:Blausen_0603_LargeIntestine_Anatomy.png)

Kidney and Nephron: "Kidney and Nephron Structures" by Wikimedia users Madhero88 and PioM (https://commons.wikimedia.org/wiki/File:KidneyAndNephron-v4_Antares42.svg)

Loop of Henle CounterCurrent Multiplier System: "Diagram" by OpenStax CNX user OpenStax College (https://cnx.org/contents/FPtK1zmh@6.27:zMTtFGyH@4/Introduction)

Male Anatomy: "Diagram" by Wikimedia user Stephanie~commonswiki (https://commons.wikimedia.org/wiki/File:Male_anatomy.png)

Female Anatomy: "Diagram" by Wikimedia user CFCF (https://commons.wikimedia.org/wiki/File:Female_Reproductive_Anterior.JPG)

Menstrual Cycle: "Diagram" by Wikimedia user Isometrik (https://commons.wikimedia.org/wiki/File:MenstrualCycle3.png)

Skeletal Muscle: "Vein Pump" by OpenStax CNX author OpenStax College (https://cnx.org/contents/FPtK1zmh@6.27:zMTtFGyH@4/Introduction)

Sarcomere: "Diagram" by Wikimedia user Slashme (https://commons.wikimedia.org/wiki/File:Sarcomere.svg)

Bone Structure: "Classification of Bones by Shape" by Wikimedia user BruceBlaus (https://commons.wikimedia.org/wiki/File:Blausen_0229_ClassificationofBones.png)

Cartilage: "Types of Cartilage" by OpenStax CNX user OpenStax College (https://cnx.org/contents/FPtK1zmh@6.27:zMTtFGyH@4/Introduction)

Epidermis: "Epidermis Structure" by Wikimedia user BruceBlaus (https://commons.wikimedia.org/wiki/File:Blausen_0353_Epidermis.png)

Sweat Gland: "Eccrine Sweat Gland" by OpenStax CNX user OpenStax College (https://cnx.org/contents/FPtK1zmh@6.27:zMTtFGyH@4/Introduction)

Licensed Under CC BY 2.5 (creativecommons.org/licenses/by/2.5/deed.en)

Synaptonemal Complex: "Recombination Hotspots" by PLOS Biology user Jody Hey (https://journals.plos.org/plosbiology/article?id=10.1371/journal.pbio.0020190)

Meiosis: "Tetrad Chromosome" by Wikimedia (https://commons.wikimedia.org/wiki/File:Tetrad.png)

Plasma: "Plasma Replication" by Wikimedia user Spaully (https://commons.wikimedia.org/wiki/File:Plasmid_replication_(english).svg)

Stomach: "Stomach Diagram" by Wikimedia user Olek Remesz (https://commons.wikimedia.org/wiki/File:Ventriculus.svg)

Uterus and Mullerian Ducts: "Diagram" by StemBook authors J. Teixeira, B.R. Rueda, and J.K. Pru (https://commons.wikimedia.org/wiki/File:The_uterus_differentiates_from_the_fetal_M%C3%BCllerian_ducts.jpg)

Bone: "Composition of Bone" by Wikimedia user BDB (https://commons.wikimedia.org/wiki/File:Composition_of_bone.png)

Licensed Under CC BY 2.0(creativecommons.org/licenses/by/2.0/deed.en)

Amino Acids: "Abbreviations for the Amino Acids" by Flickr user genomics.education (https://www.flickr.com/photos/genomicseducation/13080643615/)

DNA: "Okazaki Fragment" by Wikimedia user Gluon (https://commons.wikimedia.org/wiki/File:DNA-Okazaki-Fragment-prelim.PNG)

DNA: "Semi Conservative Replication of DNA" by Flickr user Genomics Education Programme (https://www.flickr.com/photos/genomicseducation/13081032424/)

How to Overcome Test Anxiety

Just the thought of taking a test is enough to make most people a little nervous. A test is an important event that can have a long-term impact on your future, so it is important to take it seriously and it is natural to feel anxious about performing well. But just because anxiety is normal, that doesn't mean that it is helpful in test taking, or that you should simply accept it as part of your life. Anxiety can have a variety of effects. These effects can be mild, like making you feel slightly nervous, or severe, like blocking your ability to focus or remember even a simple detail.

If you experience test anxiety—whether severe or mild—it is important to know how to beat it. To discover this, first you need to understand what causes test anxiety.

Causes of Test Anxiety

While we often think of anxiety as an uncontrollable emotional state, it can actually be caused by simple, practical things. One of the most common causes of test anxiety is that a person does not feel adequately prepared for their test. This feeling can be the result of many different issues such as poor study habits or lack of organization, but the most common culprit is time management. Starting to study too late, failing to organize your study time to cover all of the material, or being distracted while you study will mean that you're not well prepared for the test. This may lead to cramming the night before, which will cause you to be physically and mentally exhausted for the test. Poor time management also contributes to feelings of stress, fear, and hopelessness as you realize you are not well prepared but don't know what to do about it.

Other times, test anxiety is not related to your preparation for the test but comes from unresolved fear. This may be a past failure on a test, or poor performance on tests in general. It may come from comparing yourself to others who seem to be performing better or from the stress of living up to expectations. Anxiety may be driven by fears of the future—how failure on this test would affect your educational and career goals. These fears are often completely irrational, but they can still negatively impact your test performance.

Review Video: 3 Reasons You Have Test Anxiety
Visit mometrix.com/academy and enter code: 428468

Elements of Test Anxiety

As mentioned earlier, test anxiety is considered to be an emotional state, but it has physical and mental components as well. Sometimes you may not even realize that you are suffering from test anxiety until you notice the physical symptoms. These can include trembling hands, rapid heartbeat, sweating, nausea, and tense muscles. Extreme anxiety may lead to fainting or vomiting. Obviously, any of these symptoms can have a negative impact on testing. It is important to recognize them as soon as they begin to occur so that you can address the problem before it damages your performance.

Review Video: 3 Ways to Tell You Have Test Anxiety
Visit mometrix.com/academy and enter code: 927847

The mental components of test anxiety include trouble focusing and inability to remember learned information. During a test, your mind is on high alert, which can help you recall information and stay focused for an extended period of time. However, anxiety interferes with your mind's natural processes, causing you to blank out, even on the questions you know well. The strain of testing during anxiety makes it difficult to stay focused, especially on a test that may take several hours. Extreme anxiety can take a huge mental toll, making it difficult not only to recall test information but even to understand the test questions or pull your thoughts together.

Review Video: How Test Anxiety Affects Memory
Visit mometrix.com/academy and enter code: 609003

Effects of Test Anxiety

Test anxiety is like a disease—if left untreated, it will get progressively worse. Anxiety leads to poor performance, and this reinforces the feelings of fear and failure, which in turn lead to poor performances on subsequent tests. It can grow from a mild nervousness to a crippling condition. If allowed to progress, test anxiety can have a big impact on your schooling, and consequently on your future.

Test anxiety can spread to other parts of your life. Anxiety on tests can become anxiety in any stressful situation, and blanking on a test can turn into panicking in a job situation. But fortunately, you don't have to let anxiety rule your testing and determine your grades. There are a number of relatively simple steps you can take to move past anxiety and function normally on a test and in the rest of life.

Review Video: How Test Anxiety Impacts Your Grades
Visit mometrix.com/academy and enter code: 939819

Physical Steps for Beating Test Anxiety

While test anxiety is a serious problem, the good news is that it can be overcome. It doesn't have to control your ability to think and remember information. While it may take time, you can begin taking steps today to beat anxiety.

Just as your first hint that you may be struggling with anxiety comes from the physical symptoms, the first step to treating it is also physical. Rest is crucial for having a clear, strong mind. If you are tired, it is much easier to give in to anxiety. But if you establish good sleep habits, your body and mind will be ready to perform optimally, without the strain of exhaustion. Additionally, sleeping well helps you to retain information better, so you're more likely to recall the answers when you see the test questions.

Getting good sleep means more than going to bed on time. It is important to allow your brain time to relax. Take study breaks from time to time so it doesn't get overworked, and don't study right before bed. Take time to rest your mind before trying to rest your body, or you may find it difficult to fall asleep.

Review Video: The Importance of Sleep for Your Brain
Visit mometrix.com/academy and enter code: 319338

Along with sleep, other aspects of physical health are important in preparing for a test. Good nutrition is vital for good brain function. Sugary foods and drinks may give a burst of energy but this burst is followed by a crash, both physically and emotionally. Instead, fuel your body with protein and vitamin-rich foods.

Also, drink plenty of water. Dehydration can lead to headaches and exhaustion, especially if your brain is already under stress from the rigors of the test. Particularly if your test is a long one, drink water during the breaks. And if possible, take an energy-boosting snack to eat between sections.

Review Video: How Diet Can Affect your Mood
Visit mometrix.com/academy and enter code: 624317

Along with sleep and diet, a third important part of physical health is exercise. Maintaining a steady workout schedule is helpful, but even taking 5-minute study breaks to walk can help get your blood pumping faster and clear your head. Exercise also releases endorphins, which contribute to a positive feeling and can help combat test anxiety.

When you nurture your physical health, you are also contributing to your mental health. If your body is healthy, your mind is much more likely to be healthy as well. So take time to rest, nourish your body with healthy food and water, and get moving as much as possible. Taking these physical steps will make you stronger and more able to take the mental steps necessary to overcome test anxiety.

Review Video: How to Stay Healthy and Prevent Test Anxiety
Visit mometrix.com/academy and enter code: 877894

Mental Steps for Beating Test Anxiety

Working on the mental side of test anxiety can be more challenging, but as with the physical side, there are clear steps you can take to overcome it. As mentioned earlier, test anxiety often stems from lack of preparation, so the obvious solution is to prepare for the test. Effective studying may be the most important weapon you have for beating test anxiety, but you can and should employ several other mental tools to combat fear.

First, boost your confidence by reminding yourself of past success—tests or projects that you aced. If you're putting as much effort into preparing for this test as you did for those, there's no reason you should expect to fail here. Work hard to prepare; then trust your preparation.

Second, surround yourself with encouraging people. It can be helpful to find a study group, but be sure that the people you're around will encourage a positive attitude. If you spend time with others who are anxious or cynical, this will only contribute to your own anxiety. Look for others who are motivated to study hard from a desire to succeed, not from a fear of failure.

Third, reward yourself. A test is physically and mentally tiring, even without anxiety, and it can be helpful to have something to look forward to. Plan an activity following the test, regardless of the outcome, such as going to a movie or getting ice cream.

When you are taking the test, if you find yourself beginning to feel anxious, remind yourself that you know the material. Visualize successfully completing the test. Then take a few deep, relaxing breaths and return to it. Work through the questions carefully but with confidence, knowing that you are capable of succeeding.

Developing a healthy mental approach to test taking will also aid in other areas of life. Test anxiety affects more than just the actual test—it can be damaging to your mental health and even contribute to depression. It is important to beat test anxiety before it becomes a problem for more than testing.

Review Video: Test Anxiety and Depression
Visit mometrix.com/academy and enter code: 904704

Study Strategy

Being prepared for the test is necessary to combat anxiety, but what does being prepared look like? You may study for hours on end and still not feel prepared. What you need is a strategy for test prep. The next few pages outline our recommended steps to help you plan out and conquer the challenge of preparation.

Step 1: Scope Out the Test

Learn everything you can about the format (multiple choice, essay, etc.) and what will be on the test. Gather any study materials, course outlines, or sample exams that may be available. Not only will this help you to prepare, but knowing what to expect can help to alleviate test anxiety.

Step 2: Map Out the Material

Look through the textbook or study guide and make note of how many chapters or sections it has. Then divide these over the time you have. For example, if a book has 15 chapters and you have five days to study, you need to cover three chapters each day. Even better, if you have the time, leave an extra day at the end for overall review after you have gone through the material in depth.

If time is limited, you may need to prioritize the material. Look through it and make note of which sections you think you already have a good grasp on, and which need review. While you are studying, skim quickly through the familiar sections and take more time on the challenging parts. Write out your plan so you don't get lost as you go. Having a written plan also helps you feel more in control of the study, so anxiety is less likely to arise from feeling overwhelmed at the amount to cover.

Step 3: Gather Your Tools

Decide what study method works best for you. Do you prefer to highlight in the book as you study and then go back over the highlighted portions? Or do you type out notes of the important information? Or is it helpful to make flashcards that you can carry with you? Assemble the pens, index cards, highlighters, post-it notes, and any other materials you may need so you won't be distracted by getting up to find things while you study.

If you're having a hard time retaining the information or organizing your notes, experiment with different methods. For example, try color-coding by subject with colored pens, highlighters, or post-it notes. If you learn better by hearing, try recording yourself reading your notes so you can listen while in the car, working out, or simply sitting at your desk. Ask a friend to quiz you from your flashcards, or try teaching someone the material to solidify it in your mind.

Step 4: Create Your Environment

It is important to avoid distractions while you study. This includes both the obvious distractions like visitors and the subtle distractions like an uncomfortable chair (or a too-comfortable couch that makes you want to fall asleep). Set up the best study environment possible: good lighting and a comfortable work area. If background music helps you focus, you may want to turn it on, but otherwise keep the room quiet. If you are using a computer to take notes, be sure you don't have any other windows open, especially applications like social media, games, or anything else that could distract you. Silence your phone and turn off notifications. Be sure to keep water close by so you stay hydrated while you study (but avoid unhealthy drinks and snacks).

Also, take into account the best time of day to study. Are you freshest first thing in the morning? Try to set aside some time then to work through the material. Is your mind clearer in the afternoon or evening? Schedule your study session then. Another method is to study at the same time of day that you will take the test, so that your brain gets used to working on the material at that time and will be ready to focus at test time.

Step 5: Study!

Once you have done all the study preparation, it is time to settle into the actual studying. Sit down, take a few moments to settle your mind so you can focus, and begin to follow your study plan. Don't give in to distractions or let yourself procrastinate. This is your time to prepare so you'll be ready to fearlessly approach the test. Make the most of the time and stay focused.

Of course, you don't want to burn out. If you study too long you may find that you're not retaining the information very well. Take regular study breaks. For example, taking five minutes out of every hour to walk briskly, breathing deeply and swinging your arms, can help your mind stay fresh.

As you get to the end of each chapter or section, it is a good idea to do a quick review. Remind yourself of what you learned and work on any difficult parts. When you feel that you've mastered the material, move on to the next part. At the end of your study session, briefly skim through your notes again.

But while review is helpful, cramming last minute is NOT. If at all possible, work ahead so that you won't need to fit all your study into the last day. Cramming overloads your brain with more information than it can process and retain, and your tired mind may struggle to recall even previously learned information when it is overwhelmed with last-minute study. Also, the urgent nature of cramming and the stress placed on your brain contribute to anxiety. You'll be more likely to go to the test feeling unprepared and having trouble thinking clearly.

So don't cram, and don't stay up late before the test, even just to review your notes at a leisurely pace. Your brain needs rest more than it needs to go over the information again. In fact, plan to finish your studies by noon or early afternoon the day before the test. Give your brain the rest of the day to relax or focus on other things, and get a good night's sleep. Then you will be fresh for the test and better able to recall what you've studied.

Step 6: Take a Practice Test

Many courses offer sample tests, either online or in the study materials. This is an excellent resource to check whether you have mastered the material, as well as to prepare for the test format and environment.

Check the test format ahead of time: the number of questions, the type (multiple choice, free response, etc.), and the time limit. Then create a plan for working through them. For example, if you have 30 minutes to take a 60-question test, your limit is 30 seconds per question. Spend less time on the questions you know well so that you can take more time on the difficult ones.

If you have time to take several practice tests, take the first one open book, with no time limit. Work through the questions at your own pace and make sure you fully understand them. Gradually work up to taking a test under test conditions: sit at a desk with all study materials put away and set a timer. Pace yourself to make sure you finish the test with time to spare and go back to check your answers if you have time.

After each test, check your answers. On the questions you missed, be sure you understand why you missed them. Did you misread the question (tests can use tricky wording)? Did you forget the information? Or was it something you hadn't learned? Go back and study any shaky areas that the practice tests reveal.

Taking these tests not only helps with your grade, but also aids in combating test anxiety. If you're already used to the test conditions, you're less likely to worry about it, and working through tests until you're scoring well gives you a confidence boost. Go through the practice tests until you feel comfortable, and then you can go into the test knowing that you're ready for it.

Test Tips

On test day, you should be confident, knowing that you've prepared well and are ready to answer the questions. But aside from preparation, there are several test day strategies you can employ to maximize your performance.

First, as stated before, get a good night's sleep the night before the test (and for several nights before that, if possible). Go into the test with a fresh, alert mind rather than staying up late to study.

Try not to change too much about your normal routine on the day of the test. It is important to eat a nutritious breakfast, but if you normally don't eat breakfast at all, consider eating just a protein bar. If you're a coffee drinker, go ahead and have your normal coffee. Just make sure you time it so that the caffeine doesn't wear off right in the middle of your test. Avoid sugary beverages, and drink enough water to stay hydrated but not so much that you need a restroom break 10 minutes into the test. If your test isn't first thing in the morning, consider going for a walk or doing a light workout before the test to get your blood flowing.

Allow yourself enough time to get ready, and leave for the test with plenty of time to spare so you won't have the anxiety of scrambling to arrive in time. Another reason to be early is to select a good seat. It is helpful to sit away from doors and windows, which can be distracting. Find a good seat, get out your supplies, and settle your mind before the test begins.

When the test begins, start by going over the instructions carefully, even if you already know what to expect. Make sure you avoid any careless mistakes by following the directions.

Then begin working through the questions, pacing yourself as you've practiced. If you're not sure on an answer, don't spend too much time on it, and don't let it shake your confidence. Either skip it and come back later, or eliminate as many wrong answers as possible and guess among the remaining ones. Don't dwell on these questions as you continue—put them out of your mind and focus on what lies ahead.

Be sure to read all of the answer choices, even if you're sure the first one is the right answer. Sometimes you'll find a better one if you keep reading. But don't second-guess yourself if you do immediately know the answer. Your gut instinct is usually right. Don't let test anxiety rob you of the information you know.

If you have time at the end of the test (and if the test format allows), go back and review your answers. Be cautious about changing any, since your first instinct tends to be correct, but make sure you didn't misread any of the questions or accidentally mark the wrong answer choice. Look over any you skipped and make an educated guess.

At the end, leave the test feeling confident. You've done your best, so don't waste time worrying about your performance or wishing you could change anything. Instead, celebrate the successful completion of this test. And finally, use this test to learn how to deal with anxiety even better next time.

Review Video: 5 Tips to Beat Test Anxiety
Visit mometrix.com/academy and enter code: 570656

Important Qualification

Not all anxiety is created equal. If your test anxiety is causing major issues in your life beyond the classroom or testing center, or if you are experiencing troubling physical symptoms related to your anxiety, it may be a sign of a serious physiological or psychological condition. If this sounds like your situation, we strongly encourage you to seek professional help.

Thank You

We at Mometrix would like to extend our heartfelt thanks to you, our friend and patron, for allowing us to play a part in your journey. It is a privilege to serve people from all walks of life who are unified in their commitment to building the best future they can for themselves.

The preparation you devote to these important testing milestones may be the most valuable educational opportunity you have for making a real difference in your life. We encourage you to put your heart into it—that feeling of succeeding, overcoming, and yes, conquering will be well worth the hours you've invested.

We want to hear your story, your struggles and your successes, and if you see any opportunities for us to improve our materials so we can help others even more effectively in the future, please share that with us as well. **The team at Mometrix would be absolutely thrilled to hear from you!** So please, send us an email (support@mometrix.com) and let's stay in touch.

If you'd like some additional help, check out these other resources we offer for your exam: http://mometrixflashcards.com/MCAT

Additional Bonus Material

Due to our efforts to try to keep this book to a manageable length, we've created a link that will give you access to all of your additional bonus material.

Please visit https://www.mometrix.com/bonus948/mcat to access the information.